clinical
examination

Includes CD-ROM

www.studentconsult.com

delivers **Clinical Examination 5e** online and more!

online access
+
interactive
extras
studentconsult.com

Thank you for purchasing

Clinical Examination 5e

Your purchase entitles you to free online access
to Clinical Examination 5e.

Find what you need to know, right now!
Access via your home computer, the library, or on the wards!

Fully searchable text
■ Access by keyword, subject, or index

Link up
■ Integration links give bonus content from
other leading Elsevier titles

Build your online library
■ Search across all of your favourite
textbooks
■ View illustrations online and download
for your own personal use

POCKETConsult enabled
■ Enables you to download excerpts
to your handheld device

Additional features
■ Self-assessment questions
■ Heart and lung sounds
■ Image collection
■ Access to drugs database

How to register

Scratch off the sticker on the inside front cover to get your **unique** PIN number.

Connect to the internet and go to
www.studentconsult.com
for simple instructions on how to register – you'll need your PIN number for registration.

Access to and use of the online editions of textbooks through the STUDENT CONSULT
website is for individuals only; library and institutional access and use are strictly prohibited.
For information on products and services available for institutional access, please contact our
Account Support Center at (+1) 877-857-1047.

Important note: Purchase of this book includes access to the online version of this edition
for use exclusively by the individual purchaser from the launch of the site. This licence and
access to the online version operates strictly on the basis of a single user per PIN number.
*The sharing of passwords is strictly prohibited, and any attempt to do so will
invalidate the password*. Access may not be shared, resold or otherwise circulated and will
terminate on publication of the next edition of this book. Full details and terms of use are
available upon registration and access will be subject to your acceptance of these terms of use.

clinical examination

A systematic guide to physical diagnosis

Nicholas J Talley

MD, PhD, MMedSci (Epi), FRACP, FRCP (London), FRCP (Edin), FAFPHM, FACP, FACG, AGAF

Professor of Medicine, Mayo Clinic College of Medicine;
Chair, Department of Internal Medicine, Mayo Clinic, Jacksonville, FL;
Consultant Gastroenterologist, Mayo Clinic, Jacksonville, FL, USA

Simon O'Connor

FRACP, DDU, FCSANZ

Cardiologist, The Canberra Hospital;
Clinical Senior Lecturer, Australian National University Medical School,
 Canberra, ACT

CHURCHILL LIVINGSTONE

ELSEVIER

Sydney   Edinburgh   London   New York   Philadelphia   St Louis   Toronto

ELSEVIER

Churchill Livingstone
is an imprint of Elsevier

Elsevier Australia
(a division of Reed International Books Australia Pty Ltd)
30–52 Smidmore Street, Marrickville, NSW 2204
ACN 001 002 357

National Library of Australia Cataloguing-in-Publication Data

---

Talley, Nicholas Joseph.
  Clinical examination: a systematic guide to physical
  diagnosis.

  5th ed.
  Includes index.
  ISBN: 978-0-7295-3762-9.

1. Physical diagnosis. I. O'Connor, Simon. II. Title.

616.075

Publishing Director: Vaughn Curtis
Developmental Editor: Suzanne Hall
Publishing Services Manager: Helena Klijn
Edited and project managed by Carol Natsis
Proofread by Tim Learner
Designed and typeset by DiZign Pty Ltd
Photography for 5e by Glenn McCulloch
Illustrations for 5e by Shelly Communications
Indexed by Forsyth Publishing Services
Printed by Kyodo Printing

Foreword 1

Professor Talley and Dr O'Connor have updated their highly acclaimed textbook, *Clinical examination: a systematic guide to physical diagnosis*, now in its fifth edition.

The importance of a carefully obtained history and appropriately performed physical examination cannot be underestimated. These become particularly important as society calls on doctors to provide not only high-quality but safe, reliable and affordable health care. The information provided in this volume certainly goes a long way towards setting the stage for the delivery of this type of medical care.

Careful attention to application of the materials presented in this book should help ensure that the goals of high-quality, safe, reliable and affordable care can be met. The structure of the book includes general principles of history and physical examination as well as more detailed descriptions of the approach to various systems. The written material is nicely complemented by tables, illustrations and photographs, which all help to demonstrate and emphasise the important aspects of these evaluations. The rich variety of patient photographs and X-rays, as well as tabulation of findings, makes this a valuable resource for beginning students of clinical medicine as well as a handy reference source for those with more experience.

This fifth edition joins the age of electronic curricula in that the student will have access to an Elsevier Clinical Examination website that will provide more information, including video clips of the more challenging examinations. Professor Talley and Dr O'Connor are to be congratulated on this newest edition of this important resource.

Professor Keith Lindor
Dean, Mayo Medical School, Rochester MN, USA

Foreword 2

Touch is deeply embedded in the history of the healing arts of many cultures. Millions still believe that a touch by a great healer may lead to miraculous cure—the lame walk, the blind see, the deaf hear. It used to be—and still may be to some extent—an act of great courage for a doctor to touch an infectious patient. We, of course, believe none of this stuff about the meaning of touch: we are much too sophisticated. Or are we?

An elderly doctor, now himself a patient, wrote to me recently of a visit he had made to his physician. 'The doctor looked at his computer screen throughout most of our encounter and I had very little eye contact with him,' he lamented. 'He spent far more time touching the keyboard than he did touching me.' Exquisite imaging devices, genetic profiling, fully automated biochemistry—what need do we have for physical examination and speaking to the patient? Algorithms spring from hand-held computers to tell us everything we need to know and do and quite a lot more as well just to be safe. Blinking lights warn us of impending errors for which patients may sue us. The only troublesome feature in this technological fantasia is the *patient*—persistently human, unique, fearful, ill, depressed, disabled, in pain, seeking love, relief and comfort and, if possible, cure. Can we help?

It is good to know that technology has not engulfed physicians of the calibre of Talley and O'Connor, who retain their independence and passion for humane encounter in medicine.

It may well remain true that a physician can make a diagnosis from the patient's history alone in 75 per cent of cases, if he or she listens skilfully, possibly more so when the ailment is complex and tests are so annoyingly equivocal. The physical examination—apart from what it communicates of the doctor's shared humanity—remains a superb tool for making many diagnoses, and for imparting reassurance about progress throughout the course of a long illness.

Pity our patients—and us—if we ever get to the point where the skills recorded in this great little book are forgotten or suppressed in a sanitised world of scanners, keyboards and blinking screens.

Stephen R Leeder
Director, Australian Health Policy Institute, University of Sydney
Former Dean, Faculty of Medicine, University of Sydney

Contents

Foreword 1 v
Foreword 2 vi
Preface xi
Acknowledgments xii
Clinical methods: a historical perspective xiii
The Hippocratic oath xv

Chapter 1 The general principles of history taking 1
  Bedside manner and establishing rapport 1
  Obtaining the history 1
  Introductory questions 2
  The presenting (principal) symptom 3
  History of the presenting illness 3
    Current symptoms; current treatment and drug history; sexual history; menstrual history; the impact of the illness
  The past history 5
  The social and personal history 5
    Occupation and education; social habits and maintenance of good health; overseas travel and immunisation; marital status, social support and living conditions
  Activities of daily living 8
  The family history 8
  Systems review 9
  The 'uncooperative' or 'difficult' patient 9
  Cross-cultural history taking 12
  Skills in history taking 12
  The assessment 12
  References 13
  Suggested reading 14

Chapter 2 The general principles of physical examination 15
  Evidence-based clinical examination 16
  First impressions 18
  Vital signs 18
  Facies 18
    Jaundice; cyanosis; pallor; hair
  Weight, body habitus and posture 20
  Hydration 21
  The hands and nails 22
  Temperature 23
  Smell 23
  Preparing the patient for examination 24
  References 24
  Suggested reading 25

Chapter 3 The cardiovascular system 27
  The cardiovascular history 27
    Presenting symptoms; risk factors for coronary disease; treatment; past history; social history
  The cardiovascular examination 32
    Positioning the patient; general appearance; hands; arterial pulse; blood pressure; face; neck; praecordium; back; abdomen, lower limbs; peripheral vascular disease; acute arterial occlusion; deep venous thrombosis; varicose veins

Correlation of physical signs and cardiovascular disease 60
Cardiac failure; chest pain; pericardial disease; systemic hypertension; pulmonary hypertension; valve diseases of the left heart; valve diseases of the right heart; cardiomyopathy; aortic dissection; acyanotic congenital heart disease; cyanotic congenital heart disease; 'grown-up' congenital heart disease

The chest X-ray: a systematic approach 82
Frontal film; lateral film; examples of chest X-rays in cardiac disease

Summary 88
The cardiovascular examination: a suggested method

References 90

Suggested reading 91

Chapter 4 The respiratory system and breast examination 93

The respiratory history 93
Presenting symptoms; treatment; past history; occupational history; social history; family history

The respiratory examination 98
Positioning the patient; general appearance; hands; face; trachea; chest; heart; abdomen; other; bedside assessment of lung function

Correlation of physical signs and respiratory disease 110
Consolidation (lobar pneumonia); collapse; pleural effusion; pneumothorax; tension pneumothorax; bronchiectasis; bronchial asthma; chronic obstructive pulmonary disease (chronic airflow limitation); emphysema; chronic bronchitis; pulmonary fibrosis; tuberculosis; mediastinal compression; carcinoma of the lung; sarcoidosis; pulmonary embolism

The chest X-ray 118
Chest X-ray checklist

Examination of the breasts 122
Inspection; palpation; evaluation of a breast lump

Summary 124
The respiratory examination: a suggested method

References 126

Suggested reading 126

Chapter 5 The gastrointestinal system 127

The gastrointestinal history 127
Presenting symptoms; treatment; past history; social history; family history

The gastrointestinal examination 133
Positioning the patient; general appearance; the hands; the arms; the face; the neck and chest; the abdomen—inspection, palpation, percussion, auscultation; hernias; rectal examination; proctosigmoidoscopy; other

Examination of the gastrointestinal contents 162
Faeces; vomitus

Urinalysis 163

Examination of the acute abdomen 164

Correlation of physical signs and gastrointestinal disease 167
Liver disease; portal hypertension; hepatic encephalopathy; dysphagia; assessment of gastrointestinal bleeding; malabsorption; inflammatory bowel disease

The abdominal X-ray: a systematic approach 171
Radiography; bowel gas pattern; bowel dilation; calcification; ascites

Summary 174
The gastrointestinal examination: a suggested method

References 176

Suggested reading 176

Chapter 6 The genitourinary system 179

The genitourinary history 179
Presenting symptoms; menstrual and sexual history; treatment; past history; social history; family history

The genitourinary examination 184
  General appearance; hands; arms; face; neck; chest; abdominal examination; back; legs; blood pressure
The urine 188
  Colour; transparency; smell; specific gravity; chemical analysis; pH; protein; glucose and ketones; blood; nitrite; urine sediment
Male genitalia 191
  Differential diagnosis of a scrotal mass
Pelvic examination 192
Summary 194
  Examination of a patient with chronic renal failure: a suggested method
References 195
Suggested reading 195

Chapter 7 The haematological system 197
The haematological history 197
  Presenting symptoms; treatment; past history; social history; family history
The haematological examination 198
  General appearance; hands; forearms; epitrochlear nodes; axillary nodes; face; cervical and supraclavicular nodes; bone tenderness; abdominal examination; inguinal nodes; legs; fundi
Examination of the peripheral blood film 203
Correlation of physical signs and haematological disease 207
  Anaemia; pancytopenia; acute leukaemia; chronic leukaemia; myeloproliferative disease; lymphoma; multiple myeloma
Summary 211
  The haematological examination: a suggested method
References 213
Suggested reading 213

Chapter 8 The rheumatological system 215
The rheumatological history 215
  Presenting symptoms; treatment history; past history; social history; family history
The rheumatological examination 219
  General inspection; principles of joint examination—look, feel, move, measure; assessment of individual joints—hands and wrists, elbows, shoulders, temporomandibular joints, neck, thoracolumbar spine and sacroiliac joints, hips, knees, ankles and feet
Correlation of physical signs and rheumatological disease 240
  Rheumatoid arthritis; seronegative spondyloarthropathies; gouty arthritis; calcium pyrophosphate arthropathy (pseudogout); calcium hydroxyapatite arthropathy; systemic lupus erythematosus; scleroderma (progressive systemic sclerosis); the vasculitides; soft-tissue rheumatism; nerve entrapment syndromes
References 255
Suggested reading 256

Chapter 9 The endocrine system 257
The endocrine history 257
  Presenting symptoms; past history; social history; family history
The endocrine examination 259
  The thyroid—the thyroid gland, hyperthyroidism (thyrotoxicosis), hypothyroidism (myxoedema); the pituitary—panhypopituitarism, acromegaly; the adrenals—Cushing's syndrome, Addison's disease; calcium metabolism—primary hyperparathyroidism, the MEN syndromes, hypoparathyroidism; some syndromes associated with short stature; hirsutism; gynaecomastia; diabetes mellitus; Paget's disease (osteitis deformans)
Summary 280
  The endocrine system: a suggested method of examination
References 281
Suggested reading 282

Chapter 10 The nervous system 283

The neurological history 283
Headache and facial pain; faints and fits; dizziness; visual disturbances and deafness; disturbances of gait; disturbed sensation or weakness in the limbs; tremor and involuntary movements; speech and mental status; past health; social history; family history

The neurological examination 287
General signs; higher centres and speech; the cranial nerves; head and neck; medical examination of the eyes: a summary; limbs and trunk; upper limbs; lower limbs; gait

Correlation of physical signs and neurological disease 345
Upper motor neurone lesions; lower motor neurone lesions; motor neurone disease; peripheral neuropathy; Guillain-Barré syndrome; thickened peripheral nerves; spinal cord compression; important spinal cord syndromes; myopathy; dystrophia myotonica; myasthenia gravis; the cerebellum; Parkinson's disease; other extrapyramidal movement disorders

The unconscious patient 363
General inspection; level of consciousness; neck; head and face; upper and lower limbs; body; coma scale

Summary 365
Examining the nervous system: a suggested method

References 368

Suggested reading 368

Chapter 11 The psychiatric history and mental state examination 369

Obtaining the history 370
Introductory questions; history of the presenting illness; past history; family history; social and personal history

The mental state examination 377

The diagnosis 377

References 383

Suggested reading 383

Chapter 12 The skin and nails 385

The dermatological history 385

General principles of physical examination of the skin 385

How to approach the clinical diagnosis of a lump 387

Correlation of physical signs and skin disease 388
Pruritus; erythrosquamous eruptions; blistering eruptions; erythroderma; pustular and crusted lesions; dermal plaques; erythema nodosum; erythema multiforme; hyperpigmentation; flushing and sweating; skin tumours

The nails 394

Summary 395
The dermatological examination in internal medicine: a suggested method

References 397

Suggested reading 397

Chapter 13 A system for the infectious diseases examination 399

Pyrexia of unknown origin (PUO) 399
History; examination

HIV infection and the acquired immunodeficiency syndrome (AIDS) 401
Examination

References 405

Suggested reading 405

Appendix I Writing and presenting the history and physical examination 407
Appendix II A suggested method for a rapid screening physical examination 411
Appendix III The pre-anaesthetic medical evaluation (PAME) 415
Index 419

Preface

Medicine is not only a science; it is also an art. It does not consist of compounding pills and plasters; it deals with the very processes of life, which must be understood before they may be guided.

Paracelsus (ca 1493–1541)

The commission from our new publishers, Elsevier Australia, to write a new edition of *Clinical examination* has given us a major opportunity to revise and modernise this book. We hope it is already a familiar friend and guide for medical students in many countries and that the substantial changes in this new edition will widen its appeal.

The text has been thoroughly revised and updated. Many specialists have provided expert advice on changes in their own fields and their help has been invaluable to us in our efforts to maintain the relevance of the book for modern medical students.

The evidence-based approach to the usefulness of physical signs has been expanded and *Good Signs Guides* introduced to help students understand the relative values and importance of clinical findings in making a diagnosis.

New colour photographs and revised drawings have been included throughout the book. We think these will make for clearer explanations of examination techniques and of the pathophysiology of clinical signs. We have provided more detailed analyses of the anatomical and physiological bases of examination findings. This seems particularly important for graduate medical students who learn anatomy and physiology at the bedside.

By following the links from <http://www.studentconsult.com>, students using this edition of *Clinical examination* can find more information about the techniques of physical examination, including video clips demonstrating some of the more difficult examinations. The website also provides revision and examination aids. New information and updates will be posted at the site as they become available.

We are very grateful to the many Elsevier Australia staff who have worked with us with great professionalism (and patience) on this new edition.

Nicholas J Talley and Simon O'Connor

Acknowledgments

The following eminent specialists reviewed appropriate chapters of this book. We are very grateful for their comments and advice, but we take responsibility for any errors or omissions.

Dr D Coulshed FRACP, Senior Lecturer in Medicine and Staff Specialist in Cardiology, Nepean Hospital, Sydney

Dr B Frankum FRACP, Staff Specialist in Immunology, Nepean Hospital, Sydney and Lecturer in Medical Education, University of Sydney

Dr M Hurwitz FCP(SA), FRACP, FCCP, Staff Specialist in Thoracic Medicine, The Canberra Hospital, Canberra

Dr P McManis FRACP, Senior Lecturer in Medicine and Staff Specialist in Neurology, Nepean Hospital, Sydney

A/Professor N Manolias FRACP, FRCPA, Staff Specialist in Rheumatology, Westmead Hospital, Sydney and Senior Lecturer, University of Sydney

Dr L Morgan FRACP, Consultant in Respiratory Medicine, Nepean Hospital, Sydney

A/Professor J Morris FRACP, FRCP, Head of Neurology, Westmead Hospital, Sydney

Professor J Murtagh FRACGP, Adjunct Professor of General Practice, Monash University, Melbourne and Executive Director, Education, Royal Australian College of General Practitioners

Dr A Shakeshaft FRACS, Colorectal Surgeon, Nepean Hospital, Sydney

Professor J Wiley FRACP, Professor of Haematology, Nepean Hospital, Sydney

Dr G Briggs very kindly provided the original X-ray material. Professor P Boyce provided the original psychiatry chapter, and Dr A Cooper prepared the original chapter on the skin, for which we remain very grateful. Dr A Manoharan and Dr J Isbister provided the original blood film photographs and the accompanying text. A/Professor L Schreiber provided the section on soft-tissue rheumatology, which we have updated. Associate Professor S Posen, Associate Professor IPC Murray, Dr G Bauer, Dr E Wilmshurst, Dr J Stiel and Dr J Webb helped us obtain many of the original photographs. The dermatology illustrations in Chapter 12 are reproduced with permission from *Clinical dermatology illustrated: a regional approach,* 3rd edition, by John RT Reeves and Howard Maibach (MacLennan & Petty, Sydney, 2000). Professor John Reeves kindly lent us his transparencies. The retinal photographs were kindly provided by Dr Chris Kennedy and Professor Ian Constable (and all are copyright Lion's Eye Institute).

Some of the new photographs for the 5th edition have come from the Mayo Clinic library and from FS McDonald, (editor), *Mayo Clinic images in internal medicine: self-assessment for board exam review* (Mayo Clinic Scientific Press: Rochester MN & CRC Press: Boca Raton FL, 2004). We would like to thank the following from Mayo Clinic College of Medicine for their kind assistance in selecting this additional photographic material: Dr Ashok M Patel MD, Dr Ayalew Tefferi MD, Dr Mark R Pittelkow MD and Dr Eric L Matteson MD.

We are also indebted to Steven McGee, Associate Professor of Internal Medicine, University of Washington, for permission to use some of his detailed LR figures from his book, *Evidence-based physical diagnosis* (Saunders, 2001) in the *Good signs guides.*

Elsevier Australia and the authors also extend their appreciation to the following reviewers for their comments and insights on the entire manuscript:

Dr P Coleman MB, MRCPI, FRACGP, Consultant Physician, Specialist in Nephrology and Hypertension, Manly Hospital, Manly, New South Wales.

Dr S Sanders BMBS, SHO in Paediatrics, Northwick Park Hospital, Harrow, United Kingdom.

Professor I Wilson PhD, FRACGP, Department of Medical Education, University of Western Sydney, Campbelltown, New South Wales.

Clinical methods: a historical perspective

The best physician is the one who is able to differentiate the possible and the impossible.
Herophilus of Alexandria

From classical Greek times interrogation of the patient has been considered most important because disease was, and still is, viewed in terms of the discomfort it causes. However, the current emphasis on the use of history taking and physical examination for diagnosis developed only in the 19th century. Although the terms 'symptoms and signs' have been part of the medical vocabulary since the revival of classical medicine, until relatively recently they were used synonymously.

During the 19th century, the distinction between *symptoms* (subjective complaints, which the clinician learns from the patient's account of his or her feelings) and *signs* (objective morbid changes detectable by the clinician) evolved.

Until the 19th century, diagnosis was empirical and based on the classical Greek belief that all disease had a single cause, an imbalance of the four humours (yellow bile, black bile, blood and phlegm). Indeed the Royal College of Physicians, founded in London in 1518, believed that clinical experience without classical learning was useless, and physicians who were College members were fined if they ascribed to any other view.

At the time of Hippocrates (460–375 BC) observation (inspection) and feeling (palpation) had a place in the examination of patients. The ancient Greeks, for example, noticed that patients with jaundice often had an enlarged liver that was firm and irregular. Shaking a patient and listening for a fluid splash was also recognised by the Greeks.

Herophilus of Alexandria (335–280 BC) described a method of taking the pulse in the 4th century BC. However, it was Galen of Pergamum (130–200 AD) who established the pulse as one of the major physical signs, and it continued to have this important role up to the 18th century, with minute variations being recorded. These variations were erroneously considered to indicate changes in the body's harmony.

William Harvey's (1578–1657) studies of the human circulation, published in 1628, had little effect on the general understanding of the value of the pulse as a sign. Sanctorius (1561–1636) was the first to time the pulse using a clock, while John Floyer (1649–1734) invented the pulse watch in 1707 and made regular observations of the pulse rate. Abnormalities in heart rate were described in diabetes mellitus in 1776 and in thyrotoxicosis in 1786.

Fever was studied by Hippocrates and was originally regarded as an entity rather than a sign of disease. The thermoscope was devised by Sanctorius in 1625. In association with Gabriel Fahrenheit (1686–1736), Hermann Boerhaave (1668–1738) introduced the thermometer as a research instrument and this was produced commercially in the middle of the 18th century.

In the 13th century Johannes Actuarius (d. 1283) used a graduated glass to examine the urine. In Harvey's time a specimen of urine was sometimes looked at (inspected) and even tasted, and was considered to reveal secrets about the body. Harvey recorded that sugar diabetes (mellitus) and dropsy (oedema) could be diagnosed in this way. The detection of protein in the urine, which Frederik Dekkers (1644–1720) first described in 1673, was ignored until Richard Bright (1789–1858) demonstrated its importance in renal disease. Although Celsus described and valued measurements such as weighing and measuring a patient in the 1st century AD, these methods became widely used only in the 20th century.

A renaissance in clinical methods began with the concept of Battista Morgagni (1682–1771) that disease was not generalised but arose in organs, a conclusion published in 1761. Leopold Auenbrugger invented chest tapping (percussion) to detect disease in the same year. Van Swieten, his teacher, in fact used percussion to detect ascites. The technique was forgotten for nearly half a century until Jean Corvisart (1755–1821) translated Auenbrugger's work in 1808.

The next big step occurred with René Laënnec (1781–1826), a student of Corvisart. He invented the stethoscope in 1816 (at first merely a roll of stiff paper) as an aid to diagnosing heart and lung disease by listening (auscultation). This revolutionised chest examination, partly because it made the chest accessible in patients too modest to allow a direct application of the examiner's ear to the chest wall, as well as allowing accurate clinicopathological correlations. William Stokes (1804–78) published the first treatise in English on the use of the stethoscope in 1825. Josef Skoda's (1805–81) investigations of the value of these clinical methods led to their widespread and enthusiastic adoption after he published his results in 1839.

These advances helped lead to a change in the practice of medicine. Bedside teaching was first introduced in the Renaissance by Montanus (1498–1552) in Padua in 1543. In the 17th century, physicians based their opinion on a history provided by an apothecary (assistant) and rarely saw the patients themselves. Thomas Sydenham (1624–89) began to practise more modern bedside medicine, basing his treatment on experience and not theory, but it was not until a century later that the scientific method brought a systematic approach to clinical diagnosis.

This change began in the hospitals of Paris after the French Revolution, with recognition of the work of Morgagni, Corvisart, Laënnec and others. Influenced by the philosophy of the Enlightenment, which suggested that a rational approach to all problems was possible, the Paris Clinical School combined physical examination with autopsy as the basis of clinical medicine. The methods of this school were first applied abroad in Dublin, where Robert Graves (1796–1853) and William Stokes worked. Later at Guy's Hospital in London the famous trio of Richard Bright, Thomas Addison (1793–1860) and Thomas Hodgkin (1798–1866) made their important contributions. In 1869 Samuel Wilks (1824–1911) wrote on the nail changes in disease and the signs he described remain important. Carl Wunderlich's (1815–77) work changed the concept of temperature from a disease in itself to a symptom of disease.

Spectacular advances in physiology, pathology, pharmacology and the discovery of microbiology in the latter half of the 19th century led to the development of the new 'clinical and laboratory medicine', which is the rapidly advancing medicine of the present day. The modern systematic approach to diagnosis, with which this book deals, is still, however, based on taking the history and examining the patient by looking (inspecting), feeling (palpating), tapping (percussing) and listening (auscultating).

Suggested reading

Reiser SJ. The clinical record in medicine. Part I: Learning from cases. *Ann Intern Med* 1991; 114:902–907.
Bordage G. Where are the history and the physical? *Can Med Assoc J* 1995; 152:1595–1598.
McDonald C. Medical heuristics: the silent adjudicators of clinical practice. *Ann Intern Med* 1996; 124:56–62.

The Hippocratic oath

I swear by Apollo the physician, and Aesculapius, and Hygieia, and Panacea, and all the gods and goddesses that, according to my ability and judgment, I will keep this Oath and this stipulation:

To reckon him who taught me this Art equally dear to me as my parents, to share my substance with him and relieve his necessities if required; to look upon his offspring in the same footing as my own brother, and to teach them this Art, if they shall wish to learn it, without fee or stipulation, and that by precept, lecture, and every other mode of instruction, I will impart a knowledge of the Art to my own sons and those of my teachers, and to disciples bound by a stipulation and oath according to the law of medicine, but to none others.

I will follow that system of regimen which, according to my ability and judgment, I consider for the benefit of my patients, and abstain from whatever is deleterious and mischievous. I will give no deadly medicine to any if asked, nor suggest any such counsel; and in like manner I will not give a woman a pessary to produce abortion.

With purity and with holiness I will pass my life and practise my Art. I will not cut persons labouring under the stone, but will leave this to be done by men who are practitioners of this work. Into whatever houses I enter I will go into them for the benefit of the sick and will abstain from every voluntary act of mischief and corruption; and further from the seduction of females or males, of freemen and slaves.

Whatever, in connection with my professional practice, or not in connection with it, I may see or hear in the lives of men which ought not to be spoken of abroad I will not divulge, as reckoning that all such should be kept secret.

While I continue to keep this Oath unviolated may it be granted to me to enjoy life and the practice of the Art, respected by all men, in all times! But should I trespass and violate this Oath, may the reverse be my lot!

Hippocrates, born on the Island of Cos (460?–357 BC) is agreed by everyone to be the father of medicine. He is said to have lived to the age of 109.

Many of the statements in this ancient oath remain relevant today, while others, such as euthanasia and abortion, remain controversial. The seduction of slaves, however, is less of a problem.

Credits

New photography for the 5th edition by Glenn McCulloch, unless stated otherwise.

Illustrations by Shelly Communications Pty Ltd, unless stated otherwise.

Good signs guides based on detailed LR figures from McGee S. *Evidence-based physical diagnosis*, Saunders: Philadelphia, 2001, with permission.

Key

Mayo Clinic: From Mayo Clinic Library and FS McDonald, ed. *Mayo Clinic images in internal medicine: self-assessment for board exam review.* © Mayo Clinic Scientific Press: Rochester MN & CRC Press: Boca Raton FL, 2004, with permission.

Reeves & Maibach: From Reeves JT and Maibach H, *Clinical dermatology illustrated: a regional approach*, 3rd edn. McLennan & Petty: Sydney, 2000.

Page numbers shown in bold face, underlined; figure numbers shown in bold face.

Chapter 2
<u>17</u> 2.1 Adapted from Sackett DL, Richardson WS, Rosenberg W, Haynes RB. *Evidence-based medicine: how to practice and teach EBM.* Churchill-Livingstone: London, 1997, with permission.

Chapter 3
<u>41</u> 3.12b Mayo Clinic. <u>49</u> 3.25 Adapted from Swash M, ed. *Hutchison's clinical methods*, 20th edn. London: Baillière Tindall, 1995, with permission. <u>59</u> 3.31, 3.32, 3.33 Mayo Clinic. <u>64</u> 3.36 Dr Chris Kennedy & Prof. Ian Constable © Lions Eye Institute, Perth. <u>65</u> 3.37, 3.38 Dr Chris Kennedy & Prof. Ian Constable © Lions Eye Institute, Perth.

Chapter 4
<u>102</u> 4.3 Mayo Clinic. <u>114</u> 4.12 Mayo Clinic.

Chapter 5
<u>136</u> 5.3, 5.4, 5.5, 5.6 Mayo Clinic. <u>137</u> 5.7a From Jones DV et al, in Feldman M et al, *Sleisenger & Fordtran's gastrointestinal disease,* 6th edn, Chapter 112. Philadelphia: WB Saunders, 1998, with permission. 5.7b Mayo Clinic. 5.8 Mayo Clinic. <u>138</u> 5.9 Mayo Clinic. <u>139</u> 5.11 Mayo Clinic. <u>141</u> 5.14 Mayo Clinic. <u>142</u> 5.15 Mayo Clinic. <u>144</u> 5.17 Mayo Clinic. <u>147</u> 5.20 Adapted from Swash M, ed. *Hutchison's clinical methods*, 20th edn. London: Baillière Tindall, 1995, with permission. <u>171</u> 5.33, 5.34 Mayo Clinic.

Chapter 6
<u>185</u> 6.2 Mayo Clinic.

Chapter 7
<u>203</u> 7.7 Mayo Clinic.

Chapter 8
<u>244</u> 8.37 Mayo Clinic.

Chapter 9
<u>270</u> 9.9 Mayo Clinic. <u>273</u> 9.11 Mayo Clinic. <u>277</u> 9.14, 9.15 Mayo Clinic. <u>278</u> 9.17 Dr Chris Kennedy & Prof. Ian Constable © Lions Eye Institute, Perth. <u>279</u> 9.18, 9.19 Dr Chris Kennedy & Prof. Ian Constable © Lions Eye Institute, Perth.

Chapter 10
<u>355</u> 10.103a Mayo Clinic.

Chapter 12
<u>388</u> 12.2, 12.3 Reeves & Maibach. <u>389</u> 12.4, 12.5, 12.6 Reeves & Maibach. <u>390</u> 12.7, 12.8, 12.9, 12.10 Reeves & Maibach. <u>392</u> 12.11 Reeves & Maibach. <u>393</u> 12.12 Reeves & Maibach. <u>394</u> 12.13, 12.14, 12.15 Reeves & Maibach. <u>395</u> 12.16 12.17 Reeves & Maibach.

Chapter 13
<u>401</u> 13.1 Reeves & Maibach. <u>403</u> 13.2 Reeves & Maibach. 13.3 Mayo Clinic. <u>404</u> 13.4 Mayo Clinic. <u>404</u> 13.5, 13.6 Dr Chris Kennedy & Prof. Ian Constable © Lions Eye Institute, Perth.

negative. Another way of looking at this is the positive or negative predictive value of a test—that is, the probability that a positive result means the condition is present or that a negative result means it is absent.

The likelihood that a test or sign result will be a true positive or negative depends on the pre-test probability of the presence of the condition. For example, if splinter haemorrhages (page 34) are found in the nails of a well manual labourer they are likely to represent a false positive sign of infective endocarditis. This sign is not very sensitive or specific and the pre-test probability of the condition is low. If splinters are found in a sick patient with known valvular heart disease and a new murmur, the sign is likely to be a true positive in this patient with a high pre-test probability of endocarditis. This pre-test probability analysis of the false and true positive rate is based on Bayes' theorem.

A useful way to look at sensitivity and specificity is the *likelihood ratio* (LR). A positive LR,

$$\text{Positive LR} = \frac{\text{sensitivity}}{1 - \text{specificity}}$$

indicates that the presence of a sign is likely to occur that much more often in an individual with the disease than in one without it. The higher the positive LR, the more useful is a positive sign. A negative likelihood ratio increases the likelihood that the disease is absent if the sign is not present.

$$\text{Negative LR} = \frac{1 - \text{sensitivity}}{\text{specificity}}$$

Remember that if the LR is greater than 1 there is an increased probability of disease; if the LR is between 1 and 0 there is a decreased probability of disease.

For example, the presence of a third heart sound in a patient who might have heart failure (e.g. breathlessness on exertion) has a positive likelihood ratio of 3.8 and a negative LR around 1. This means that a third heart sound is specific for heart failure (increases likelihood of the condition nearly four times) but not sensitive (the absence of a third heart sound does not reduce the likelihood).

All these figures are calculated on a population suspected of disease; it would be quite incorrect to apply them to an asymptomatic group of people. Fagan's nomogram (Figure 2.1) can be used to apply LRs to clinical problems if the pre-test probability of the condition is known or can be estimated. When the pre-test probability is very low, even a high positive LR does not make the disease very likely. A line is drawn from the pre-test probability number through the known LR and ends up on the post-test

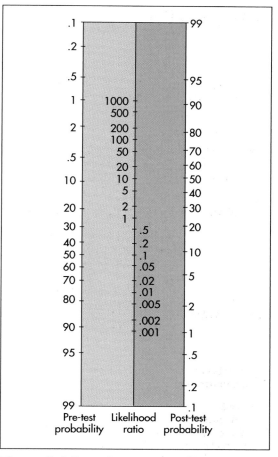

Figure 2.1 Fagan's nomogram for interpreting a diagnostic test result

(Adapted from Sackett DL, Richardson WS, Rosenberg W, Haynes RB. *Evidence-based medicine: how to practice and teach EBM*. Churchill-Livingstone: London, 1997.)

probability number. For example, if the pre-test probability of the condition is low, say 10 (10%) and a sign is present which has an LR of 2, the post-test probability of the condition being present is about 20%. We have included LRs in a selection of *Good signs guides* in some chapters of this book.

In medical practice multiple factors are taken into account when diagnostic decisions are made. Only very rarely is one symptom or sign or test diagnostic of a condition. The skilled and experienced clinician uses many pieces of information and is sceptical when an unexpected or illogical finding or test result is obtained for a patient.

First impressions

First impressions of a patient's condition must be deliberately sought; they cannot be passively acquired. The specific changes that occur in particular illnesses (e.g. myxoedema) will be discussed in detail in the appropriate chapters. However, certain abnormalities should be obvious to the trained or training doctor.

First, decide how sick the patient seems to be: that is, does he or she look generally ill or well? The cheerful person sitting up in bed reading Proust (Figure 2.2) is unlikely to require urgent attention to save his life. At the other extreme, the patient on the verge of death may be described as *in extremis* or moribund. The patient in this case may be lying still in bed and seem unaware of the surroundings. The face may be sunken and expressionless, respiration may be shallow and laboured; at the end of life, respiration often becomes slow and intermittent, with longer and longer pauses between rattling breaths.

Apart from gaining a general impression of a patient's state of health, certain general physical signs must be sought.

Vital signs

Certain important measurements must be made during the assessment of the patient. These relate primarily to cardiac and respiratory function and include pulse, blood pressure, temperature and respiratory rate. These vital signs must be assessed at once if a patient appears unwell. Patients in hospital have these measurements taken regularly and charted. They provide important basic physiological information.

Figure 2.2 'For a long time I used to go to bed early.'

Facies

A specific diagnosis can sometimes be made by inspecting the face, its appearance giving a clue to the likely diagnosis. Other physical signs must usually be sought to confirm the diagnosis. Some facial characteristics are so typical of certain diseases that they immediately suggest the diagnosis and are called the diagnostic facies (Table 2.2). Apart from these, there are several other important abnormalities that must be looked for in the face.

Jaundice

When the serum bilirubin level rises to about twice the upper limit of normal, bilirubin is deposited in the tissues of the body. It then causes yellow discoloration of the skin (*jaundice*) and more dramatically, the apparent discoloration of the sclerae. The usual term *scleral icterus* is misleading, since the bilirubin is actually deposited in the vascular conjunctiva rather than the avascular sclerae. The sclerae (conjunctivae) are rarely affected by other pigment changes. In fact, jaundice is the only condition causing yellow sclerae. Other causes of yellow discoloration of the skin, but where the sclerae remain normal, are carotenaemia (usually due to excess consumption of carotene, often from

---

Table 2.2 Some important diagnostic facies

Amiodarone (anti-arrhythmic drug)—deep blue discoloration around malar area and nose
Acromegalic (page 267)
Cushingoid (page 269)
Down syndrome (page 273)
Hippocratic (advanced peritonitis)—eyes are sunken, temples collapsed, nose is pinched with crusts on the lips and the forehead is clammy (page 21)
Marfanoid (page 34)
Mitral (page 41)
Myopathic (page 355)
Myotonic (page 356)
Myxoedematous (page 265)
Pagetic (page 279)
Parkinsonian (page 361)
Ricketic (page 274)
Thyrotoxic (page 263)
Turner's syndrome (page 273)
Uraemic (page 184)
Virile facies (page 274)

intemperate eating of carrots or mangoes), acri-flavine, fluorescein and picric acid ingestion.

Jaundice may be the result of excess production of bilirubin, usually from excessive destruction of red blood cells (termed haemolytic anaemia), when it can produce a pale lemon-yellow scleral discoloration. Alternatively, jaundice may be due to obstruction to bile flow from the liver, which, if severe, produces a dark yellow or orange tint. Scratch marks may be prominent due to associated itching (pruritus). The other main cause of jaundice is hepatocellular failure. Jaundice is discussed in more detail in Chapter 5.

Cyanosis

This refers to a blue discoloration of the skin and mucous membranes; it is due to the presence of deoxygenated haemoglobin in superficial blood vessels. The haemoglobin molecule changes colour from blue to red when oxygen is added to it in the lungs. If more than about 50 g/L of deoxygenated haemoglobin is present in the capillary blood, the skin will have a bluish tinge.[7] Cyanosis does *not* occur in anaemic hypoxia because the total haemoglobin content is low. Cyanosis is more easily detected in fluorescent light than in daylight.

Central cyanosis means that there is an abnormal amount of deoxygenated haemoglobin in the arteries and that a blue discoloration is present in parts of the body with a good circulation, such as the tongue. This must be distinguished from *peripheral cyanosis*, which occurs when the blood supply to a certain part of the body is reduced and the tissues extract more oxygen than normal from the circulating blood: for example, the lips in cold weather are often blue, but the tongue is spared. The presence of central cyanosis should lead one to a careful examination of the cardiovascular (Chapter 3) and respiratory (Chapter 4) systems (see also Table 2.3).

Pallor

A deficiency of haemoglobin (*anaemia*) can produce pallor of the skin and should be noticeable, especially in the mucous membranes of the sclerae if the anaemia is severe (less than 70 g/L of haemoglobin). Pull the lower eyelid down and compare the colour of the anterior part of the palpebral conjunctiva (attached to the inner surface of the eyelid) with the posterior part where it reflects off the sclera. There is usually a marked difference between the red anterior and creamy posterior parts. This difference is absent when significant anaemia is present. Although this is at best a crude way of screening for

---

Table 2.3 Causes of cyanosis

Central cyanosis

1 Decreased arterial oxygen saturation
   • Decreased concentration of inspired oxygen: high altitude
   • Lung disease: chronic obstructive pulmonary disease with cor pulmonale, massive pulmonary embolism
   • Right-to-left cardiac shunt (cyanotic congenital heart disease)
2 Polycythaemia
3 Haemoglobin abnormalities (rare)
   • Methaemoglobinaemia
   • Sulphaemoglobinaemia

Peripheral cyanosis

1 All causes of central cyanosis cause peripheral cyanosis
2 Exposure to cold
3 Reduced cardiac output: left ventricular failure or shock
4 Arterial or venous obstruction

GOOD SIGNS GUIDE 2.1
Anaemia

Sign	Positive LR*	Negative LR†
Pallor at multiple sites	4.5	0.7
Facial pallor	3.8	0.6
Palm crease pallor	7.9	NS
Conjunctival pallor	16.7	–

* Positive likelihood ratio: when the finding is *present*, describes the probability change. The higher the LR is above 1, the more likely there is disease.
† Negative likelihood ratio: when the finding is *absent*, describes the probability change. The closer the LR is to 0, the more likely there is *not* disease.
NS = not significant.
From McGee S, *Evidence-based physical diagnosis*, Saunders, 2001.

---

anaemia, it can be specific (though not sensitive) when anaemia is suspected for other reasons as well (*Good signs guide 2.1*). It should be emphasised that pallor is a sign, while anaemia is a diagnosis based on laboratory results.

Facial pallor may also be found in *shock*, which is usually defined as a reduction of cardiac output, such that the oxygen demands of the tissues are not being met (Table 2.4). These patients usually appear clammy and cold and are significantly hypotensive (have low blood pressure) (page 21). Pallor may also be a normal variant due to a deep-lying venous system and opaque skin.

Hair

Bearded or bald women and hairless men not uncommonly present to doctors. These conditions may be a result of more than the rich normal variations of life, and occasionally are due to endocrine disease (Chapter 9).

Weight, body habitus and posture

Look specifically for obesity. This is most objectively assessed by calculation of the body mass index (BMI), where the weight in kilograms is divided by the height in metres squared. Normal is less than 25 kg/m^2. A BMI of ≥30 indicates frank obesity. *Morbid* obesity is a weight of more than twice the ideal (BMI >45–50). Medical risks are increasingly recognised in association with obesity (Table 2.5). There are racial differences in BMIs associated with medical risk. Australian Aboriginals and Asians may have increased medical risk once the BMI exceeds 20.

The waist–hip ratio (WHR) is also predictive of health risk. This measurement is of the circumference of the waist (at the midpoint between the costal margin and the iliac crest) divided by that at the hips (at the widest part around the buttocks). Increased risk occurs when this exceeds 1.0 for men and 0.85 for women.

Severe underweight (BMI <18.5) is called cachexia.[8] Look for wasting of the muscles, which may be due to neurological or debilitating disease, such as malignancy.

Note excessively short or tall stature, which may be rather difficult to judge when the patient is lying in bed (page 273). Inspect for limb deformity or missing limbs (rather embarrassing if missed in viva voce examinations) and observe if the physique is consistent with the patient's stated chronological age.

Table 2.4 Causes of shock

1 Hypovolaemia
  - External fluid loss, e.g. blood, vomitus, diarrhoea, urine, burns, excess sweating
  - Sequestration of body fluids in the abdomen (e.g. ascites), chest (e.g. haemothorax) or limbs (e.g. fracture)
2 Cardiac
  - Pump failure, e.g. myocardial infarction, acute mitral regurgitation
  - Cardiac tamponade
  - Dissecting aortic aneurysm
  - Arrhythmia
3 Massive pulmonary embolus
4 Sepsis, e.g. gram-negative bacteria (endotoxin)
5 Anaphylaxis
6 Endocrine failure, e.g. adrenal failure, hypothyroidism
7 Neuropathic—from drugs (e.g. antihypertensives, anaesthesia), spinal cord injury of autonomic neuropathy

---

Table 2.5 Medical conditions associated with obesity (BMI ≥30)

Endocrine
Type 2 diabetes
Amenorrhoea
Dyslipidaemia
Infertility
Polycystic ovary syndrome
Hypogonadism

Respiratory
Sleep apnoea
Dyspnoea

Cardiovascular
Hypertension
Cardiac failure
Ischaemic heart disease
Cor pulmonale (right heart failure secondary to lung disease)
Pulmonary embolism

Musculoskeletal
Arthritis
Immobility

Skin
Skin abscesses
Cellulitis
Venous stasis
Fungal infections

Gut
Gastro-oesophageal reflux disease
Non-alcoholic steatohepatitis
Hernias

Table 2.6 Some body habitus syndromes
Endocrine
Acromegaly (Figure 9.6) Cushing's syndrome (Figure 9.9) Hypopituitarism (page 266) Pseudohypoparathyroidism (Figure 9.11) Rickets Paget's disease (Figure 9.20)
Musculoskeletal
Marfan's syndrome (Figure 3.2) Turner's syndrome Klinefelter's syndrome (page 274) Achondroplasia (page 274)

A number of body shapes are almost diagnostic of different conditions (Table 2.6). If the patient walks into the examining room, the opportunity to examine gait should not be lost: the full testing of gait is described in Chapter 10.

Hydration

Although this is not easy to assess, all doctors must be able to estimate the approximate state of *hydration* of a patient.[9–11] For example, a severely dehydrated patient is at risk of death from developing acute renal failure, while an overhydrated patient may develop pulmonary oedema.

To assess dehydration (Table 2.7), inspect for sunken orbits, dry mucous membranes and the moribund appearance of severe dehydration. Reduced skin turgor (pinch the skin: normal skin returns immediately on being released) occurs in moderate and severe dehydration (this traditional test is not of proven value, especially in the elderly, whose skin may always be like that). The presence of dry axillae increases the likelihood of dehydration and a moist tongue reduces the likelihood, but the other signs are in fact of little proven value (*Good signs guide 2.2*).

Take the blood pressure (page 38) and look for a fall in blood pressure when the patient sits or stands up after lying down. The patient should stand, if he or she can, for at least 1 minute before the blood pressure is taken again (the inability of the patient to stand because of postural dizziness is probably a more important sign than the blood pressure difference). This is called postural hypotension. An increase in the pulse rate of 30 or more, when the patient stands is also a sign of *hypovolaemia*.

Table 2.7 Physical signs of dehydration (of variable reliability—see *Good signs guide 2.2*)
Mild (<5%): = 2.5 L deficit
Mild thirst Dry mucous membranes Concentrated urine
Moderate (5%–8%): = 4 L deficit
As above Moderate thirst Reduced skin turgor (elasticity), especially arms, forehead, chest, abdomen Tachycardia
Severe (9%–12%): = 6 L deficit
As above Great thirst Reduced skin turgor and decreased eyeball pressure Collapsed veins, sunken eyes, 'gaunt' face Postural hypotension Oliguria (<400 mL urine/24 hours)
Very severe (>12%): >6 L deficit
As above Comatose Moribund Signs of shock
Note: Total body water in a man of 70 kg is about 40 L.

GOOD SIGNS GUIDE 2.2 Hypovolaemia		
Sign	**Positive LR**	**Negative LR**
Dry axillae	2.8	NS
Dry mucous membranes; nose and mouth	NS	0.3
Sunken eyes	NS	0.5
Confusion	NS	NS
Speech not clear	NS	0.5
NS = not significant.		
From McGee S, *Evidence-based physical diagnosis*, Saunders, 2001.		

Weigh the patient. Following the body weight daily is the best way to determine changes in hydration over time. For example, a 5% decrease in body weight over 24 hours indicates that about 5% of body water has been lost (use the same set of scales).

Assessment of the patient's jugular venous pressure is one of the most sensitive ways of judging intravascular volume overload, or overhydration (see Chapter 3).

The hands and nails

Changes occur in the hands in many different diseases. It is useful as an introduction to shake a patient's hand when meeting him or her. Apart from being polite, this may help make the diagnosis of dystrophia myotonica, a rare muscle disease in which the patient may be unable to let go. Shaking hands is also an acceptable and gentle way of introducing the physical examination. Physical examination is an intrusive event that is tolerated only because of the doctor's (and even the medical student's) professional and cultural standing.

There is probably no subspecialty of internal medicine in which examination of the hands is not rewarding. The shape of the nails may change in some cardiac and respiratory diseases, the whole size of the hand may increase in acromegaly (page 267), gross distortion of the hands' architecture occurs in some forms of arthritis (page 216), tremor or muscle wasting may represent neurological disease (page 322), and pallor of the palmar creases may indicate anaemia (Table 2.8). These and other changes in the hands await you later in the book.

Table 2.8 Nail signs in systemic disease

Nail sign	Some causes	Page no.
Blue nails	Cyanosis, Wilson's disease, ochronosis	19
Red nails	Polycythaemia (reddish-blue), carbon monoxide poisoning (cherry-red)	209
Yellow nails	Yellow nail syndrome	113
Clubbing	Lung cancer, chronic pulmonary suppuration, infective endocarditis, cyanotic heart disease, congenital, HIV infection, chronic inflammatory bowel disease	33
Splinter haemorrhages	Infective endocarditis, vasculitis	34
Koilonychia (spoon-shaped nails)	Iron deficiency, fungal infection, Raynaud's disease	198
Pale nail bed	Anaemia	198
Onycholysis	Thyrotoxicosis, psoriasis	262
Non-pigmented transverse bands (Beau's lines)	Fever, cachexia, malnutrition	184
Leuconychia (white nails)	Hypoalbuminaemia	139
Transverse opaque white bands (Muehrcke's lines)	Hypoalbuminaemia (also caused by chemotherapy or severe illness)	184
Single transverse white band (Mees' lines)	Arsenic poisoning, renal failure (also caused by chemotherapy or severe illness)	184
Nailfold erythema and telangiectasia	Systemic lupus erythematosus	245
'Half and half nails' (proximal portion white to pink and distal portion red or brown: Terry's nails)	Chronic renal failure, cirrhosis	184

Temperature

The temperature should always be recorded as part of the initial clinical examination of the patient. The normal temperature ranges from 36.6°C to 37.2°C (98°F to 99°F) (Table 2.9). In very hot weather the temperature may rise by up to 0.5°C. Patients who report they have a fever are usually correct, as is a mother who reports that her child's forehead is warm and that fever is present (*Good signs guide 2.3*).

Table 2.9 Average temperature values

	Normal	Fever
Mouth	36.8°C	>37.3°C
Axilla	36.4°C	>36.9°C
Rectum	37.3°C	>37.7°C

GOOD SIGNS GUIDE 2.3 Fever		
Sign	**Positive LR**	**Negative LR**
Patient says has fever	4.9	0.2
Warm forehead	2.5	0.4
From McGee S, *Evidence-based physical diagnosis*, Saunders, 2001.		

There is a diurnal variation; body temperature is lowest in the morning and reaches a peak between 6.00 and 10.00 p.m. The febrile pattern of most diseases follows this diurnal variation. The pattern of the fever (pyrexia) may be helpful in diagnosis (Table 2.10).

Very high temperatures (*hyperpyrexia*, defined as above 41.6°C) are a serious problem and may result in death. The causes include heat stroke from exposure or excessive exertion (e.g. in marathon runners), malignant hyperthermia (a group of genetically determined disorders in which hyperpyrexia occurs in response to various anaesthetic agents [e.g. halothane] or muscle relaxants [e.g. suxamethonium]), the neuroleptic malignant syndrome, and hypothalamic disease.

Hypothermia is defined as a temperature of less than 35°C. Normal thermometers do not record below 35°C and therefore special low-reading thermometers must be used if hypothermia is suspected. Causes of hypothermia include hypothyroidism and prolonged exposure to cold (page 264).

Smell

Certain medical conditions are associated with a characteristic odour.[12] These include the sweet smell of the breath in patients with liver failure, the ammoniacal fish breath ('uraemic fetor') of kidney failure and, of course, the stale cigarette smell of the patient who smokes. This smell will be on his or her

Table 2.10 Types of fever

Type	Character	Examples
Continued	Does not remit	Typhoid fever, typhus, drug fever, malignant hyperthermia
Intermittent	Temperature falls to normal each day	Pyogenic infections, lymphomas, miliary tuberculosis
Remittent	Daily fluctuations >2°C, temperature does not return to normal	Not characteristic of any particular disease
Relapsing	Temperature returns to normal for days before rising again	Malaria: Tertian—3-day pattern, fever peaks every other day (*Plasmodium vivax, P. ovale*); Quartan—4-day pattern, fever peaks every 3rd day (*P. malariae*) Lymphoma: Pel-Ebstein* fever of Hodgkin's disease (very rare) Pyogenic infection

* Pieter Pel (1859–1919), Professor of Medicine, Amsterdam; Wilhelm Ebstein (1836–1912), German physician
Note: The use of antipyretic and antibiotic drugs has made these patterns unusual today.

clothes and even on the referral letter kept in a bag or pocket next to a packet of cigarettes. The recent consumption of alcoholic drinks may be obvious and 'bad breath', although often of uncertain cause, may be related to poor dental hygiene, gingivitis (infection of the gums) or nasopharyngeal tumours. Chronic suppurative infections of the lung can make the breath and saliva foul smelling. Skin abscesses may be very offensive, especially if caused by anaerobic organisms or *Pseudomonas* spp. Urinary incontinence is associated with the characteristic smell of stale urine, which is often more offensive if the patient has a urinary tract infection. Severe bowel obstruction and the rare gastrocolic fistula can cause faecal contamination of the breath when the patient belches. The black faeces (*melaena*) caused by gastric bleeding and the breakdown of blood in the gut has a strong smell, familiar to anyone who has worked in a ward for patients with gastrointestinal illnesses. The metallic smell of fresh blood, sometimes detectable during invasive cardiological procedures, is very mild by comparison.

Preparing the patient for examination

An accurate physical examination is best performed when the examining conditions are ideal. This means that, if possible, the patient should be in a well-lit room (preferably daylight) from which distracting noises and interruptions have been excluded (rarely possible in busy hospital wards). Screens must be drawn around patients before they are examined. Consulting rooms and outpatient clinics should be set up to ensure privacy and comfort for patients.

The patient must be undressed so that the parts to be examined are accessible. Modesty requires that a woman's breasts be covered temporarily with a towel or sheet while other parts of the body are being examined. Male doctors and students should be accompanied by a female *chaperone* when they examine a woman's pelvis or rectum. Both men and women should have the groin covered—for example, during the examination of the legs. Outpatients should be provided with a gown to wear. However, important physical signs will be missed in some patients if excessive attention is paid to modesty. The position of the patient in bed or elsewhere should depend on what system is to be examined. For example, a patient's abdomen is best examined if he or she lies flat with one pillow so that the abdominal muscles are relaxed. This is discussed in detail in subsequent chapters.

Within each of the examining systems, four elements comprise the main parts of the physical examination: looking—*inspection*; feeling—*palpation*; tapping—*percussion*; and listening—*auscultation*. For many systems a fifth element, *assessment of function*, is added. *Measuring* is also relevant in some systems. Each of these will be discussed in detail in the following chapters.

References

1. Sacket DL. The science of the art of clinical examination. *JAMA* 1992; 267:2650–2652. Examines the limitations of current research in the field of clinical examination.
2. Sackett DL. A primer on the precision and accuracy of the clinical examination (the rational clinical examination). *JAMA* 1992; 267:2638–2644. An important article examining the relevance of understanding both precision (reproducibility among various examiners) and accuracy (determining the truth) in clinical examination.
3. Wiener S, Nathanson M. Physical examination: frequently observed errors. *JAMA* 1976; 236:852–855. This article categorises errors, including poor skills, under-reporting and over-reporting of signs, use of inadequate equipment and inadequate recording.
4. Fitzgerald FT, Tierney LM Jr. The bedside Sherlock Holmes. *West J Med* 1982; 137:169–175. Here deductive reasoning is discussed as a tool in clinical diagnosis.
5. Sackett DL, Haynes RB, Tugwell P. *Clinical epidemiology. A basic science for clinical medicine*. Boston: Little, Brown & Co, 1985. The perceived commonness of diseases affects our approach to their diagnosis.
6. Oxman AD and the GRADE working group. Grading quality of evidence and strength of recommendations. *BMJ* 2004; 328:1490–1494.
7. Martin L, Khalil H. How much reduced hemoglobin is necessary to generate central cyanosis? *Chest* 1990; 97:182–185. This useful article explains the chemistry of haemoglobin and its colour change.
8. Detsky AS, Smalley PS, Chang J. Is this patient malnourished? *JAMA* 1994; 271:54–58. Assessment of nutrition is an important part of the examination but needs a scientific approach.
9. Gross CR, Lindquist RD, Woolley AC, et al. Clinical indicators of dehydration severity in elderly patients. *J Emerg Med* 1992; 10:267–274. This important and urgent assessment is more difficult in elderly sick patients.
10. Koziol-McLain J, Lowenstein SR, Fuller B. Orthostatic vital signs in emergency medicine department patients. *Ann Emerg Med* 1991; 20:606–610. These signs help in the assessment of the severity of illness in emergency patients but there is a wide range of normal.

11. McGee S, Abernethy WB III, Simel DL. Is this patient hypovolemic? *JAMA* 1999; 281:1022–1029. The most sensitive clinical features for large-volume blood loss are severe postural dizziness and a postural rise in pulse rate of >30 beats a minute, not tachycardia or supine hypotension. A dry axilla supports dehydration. Moist mucous membranes and a tongue without furrows make hypovolaemia unlikely; assessing skin turgor, surprisingly, is not of proven value.
12. Hayden GF. Olfactory diagnosis in medicine. *Postgrad Med* 1980; 67:110–115, 118. Describes characteristic patient odours and their connections with disease, although the diagnostic accuracy is uncertain.

Suggested reading

Original article

Joshua AM, Celermajer DS, Stockler MR. Beauty is in the eye of the examiner: reaching agreement about physical signs and their value. *Intern Med J* 2005; 35:178–187.

Textbooks

Beaven DW, Brooks SE. *Color atlas of the nail in clinical diagnosis*, 2nd edn. Chicago: Year Book Medical Publishers, 1994.

Browse NL. *An introduction to the symptoms and signs of surgical disease*, 3rd edn. London: Edward Arnold, 1997.

Lumley JJP, ed. *Hamilton Bailey's demonstrations of physical signs in clinical surgery*, 18th edn. Oxford: Butterworth-Heinemann, 1997.

McGee S. *Evidence-based physical diagnosis*. Philadelphia: Saunders, 2001.

McHardy KC et al. *Illustrated signs in clinical medicine*. Edinburgh: Churchill-Livingstone, 1997.

Orient JM. *Sapira's art and science of bedside diagnosis*, 2nd edn. Baltimore: Lippincott, Williams & Wilkins, 2000.

Schneiderman H, Peixoto AJ. *Bedside diagnosis. An annotated bibliography of literature on physical examination and interviewing*, 3rd edn. Philadelphia: American College of Physicians, 1997. A superb summary of the evidence base for clinical examination.

Zatouroff M. *Color atlas of physical signs in general medicine*, 2nd edn. Chicago: Mosby Year Book, 1996.

chapter 3

The cardiovascular system

The heart...moves of itself and does not stop unless for ever.

Leonardo da Vinci (1452–1519)

This chapter deals with the history and the examination of the heart and blood vessels, as well as other parts of the body where symptoms and signs of heart disease may appear. Not only is this fundamental to the assessment of any patient, but it is also an extremely common system tested in viva voce examinations. It is believed by cardiologists to be the most important system in the body.

The cardiovascular history

Presenting symptoms (Table 3.1)

Chest pain

The mention of chest pain by a patient tends to provoke more urgent attention than other symptoms (Table 3.2). The surprised patient may find himself whisked into an emergency ward with the rapid appearance of worried-looking doctors. This is because ischaemic heart disease, which may be a life-threatening condition, often presents in this manner. The pain of *angina* and *myocardial infarction* tends to be similar in character; it may be due to the accumulation of metabolites from ischaemic muscle following complete or partial obstruction of a coronary artery, leading to stimulation of the cardiac sympathetic nerves.[1,2] Patients with cardiac transplants who develop coronary disease in the transplanted heart may not feel angina, presumably because the heart is denervated. Similarly, patients

with diabetes are more likely to be diagnosed with 'silent infarcts'.

To help determine the cause of chest pain, it is important to ascertain the duration, location, quality, and precipitating and aggravating factors (the four cardinal features), as well as means of relief and accompanying symptoms.[3]

Angina[a] comes from the Latin word meaning 'choking', and the patient may complain of crushing pain, heaviness, discomfort or a choking sensation in the retrosternal area or in the throat. It is best to ask if the patient experiences chest 'discomfort' rather than 'pain', because angina is often dull and aching in character and may not be perceived as pain. The pain or discomfort is usually central rather than left-sided. The patient may dismiss his or her pain as non-cardiac because it is not felt over the heart on the left side. It may radiate to the jaw or to the arms, but very rarely travels below the umbilicus. The severity of the pain varies. Angina characteristically occurs with exertion, with rapid relief once the patient rests or slows down. The amount of exertion necessary to produce the pain may be predictable to the patient. A change in the pattern of onset of previously stable angina must be taken very seriously. Although angina typically

---

[a] William Heberden's (1710–1801) description of angina (1768) is difficult to improve upon: 'They who are afflicted with it, are seized while they are walking (more especially if it be up hill and soon after eating) with a painful and most disagreeable sensation in the breast, which seems as if it would extinguish life, if it were to increase or continue; but the moment they stand still, all this uneasiness vanishes.'

Table 3.1 Cardiovascular history

Major symptoms

Chest pain or heaviness
Dyspnoea: exertional (note degree of exercise necessary), orthopnoea, paroxysmal nocturnal dyspnoea
Ankle swelling
Palpitations
Syncope
Intermittent claudication
Fatigue

Past history

History of ischaemic heart disease: myocardial infarction, coronary artery bypass grafting
Rheumatic fever, chorea, sexually transmitted disease, recent dental work, thyroid disease
Prior medical examination revealing heart disease (e.g. military, school, insurance)
Drugs

Social history

Tobacco and alcohol use
Occupation

Family history

Myocardial infarcts, cardiomyopathy, congenital heart disease, mitral valve prolapse, Marfan's syndrome

Coronary artery disease risk factors

Previous coronary disease
Smoking
Hypertension
Hyperlipidaemia
Family history of coronary artery disease
Diabetes mellitus
Obesity and physical inactivity
Male sex and advanced age
Raised homocysteine levels

Functional status in established heart disease*

Class I—disease present but no symptoms, or angina or dyspnoea during unusually intense activity
Class II—angina or dyspnoea during ordinary activity
Class III—angina or dyspnoea during less than ordinary activity
Class IV—angina or dyspnoea at rest

* New York Heart Association classification

Table 3.2 Causes of chest pain

Cardiac pain	Myocardial ischaemia or infarction
Vascular pain	Aortic dissection Aortic aneurysm
Pleuropericardial pain	Pericarditis Infective pleurisy Pneumothorax Pneumonia Autoimmune disease Mesothelioma Metastatic tumour
Chest wall pain	Persistent cough Muscular strains, trauma Intercostal myositis Thoracic herpes zoster Coxsackie B infection Thoracic nerve compression or infiltration Rib fracture Rib tumour, primary or metastatic Tietze's syndrome Slipping rib syndrome
Gastrointestinal pain	Gastroesophageal reflux (common) Oesophageal spasm (rare)
Airway pain	Tracheitis Intubation Central bronchial carcinoma Inhaled foreign body
Mediastinal pain	Oesophageal spasm Oesophagitis Mediastinitis Sarcoid adenopathy Lymphoma

occurs on exertion, it may also occur at rest or wake a patient from sleep. Ischaemic chest pain is usually unaffected by respiration. The use of sublingual nitrates characteristically brings relief within a couple of minutes, but this is not specific as nitrates may also relieve oesophageal spasm and also have a pronounced placebo effect.

The pain of myocardial infarction often comes on at rest, is usually more severe and lasts much longer. Pain present for more than half an hour is more likely to be due to myocardial infarction than to angina, but pain present continuously for many days is unlikely to be either. Associated symptoms of myocardial infarction include dyspnoea, sweating, anxiety, nausea and faintness.

Other causes of retrosternal pain are listed in Table 3.2. Chest pain made worse by inspiration is called *pleuritic pain*. This may be due to pleurisy (page 96) or pericarditis (page 63). This pain is not usually brought on by exertion and is often relieved by sitting up and leaning forwards. It is caused by the movement of inflamed pleural or pericardial surfaces on one another.

Chest wall pain is usually localised to a small area of the chest wall, is sharp and is associated with respiration or movement of the shoulders rather than with exertion. It may last only a few seconds or be present for prolonged periods. Disease of the *cervical or upper thoracic spine* may also cause pain associated with movement. This pain tends to radiate around from the back towards the front of the chest.

Pain due to a *dissecting aneurysm* of the aorta is usually very severe and may be described as tearing. This pain is usually greatest at the moment of onset and radiates to the back. These three features—quality, rapid onset and radiation—are very specific for aortic dissection. A history of hypertension or of a connective tissue disorder such as Marfan's syndrome or Ehlers-Danlos syndrome puts the patient at increased risk of this condition.

Massive pulmonary embolism causes pain of very sudden onset which may be retrosternal and associated with collapse, dyspnoea and cyanosis (page 117). It is often pleuritic, but can be identical to anginal pain, especially if associated with right ventricular ischaemia.

Spontaneous pneumothorax may result in pain and severe dyspnoea (page 113). The pain is sharp and localised to one part of the chest.

Gastro-oesophageal reflux can quite commonly cause angina-like pain without heartburn. It is important to remember that these two relatively common conditions may co-exist. *Oesophageal spasm* may cause retrosternal chest pain or discomfort and can be quite difficult to distinguish from angina, but is rare. The pain may come on after eating or drinking hot or cold fluids, may be associated with dysphagia (difficulty swallowing) and may be relieved by nitrates.

Cholecystitis can cause chest pain and be confused with myocardial infarction. Right upper quadrant abdominal tenderness is usually present (page 151).

Dyspnoea

Shortness of breath may be due to cardiac disease. Dyspnoea (Greek *dys* 'bad', *pnoia* 'breathing') is often defined as an unexpected awareness of breathing. It occurs whenever the work of breathing is excessive, but the mechanism is uncertain. It is probably due to a sensation of increased force required of the respiratory muscles to produce a volume change in the lungs, because of a reduction in compliance of the lungs or increased resistance to air flow. Cardiac dyspnoea is typically chronic and occurs with exertion because of failure of the left ventricular output to rise with exercise; this in turn leads to an acute rise in left ventricular end-diastolic pressure, raised pulmonary venous pressure, interstitial fluid leakage and thus reduced lung compliance. However, the dyspnoea of chronic cardiac failure does not correlate well with measurements of pulmonary artery pressures, and clearly the origin of the symptom of cardiac dyspnoea is complicated.[4] Left ventricular function may be impaired because of ischaemia (temporary or permanent reduction in myocardial blood supply), previous infarction (damage) or hypertrophy (often related to hypertension). As it becomes more severe, cardiac dyspnoea occurs at rest.

Orthopnoea (from the Greek *ortho* 'straight'; see Table 3.3), or dyspnoea that develops when a patient is supine, occurs because in an upright position the patient's interstitial oedema is redistributed; the lower zones of the lungs become worse and the upper zones better. This allows improved overall blood oxygenation. Patients with severe orthopnoea spend the night sitting up in a chair or propped up on numerous pillows in bed. The absence of orthopnoea suggests that left ventricular failure is unlikely to be the cause of a patient's dyspnoea (negative LR = 0.04).

Paroxysmal nocturnal dyspnoea (PND) is severe dyspnoea that wakes the patient from sleep so that he or she is forced to get up gasping for breath. This occurs because of a sudden failure of left ventricular output with an acute rise in pulmonary venous and capillary pressures; this leads to transudation of fluid into the interstitial tissues, which increases the work of breathing. The sequence may be precipitated by resorption of peripheral oedema at night while supine. Acute cardiac dyspnoea may also occur with acute pulmonary oedema or a pulmonary embolus.

Cardiac dyspnoea can be difficult to distinguish from that due to lung disease or other causes (page 94). One should inquire particularly about a history

Table 3.3 Causes of orthopnoea
Cardiac failure
Uncommon causes Massive ascites Pregnancy Bilateral diaphragmatic paralysis Large pleural effusion Severe pneumonia

of any cardiac disease that could be responsible for the onset of cardiac failure. For example, a patient with a number of known previous myocardial infarctions who develops dyspnoea is more likely to have decreased left ventricular contractility. A patient with a history of hypertension or a very heavy alcohol intake may have hypertensive heart disease or an alcoholic cardiomyopathy. The presence of orthopnoea or paroxysmal nocturnal dyspnoea is more suggestive of cardiac failure than of lung disease.

Dyspnoea is also a common symptom of anxiety. These patients often describe an inability to take a big enough breath to fill the lungs in a satisfying way. Their breathing may be deep and punctuated with sighs.

Ankle swelling

Some patients present with bilateral ankle swelling due to *oedema* from cardiac failure. Patients with the recent onset of oedema and who take a serious interest in their weight may have noticed a gain in weight of 3 kg or more. Ankle oedema of cardiac origin is usually symmetrical and worst in the evenings, with improvement during the night. It may be a symptom of biventricular failure or right ventricular failure secondary to a number of possible underlying aetiologies. As failure progresses, oedema ascends to involve the legs, thighs, genitalia and abdomen. There are usually other symptoms or signs of heart disease. It is important to find out whether the patient is taking a vasodilating drug (e.g. a calcium channel blocker), which can cause peripheral oedema. There are other (more) common causes of ankle oedema than heart failure that also need to be considered (page 56). Oedema that affects the face is more likely to be related to nephrotic syndrome (page 180).

Palpitations

This is not a very precise term. It is usually taken to mean an unexpected awareness of the heartbeat.[5] Ask the patient to describe exactly what he or she notices and whether the palpitations are slow or fast, regular or irregular, and how long they last. There may be the sensation of a missed beat followed by a particularly heavy beat; this can be due to an *atrial* or *ventricular premature contraction* (which produces little cardiac output) followed by a compensating pause and then a normally conducted beat (which is more forceful than usual because there has been a longer diastolic filling period for the ventricle). If the patient complains of a rapid heartbeat, it is important to find out whether the palpitations are of sudden or gradual onset and offset. Cardiac arrhythmias are usually instantaneous in onset and offset, whereas the onset and offset of *sinus tachycardia* is more gradual. A completely irregular rhythm is suggestive of *atrial fibrillation*, particularly if it is rapid. It may be helpful to ask the patient to tap the rate and rhythm of the palpitations with his or her finger. Associated features including pain, dyspnoea or faintness must be inquired about. The awareness of rapid palpitations followed by syncope suggests *ventricular tachycardia*. These patients usually have a past history of significant heart disease. Any rapid rhythm may precipitate angina in a patient with ischaemic heart disease.

Patients may have learned manoeuvres that will return the rhythm to normal. Attacks of *supraventricular tachycardia* may be suddenly terminated by increasing vagal tone with the Valsalva manoeuvre (page 54), carotid massage, by coughing, or by swallowing cold water or ice cubes.

Syncope, presyncope and dizziness

Syncope is a transient loss of consciousness resulting from cerebral anoxia, usually due to inadequate blood flow. Presyncope is a transient sensation of weakness without loss of consciousness.

Syncope may represent a simple faint or be a symptom of cardiac or neurological disease. One must establish whether the patient actually loses consciousness and under what circumstances the syncope occurs (e.g. on standing for prolonged periods or standing up suddenly (*postural syncope*), while passing urine (*micturition syncope*), on coughing (*tussive syncope*) or with sudden emotional stress (*vasovagal syncope*). Find out whether there is any warning, such as dizziness or palpitations, and how long the episodes last. Recovery may be spontaneous or the patient may require attention from bystanders. Bystanders may also have noticed abnormal movements if the patient has epilepsy (page 284), but these can also occur in primary syncope. If the patient's symptoms appear to be postural, inquire about the use of antihypertensive or anti-anginal drugs and other medications that may induce postural hypotension. If the episode is vasovagal, it may be precipitated by something unpleasant like the sight of blood, or occur in a crowded, hot room; patients often sigh and yawn and feel nauseated and sweaty before fainting and may have previously had similar episodes, especially during adolescence and young adulthood.

If syncope is due to an arrhythmia there is often a sudden loss of consciousness regardless of the patient's posture; chest pain may also occur if the patient has ischaemic heart disease or aortic stenosis.[6] Exertional syncope may occur with obstruction to left ventricular outflow by *aortic stenosis* or *hypertrophic cardiomyopathy*.

Dizziness that occurs even when the patient is lying down or which is made worse by movements of the head is more likely to be of neurological origin, although recurrent tachyarrhythmias may occasionally cause dizziness in any position. One should attempt to decide whether the dizziness is really *vertiginous* (where the world seems to be turning around), or whether it is a presyncopal feeling.

Intermittent claudication

The word claudication[b] comes from the Latin meaning to limp. Patients with claudication notice pain in one or both calves, thighs or buttocks when they walk more than a certain distance. This distance is called the 'claudication distance'. The claudication distance may be shorter when patients walk up hills. A history of claudication suggests peripheral vascular disease with a poor blood supply to the affected muscles. The most important risk factor is smoking, and a history of vascular disease elsewhere in the body, including cerebrovascular disease and ischaemic heart disease, is common.

Fatigue

Fatigue is a common symptom of cardiac failure. It may be associated with a reduced cardiac output and poor blood supply to the skeletal muscles. There are many other causes of fatigue, including lack of sleep, anaemia and depression (page 197).

Risk factors for coronary artery disease

An essential part of the cardiac history involves obtaining detailed information about a patient's risk factors—the patient's *cardiovascular risk factor profile*.

Previous ischaemic heart disease is the most important risk factor for further ischaemia. The patient may know of previous infarcts or have had a diagnosis of angina in the past.

Hypercholesterolaemia is the next most important risk factor for ischaemic heart disease. Many patients now know their serum cholesterol levels because widespread testing has become fashionable. The total serum cholesterol is a useful screening test, and levels above 5.2 mmol/L are considered undesirable. Patients with established coronary artery disease benefit from lowering of total cholesterol to below 4 mmol/L. An elevated total cholesterol level is even more significant if the high-density lipo-

protein (HDL) level is low (less than 1.0 mmol/L). Significant elevation of the triglyceride level is a coronary risk factor in its own right and also adds further to the risk if the total cholesterol is high. If a patient already has coronary disease, hyperlipidaemia is even more important. Control of risk factors for these patients is called 'secondary prevention'. Patients who have multiple risk factors for ischaemic heart disease (e.g. diabetes and hypertension) should have their cholesterol controlled aggressively. If the patient's cholesterol is known to be high, it is worth obtaining a dietary history. This can be very trying. It is important to remember that not only foods containing cholesterol but those containing saturated fats contribute to the serum cholesterol level. High alcohol consumption and obesity are associated with hypertriglyceridaemia.

Smoking is probably the next most important risk factor for cardiovascular disease and peripheral vascular disease. Some patients describe themselves as non-smokers even though they stopped smoking only a few hours before. The number of years the patient has smoked and the number of cigarettes smoked per day are both very important (and are recorded as packet years). The significance of a history of smoking for a patient who has not smoked for many years is controversial. The risk of symptomatic ischaemic heart disease falls gradually over the years after smoking has been stopped. After about 2 years the risk of myocardial infarction falls to the same level as for those who have never smoked. After 10 years the risk of developing angina falls close to that of non-smokers.

Hypertension is another important risk factor for coronary artery disease. Find out when hypertension was first diagnosed and what treatment, if any, has been instituted. The treatment of hypertension probably does reduce the risk of ischaemic heart disease, and certainly reduces the risk of hypertensive heart disease, cardiac failure and cerebrovascular disease. Treatment of hypertension has also been shown to reverse left ventricular hypertrophy.

A family history of coronary artery disease increases a patient's risk, particularly if it has been present in first-degree relatives (parents or siblings) and if it has affected these people below the age of 60. Not all heart disease, however, is ischaemic; a patient whose relatives suffered from rheumatic heart disease is at no greater risk of ischaemic heart disease than anybody else.

A history of *diabetes mellitus* increases the risk of ischaemic heart disease very substantially. A diabetic without a history of ischaemic heart disease has the same risk of myocardial infarction as a non-diabetic who has had an infarct. It is important to find out how long a patient has been diabetic and whether insulin treatment has been required. Good control

---

[b] The Roman Emperor Tiberius Claudius Drusus Nero Germanicus (10 BC–54 AD) limped owing to some form of paralysis. 'Claudication' and 'Claudius', however, are etymologically unrelated, which seems rather a cruel coincidence for Claudius. 'Claudicant' first appeared in English in 1624.

of the blood sugar level of diabetics reduces this risk. An attempt should therefore be made to find out how well a patient's diabetes has been controlled.

Renal failure is associated with a very high risk of vascular disease. This is possibly related to high calcium times phosphate product and may be reduced by dietary intervention, 'phosphate binders', efficient dialysis or renal transplant. Ischaemic heart disease is the most common cause of death for renal failure patients on dialysis.

The presence of multiple risk factors makes control of each one more important. Aggressive control of risk factors is often indicated in these patients.

Teeth

A history of dental decay or infection is important for patients with valvular heart disease since it puts them at risk of infective endocarditis. Dental caries may also be associated with an increased risk of ischaemic heart disease. Ask about the regularity of visits to the dentist and the patient's awareness of the need for antibiotic prophylaxis before dental (and some surgical) procedures.

Treatment

The medications a patient is taking often give a good clue to the diagnosis. Find out about any ill-effects from current or previous medications. The surgical history must also be elicited. The patient may have had a previous angioplasty or coronary artery bypass grafting, and may know how many arteries were dilated or bypassed. If the patient is unable to provide a history, a midline sternotomy scar and scars consistent with previous saphenous vein harvesting support this diagnosis.

Past history

Patients with a history of definite previous angina or myocardial infarction remain at high risk for further ischaemic events. It is very useful at this stage to find out how a diagnosis of ischaemic heart disease was made and in particular what investigations were undertaken. The patient may well remember exercise testing or a coronary angiogram, and some patients can even remember how many coronary arteries were narrowed, how many coronary bypasses were performed (having more than three grafts often leads to a certain amount of boasting). The angioplasty patient may know how many arteries were dilated and whether *stents* (often called coronary stunts by patients and cardiac surgeons) were inserted.

Patients may recall a diagnosis of rheumatic fever in their childhood, but many were labelled as having 'growing pains'.[7] A patient who was put to bed for a long period as a child may well have had rheumatic fever. A history of rheumatic fever places patients at risk of rheumatic valvular disease.

Social history

Both ischaemic heart disease and rheumatic heart disease are chronic conditions that may affect a patient's ability to function normally. It is therefore important to find out whether the patient's condition has prevented him or her from working and over what period. Patients with severe cardiac failure, for example, may need to make adjustments to their living arrangements so that they are not required to walk up and down stairs at home.

The cardiovascular examination

The cardiovascular system lends itself particularly well to the formal examination approach. There are a number of equally satisfactory methods, but the precise approach used is not as important as having a method which is comprehensive, gives the impression of being (and is) proficient, and ensures that no important part of the examination is omitted.

First, one should appropriately expose and position the patient properly and pause to get an impression of the general appearance. Then detailed examination begins with the hands and pulses and progresses smoothly to the neck, face, and then on to the *praecordium* (from the Latin *prae* 'in front of', and *cor* 'heart'). A summary of a suggested method of examination is found at the end of this chapter.

Positioning the patient

It is important to have the patient lying in bed with enough pillows to support him or her at 45 degrees (Figure 3.1). This is the usual position in which the jugular venous pressure is assessed. During auscultation, optimal examination requires further positioning of the patient, as will be discussed later.

General appearance

Look at the general state of health. Does the patient appear to be ill? If he or she looks ill try to decide why you have formed that impression. Note whether the patient at rest has rapid and laboured respiration, suggesting dyspnoea (Table 4.3).

The patient may look *cachectic*: that is, there may be severe loss of weight and muscle wasting. This is commonly caused by malignant disease, but

Figure 3.1 Cardiovascular examination: positioning the patient

severe cardiac failure may also have this effect (*cardiac cachexia*). It probably results from a combination of anorexia (due to congestive enlargement of the liver), impaired intestinal absorption (due to congested intestinal veins) and increased levels of inflammatory cytokines such as TNF-α.

There are also some syndromes that are associated with specific cardiac disease. Marfan's syndrome[c] (Figure 3.2), Down syndrome[d] (page 273) and Turner's syndrome[e] (page 273) are important examples.

The hands

Pick up the right hand. Look first at the nails. Now is the time for a decision as to the presence or absence of *clubbing*. Clubbing is an increase in the soft tissue of the distal part of the fingers or toes. The causes of clubbing are surprisingly varied (Table 3.4). The mechanism is unknown but there are, of course, several theories. One current theory is that platelet-derived growth factor (PDGF), released from megakaryocyte and platelet emboli in the nail beds,

cause fibrovascular proliferation. Megakaryocytes and clumps of platelets do not normally reach the arterial circulation. Their large size (up to 50 μm) prevents their passing through the pulmonary capillaries when they are released from the bone marrow. In conditions where platelets may clump in the arterial circulation (infected cardiac valve) or bypass the pulmonary capillaries (right to left shunt associated with congenital heart disease) they can reach the systemic circulation and become trapped in the terminal capillaries of the fingers and toes. Damage to pulmonary capillaries from various lung disorders can have the same effect.

Proper examination for clubbing involves inspecting the fingernails (and toenails) from the side to determine if there is loss of the angle between the nail bed and the finger—the *hyponychial angle* (Figure 3.3 a & b). One tested measurement is the *interphalangeal depth ratio*. The anteroposterior (AP) dimension of the finger is measured at the distal interphalangeal joint and compared with the AP diameter at the level of the point where the skin joins the nail. A ratio of more than 1 means clubbing.[8,f] Eventually, the distal phalanx becomes

---

[c] Bernard-Jean Antonin Marfan (1858–1942), French physician and first professor of hygiene in Paris.

[d] John Langdon Down (1828–96), Assistant Physician to the London Hospital and founder of the Normansfield Mental Hospital. He described the clinical picture of mongolism in 1866.

[e] Henry Hubert Turner (1892–1970), Clinical Professor of Medicine, Oklahoma University. He described the syndrome in 1938.

---

[f] The eminent South African cardiologist Leo Schamroth developed clubbing as a result of endocarditis in 1976. As the condition advanced, he observed in his own fingers that the diamond-shaped space formed when the nails of two similar fingers were held facing each other disappeared, only to reappear as he improved.

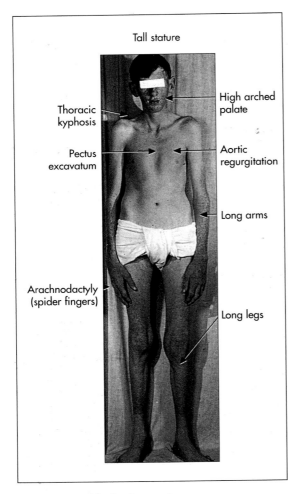

Tall stature

Thoracic kyphosis

High arched palate

Pectus excavatum

Aortic regurgitation

Long arms

Arachnodactyly (spider fingers)

Long legs

Figure 3.2 Marfan's syndrome

Tall stature, thoracic kyphosis, pectus excavatum, arachnodactyly (spider fingers), long limbs, aortic regurgitation and a high, arched palate.

Table 3.4 Causes of clubbing

Common

Cardiovascular
Cyanotic congenital heart disease
Infective endocarditis

Respiratory
Lung carcinoma (usually *not* small cell carcinoma)
Chronic pulmonary suppuration:
- Bronchiectasis
- Lung abscess
- Empyema
Idiopathic pulmonary fibrosis

Uncommon

Respiratory
Cystic fibrosis
Asbestosis
Pleural mesothelioma (benign fibrous type) or pleural fibroma

Gastrointestinal
Cirrhosis (especially biliary cirrhosis)
Inflammatory bowel disease
Coeliac disease

Thyrotoxicosis
Familial (usually before puberty) or idiopathic

Rare
Neurogenic diaphragmatic tumours
Pregnancy
Secondary hyperparathyroidism

Unilateral clubbing
Bronchial arteriovenous aneurysm
Axillary artery aneurysm

enlarged, due to soft-tissue swelling. This angle can be measured with a *shadowgraph*, which projects the silhouette of the finger so that it can be measured with a protractor. It is not in common use. If the angle is greater than 190°, clubbing is generally agreed to be present. Patients hardly ever notice that they have clubbing, even when it is severe. They often express surprise at their doctor's interest in such an unlikely part of their anatomy.

Before leaving the nails, look for *splinter haemorrhages* in the nail beds (Figure 3.4). These are linear haemorrhages lying parallel to the long axis of the nail. They are most often due to trauma, particularly in manual workers. However, an important cause is infective endocarditis (page 64), which is a bacterial or other infection of the heart valves or part of the endocardium. In this disease splinter haemorrhages are probably the result of a vasculitis in the nail bed, but this is controversial. Other rare causes of splinter haemorrhages include vasculitis, as in rheumatoid arthritis, polyarteritis nodosa or the antiphospholipid syndrome, sepsis elsewhere in the body, haematological malignancy or profound anaemia.

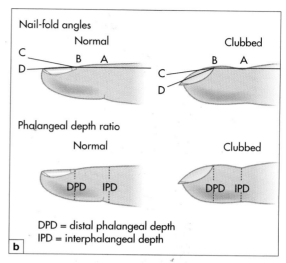

Figure 3.3 Finger clubbing: (a) appearance; (b) phalangeal depth ratio

Figure 3.4 Splinter haemorrhages—ring and little fingers of left hand. Note that the fingers are clubbed (inset)

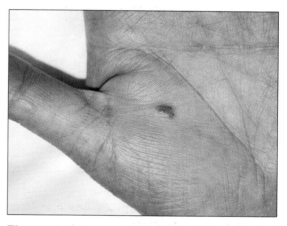

Figure 3.5 Janeway lesion

Osler's nodes[g] are a rare manifestation of infective endocarditis. These are red, raised tender nodules on the pulps of the fingers (or toes), or on the thenar or hypothenar eminences. They are reported to have occurred in 50% of patients before antibiotic treatment of endocarditis became available. Currently they are seen in fewer than 5% of patients. *Janeway*

lesions[h] (Figure 3.5) are non-tender erythematous maculopapular lesions containing bacteria, which occur very rarely on the palms or pulps of the fingers in patients with infective endocarditis.

Tendon xanthomata are yellow or orange deposits of lipid in the tendons that occur in type II hyperlipidaemia. These can be seen over the tendons of the hand and arm. *Palmar xanthomata*, and *tuboeruptive xanthomata* over the elbows and knees, are characteristic of type III hyperlipidaemia (Figure 3.6).

[g] Sir William Osler (1849–1919), Canadian physician, Professor of Medicine at McGill University at 25, and later famous Regius Professor of Medicine at Oxford and renowned medical historian. He was made a baronet. His only son was killed at Ypres.

[h] Edward Janeway (1841–1911), American physician.

Figure 3.6 Tuboeruptive xanthomata of the knee

The arterial pulse

The accomplished clinician is able, while inspecting the hands, to palpate the radial artery at the wrist. Patients expect to have the pulse taken as part of a proper medical examination. The clinician can feel the pulse while talking to the patient and while looking for other signs. When this traditional part of the examination is performed with some ceremony, it may help to establish rapport between patient and doctor. Although the radial pulse is distant from the central arteries, certain useful information may be gained from examining it. The pulse is usually felt just medial to the radius, using the forefinger and middle finger pulps of the examining hand (Figure 3.7). The following obser-

Figure 3.7 Taking the radial pulse

vations should be made: (i) rate of pulse, (ii) rhythm and (iii) presence or absence of delay of the femoral pulse compared with the radial pulse (*radiofemoral delay*). The character and volume of the pulse are better assessed from palpation of the brachial or carotid arteries.

Rate of pulse

Practised observers can estimate the rate quickly. Formal counting over 30 seconds is accurate and requires only simple mathematics to obtain the rate per minute. The normal resting heart rate in adults is usually said to be between 60 and 100 beats per minute but a more sensible range is probably 55 to 95 (95% of normal people). Bradycardia (Greek *bradys* 'slow', *kardia* 'heart') is defined as a heart rate of less than 60 beats per minute. Tachycardia (Greek *tachys* 'swift', *kardia* 'heart') is defined as a heart rate over 100 beats per minute. The causes of bradycardia and tachycardia are listed in Table 3.5.

Rhythm

The rhythm of the pulse can be regular or irregular. An irregular rhythm can be completely irregular with no pattern (*irregularly irregular* or *chaotic rhythm*); this is usually due to atrial fibrillation (Table 3.5). In atrial fibrillation coordinated atrial contraction is lost, and chaotic electrical activity occurs with bombardment of the atrioventricular (AV) node with impulses at a rate of over 600 per minute. Only a variable proportion of these is conducted to the ventricles because (fortunately) the AV node is unable to conduct at such high rates. In this way, the ventricles are protected from very rapid rates, but beat irregularly, usually at rates between 150 and 180 a minute (unless the patient is being treated with drugs to slow the heart rate). The pulse also varies in amplitude from beat to beat in atrial fibrillation because of differing diastolic filling times. This type of pulse can occasionally be simulated by frequent irregularly occurring supraventricular or ventricular extrasystoles (ectopic beats).

An irregular rhythm can also be *regularly irregular*. For example, in patients with *sinus arrhythmia* the pulse rate increases with each inspiration and decreases with each expiration; this is a normal finding. It is associated with changes in venous return to the heart. A pattern of irregularity is also detectable in the Wenckebach phenomenon.[i] Here the AV nodal conduction time increases progressively until a non-conducted atrial systole occurs. Following this the AV conduction time shortens and the cycle begins again.

---

[i] Marel Frederik Wenckebach (1864–1940), Dutch physician who practised in Vienna.

Table 3.5 Causes of bradycardia and tachycardia

Bradycardia

Regular rhythm

Physiological (athletes, during sleep: due to increased vagal tone)

Drugs (e.g. beta-blockers, digoxin, amiodarone)

Hypothyroidism (decreased sympathetic activity secondary to thyroid hormone deficiency)

Hypothermia

Raised intracranial pressure (due to an effect on central sympathetic outflow)—a late sign

Third degree atrioventricular (AV) block, or second degree (type 2) AV block

Myocardial infarction

Paroxysmal bradycardia: vasovagal syncope

Jaundice (in severe cases only, due to deposition of bilirubin in the conducting system)

Irregular rhythm

Irregularly irregular

Atrial fibrillation (in combination with conduction system disease or AV nodal blocking drugs) due to:
- alcohol, post-thoracotomy, idiopathic
- mitral valve disease or any cause of left atrial enlargement

Frequent extrasystoles

Regularly irregular rhythm

Sinus arrhythmia (normal slowing of the pulse with expiration)

Second degree AV block (type 1)

Apparent

Pulse deficit* (atrial fibrillation, ventricular bigeminy)

Tachycardia

Regular rhythm

Hyperdynamic circulation, due to:
- exercise or emotion (e.g. anxiety)
- fever (allow 15–20 beats per minute per °C above normal)
- pregnancy
- thyrotoxicosis
- anaemia
- arteriovenous fistula (e.g. Paget's disease or hepatic failure)
- beri beri (thiamine deficiency)

Congestive cardiac failure

Constrictive pericarditis

Drugs (e.g. salbutamol and other sympathomimetics, atropine)

Normal variant

Denervated heart e.g. diabetes (resting rate of 106–120 beats per minute)

Hypovolaemic shock

Supraventricular tachycardia (usually >150)

Atrial flutter with regular 2:1 AV block (usually 150)

Ventricular tachycardia (often >150)
- thyrotoxicosis
- sick sinus syndrome
- pulmonary embolism
- myocarditis
- myocardial ischaemia
- fever, acute hypoxia or hypercapnia (paroxysmal)

Multifocal atrial tachycardia

Atrial flutter with variable block

Irregular rhythm

Atrial fibrillation, due to:
- myocardial ischaemia
- mitral valve disease or any cause of left atrial enlargement
- thyrotoxicosis
- hypertensive heart disease
- sick sinus syndrome
- pulmonary embolism
- myocarditis
- fever, acute hypoxia or hypercapnia (paroxysmal)
- other: alcohol, post-thoracotomy, idiopathic

Multifocal atrial tachycardia

Atrial flutter with variable block

---

* This is the difference between the heart rate counted over the praecordium and that observed at the periphery. In beats where diastole is too short for adequate filling of the heart, too small a volume of blood is ejected during systole for a pulse to be appreciated at the wrist.

Figure 3.8 Feeling for the radiofemoral delay

Radiofemoral delay

This is an important sign and often neglected. While palpating the radial pulse, the clinician places the fingers of the other hand over the femoral pulse, which is situated below the inguinal ligament, one-third of the way up from the pubic tubercle (Figure 3.8). A noticeable delay in the arrival of the femoral pulse wave suggests the diagnosis of *coarctation of the aorta*, where a congenital narrowing in the aortic isthmus occurs at the level where the ductus arteriosus joins the descending aorta. This is just distal to the origin of the subclavian artery. This lesion can cause upper limb hypertension (page 65).

It can also be useful to palpate both radial pulses together to detect radial–radial inequality in timing or volume, usually due to a large arterial occlusion by an atherosclerotic plaque or aneurysm, or to subclavian artery stenosis on one side.

Character and volume

These are poorly assessed by palpating the radial pulse; the carotid or brachial arteries should be used to determine the character and volume of the pulse, as these more accurately reflect the form of the aortic pressure wave. However, the collapsing (bounding) pulse of *aortic regurgitation*, and *pulsus alternans* (alternating strong and weak pulse) of advanced left ventricular failure, may be readily apparent in the radial pulse.

Condition of the vessel wall

Only changes in the medial layer of the radial artery can be assessed by palpation. Thickening or tortuosity will be detected commonly in the arteries of elderly people. These changes, however, do not indicate the presence of luminal narrowing due to atherosclerosis. Therefore, this sign is of little clinical value.

The blood pressure

Measurement of the arterial blood pressure[j] is an essential part of the examination of almost any patient. Usually indirect measurements of the systolic and diastolic pressures are obtained with a *sphygmomanometer* (Greek *sphygmos* 'pulsing', *manos* 'thin').[9] The systolic blood pressure is the peak pressure that occurs in the artery following ventricular systole, and the diastolic blood pressure is the level to which the arterial blood pressure falls during ventricular diastole. Normal blood pressure is defined as a systolic reading of less than 140 mmHg *and* a diastolic reading of less than 90 mmHg. In some circumstances, lower pressures may be considered normal (e.g. in pregnancy) or desirable (e.g. for diabetics).

Measuring the blood pressure with the sphygmomanometer

The usual blood pressure cuff width is 12.5 cm. This is suitable for a normal-sized adult forearm. However, in obese patients with large arms the normal-sized cuff will overestimate the blood pressure and therefore a large cuff must be used. A range of smaller sizes are available for children.

The cuff is wrapped around the upper arm with the bladder centred over the brachial artery (Figure 3.9). This is found in the antecubital fossa, one-third of the way over from the medial epicondyle. For an approximate estimation of the systolic blood pressure, the cuff is fully inflated and then deflated slowly (3–4 mmHg per second) until the radial pulse returns. Then for a more accurate estimation of the blood pressure, this manoeuvre is repeated with the diaphragm of the stethoscope placed over the brachial artery, slipped underneath the distal end of the cuff's bladder.

Five different sounds will be heard as the cuff is slowly released (Figure 3.10). These are called the Korotkoff[k] sounds. The pressure at which a sound is first heard over the artery is the systolic blood pressure (Korotkoff I). As deflation of the cuff continues the sound increases in intensity (KII), then decreases (KIII), becomes muffled (KIV) and then disappears (KV). Different observers have used

---

[j] Blood pressure was first measured in a horse in 1708 by Stephen Hales, an English clergyman. Measurement of the blood pressure was the last of the traditional vital signs measurements to come into regular use. It wasn't until early in the 20th century that work by Korotkoff and Janeway led to its routine use.

[k] Nikolai Korotkoff (1874–1920), a St Petersburg surgeon, described the auscultatory method of determining blood pressure in 1905, although his findings were scoffed at.

Figure 3.9 Measuring the blood pressure, with patient lying at 45 degrees

Phase	Korotkoff sounds	
		120 mmHg systolic
1	A thud	
		110 mmHg
2	A blowing noise	
		100 mmHg
3	A softer thud	
		90 mmHg diastolic (1st)
4	A disappearing blowing noise	
		80 mmHg diastolic (2nd)
5	Nothing	

Figure 3.10 Korotkoff sounds

Systolic pressure is determined by the appearance of the first audible sound, and diastolic pressure is determined by its disappearance.

KIV and KV to indicate the level of the diastolic pressure. KV is probably the best measure. However, this provides a slight underestimate of the arterial diastolic blood pressure. Although diastolic pressure usually corresponds most closely to KV, in severe aortic regurgitation KIV is a more accurate indication (page 72). KV is absent in some normal people and KIV must be used.

Occasionally, there will be an auscultatory gap (the sounds disappear just below the systolic pressure and reappear before the diastolic pressure) in healthy people.

The systolic blood pressure may normally vary between the arms by up to 10 mmHg; in the legs the blood pressure is normally up to 20 mmHg higher than in the arms, unless the patient has coarctation of the aorta. Measurement of the blood pressure in the legs is more difficult than in the arms. It requires a large cuff that is placed over the mid-thigh. The patient lies prone and the stethoscope is placed in the popliteal fossa, behind the knee.

During inspiration, the systolic and diastolic blood pressures normally decrease (because intrathoracic pressure becomes more negative, blood pools in the pulmonary vessels, so left-heart filling is reduced). When this normal reduction in blood pressure with inspiration is *exaggerated*, it is termed *pulsus paradoxus*. Kussmaul meant by this that there was a fall in blood pressure and a paradoxical rise in pulse rate. A fall in arterial pulse pressure on inspiration of more than 10 mmHg is abnormal and may occur with *constrictive pericarditis, pericardial effusion*, or severe asthma. To detect this; lower the cuff pressure slowly until K1 sounds are heard intermittently (expiration) and then until K1 is audible with every beat. The difference between the two readings represents the level of the pulsus paradoxus.

Variations in blood pressure

When blood pressure is measured with an intra-arterial catheter it becomes clear that blood pressure varies from minute to minute in normal people. Short-term changes of 4 mmHg in the systolic and 3 mmHg in the diastolic readings are common. Hour-to-hour and day-to-day variations are even greater. The standard deviation between visits is up to 12 mmHg for systolic pressure and 8 mmHg for diastolic. This means that when there is concern about an abnormal reading, repeat measurements are necessary.

When the heart is very irregular (most often because of atrial fibrillation), the cuff should be deflated slowly and the point at which most of the cardiac contractions are audible (KI) taken as the systolic pressure and the point at which most have disappeared (KV) taken as diastole.

High blood pressure

This is difficult to define.[9] The most helpful definitions of hypertension are based on an estimation of the level associated with an increased risk of vascular disease. In this case, recordings above 145/90 mmHg may be considered abnormal; such levels may occur in up to 20% of the adult population.[l] Blood pressure measured by the patient at home, or by a 24-hour monitor, should be up to 10/5 mmHg less than that measured in the surgery.

Postural blood pressure

The blood pressure should routinely be taken with the patient both lying down and standing (Figure 3.11).[11] A fall of more than 15 mmHg in systolic blood pressure or 10 mmHg in diastolic blood pressure on standing is abnormal and is called *postural hypotension* (Table 3.6). It may cause dizziness or not be associated with symptoms. The most common cause is the use of antihypertensive drugs, α-adrenergic antagonists in particular.

---

[l] In pseudohypertension the blood pressure, as measured by the sphygmomanometer, is artificially high because of arterial wall calcification. Osler's manoeuvre traditionally detects this condition: inflate the cuff above systolic pressure and palpate the radial artery, which in pseudohypertension may be palpable despite being pulseless. However, the value of Osler's manoeuvre has been questioned.[10]

Figure 3.11 Measuring the blood pressure, with patient standing

---

Table 3.6 Causes of postural hypotension

Hypovolaemia (e.g. dehydration, bleeding)
Drugs (e.g. vasodilators and other anti-hypertensives, tricyclic antidepressants, diuretics, antipsychotics)
Addison's* disease
Hypopituitarism
Autonomic neuropathy (e.g. diabetes mellitus, amyloidosis, Shy-Drager syndrome)
Idiopathic orthostatic hypotension (rare progressive degeneration of the autonomic nervous system, usually in elderly men)

* Thomas Addison (1793–1860), London physician.

The face

Inspect the sclerae for *jaundice* (page 18). This can occur with severe congestive cardiac failure and hepatic congestion. Prosthetic heart valve-induced haemolysis of red blood cells, due to excessive turbulence, is an uncommon but cardiac cause of jaundice. *Xanthelasmata* (Figure 3.12 a & b) are intracutaneous yellow cholesterol deposits around the eyes and are relatively common. These may be a normal variant or may indicate type II or III hyperlipidaemia. They are not always associated with hyperlipidaemia.

Figure 3.12 Xanthelasmata
(Figure 3.12b from FS McDonald, ed., *Mayo clinic images in internal medicine*, with permission. © Mayo Clinic Scientific Press and CRC Press.)

Next look for the presence of a *mitral facies*, which refers to rosy cheeks with a bluish tinge, due to dilatation of the malar capillaries. This is associated with pulmonary hypertension and a low cardiac output such as occurs in severe mitral stenosis.

Now look in the mouth using a torch to see if there is a *high arched palate*. This occurs in Marfan's syndrome, a condition that is associated with congenital heart disease, including aortic regurgitation secondary to aortic root dilatation, and also mitral regurgitation due to mitral valve prolapse. Notice whether the teeth look diseased, as they can be a source of organisms responsible for infective endocarditis. Look at the tongue and lips for central cyanosis. Inspect the mucosa for petechiae that may indicate infective endocarditis.

The neck

Oddly enough this small area of the body is packed with cardiovascular signs, which must be elicited with great care and skill.

Figure 3.13 Palpating the carotid pulse

Carotid arteries

The carotids are not only easily accessible, medial to the sternomastoid muscles (Figure 3.13), but provide a great deal of information about the wave form of the aortic pulse, which is affected by many cardiac abnormalities. Never palpate both carotid arteries simultaneously as they provide much of the blood supply to the *brain* (a vital organ). Evaluation of the pulse wave form (the amplitude, shape and volume) is important in the diagnosis of various underlying cardiac diseases and in assessing their severity. It takes considerable practice to distinguish the different important types of carotid wave forms (Table 3.7).

Table 3.7 Arterial pulse character

Type of pulse	Cause(s)
Anacrotic	Aortic stenosis
	Small volume, slow uptake, notched wave on upstroke
Plateau	Aortic stenosis
	Slow upstroke
Bisferiens	Aortic stenosis *and* regurgitation
	Anacrotic and collapsing
Collapsing	Aortic regurgitation
	Hyperdynamic circulation (page 38)
	Patent ductus arteriosus
	Peripheral arteriovenous fistula
	Arteriosclerotic aorta (elderly patients in particular)
Small volume	Aortic stenosis
	Pericardial effusion
Alternans	Left ventricular failure
	Alternating strong and weak beats
Jerky	Hypertrophic cardiomyopathy

Jugular venous pressure (JVP)—pulsation

Just as the carotid pulse tells us about the aorta and left ventricular function, the *jugular venous pressure* (JVP) (Figure 3.14) tells us about right atrial and right ventricular function.[12] The positioning of the patient and lighting are important for this examination to be done properly. The patient must be lying down at 45 degrees to the horizontal with his or her head on pillows and in good lighting conditions. The internal jugular vein is deep in the sternomastoid muscle, while the external jugular vein is lateral to it. Traditionally, use of the external jugular vein to estimate venous pressure is discouraged, but the right internal and external jugular veins usually give consistent readings. The left-sided veins are less accurate because they cross from the left side of the chest before entering the right atrium. Pulsations that occur in the right-sided veins reflect movements of the top of a column of blood that extends directly into the right atrium. The column of blood may be used as a manometer and enables us to observe pressure changes in the right atrium. By convention, the sternal angle is taken as the zero point and the maximum height of pulsations in the internal jugular vein, which are visible above this level when the patient is at 45 degrees, is measured in centimetres. In the average person the centre of the right atrium lies 5 cm below this zero point.

When the patient is lying at 45 degrees, the sternal angle is also roughly in line with the base of the neck (Figure 3.14). This provides a convenient zero point from which to measure the vertical height of the column of blood in the jugular vein. The jugular venous pulsation can be distinguished from the

Figure 3.14 Assessment of the JVP

The patient should lie at 45 degrees. The relationships between the sternomastoid muscle, the JVP, the sternal angle and the mid right atrium are shown.

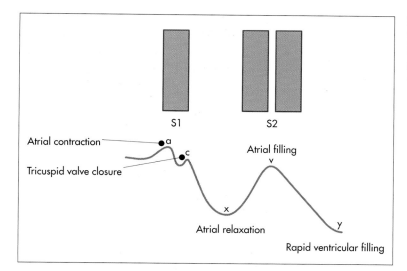

Figure 3.15 The jugular venous pressure, and its relationship to the first (S1) and second (S2) heart sounds

arterial pulse because: (i) it is visible but not palpable and has a more prominent *inward* movement than the artery; (ii) it has a complex wave form, usually seen to flicker twice with each cardiac cycle (if the patient is in sinus rhythm); (iii) it moves on respiration—normally the JVP decreases on inspiration; and (iv) it is at first obliterated and then filled from above when light pressure is applied at the base of the neck.

The JVP must be assessed for *height* and *character*. When the JVP is more than 3 cm above the zero point, the right-heart filling pressure is raised (a normal reading is less than 8 cm of water: 5 cm + 3 cm). This is a sign of right ventricular failure, volume overload or of some types of pericardial disease.

The assessment of the *character* of JVP is difficult even for experienced clinicians. There are two positive waves in the normal JVP. The first is called the *a wave* and coincides with right atrial systole.[m] It is due to atrial contraction. The *a wave* also coincides with the first heart sound and precedes the carotid pulsation. The second impulse is called the *v wave* and is due to atrial filling, in the period when the tricuspid valve remains closed during ventricular systole. Between the *a* and *v* waves there is a trough caused by atrial relaxation. This is called the *x descent*. It is interrupted by the *c point,* which is due to transmitted carotid pulsation and coincides with tricuspid valve closure. It is not usually visible. Following the *v* wave, the tricuspid valve opens and rapid ventricular filling occurs; this results in the *y descent* (Figure 3.15).

In Table 3.8, characteristic changes in the JVP are described. Any condition in which right ventricular filling is limited (e.g. *constrictive pericarditis, cardiac tamponade* or *right ventricular infarction*) can cause elevation of the venous pressure, which is more marked on inspiration when venous return to the heart increases. This rise in the JVP on inspiration, called *Kussmaul's*[n] sign, is the opposite of what normally happens. This sign is best elicited with the patient sitting up at 90 degrees and breathing quietly through the mouth.

The abdominojugular reflux test *(hepatojugular reflux)* is a way of testing for right or left ventricular failure or reduced right ventricular compliance.[13] Pressure exerted over the liver or middle of the abdomen for 10 seconds will increase venous return to the right atrium. The JVP normally rises transiently following this manoeuvre.[o] If there is right ventricular failure or left atrial pressures are elevated (left ventricular failure), it may remain elevated (>4 cm) for the duration of the compression—a positive hepatojugular reflux. The sudden fall in the JVP (> 4 cm) as the pressure is released may be easier to see than the initial rise. It is not necessary to compress the liver and so the older name, *hepatojugular reflux*, is not so appropriate. It is important that the patient be relaxed, breathe through the mouth and not perform a Valsalva manoeuvre. The

---

[m] Sir James Mackenzie first applied these labels to the jugular waveforms in the late 19th century.

[n] Adolf Kussmaul (1822–1909), German physician who also described laboured breathing ('air hunger') in diabetic coma (1874) and was the first to use an oesophagoscope. He coined the word 'hemiballismus'.

[o] First described by Louis Pasteur in 1885.

Table 3.8 Jugular venous pressure (pulse)

Causes of an elevated central venous pressure

Right ventricular failure
Tricuspid stenosis or regurgitation
Pericardial effusion or constrictive pericarditis
Superior vena caval obstruction
Fluid overload
Hyperdynamic circulation

Wave form

*Causes of a **dominant a wave***
Tricuspid stenosis (also causing a slow *y* descent)
Pulmonary stenosis
Pulmonary hypertension
*Causes of **cannon a waves***
Complete heart block
Paroxysmal nodal tachycardia with retrograde atrial conduction
Ventricular tachycardia with retrograde atrial conduction or atrioventricular dissociation
*Cause of a **dominant v wave***
Tricuspid regurgitation
***x* descent**
Absent: atrial fibrillation
Exaggerated: acute cardiac tamponade, constrictive pericarditis
***y* descent**
Sharp: severe tricuspid regurgitation, constrictive pericarditis
Slow: tricuspid stenosis, right atrial myxoma

examiner should press firmly with the palm over the middle of the abdomen. It is not necessary to apply pressure for more than 10 seconds.

Cannon a waves occur when the right atrium contracts against the closed tricuspid valve. This occurs intermittently in complete heart block where the two chambers beat independently.

Giant a waves are large but not explosive *a* waves with each beat. They occur when right atrial pressures are raised because of elevated pressures in the pulmonary circulation or obstruction to outflow (tricuspid stenosis).

The *large v waves* of tricuspid regurgitation should never be missed. They are a reliable sign of tricuspid regurgitation and are visible welling up into the neck during each ventricular systole.

The praecordium

Now at last the examiner has reached the praecordium.

Inspection

Inspect first for scars. Previous cardiac operations will have left scars on the chest wall. The position of the scar can be a clue to the valve lesion that has been operated on. Most valve surgery requires cardio-pulmonary bypass and for this a *median sternotomy* (a cut down the middle of the sternum) is very commonly used. This type of scar is occasionally hidden under a forest of chest hair. It is not specifically helpful, as it may also be a result of previous coronary artery bypass grafting. Alternatively, left- or even right-sided lateral thoracotomy scars, which may be hidden under a pendulous breast, may indicate a previous closed mitral valvotomy. In this operation a stenosed mitral valve is opened through an incision made in the left atrial appendage; cardiopulmonary bypass is not required. Coronary artery bypass grafting and even valve surgery are now performed using small lateral 'port' incisions for video-assisted instruments.

Skeletal abnormalities such as *pectus excavatum* (funnel chest (page 102) or *kyphoscoliosis* (Greek *kyphos* 'hunchbacked', *skolios* 'curved'), a curvature of the vertebral column (page 102), may be present. Skeletal abnormalities such as these, which may be part of Marfan's syndrome, can cause distortion of the position of the heart and great vessels in the chest and thus alter the position of the apex beat. Severe deformity can interfere with pulmonary function and cause pulmonary hypertension (page 66).

Another surgical 'abnormality' that must not be missed, if only to avoid embarrassment, is a pacemaker or cardioverter-defibrillator box. These are usually under the right or left pectoral muscle just below the clavicle, are usually easily palpable and obviously metallic. The pacemaker leads may be palpable under the skin, leading from the top of the box. The box is normally mobile under the skin. Fixation of the skin to the box or stretching of the skin over the box may be an indication for repositioning. Erosion of the box through the skin is a serious complication because of the inevitable infection that will occur around this foreign body. Rarely a loose lead connection will lead to twitching of the muscles of the chest wall around the box. Penetration of the right ventricular lead into or through the right ventricular wall may lead to disconcerting paced diaphragmatic contractions (hiccups) at whatever rate the pacemaker is set. Defibrillator boxes are

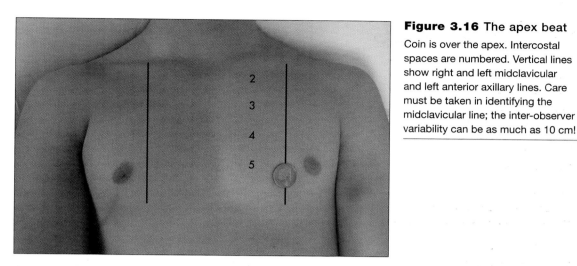

Figure 3.16 The apex beat

Coin is over the apex. Intercostal spaces are numbered. Vertical lines show right and left midclavicular and left anterior axillary lines. Care must be taken in identifying the midclavicular line; the inter-observer variability can be as much as 10 cm!

larger than pacemakers. They are currently about 10×5 cm and a little less than 1 cm thick.

Look for the apex beat. Its normal position is in the fifth left intercostal space, 1 cm medial to the midclavicular line (Figure 3.16). It is due primarily to recoil of the heart as blood is expelled in systole. There may be other visible pulsations—for example, over the pulmonary artery in cases of severe pulmonary hypertension.

Palpation

The *apex beat* must be palpated (Figures 3.16 and 3.17).[14] It is important to count down the number of interspaces. The first palpable interspace is the second. It lies just below the manubriosternal angle. The position of the apex beat is defined as the most lateral and inferior point at which the palpating fingers are raised with each systole. The normal apex is felt over an area the size of a 20 cent (50 p) coin (Figure 3.16). Note that the apex beat is palpable in only about 50% of adults.

It is worth noting that the palpable apex beat is not the anatomical apex of the heart but a point above it. At the time the apex beat is palpable,[p] the heart is assuming a more spherical shape and the apex is twisting away from the chest wall. The area above the apex, however, is moving closer to the chest and is

Figure 3.17 Feeling for the apex beat

palpable. If the apex beat is displaced laterally or inferiorly, or both, this usually indicates enlargement,[14] but may sometimes be due to chest wall deformity, or pleural or pulmonary disease (page 102).

The character of the apex beat may provide the examiner with vital diagnostic clues. The normal apex beat gently lifts the palpating fingers. There are a number of types of abnormal apex beats. The *pressure loaded* (heaving, hyperdynamic or systolic overloaded) apex beat is a forceful and sustained impulse. This occurs with aortic stenosis or hypertension. The *volume loaded* (thrusting) apex beat is a displaced, diffuse, non-sustained impulse. This occurs most commonly in advanced mitral regurgitation or dilated cardiomyopathy. The *dyskinetic* apex beat is an uncoordinated impulse felt over a

---

[p] James Hope was the first to demonstrate (in 1830) that the apex beat was caused by ventricular contraction. Jean-Nicholas Corvisant (Napoleon's personal doctor) was the first to associate abnormal palpation of the heart with cardiac chamber enlargements.

Figure 3.18 Feeling for the parasternal impulse

Figure 3.19 Palpating the base of the heart

larger area than normal in the praecordium and is usually due to left ventricular dysfunction (e.g. in anterior myocardial infarction). The *double impulse* apex beat, where two distinct impulses are felt with each systole, is characteristic of hypertrophic cardio-myopathy (page 77). The *tapping* apex beat will be felt when the first heart sound is actually palpable (heart sounds are not palpable in health) and indicates mitral or very rarely tricuspid stenosis. The character, but not the position, of the apex beat may be more easily assessed when the patient lies on the left side.

In many patients the apex beat may not be palpable. This is most often due to a thick chest wall, emphysema, pericardial effusion, shock (or death) and rarely to dextrocardia (where there is inversion of the heart and great vessels). The apex beat will be palpable to the right of the sternum in many cases of dextrocardia.

Other praecordial impulses may be palpable in patients with heart disease. A *parasternal impulse* may be felt when the heel of the hand is rested just to the left of the sternum with the fingers lifted slightly off the chest (Figure 3.18). Normally no impulse or a slight inward impulse is felt. In cases of right ventricular enlargement or severe left atrial enlargement, where the right ventricle is pushed anteriorly, the heel of the hand is lifted off the chest wall with each systole. Palpation with the fingers over the pulmonary area may reveal the palpable tap of pulmonary valve closure (*palpable P2*) in cases of pulmonary hypertension (Figure 3.19).

Turbulent blood flow, which causes cardiac murmurs on auscultation, may sometimes be palpable. These palpable murmurs are called *thrills*. The praecordium should be systematically palpated for thrills with the flat of the hand, first over the apex and left sternal edge, and then over the *base of the heart* (this is the upper part of the chest and includes the aortic and pulmonary areas) (Figure 3.19).

Apical thrills can be more easily felt with the patient rolled over to the left side (the left lateral position) as this brings the apex closer to the chest wall. Thrills may also be palpable over the base of the heart. These may be maximal over the pulmonary or aortic areas, depending on the underlying cause, and are best felt with the patient sitting up, leaning forwards and in full expiration. In this position the base of the heart is moved closer to the chest wall. A thrill that coincides in time with the apex beat is called a *systolic thrill*; one that does not coincide with the apex beat is called a *diastolic thrill*.

The presence of a thrill usually indicates an organic lesion. Careful palpation for thrills is a useful, but often neglected, part of the cardiovascular examination.

Percussion

It is possible to define the cardiac outline by means of percussion[q] but this is not routine (page 105).[15] Percussion is most accurate when performed in the fifth intercostal space. The patient should lie supine and the examiner percusses from the anterior axillary line towards the sternum. The point at which the percussion note becomes dull represents the left heart border. A distance of more than 10.5 cm between the border of the heart and the middle of the sternum indicates cardiomegaly. The sign is not useful in the presence of lung disease.

---

[q] Percussion of the heart and other organs was enthusiastically promoted by Pierre Poiry, a student of Laënnec, in the early 19th century. He performed indirect percussion using an ivory plate instead of his left middle finger.

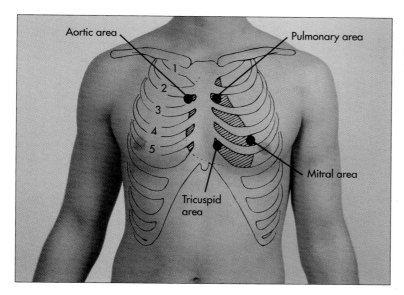

Figure 3.20 The areas best for auscultation do not exactly correlate with the anatomical location of the valves.

Auscultation

Now at last the stethoscope is required.[16] However, in some cases the diagnosis should already be fairly clear. In the viva voce examination, the examiners will occasionally stop a candidate before auscultation and ask for an opinion.

Auscultation of the heart begins in the mitral area with the bell of the stethoscope (Figures 3.20 and 3.21). The bell is designed as a resonating chamber and is particularly efficient in amplifying low-pitched sounds, such as the diastolic murmur of mitral stenosis or a third heart sound. It must be applied to the chest wall lightly, because forceful application will stretch the skin under the bell so that it forms a diaphragm. Some modern stethoscopes do not have a separate bell; the effect of a bell is produced when the diaphragm is placed lightly on the chest, and of a diaphragm when it is pushed more firmly. Next, listen in the mitral area with the diaphragm of the stethoscope (Figure 3.22), which best reproduces higher-pitched sounds, such as the systolic murmur of mitral regurgitation or a fourth heart sound. Then place the stethoscope in the tricuspid area (fifth left intercostal space) and listen. Next inch up the left sternal edge to the pulmonary (second left intercostal space) and aortic (second right intercostal space) areas (Figures 3.23 and 3.24), listening carefully in each position with the diaphragm.

For accurate auscultation, experience with what is normal is important. This can be obtained only through constant practice. Auscultation of the normal heart reveals two sounds called, not surprisingly, the first and second heart sounds. The explanation for the origin of these noises changes from year to year; the sounds are probably related to vibrations caused by the closing of the heart valves in combination with rapid changes in blood flow and tensing within cardiac structures that occur as the valves close.

The *first heart sound* (S1) has two components: mitral and tricuspid valve closure. Mitral closure occurs slightly before tricuspid, but usually only one sound is audible. The first heart sound indicates the beginning of ventricular systole.

The *second heart sound* (S2), which is softer, shorter and at a slightly higher pitch than the first and marks the end of systole, is made up of sounds arising from aortic and pulmonary valve closures. In normal cases, although left and right ventricular systole end at the same time, the lower pressure in the pulmonary circulation compared with the aorta means that flow continues into the pulmonary artery after the end of right ventricular systole. As a result, closure of the pulmonary valve occurs later than that of the aortic valve. These components are usually (in 70% of normal adults) sufficiently separated in time so that splitting of the second heart sound is audible. Because the pulmonary component of the second heart sound (P2) may not be audible throughout the praecordium, splitting of the second heart sound may best be appreciated in the pulmonary area and

Figure 3.21 Auscultation in the mitral area with the bell of the stethoscope

Listening for mitral stenosis in the left lateral position

Figure 3.23 Auscultation at the base of the heart (pulmonary area)

Figure 3.22 Auscultation at the apex with the diaphragm of the stethoscope

Figure 3.24 Auscultation at the base of the heart (aortic area)

along the left sternal edge. Pulmonary valve closure is further delayed (by 20 or 30 milliseconds) with inspiration because of increased venous return to the right ventricle; thus, splitting of the second heart sound is wider on inspiration. The second heart sound marks the beginning of diastole, which is usually longer than systole.

It can be difficult to decide which heart sound is which. Palpation of the carotid pulse will indicate the timing of systole and enable the heart sounds to be more easily distinguished. It is obviously crucial to define systole and diastole during auscultation so that cardiac murmurs and abnormal sounds can be placed in the correct part of the cardiac cycle. Students are often asked to time a cardiac murmur; this is not a request to measure its length, but rather to say in which part of the cardiac cycle it occurs.

Even the experts can mistake a murmur if they do not time it. It is important, during auscultation, to concentrate separately on the components of the cardiac cycle. The clinician should attempt to identify each and listen for abnormalities. There can be more than 12 components to identify in patients with heart disease. An understanding of the cardiac cycle is helpful when interpreting the auscultatory findings (Figure 3.25).

Abnormalities of the heart sounds

Alterations in intensity. The first heart sound (S1) is *loud* when the mitral or tricuspid valve cusps remain wide open at the end of diastole and shut forcefully with the onset of ventricular systole. This occurs in mitral stenosis because the narrowed valve orifice limits ventricular filling, so that there is no

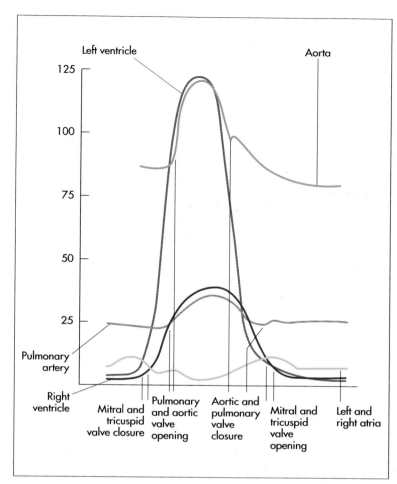

Figure 3.25 The cardiac cycle

Normally the onset of left ventricular systole precedes the onset of pressure rise in the right ventricle. The mitral valve, therefore, closes before the tricuspid valve. Because the pulmonary artery diastolic pressure is lower than aortic diastolic pressure, the pulmonary valve opens before the aortic valve. Therefore, pulmonary ejection sounds occur closer to the first heart sound than do aortic ejection sounds. During systole the pressure in the ventricles slightly exceeds the pressure in the corresponding great arteries. Towards the end of systole, the ventricular pressure falls below the pressure in the great arteries, and when diastolic pressure is reached the semilunar valves close. Normally, aortic valve closure precedes pulmonary valve closure. The mitral and tricuspid valves begin to open at the point at which the ventricular pressures fall below the corresponding atrial pressures.
(Adapted from Swash M, ed. *Hutchison's clinical methods*, 20th edn. Philadelphia: Baillière Tindall, 1995, with permission.)

diminution in flow towards the end of diastole. The normal mitral valve cusps drift back towards the closed position at the end of diastole as ventricular filling slows down. Other causes of a loud S1 are related to reduced diastolic filling time (e.g. tachycardia or any cause of a short atrioventricular conduction time).

Soft first heart sounds can be due to a prolonged diastolic filling time (as with first-degree heart block) or a delayed onset of left ventricular systole (as with left bundle branch block), or to failure of the leaflets to coapt normally (as in mitral regurgitation).

The **second heart sound** (S2) will have a *loud* aortic component (A2) in patients with systemic hypertension. This results in forceful aortic valve closure secondary to high aortic pressures. Congenital aortic stenosis is another cause, because the valve is mobile but narrowed, and closes suddenly

at the end of systole. The pulmonary component of the second heart sound (P2) is *loud* in pulmonary hypertension, where the valve closure is forceful because of the high pulmonary pressure.

A *soft* A2 will be found when the aortic valve is calcified and leaflet movement is reduced, and in aortic regurgitation when the leaflets cannot coapt.

Splitting. Splitting of the **first heart sound** is usually not detectable clinically; however, when it occurs it is most often due to the cardiac conduction abnormality known as complete right bundle branch block.

Increased normal splitting (wider on inspiration) of the **second heart sound** occurs when there is any delay in right ventricular emptying, as in right bundle branch block (delayed right ventricular depolarisation), pulmonary stenosis (delayed right ventricular ejection), ventricular septal defect (increased right ventricular volume load), and mitral regurgitation (because of earlier aortic valve closure, due to more rapid left ventricular emptying).

In the case of *fixed splitting* of the second heart sound, there is no respiratory variation (as is normal) and splitting tends to be wide. This is caused by an atrial septal defect where equalisation of volume loads between the two atria occurs through the defect. This results in the atria acting as a common chamber.

In the case of *reversed splitting* P2 occurs first and splitting occurs in expiration. This can be due to delayed left ventricular depolarisation (left bundle branch block), delayed left ventricular emptying (severe aortic stenosis, coarctation of the aorta) or increased left ventricular volume load (large patent ductus arteriosus). However, in the last-mentioned, the loud machinery murmur means that the second heart sound is usually not heard.

Extra heart sounds. The **third heart sound** (S3) is a low-pitched mid-diastolic sound that is best appreciated by listening for a triple rhythm.[17] It has been likened (rather accurately) to the galloping of a horse and is often called a *gallop rhythm*. It is more likely to be appreciated if the clinician listens not to the individual heart sounds but to the rhythm of the heart. It is probably caused by tautening of the mitral or tricuspid papillary muscles at the end of rapid diastolic filling, when blood flow temporarily stops. A physiological left ventricular S3 sometimes occurs in children and young people and is due to very rapid diastolic filling. A pathological S3 is due to reduced ventricular compliance, so that a filling sound is produced even when diastolic filling is not especially rapid. It is strongly associated with increased atrial pressure.

A *left ventricular* S3 is louder at the apex than at the left sternal edge, and is louder on expiration. It can be associated with an increased cardiac output, as occurs in pregnancy and thyrotoxicosis. Otherwise, it is an important sign of left ventricular failure and dilatation, but may also occur in aortic regurgitation, mitral regurgitation, ventricular septal defect and patent ductus arteriosus.[18]

A *right ventricular* S3 is louder at the left sternal edge and with inspiration. It occurs in right ventricular failure or constrictive pericarditis.

The **fourth heart sound** (S4) is a late diastolic sound pitched slightly higher than the S3.[19] Again, this is responsible for the impression of a triple (gallop) rhythm. It is due to a high-pressure atrial wave reflected back from a poorly compliant ventricle. It does not occur if the patient is in atrial fibrillation, because the sound depends on effective atrial contraction, which is lost when the atria fibrillate.

A *left ventricular* S4 occurs whenever left ventricular compliance is reduced due to aortic stenosis, acute mitral regurgitation, systemic hypertension, ischaemic heart disease or advanced age. It is often present during an episode of angina or with a myocardial infarction, and may be the only physical sign of that condition.

A *right ventricular* S4 occurs when right ventricular compliance is reduced in pulmonary hypertension or pulmonary stenosis.

If the heart rate is greater than 120 per minute, S3 and S4 may be superimposed, resulting in a **summation gallop**. In this case, two inaudible sounds may combine to produce an audible one. This does not necessarily imply ventricular stress, unless one or both of the extra heart sounds persists when the heart rate slows or is slowed by carotid sinus massage. When both S3 and S4 are present, the rhythm is described as a quadruple rhythm. It usually implies severe ventricular dysfunction.

Additional sounds. An **opening snap** is a high-pitched sound that occurs in mitral stenosis at a variable distance after S2. It is due to the sudden opening of the mitral valve and is followed by the diastolic murmur of mitral stenosis. It can be difficult to distinguish from a widely split S2, but normally occurs rather later in diastole than the pulmonary component of the second heart sound. It is pitched higher than a third heart sound and so is not usually confused with this. It is best heard at the lower left sternal edge with the diaphragm of the stethoscope. Use of the term 'opening snap' implies the diagnosis of mitral or rarely of tricuspid stenosis.

A **systolic ejection click** is an early systolic high-pitched sound that is heard over the aortic or pulmonary and left sternal edge area, and which may occur in cases of congenital aortic or pulmonary stenosis where the valve remains mobile; it is followed by the systolic ejection murmur of aortic or pulmonary stenosis. It is due to the abrupt doming of the abnormal valve early in systole.

A **non-ejection systolic click** is a high-pitched sound heard during systole and is best appreciated at the mitral area. It is a common finding. It may be followed by a systolic murmur. The click may be due to prolapse of one or more redundant mitral valve leaflets during systole. Non-ejection clicks may also be heard in patients with *atrial septal defects* or *Ebstein's anomaly* (page 78).

An **atrial myxoma** is a very rare tumour which may occur in either atrium. During atrial systole a loosely pedunculated tumour may be propelled into the mitral or tricuspid valve orifice causing an early diastolic plopping sound, a **tumour plop**. This sound is only rarely heard even in patients with a myxoma (about 10%).

A **diastolic pericardial knock** may occur when there is sudden cessation of ventricular filling because of constrictive pericardial disease.[20]

Prosthetic heart valves produce characteristic sounds (page 76). Rarely, a right ventricular pacemaker produces a late diastolic high-pitched click due to contraction of the chest wall muscles (the **pacemaker sound**).[21]

Murmurs of the heart

In deciding the origin of a cardiac murmur, a number of different features must be considered. These are: associated features (peripheral signs), timing, the area of greatest intensity, the loudness and pitch, and the effect of dynamic manoeuvres, including respiration and the Valsalva manoeuvre (Figure 3.26 a & b). The presence of a characteristic murmur is very reliable for the diagnosis of certain valvular abnormalities, but for others less so (*Good signs guide 3.1*).

Associated features. As already mentioned, the cause of a cardiac murmur can sometimes be elicited by careful analysis of the peripheral signs.

Timing (Table 3.9). **Systolic murmurs** (which occur during ventricular systole) may be pansystolic, ejection systolic or late systolic.

The *pansystolic murmur* extends throughout systole, beginning with the first heart sound, then going right up to the second heart sound. Its loudness and pitch vary during systole. Pansystolic murmurs occur when a ventricle leaks to a lower pressure chamber or vessel. As there is a pressure gradient from the moment the ventricle begins to contract (S1), blood flow and the murmur both begin at the first heart sound and continue until the pressures equalise (S2). Causes of pansystolic murmurs include mitral regurgitation,[r] tricuspid regurgitation and ventricular septal defect.

With an *ejection (mid)systolic* murmur, the murmur does not begin right at the first heart sound; its intensity is greatest in midsystole or later, and wanes again late in systole. This is described as a *crescendo-decrescendo* murmur. These murmurs are usually caused by turbulent flow through the aortic or pulmonary valve orifices or by greatly increased flow through a normal-sized orifice or outflow tract.

---

[r] The term incompetence is synonymous with regurgitation, but the latter better describes the pathophysiology.

Table 3.9 Cardiac murmurs

Timing	Lesion
Pansystolic	Mitral regurgitation Tricuspid regurgitation Ventricular septal defect Aortopulmonary shunts
Midsystolic	Aortic stenosis Pulmonary stenosis Hypertrophic cardiomyopathy Pulmonary flow murmur of an atrial septal defect
Late systolic	Mitral valve prolapse Papillary muscle dysfunction (due usually to ischaemia or hypertrophic cardiomyopathy)
Early diastolic	Aortic regurgitation Pulmonary regurgitation
Mid-diastolic	Mitral stenosis Tricuspid stenosis Atrial myxoma Austin Flint* murmur of aortic regurgitation Carey Coombs[†] murmur of acute rheumatic fever
Presystolic	Mitral stenosis Tricuspid stenosis Atrial myxoma
Continuous	Patent ductus arteriosus Arteriovenous fistula (coronary artery, pulmonary, systemic) Aortopulmonary connection (e.g. congenital, Blalock[‡] shunt) Venous hum (usually best heard over right supraclavicular fossa and abolished by ipsilateral internal jugular vein compression) Rupture of sinus of Valsalva into right ventricle or atrium 'Mammary souffle' (in late pregnancy or early postpartum period)

Note: The combined murmurs of aortic stenosis and aortic regurgitation, or mitral stenosis and mitral regurgitation, may sound as if they fill the entire cardiac cycle, but are not continuous murmurs by definition.

* See footnote gg, page 72.
[†] Carey F Coombs (b. 1879), Bristol physician.
[‡] Alfred Blalock (1899–1965), Baltimore physician.

Figure 3.26 Sites of maximum intensity and radiation of murmurs and heart sounds

(a) Systolic murmurs:
   AS = aortic stenosis;
   MR = mitral regurgitation;
   HCM = hypertrophic
      cardiomyopathy;
   PS = pulmonary stenosis;
   VSD = ventricular septal defect;
   I = innocent.
(b) Diastolic murmurs and sounds:
   AR = aortic regurgitation;
   MS = mitral stenosis;
   S3 = third heart sound;
   PR = pulmonary regurgitation;
   PDA = patent ductus arteriosus
      (continuous murmur).

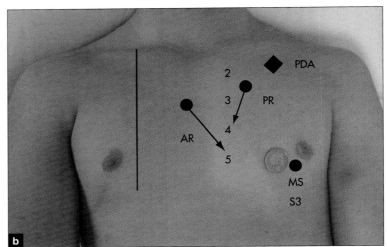

GOOD SIGNS GUIDE 3.1 Characteristic murmurs and valvular heart disease		
Sign	Positive LR	Negative LR
Characteristic systolic murmur		
Aortic stenosis	3.3	0.1
Mild mitral regurgitation or worse (moderate or severe)	5.4	0.4
Mild tricuspid regurgitation or worse	14.6	0.8
Moderate to severe tricuspid regurgitation	10.1	0.4
Characteristic diastolic murmur		
Mild aortic regurgitation or worse	9.9	0.3
Pulmonary regurgitation	17.4	NS

NS = not significant.
From McGee S, *Evidence-based physical diagnosis*, Saunders, 2001.

With a *late systolic* murmur it is possible to distinguish an appreciable gap between the first heart sound and the murmur, which then continues right up to the second heart sound. This is typical of mitral valve prolapse or papillary muscle dysfunction where mitral regurgitation begins in midsystole.

Diastolic murmurs occur during ventricular diastole.

The *early diastolic* murmur begins immediately with the second heart sound and has a decrescendo quality (it is loudest at the beginning and extends for a variable distance into diastole). These early diastolic murmurs are typically high pitched and are due to regurgitation through leaking aortic or pulmonary valves. The murmur is loudest at the beginning because this is when aortic and pulmonary artery pressures are highest.

Mid-diastolic murmurs begin later in diastole and may be short or extend right up to the first heart sound. They have a much lower pitched quality than early diastolic murmurs. They are due to impaired flow during ventricular filling and can be caused by mitral stenosis and tricuspid stenosis, where the valve is narrowed, or rarely by an atrial myxoma, where the tumour mass obstructs the valve orifice. In severe aortic regurgitation, the regurgitant jet from the aortic valve may cause the anterior leaflet of the mitral valve to shudder, producing a diastolic murmur. Occasionally, normal mitral or tricuspid valves can produce flow murmurs, which are short and mid-diastolic, and occur when there is torrential flow across the valve. Causes include a high cardiac output or intracardiac shunting (atrial or ventricular septal defects).

Presystolic murmurs may be heard when atrial systole increases blood flow across the valve just before the first heart sound. They are extensions of the mid-diastolic murmurs of mitral stenosis and tricuspid stenosis, and usually do not occur when atrial systole is lost in atrial fibrillation.

As the name implies, **continuous murmurs** extend throughout systole and diastole. They are produced when a communication exists between two parts of the circulation with a permanent pressure gradient so that blood flow occurs continuously. They can usually be distinguished from combined systolic and diastolic murmurs (due, for example, to aortic stenosis and aortic regurgitation), but this may sometimes be difficult. The causes are presented in Table 3.9.

A **pericardial friction rub** is a superficial scratching sound; there may be up to three distinct components occurring at any time during the cardiac cycle. They are not confined to systole or diastole. A rub is caused by movement of inflamed pericardial surfaces. It is a result of pericarditis. The sound can vary with respiration and posture; it is often louder when the patient is sitting up and breathing out. It tends to come and go, and is often absent by the time students can be found to come and listen for it. It has been likened to the crunching sound made when *walking on snow*.

A **mediastinal crunch** (Hamman's sign[s]) is a crunching sound heard in time with the heart beat but with systolic and diastolic components. It is caused by the presence of air in the mediastinum, and once heard it is not forgotten. It is very often present after cardiac surgery and may occur associated with a pneumothorax or after aspiration of a pericardial effusion.

Area of greatest intensity. Although the place on the praecordium where a murmur is heard most easily is a guide to its origin, this is not a particularly reliable physical sign. For example, mitral regurgitation murmurs (*Good signs guide 3.1*) are usually loudest at the apex, over the mitral area, and tend to radiate towards the axillae, but they may be heard widely over the praecordium and even right up into the aortic area or over the back. Conduction of an ejection murmur up into the carotid arteries strongly suggests that this arises from the aortic valve.

Loudness and pitch. Unfortunately, the *loudness* of the murmur is not always helpful in deciding the severity of the valve lesion. For example, in the severest forms of valve stenosis, murmurs may be soft. However, murmurs are usually graded according to loudness. Cardiologists most often use a classification with six grades (Levine's grading system):[22]

Grade 1/6: very soft and not heard at first (often audible only to consultants and to those students who have been told the murmur is present)
Grade 2/6: soft, but can be detected almost immediately by an experienced auscultator
Grade 3/6: moderate; there is no thrill
Grade 4/6: loud; thrill just palpable
Grade 5/6: very loud; thrill easily palpable
Grade 6/6: very, very loud; can be heard even without placing the stethoscope right on the chest

This grading is useful, particularly because a change in the intensity of a murmur may be of great significance—for example, after a myocardial infarction.

---

[s] Louis Hamman (1877–1946), physician, Johns Hopkins Hospital, Baltimore.

GOOD SIGNS GUIDE 3.2
Dynamic auscultation

Sign	Positive LR	Negative LR
Louder on inspiration—right-sided murmur	7.8	0.2
Louder with Valsalva strain—hypertrophic cardiomyopathy	14.0	0.3
Louder squatting to standing—hypertrophic cardiomyopathy	6.0	0.1
Softer with isometric handgrip—hypertrophic cardiomyopathy	3.6	0.1
Louder with isometric handgrip—mitral regurgitation	5.8	0.3

From McGee S, *Evidence-based physical diagnosis*, Saunders, 2001.

Table 3.10 Dynamic manoeuvres and systolic cardiac murmurs

Manoeuvre	Lesion			
	Hypertrophic cardiomyopathy	Mitral valve prolapse	Aortic stenosis	Mitral regurgitation
Valsalva strain phase (decreases preload)	Louder	Longer	Softer	Softer
Squatting or leg raise (increases preload)	Softer	Shorter	Louder	Louder
Hand grip (increases afterload)	Softer	Shorter	Softer	Louder

It requires practice to appreciate the *pitch* of the murmur, but this may be of use in identifying its type. In general, low-pitched murmurs indicate turbulent flow under low pressure, as in mitral stenosis, and high-pitched murmurs indicate a high velocity of flow, as in mitral regurgitation.

Dynamic manoeuvres (*Good signs guide 3.2*). All patients with a newly diagnosed murmur should undergo dynamic manoeuvre testing (Table 3.10).[23]

■ **Respiration.** Murmurs that arise on the right side of the heart become louder during inspiration as this increases venous return and therefore blood flow to the right side of the heart. Left-sided murmurs are either unchanged or become softer. Expiration has the opposite effect. This can be a sensitive and specific way of differentiating right- and left-sided murmurs.

■ **Deep expiration.** A routine part of the examination of the heart (Figure 3.27) includes leaning a patient forward in full expiration and listening to the base of the heart for aortic regurgitation, which may otherwise be missed. In this case the manoeuvre brings the base of the heart closer to the chest wall. The scraping sound of a pericardial friction rub is also best heard in this position.

■ **The Valsalva manoeuvre.**[t] This is a forceful expiration against a closed glottis. One should ask the patient to hold his or her nose with the fingers, close the mouth, breathe out hard and completely so as to pop the eardrums, and hold this for as long as possible. Listen over the left sternal edge during this manoeuvre for changes in the systolic murmur of hypertrophic cardiomyopathy, and over the apex for changes when mitral valve prolapse is suspected.

The Valsalva manoeuvre has four phases. In phase 1 (beginning the manoeuvre) a rise in intrathoracic pressure and a transient increase in left ventricular output and blood pressure occurs. In phase 2 (the straining phase) systemic venous return falls, filling of the right and then the left side of the heart is reduced, and stroke volume and blood

---

[t] Antonio Valsalva (1666–1723), Professor of Anatomy at Bologna, was noted for his studies of the ear. He described his manoeuvre in 1704. Forced expiration against the closed glottis causes discharge of pus into the external auditory canal in cases of chronic otitis media. Friedrich Weber rediscovered the manoeuvre in 1859 and demonstrated that he could slow his pulse at will. He stopped demonstrating this after he caused himself to faint and have convulsions.

Figure 3.27 Dynamic auscultation for aortic regurgitation or a pericardial friction rub; patient in deep expiration

pressure fall while the heart rate increases. As stroke volume and arterial blood pressure fall, most cardiac murmurs become softer; however, because the left ventricular volume is reduced, the systolic murmur of hypertrophic cardiomyopathy becomes louder and the systolic click and murmur of mitral valve prolapse begins earlier. In phase 3 (the release of the manoeuvre) first right-sided and then left-sided cardiac murmurs become louder briefly before returning to normal. Blood pressure falls further because of pooling of blood in the pulmonary veins. In phase 4 the blood pressure overshoots as a result of increased sympathetic activity as a response to the previous hypotension. Changes in heart rate are opposite to the blood pressure changes.

The blood pressure responses can be measured by inflating a cuff to 15 mmHg over the systolic pressure before the manoeuvre. Korotkoff sounds will then appear in phases 1 and 4 in a normal patient. Absence of the phase 4 overshoot is a sign of cardiac failure. The left ventricle is unable to increase cardiac output despite increased sympathetic activity.

- **Standing to squatting.** When the patient squats rapidly from the standing position, venous return and systemic arterial resistance increase simultaneously, causing a rise in stroke volume and arterial pressure. This makes most murmurs louder. However, left ventricular size is increased, which reduces the obstruction to outflow and therefore reduces the intensity of the systolic murmur of hypertrophic cardiomyopathy, while the midsystolic click and murmur of mitral valve prolapse are delayed.
- **Squatting to standing.** When the patients stands up quickly after squatting the opposite changes in the loudness of these murmurs occurs.
- **Isometric exercise.** Sustained hand grip or repeated sit-ups for 20 for 30 seconds increases systemic arterial resistance, blood pressure and heart size. The systolic murmur of aortic stenosis may become softer because of a reduction in the pressure gradient across the valve but often remains unchanged. Most other murmurs become louder, except the systolic murmur of hypertrophic cardiomyopathy, which is softer, and the mitral valve prolapse murmur, which is delayed because of an increased ventricular volume.

Auscultation of the neck

This is often performed as a part of dynamic auscultation for valvular heart disease (page 54), but certain aspects of the examination may be considered here. Abnormal sounds heard over the arteries are called *bruits*. These sounds are low pitched and may be more easily heard with the bell of the stethoscope. Carotid artery bruits are most easily heard over the anterior part of the sternomastoid muscle above the medial end of the clavicle. Ask the patient to stop breathing for a brief period to remove the competing noise of breath sounds. It may be prudent to ask the patient not to speak. The amplified voice is often painfully loud when heard through the stethoscope.

A systolic bruit may be a conducted sound from the heart. The murmur of aortic stenosis is always audible in the neck and a soft carotid bruit is sometimes audible in patients with severe mitral regurgitation or pulmonary stenosis. A bruit due to carotid stenosis will not be audible over the base of the heart. Move the stethoscope from point to point onto the chest wall; if the bruit disappears, it is likely the sound arises from the carotid. It is not possible to exclude a carotid bruit in a patient with a murmur of aortic stenosis that radiates to the neck. Carotid artery stenosis is an important cause of a carotid bruit. More severe stenosis is associated with a noise that is longer and of increased pitch. Total obstruction of the vessel leads to disappearance of the bruit. It is not possible to make a diagnosis of significant (>50% obstruction) carotid stenosis clinically, but the presence of a bruit is often the indication for investigations. Thyrotoxicosis can result in a systolic bruit (page 261) due to the increased vascularity of the gland.

A continuous noise is sometimes audible at the base of the neck. This is usually a venous hum, a result of audible venous flow. It disappears if light pressure is applied to the neck just above the stethoscope. Occasionally a loud machinery murmur (page 79) or severe aortic regurgitation (page 73) may cause a similar sound. Haemodialysis patients frequently have an audible bruit transmitted from their arterio-venous fistula.

The back

It is now time to leave the praecordium. Percussion and auscultation of the *lung bases* (Chapter 4) are also part of the cardiovascular examination. Signs of cardiac failure may be detected in the lungs; in particular late or pan-inspiratory crackles or a pleural effusion may be present. The murmur associated with coarctation of the aorta may be prominent over the upper back.

While the patient is sitting up, feel for pitting oedema of the sacrum, which occurs in severe right heart failure, especially in patients who have been in bed. This is because the sacrum then becomes a dependent area and oedema fluid tends to settle under the influence of gravity.

Figure 3.28 Severe pitting oedema of the legs

The abdomen

Lay the patient down flat (on one pillow) and examine the abdomen (Chapter 5). You are looking particularly for an enlarged tender *liver* which may be found when the hepatic veins are congested in the presence of right heart failure. Distension of the liver capsule is said to be the cause of liver tenderness in these patients. When tricuspid regurgitation is present the liver may be *pulsatile* as the right ventricular systolic pressure wave is transmitted to the hepatic veins. Test for hepatojugular reflux (page 43).[13,24] *Ascites* may occur with severe right heart failure. *Splenomegaly*, if present, may indicate infective endocarditis.

Feel for the pulsation of the abdominal aorta, to the left of the middle line. It is often palpable in normal thin people but the possibility of an abdominal aortic aneurysm should always be considered when the aorta's pulsations are palpable and expansile (page 153).[25,26]

The lower limbs

Palpate behind the medial malleolus of the tibia and the distal shaft of the tibia for *oedema* by compressing the area for at least 15 seconds with the thumb. This latter area is often tender in normal people and gentleness is necessary. Oedema may be pitting (the skin is indented and only slowly refills—Figure 3.28), or non-pitting. Pitting oedema occurs in cardiac failure unless the condition has been present for a long time and secondary changes in the lymphatic vessels have occurred. If oedema is present, note its upper level (e.g. 'pitting oedema to mid-calf' or 'pitting oedema to mid-thigh'). Severe oedema can involve the skin of the abdominal wall and the scrotum as well as the lower limbs. Causes of oedema are listed in Table 3.11.

Look for evidence of Achilles[u] tendon xanthomata due to hyperlipidaemia. Also look for cyanosis and clubbing of the toes (this may occur without finger clubbing in a patient with a patent ductus arteriosus, because a rise in pulmonary artery pressures, sufficient to reverse the direction of flow in the shunt, has occurred).

[u] Achilles, mythical Greek hero, whose body was invulnerable except for his heels, by which he was held when dipped in the River Styx as a baby to make him immortal. He was killed by Paris, who shot an arrow into his heel.

Table 3.11 Causes of oedema

Pitting lower limb oedema

Cardiac: congestive cardiac failure, constrictive pericarditis

Drugs: calcium antagonists

Hepatic: cirrhosis causing hypoalbuminaemia

Renal: nephrotic syndrome causing hypoalbuminaemia

Gastrointestinal tract: malabsorption, starvation, protein-losing enteropathy causing hypoalbuminaemia

Beri-beri (wet)

Cyclical oedema

Pitting unilateral lower limb oedema

Deep venous thrombosis

Compression of large veins by tumour or lymph nodes

Non-pitting lower limb oedema

Hypothyroidism

Lymphoedema

- Infectious (e.g. filariasis)
- Malignant (tumour invasion of lymphatics)
- Congenital (lymphatic development arrest)
- Allergy
- Milroy's* disease (unexplained lymphoedema which appears at puberty and is more common in females)

* William Milroy (1855–1914), Professor of Medicine, University of Nebraska, described the disease in 1928.

GOOD SIGNS GUIDE 3.3
Peripheral vascular disease

Sign	Positive LR	Negative LR
Sores or ulcers on feet	7.0	NS
Feet pale, red or blue	2.8	0.7
Atrophic skin	1.7	NS
Absent hair	1.7	NS
One foot cooler	6.1	0.9
Absent femoral pulse	6.1	NS
Absent dorsalis pedis and posterior tibial pulses	14.9	0.3
Limb bruit present	7.3	0.7
Capillary refill time >5 seconds	1.9	NS
Capillary refill >20 seconds	3.6	NS

NS = not significant.

From McGee S, *Evidence-based physical diagnosis*, Saunders, 2001.

Peripheral vascular disease

Examine both *femoral arteries* by palpating and then auscultating them. A bruit may be heard if the artery is narrowed. Next palpate the following pulses: *popliteal* (behind the knee—Figure 3.29a: if this is difficult to feel when the patient is supine, try the method shown in Figure 3.29b), *posterior tibial* (under the medial malleolus, Figure 3.30a) and *dorsalis pedis* (on the forefoot, Figure 3.30b) on both sides.[27]

Patients with exertional calf pain (intermittent claudication) are likely to have disease of the peripheral arteries. More severe disease can lead to pain even at rest and to ischaemic changes in the legs and feet (*Good signs guide 3.3*). Look for atrophic skin and loss of hair, colour changes of the feet (blue or red) and ulcers at the lower end of the tibia. Venous and diabetic ulcers can be distinguished from arterial ulcers (Figures 3.31–3.33).

Look for reduced capillary return (compress the toenails—the return of the normal red colour is slow).[28] In such cases, perform *Buerger's test*[v] to help confirm your diagnosis: elevate the legs to 45 degrees (pallor is rapid if there is a poor arterial supply), then place them dependent at 90 degrees over the edge of the bed (cyanosis occurs if the arterial supply is impaired).

Acute arterial occlusion

Acute arterial occlusion of a major peripheral limb artery results in a painful, pale, pulseless and 'paralysed' limb (the four Ps). It can be the result of embolism, thrombosis or injury. Peripheral arterial embolism usually arises from thrombus in the heart, where it is often secondary to (i) myocardial infarction, (ii) dilated cardiomyopathy, (iii) atrial fibrillation or (iv) infective endocarditis.[29]

---

v Leo Buerger (1879–1943), New York physician, born in Vienna, who described thromboangiitis obliterans. He was obsessed with expensive motor cars.

Figure 3.29 Palpating the popliteal artery: (a) patient supine; (b) patient prone

Figure 3.30 Feeling (a) the posterior tibial artery and (b) the dorsalis pedis artery

Deep venous thrombosis

Deep venous thrombosis is a difficult clinical diagnosis (*Good signs guide 3.4*).[30] The patient may complain of calf pain. On examination, the clinician should look for swelling of the calf and the thigh, and dilated superficial veins. Feel then for increased warmth and squeeze the calf (gently) to determine if the area is tender. Homans' sign[w] (pain in the calf when the foot is sharply dorsiflexed) is of limited diagnostic value and is theoretically dangerous because of the possibility of dislodgment of loose thrombus. The causes of thrombosis were described by Virchow[x] in 1856 under three broad headings (the famous *Virchow's triad*): (i) changes in the vessel wall, (ii) changes in blood flow and (iii) changes in the constitution of the blood. Deep venous thrombosis is usually caused by prolonged immobilisation, cardiac failure (stasis) or trauma (vessel wall damage), but may also result from occult neoplasm, disseminated intravascular coagulation, the contraceptive pill, pregnancy and a number of inherited defects of coagulation (the *thrombophilias*: e.g. Factor V Leiden deficiency, anti-thrombin III deficiency).

[w] John Homans (1877–1954), Professor of Surgery, Harvard University, Boston. He described his sign in 1941, originally in cases of thrombophlebitis.

[x] Rudolph Virchow (1821–1902), brilliant German pathologist, regarded as the founder of modern pathology. Professor of Pathological Anatomy in Berlin. He provided the first description of leukaemia. He died at 81 after fracturing his femur jumping from a moving tram.

GOOD SIGNS GUIDE 3.4 Deep venous thrombosis		
Sign	**Positive LR**	**Negative LR**
Asymmetrical calf swelling >2 cm difference	2.1	0.6
Thigh swelling	2.5	0.6
Superficial venous dilatation	1.9	NS
Tenderness and erythema	NS	NS
Asymmetrical skin warmth	1.4	NS
Homans' sign	NS	NS

NS = not significant.
From McGee S, *Evidence-based physical diagnosis*, Saunders, 2001.

Figure 3.31 Venous ulcer

This venous ulcer has an irregular margin, pale surrounding neo-epithelium (new skin), and a pink base of granulation tissue. There is often a history of deep venous thrombosis. The skin is warm and oedema is often present. (See Table 3.12.)
(From FS McDonald, ed., *Mayo clinic images in internal medicine*, with permission. © Mayo Clinic Scientific Press and CRC Press.)

Figure 3.32 Arterial ulcer

This arterial ulcer has a regular margin and 'punched out' appearance. The surrounding skin is cold. The peripheral pulses are absent. (See Table 3.12.)
(From FS McDonald, ed., *Mayo clinic images in internal medicine*, with permission. © Mayo Clinic Scientific Press and CRC Press.)

Figure 3.33 Diabetic (neuropathic) ulcer

Neuropathic ulcers are painless and are associated with reduced sensation in the surrounding skin. (See Table 3.12.)
(From FS McDonald, ed., *Mayo clinic images in internal medicine*, with permission. © Mayo Clinic Scientific Press and CRC Press.)

Varicose veins

If a patient complains of 'varicose veins', ask him or her to *stand* with the legs fully exposed.[31] *Inspect* the front of the whole leg for tortuous, dilated branches of the long saphenous vein (below the femoral vein in the groin to the medial side of the lower leg). Then inspect the back of the calf for varicosities of the short saphenous vein (from the popliteal fossa to the back of the calf and lateral malleolus). Look to see if the leg is inflamed, swollen or pigmented (subcutaneous haemosiderin deposition secondary to venous stasis).

Palpate the veins. Hard leg veins suggest thrombosis, while tenderness indicates thrombophlebitis. Perform the *cough impulse test*. Put the fingers over the long saphenous vein opening in the groin, medial to the femoral vein. (Don't forget the anatomy—femoral vein (medial), artery (your landmark), nerve (lateral).) Ask the patient to cough: a fluid thrill is felt if the saphenofemoral valve is incompetent.

The following supplementary tests are occasionally helpful (and surgeons like to quiz students on them in examinations).

Trendelenburg test:[y] with the patient lying down, the leg is elevated. Firm pressure is placed on the saphenous opening in the groin, and the patient is instructed to stand. The sign is positive if the veins stay empty until the groin pressure is released (incompetence at the saphenofemoral valve). If the veins fill despite groin pressure, the incompetent valves are in the thigh or calf, and Perthes' test[z] is performed.

Perthes' test: repeat the Trendelenburg test, but when the patient stands, allow some blood to be released and then get him or her to stand up and down on the toes a few times. The veins will become less tense if the perforating calf veins are patent and have competent valves (the muscle pump is functioning).

If the pattern of affected veins is unusual (e.g. pubic varices), the clinician should try to exclude secondary varicose veins. These may be due to an intrapelvic neoplasm which has obstructed deep venous return. Rectal (page 160) and pelvic (page 192) examinations should then be performed.

Finally, chronic venous stasis is one cause of ulceration of the lower leg. This is often associated with pigmentation and eczema, which are due to venous stasis. The differential diagnosis of leg ulcers is summarised in Table 3.12.

---

[y] Friedrich Trendelenburg (1844–1924), Professor of Surgery, Leipzig.
[z] Georg Clemens Perthes (1869–1927), German surgeon, Professor of Surgery at Tübingen. He was the first to use radiotherapy for the treatment of cancer (in 1903).

Table 3.12 Causes of leg ulcers

1 Venous stasis ulcer—most common (Figure 3.31)
   Site: around malleoli
   Associated pigmentation, stasis eczema
2 Ischaemic ulcer (Figure 3.32)
   • Large artery disease (atherosclerosis, thromboangiitis obliterans): usually lateral side of leg (pulses absent)
   • Small vessel disease (e.g. leucocytoclastic vasculitis, palpable purpura)
3 Malignant ulcer, e.g. basal cell carcinoma (pearly translucent edge), squamous cell carcinoma (hard everted edge), melanoma, lymphoma, Kaposi's sarcoma
4 Infection, e.g. *Staphylococcus aureus*, syphilitic gumma, tuberculosis, atypical *Mycobacterium*, fungal
5 Neuropathic (painless penetrating ulcer on sole of foot: peripheral neuropathy, e.g. diabetes mellitus, tabes, leprosy) (Figure 3.33)
6 Underlying systemic disease
   • Diabetes mellitus: vascular disease, neuropathy or necrobiosis lipoidica (front of leg)
   • Pyoderma gangrenosum
   • Rheumatoid arthritis
   • Lymphoma
   • Haemolytic anaemia (small ulcers over malleoli), e.g. sickle cell anaemia

Correlation of physical signs and cardiovascular disease

When a disease is named after some author, it is very likely that we don't know much about it.

August Bier (1861–1949)

Cardiac failure

This is one of the commonest syndromes: the signs of cardiac failure should be sought in all patients admitted to hospital, especially if there is a complaint of dyspnoea.[32] Cardiac failure has been defined as a reduction in cardiac function such that cardiac output is reduced relative to the metabolic demands

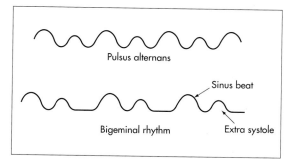

Figure 3.34 Pulsus alternans

of the body and compensating mechanisms have occurred. The specific signs depend on whether the left, right or both ventricles are involved. It is important to note that the absence of definite signs of cardiac failure may not exclude the diagnosis. Patients with compensated, chronic cardiac failure may be normal on cardiac examination.

Left ventricular failure (LVF)

- **Symptoms:** exertional dyspnoea, orthopnoea, paroxysmal nocturnal dyspnoea.
- **General signs:** tachypnoea, due to raised pulmonary pressures; central cyanosis, due to pulmonary oedema; Cheyne-Stokes breathing (see Table 4.4), especially in sedated elderly patients; peripheral cyanosis, due to low cardiac output; hypotension, due to low cardiac output; cardiac cachexia.
- **Arterial pulse:** sinus tachycardia, due to increased sympathetic tone; low pulse pressure (low cardiac output); pulsus alternans (alternate strong and weak beats; it is unlike a bigeminal rhythm caused by regular extrasystoles, in that the beats are regular; see Figure 3.34)—this is an uncommon but specific sign of unknown aetiology.
- **Apex beat:** displaced, with dilatation of the left ventricle; dyskinetic in anterior myocardial infarction or dilated cardiomyopathy; palpable gallop rhythm. The absence of these signs does not exclude left ventricular failure.
- **Auscultation:** left ventricular S3 (an important sign); functional mitral regurgitation (secondary to valve ring dilatation).
- **Lung fields:** signs of pulmonary congestion (basal inspiratory crackles) or pulmonary oedema (crackles and wheezes throughout the lung fields), due to raised venous pressures (increased preload). The typical middle to late inspiratory crackles at the lung bases may be absent in chronic,

compensated heart failure and there are many other causes of basal inspiratory crackles. This makes crackles a rather non-specific and insensitive sign of heart failure.
- **Other signs:** abnormal Valsalva response (page 54), positive abdominojugular reflux test, right ventricular failure may complicate left ventricular failure, especially if this is severe and chronic.
- **Signs of the underlying or precipitating cause:** *Causes of LVF:* (i) myocardial disease (ischaemic heart disease, cardiomyopathy); (ii) volume overload (aortic regurgitation, mitral regurgitation, patent ductus arteriosus); (iii) pressure overload (systolic hypertension, aortic stenosis).

Signs of a precipitating cause: anaemia (page 198), thyrotoxicosis (page 261), rapid arrhythmia (usually atrial fibrillation). (See *Good signs guide 3.5*.)

GOOD SIGNS GUIDE 3.5 Left ventricular failure		
General signs	**Positive LR**	**Negative LR**
Heart rate >100 beats per minute at rest	5.5	NS
Valsalva manoeuvre abnormal	7.6	0.1
Lungs		
Crackles	NS	NS
Cardiac examination		
JVP elevated	3.9	NS
Abdominojugular test positive	8.0	0.3
Apex displaced lateral to midclavicular line	5.8	NS
S3	5.7	NS
S4	NS	NS
Other findings		
Oedema	NS	NS
NS = not significant.		
From McGee S, *Evidence-based physical diagnosis*, Saunders, 2001.		

Right ventricular failure (RVF)

- **Symptoms:** ankle, sacral or abdominal swelling, anorexia, nausea.
- **General signs:** peripheral cyanosis, due to low cardiac output.

- **Arterial pulse:** low volume, due to low cardiac output.
- **Jugular venous pulse:** raised, due to the raised venous pressure (right heart preload); Kussmaul's sign, due to poor right ventricular compliance (e.g. right ventricular myocardial infarction); large *v* waves (functional tricuspid regurgitation secondary to valve ring dilatation).
- **Apex beat:** right ventricular heave.
- **Auscultation:** right ventricular S3; pansystolic murmur of functional tricuspid regurgitation (absence of a murmur does not exclude tricuspid regurgitation).
- **Abdomen:** *tender hepatomegaly*, due to increased venous pressure transmitted via the hepatic veins; *pulsatile liver* (a useful sign), if tricuspid regurgitation is present.
- **Oedema**, due to sodium and water retention plus raised venous pressure, may be manifested by pitting ankle and sacral oedema, ascites, or pleural effusions (small).
- **Signs of the underlying cause:**
  Causes of RVF: (i) left ventricular failure (severe chronic LVF causes raised pulmonary pressures resulting in secondary right ventricular failure); (ii) volume overload (atrial septal defect, primary tricuspid regurgitation); (iii) pressure overload (pulmonary stenosis, pulmonary hypertension); (iv) myocardial disease (right ventricular myocardial infarction, cardiomyopathy).

Chest pain

Many of the causes of chest pain represent a medical (or surgical) emergency. The appropriate diagnosis or differential diagnosis is often suggested by the history and urgent investigations (e.g. ECG, chest X-ray, lung scan or pulmonary angiogram) may be indicated. However, a careful and rapid physical examination may add important information in many cases. In all cases the general inspection and measurement of the vital signs will help with the assessment of the severity and urgency of the problem. Certain specific signs may help with the diagnosis.[33,34]

Myocardial infarction

- **General signs:** there are few specific signs of myocardial infarction but many patients appear obviously unwell and in distress from their chest pain. Sweating (often called diaphoresis by accident and emergency staff), an appearance of anxiety (angor animi or sense of impending

doom) and restlessness may be obvious. It is important that all this information be recorded so that changes to the patient's condition can be assessed as the infarct evolves.
- **Pulse and blood pressure:** tachycardia and/or hypotension (25% with anterior infarction from sympathetic hyperactivity; bradycardia and/or hypotension (up to 50% with inferior infarction from parasympathetic hyperactivity). Other arrhythmias including atrial fibrillation (due to atrial infarction), ventricular tachycardia and heart block may be present.
- **The JVP:** increased with right ventricular infarction; Kussmaul's sign is a specific and sensitive sign of right ventricular infarction in patients with a recent inferior infarct.
- **Apex beat:** dyskinetic in patients with large anterior infarction.
- **Auscultation:** S4; S3; decreased intensity of heart sounds; transient apical midsystolic or late-systolic murmur (in 25% from mitral regurgitation secondary to papillary muscle dysfunction), or a pericardial friction rub (with transmural infarction).
- **Complications:** arrhythmias (ventricular tachycardia, atrial fibrillation, ventricular fibrillation or heart block); heart failure; cardiogenic shock; rupture of a papillary muscle; perforation of the ventricular septum; ventricular aneurysm; thromboembolism or cardiac rupture. Signs of these complications (which do not usually occur for a few days after the infarct) include the development of a new murmur, recurrent chest pain, dyspnoea, sudden hypotension or sudden death.

The **Killip Class**[aa] can be calculated from the examination. It gives considerable prognostic information.[33]

Killip Class I	no evidence of heart failure
Killip Class II	mild heart failure; crackles over lower third or less of the lungs; systolic BP >90 mmHg
Killip Class III	pulmonary oedema, crackles more than one-third of chest; systolic BP >90 mmHg
Killip Class IV	cardiogenic shock, pulmonary oedema, crackles more than one-third of chest, systolic BP <90 mmHg

---

[aa] T. Killip, a New Zealand cardiologist, published his classification in 1967.

Killip Class III or IV is associated with a >5-fold mortality risk and Class II with a >3-fold risk compared with Class I.

Pulmonary embolism

There may be no physical signs of this condition, but dyspnoea which may be profound and make the patient exhausted is often the most obvious indication of a large pulmonary embolism. There is usually a resting tachycardia. Signs of shock—hypotension and cyanosis—indicate a very large and life-threatening embolus. There may be signs of a DVT in the legs but absence of these by no means excludes the diagnosis.

Acute aortic dissection

This is a difficult diagnosis which cannot usually be excluded on clinical grounds. A tear in the intima leads to blood surging into the aortic media, separating the intima and adventitia; this may present acutely or chronically. There are three different types: *type I* begins in the ascending aorta and extends proximally and distally; *type II* is limited to the ascending aorta and aortic arch (this is particularly associated with Marfan's syndrome); *type III* begins distal to the left subclavian artery and has the best prognosis.

- **Symptoms:** chest pain (typically very severe, it radiates to the back and is maximal in intensity at the time of onset due to either the aortic tear or associated myocardial infarction); stroke; syncope (associated with tamponade); symptoms of left ventricular failure; and, rarely, limb pain (ischaemia), paraplegia (spinal cord ischaemia), or abdominal pain (mesenteric ischaemia).
- **Signs:** The examination can reveal signs that make the diagnosis very likely (specific but not sensitive). There may be signs of a body habitus associated with dissection (e.g. Marfan's, Ehlers-Danlos syndromes). The pulses and blood pressures in the two arms must be assessed. A diminution of the radial pulse on one side or difference in blood pressure of 20 mmHg or more between the two arms is significant and suggests dissection has progressed to involve the origin of the arm vessels. Examine the patient for signs of pericardial tamponade (page 63), which occurs if the aorta ruptures into the pericardial sac. Examine the heart for signs of aortic regurgitation caused by disruption of the aortic valve annulus. A neurological examination may reveal signs of hemiplegia,

due to dissection of one of the carotid arteries. Rare signs that have been described include a pulsatile sternoclavicular joint, hoarseness (recurrent laryngeal nerve compression) and dysphagia (oesophageal compression).

Pericardial disease

Acute pericarditis

- **Signs:** fever; dyspnoea; pericardial friction rub—sit the patient up and listen to the heart with the patient holding the breath in deep expiration.
- **Causes of acute pericarditis:** (i) viral infection (coxsackievirus A or B, influenza); (ii) after myocardial infarction: early, or late (10–14 days, termed Dressler's syndrome[bb]); (iii) after pericardiotomy (cardiac surgery); (iv) uraemia; (v) neoplasia—tumour invasion (e.g. bronchus, breast, lymphoma) or after irradiation for tumour; (vi) connective tissue disease (e.g. systemic lupus erythematosus, rheumatoid arthritis); (vii) hypothyroidism; (viii) other infections (e.g. tuberculosis, pyogenic pneumonia or septicaemia); (ix) acute rheumatic fever.

Chronic constrictive pericarditis

- **General signs:** cachexia.
- **Pulse and blood pressure:** pulsus paradoxus (more than the normal 10 mmHg fall in the arterial pulse pressure on inspiration, because increased right ventricular filling compresses the left ventricle); low blood pressure.
- **The JVP:** raised; Kussmaul's sign (50%); prominent *x* and *y* descents.
- **Apex beat:** impalpable.
- **Auscultation:** heart sounds distant, early S3; early pericardial knock (rapid ventricular filling abruptly halted).
- **Abdomen:** hepatomegaly, due to raised venous pressure; splenomegaly, due to raised venous pressure; ascites.
- **Peripheral oedema.**
- **Causes of chronic constrictive pericarditis:** (i) cardiac operation or trauma; (ii) tuberculosis, histoplasmosis or pyogenic infection; (iii) neoplastic disease; (iv) mediastinal irradiation; (v) connective tissue disease (especially rheumatoid arthritis); (vi) chronic renal failure.

[bb] William Dressler (1890–1969), a New York cardiologist, described this syndrome in 1956.

Figure 3.35 Example of an intravenous drug addict's forearm

Figure 3.36 A Roth's spot on fundoscopy

Acute cardiac tamponade

- **General signs:** tachypnoea; anxiety and restlessness; syncope. Patients look very ill.
- **Pulse and blood pressure:** rapid pulse rate; pulsus paradoxus; hypotension.
- **The JVP:** raised; prominent *x* but an absent *y* descent.
- **Apex beat:** impalpable.
- **Auscultation:** quiet heart sounds.
- **Lungs:** dullness and bronchial breathing at the left base, due to lung compression by the distended pericardial sac.

Infective endocarditis

- **General signs:** fever; weight loss; pallor (anaemia).
- **Hands:** splinter haemorrhages; clubbing (within six weeks of onset); Osler's nodes (rare); Janeway lesions (very rare).
- **Arms:** evidence of intravenous drug use (Figure 3.35)—right (and left) heart endocarditis can result from this.
- **Eyes:** pale conjunctivae (anaemia); retinal or conjunctival haemorrhages—Roth's spots[cc] are fundal vasculitic lesions with a yellow centre surrounded by a red ring (Figure 3.36).
- **Heart**—signs of *underlying heart disease*: (i) acquired (mitral regurgitation, mitral stenosis, aortic stenosis, aortic regurgitation); (ii) congenital (patent ductus arteriosus, ventricular septal defect, coarctation of the aorta); (iii) prosthetic valves.

- **Abdomen:** splenomegaly.
- **Peripheral evidence of embolisation** to limbs or central nervous system.
- **Urinalysis:** haematuria (a fresh urine specimen will then show dysmorphic red cells and red cell casts on microscopy).

Systemic hypertension

It is important to have in mind a method for the examination of a patient with systemic hypertension. The examination aims to measure the blood pressure level, determine if there is an underlying cause present, and assess the severity as determined by signs of end-organ damage. It is a common clinical problem.

On general inspection the signs of the rare causes of secondary hypertension must be sought: for example, Cushing's syndrome,[dd] acromegaly, polycythaemia (page 209) or chronic renal failure.

Take the blood pressure, with the patient lying and standing, using an appropriately sized cuff (page 40). A rise in diastolic pressure on standing occurs typically in essential hypertension; a fall on standing may suggest a secondary cause, but is usually an effect of antihypertensive medications. Palpate for radiofemoral delay, and check the blood pressure in the legs if coarctation of the aorta is suspected or if severe hypertension is discovered before 30 years of age.

Next examine the fundi for Keith-Wagener retinal changes of hypertension (Figures 3.37 and 3.38) which can be classified from grades 1 to 4: **grade 1**—

[cc] Moritz von Roth (1839–1914), Swiss physician and pathologist, described these changes in 1872.

[dd] Harvey Cushing (1869–1939), Professor of Surgery, Harvard University, and 'founder of neurosurgery'. Friend of Osler and prize-winning writer of Osler's biography in 1925.

Figure 3.37 Hypertensive retinopathy grade 3
Note flame-shaped haemorrhages and cottonwool spots.

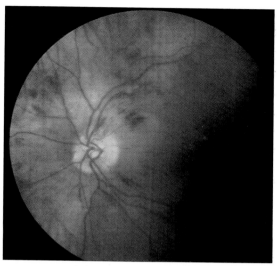

Figure 3.38 Hypertensive retinopathy grade 4
Note AV nipping, silver wiring and papilloedema.

'silver wiring' of the arteries only (sclerosis of the vessel wall reduces its transparency so that the central light streak becomes broader and shinier); **grade 2**—grade 1 plus arteriovenous nipping or nicking (indentation or deflection of the veins where they are crossed by the arteries); **grade 3**—grade 2 plus haemorrhages (flame-shaped) and exudates (soft—cottonwool spots due to ischaemia, or hard—lipid residues from leaking vessels); **grade 4**—grade 3 plus papilloedema (page 298). It is important to describe the changes present rather than just give a grade.

Now examine the rest of the cardiovascular system for signs of left ventricular failure secondary to hypertension, and for coarctation of the aorta. A fourth heart sound is frequently detectable if the blood pressure is greater than 180/110 mmHg.

Then go to the abdomen to palpate for renal or adrenal masses (possible causes), and for the presence of an abdominal aortic aneurysm (a possible complication). Auscultate for a renal bruit (page 187) due to renal artery stenosis.[35] Remember that most left sided abdominal bruits arise from the splenic artery and are of no significance. A bruit is less likely to be significant if it is short, soft and midsystolic. A loud systolic–diastolic bruit that is prominent in the epigastrium is more likely to be associated with renal artery stenosis.

Examine the central nervous system for signs of previous cerebrovascular accidents, and palpate and auscultate the carotid arteries for bruits (stenosis may be a manifestation of vascular disease, and may be associated with renal artery stenosis). Urinalysis should also be performed to look for evidence of renal disease (page 189).

Causes of systemic hypertension

Hypertension may be essential or idiopathic (more than 95% of cases), or secondary (less than 5%). Immoderate alcohol and salt consumption and obesity are associated with hypertension. Obstructive sleep apnoea is also an association.

Secondary causes include: (i) renal disease—renal artery stenosis, chronic pyelonephritis, analgesic nephropathy, connective tissue disease, glomerulonephritis, polycystic disease, diabetic nephropathy, reflux nephropathy; (ii) endocrine disorders—Cushing's syndrome, Conn's syndrome (primary aldosteronism), phaeochromocytoma, acromegaly, thyrotoxicosis, hypothyroidism, hyperparathyroidism; (iii) coarctation of the aorta; and (iv) other, such as the contraceptive pill, polycythaemia rubra vera, toxaemia of pregnancy, neurogenic causes (increased intracranial pressure, lead poisoning, acute porphyria), or hypercalcaemia.

Complications of hypertension

These include left ventricular failure, cerebrovascular ischaemic events (strokes), renal failure, and eye disease (blindness). Hypertension is also a risk factor for ischaemic heart disease and peripheral vascular disease including abdominal aortic aneurysm and arterial dissections.

Malignant (accelerated) hypertension

This can be defined as the presence of flame-shaped haemorrhages, cottonwool spots and/or papilloedema (≥grade 3 Keith-Wagener retinal changes) as a result of severe hypertension. These patients need admission to hospital for urgent treatment.

Pulmonary hypertension

Systolic pulmonary artery pressures higher than 30 mmHg are abnormal and constitute pulmonary hypertension. Symptoms of pulmonary hypertension do not usually occur until the pressures are about twice normal (i.e. >50 mmHg). Exertional dyspnoea and fatigue are then common and chest pain probably due to right ventricular ischaemia occurs in up to 50% of patients. It is important to know what signs to look for in a patient who may have pulmonary hypertension.

- **General signs** (usually only in patients with severe hypertension): tachypnoea; peripheral cyanosis and cold extremities, due to low cardiac output; hoarseness (very rare, due to pulmonary artery compression of the left recurrent laryngeal nerve).
- **The pulse:** usually of small volume, due to the low cardiac output (only in severe disease).
- **The JVP:** prominent *a* wave, due to forceful right atrial contraction.
- **Apex beat/praecordium:** right ventricular heave; palpable P2.
- **Auscultation:** systolic ejection click, due to dilatation of the pulmonary artery; loud P2, due to forceful valve closure because of high pulmonary artery pressures; S4; pulmonary ejection murmur, due to dilatation of the pulmonary artery resulting in turbulent blood flow; murmur of pulmonary regurgitation if dilatation of the pulmonary artery occurs.
- **Signs of right ventricular failure** (late: termed *cor pulmonale*).

Causes of pulmonary hypertension

Pulmonary hypertension may be primary (idiopathic) or secondary.

Secondary causes include: (i) pulmonary emboli—e.g. blood clots, tumour particles, fat globules; (ii) lung disease—chronic obstructive pulmonary disease (page 115), obstructive sleep apnoea, interstitial lung disease (e.g. pulmonary fibrosis); (iii) left ventricular failure resulting in back-pressure into the pulmonary circulation; (iv) congenital heart disease causing a left-to-right shunt—atrial septal defect, ventricular septal defect, patent ductus arteriosus; and (v) severe kyphoscoliosis.

Innocent murmurs

The detection of a systolic murmur on routine examination is a common problem. It can cause considerable alarm to both the patient and the examining clinician. These murmurs in asymptomatic people are often the result of normal turbulence within the heart and great vessels. When no structural abnormality of the heart or great vessels is present these are called *innocent, functional* or *organic* murmurs. They probably arise from vibrations within the aortic arch near the origins of the head and neck vessels or from the right ventricular outflow tract. They are more common in children and young adults.

Innocent murmurs are always systolic. (A venous hum, which is not really a murmur, has both systolic and diastolic components.) They are usually soft and ejection-systolic in character. Those arising from the aortic arch may radiate to the carotids and be heard in the neck. Those arising from the right ventricular outflow tract are loudest in the pulmonary area and may have a scratchy quality.

These outflow tract murmurs must be distinguished from the pulmonary flow murmur of an atrial septal defect (page 79). Therefore it is important to listen carefully for wide or fixed splitting of the second heart sound before pronouncing a murmur innocent.

Valve diseases of the left heart

Mitral stenosis

The normal area of the mitral valve is 4 to 6 cm². Reduction of the valve area to half normal or less causes significant obstruction to left ventricular filling, and blood will flow from the left atrium to the left ventricle only if the left atrial pressure is raised.

- **Symptoms:** dyspnoea, orthopnoea, paroxysmal nocturnal dyspnoea (increased left atrial pressure); haemoptysis (ruptured bronchial veins); ascites, oedema, fatigue (pulmonary hypertension).
- **General signs:** tachypnoea; 'mitral facies'; peripheral cyanosis (severe mitral stenosis).
- **Pulse and blood pressure:** normal or reduced in volume, due to a reduced cardiac output; atrial fibrillation may be present because of left atrial enlargement.
- **The JVP:** normal; prominent *a* wave if pulmonary hypertension is present; loss of the *a* wave if the patient is in atrial fibrillation.
- **Palpation:** tapping quality of the apex beat (palpable S1); right ventricular heave and palpable P2 if pulmonary hypertension is present; diastolic thrill rarely (lay patient on the left side).

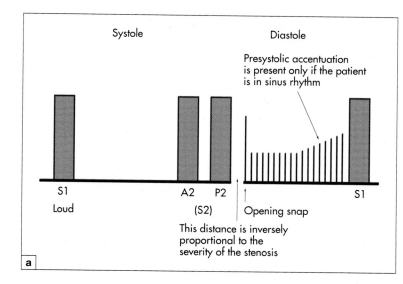

Systole   Diastole

Presystolic accentuation
is present only if the patient
is in sinus rhythm

S1   A2   P2   S1
Loud   (S2)

Opening snap

This distance is inversely
proportional to the
severity of the stenosis

a

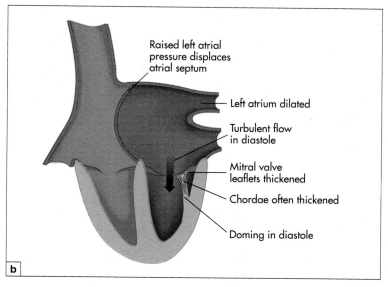

Raised left atrial
pressure displaces
atrial septum

Left atrium dilated

Turbulent flow
in diastole

Mitral valve
leaflets thickened

Chordae often thickened

Doming in diastole

b

Figure 3.39 Mitral stenosis, at the apex: (a) murmur; (b) anatomy

■ **Auscultation** (Figure 3.39 a & b): loud S1 (valve cusps widely apart at the onset of systole)—this also indicates that the valve cusps remain mobile; loud P2 if pulmonary hypertension is present; opening snap (high left atrial pressure forces the valve cusps apart, but the valve cone is halted abruptly); low-pitched rumbling diastolic murmur (best heard with the bell of the stethoscope with the patient in the left lateral position, and quite different in quality and timing from the murmur of aortic regurgitation); a late diastolic accentuation of the diastolic murmur may occur if the patient is in sinus rhythm, but is usually absent if atrial fibrillation has supervened—this is best heard in the left lateral position; exercise accentuates the murmur (ask the patient to sit up and down quickly in bed several times).

■ **Signs indicating severe mitral stenosis** (valve area less than 1 cm²): small pulse pressure; soft first heart sound (immobile valve cusps); early opening snap (due to increased left atrial pressure); long diastolic murmur (persists as long as there is a gradient); diastolic thrill at the apex; signs of pulmonary hypertension.

■ **Causes of mitral stenosis:** (i) rheumatic (following acute rheumatic fever); (ii) congenital parachute valve (all chordae insert into one papillary muscle—rare).

Figure 3.40 Mitral regurgitation: (a) murmur, at the apex; (b) anatomy

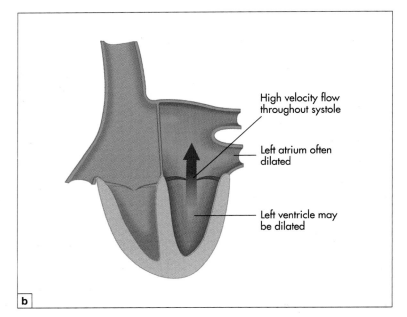

Mitral regurgitation (chronic)

A regurgitant mitral valve allows part of the left ventricular stroke volume to regurgitate into the left atrium, imposing a volume load on both the left atrium and the left ventricle.

- **Symptoms:** dyspnoea (increased left atrial pressure); fatigue (decreased cardiac output).
- **General signs:** tachypnoea.
- **Pulse:** normal, or sharp upstroke due to rapid left ventricular decompression; atrial fibrillation is relatively common.
- **Palpation:** the apex beat is displaced, diffuse and hyperdynamic; a pansystolic thrill is occasionally present at the apex; a parasternal impulse (due to left atrial enlargement behind the right ventricle—the left atrium is often larger in mitral regurgitation than in mitral stenosis and can be enormous).
- **Auscultation** (Figure 3.40 a & b): soft or absent S1 (by the end of diastole, atrial and ventricular pressures have equalised and the valve cusps have drifted back together); left ventricular S3, which is due to rapid left ventricular filling in early diastole and, when soft, does not imply severe regurgitation; pansystolic murmur maximal at the apex and usually radiating towards the axilla.
- **Signs indicating severe chronic mitral regurgitation:** small volume pulse; enlarged left ventricle; loud S3; soft S1; A2 is early, because rapid left ventricular decompression into the left atrium causes

> **GOOD SIGNS GUIDE 3.6**
> **Moderate to severe mitral regurgitation**
>
> | | Positive LR | Negative LR |
> |---|---|---|
> | Characteristic murmur grade 3 or more | 4.4 | 0.2 |
> | S3 (third heart sound) | 1.8 | 0.8 |
>
> From McGee S, *Evidence-based physical diagnosis*, Saunders, 2001.

the aortic valve to close early; early diastolic rumble; signs of pulmonary hypertension; signs of left ventricular failure (*Good signs guide 3.6*).

- **Causes of chronic mitral regurgitation:** (i) mitral valve prolapse; (ii) 'degenerative'—associated with ageing; (iii) rheumatic; (iv) papillary muscle dysfunction, due to left ventricular failure or ischaemia; (v) cardiomyopathy—hypertrophic, dilated or restrictive cardiomyopathy; (vi) connective tissue disease—e.g. Marfan's syndrome, rheumatoid arthritis, ankylosing spondylitis; (vii) congenital (e.g. atrioventricular canal defect).

Acute mitral regurgitation

In this case patients can present with pulmonary oedema and cardiovascular collapse. There is usually a systolic apical thrill and a loud apical systolic murmur present (it is short because atrial pressure is increased). With anterior leaflet chordae rupture the murmur radiates to the axilla and back; with posterior leaflet rupture the murmur radiates to the cardiac base and carotids.

- **Causes:** (i) myocardial infarction (dysfunction or rupture of papillary muscles); (ii) infective endocarditis; (iii) trauma or surgery; (iv) spontaneous rupture of a myxomatous chord (sometimes during exercise).

Mitral valve prolapse (systolic-click murmur syndrome)

This syndrome can cause a systolic murmur or click or both at the apex. The presence of the murmur indicates that there is some mitral regurgitation present.

- **Auscultation** (Figure 3.41 a & b): systolic click or clicks at a variable time (usually midsystolic) may be the only abnormality audible, but a click is not always audible; systolic murmur—high-pitched late systolic murmur, commencing with the click and extending throughout the rest of systole.
- **Dynamic auscultation:** murmur and click occur earlier and may become louder with the Val-

salva manoeuvre and with standing, but both occur later and may become softer with squatting and isometric exercise.

- **Causes of mitral valve prolapse:** (i) myxomatous degeneration of the mitral valve tissue—it is very common, especially in women, and the severity may increase with age, particularly in men, so that significant mitral regurgitation may supervene; (ii) may be associated with atrial septal defect (secundum), hypertrophic cardiomyopathy, or Marfan's syndrome.

Aortic stenosis

The normal area of the aortic valve is more than 2 cm². Significant narrowing of this valve restricts left ventricular outflow and imposes a pressure load on the left ventricle.

- **Symptoms:** exertional chest pain (50% do not have coronary artery disease), exertional dyspnoea and exertional syncope.
- **General signs:** usually there is nothing remarkable about the general appearance.
- **The pulse:** there may be a plateau or anacrotic pulse, or the pulse may be late peaking (tardus) and of small volume (parvus).[36]
- **Palpation:** the apex beat is hyperdynamic and may be slightly displaced; systolic thrill at the base of the heart (aortic area).
- **Auscultation** (Figure 3.42 a & b): a narrowly split or reversed S2 because of delayed left ventricular ejection; a harsh midsystolic ejection murmur, maximal over the aortic area and

> **GOOD SIGNS GUIDE 3.7**
> **Severe aortic stenosis**
>
> | Sign | Positive LR | Negative LR |
> |---|---|---|
> | Delayed carotid upstroke | 3.7 | 0.4 |
> | Diminished carotid pulse on palpation | 2.3 | 0.3 |
> | Apical impulse sustained (pressure loaded) | 4.1 | 0.3 |
> | Absent or decreased A2 | 3.6 | 0.4 |
> | S4 gallop | NS | NS |
> | Late peaking murmur | 4.4 | 0.2 |
> | Long murmur | 3.9 | 0.2 |
> | Murmur radiates to the neck | 1.4 | 0.1 |
>
> NS = not significant.
> From McGee S, *Evidence-based physical diagnosis*, Saunders, 2001.

Figure 3.41 Mitral valve prolapse (MVP): (a) murmur, at the apex; (b) anatomy

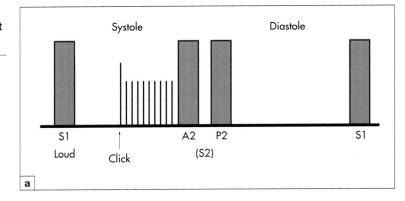

Systole Diastole

S1
Loud
Click
A2 P2
(S2)
S1

a

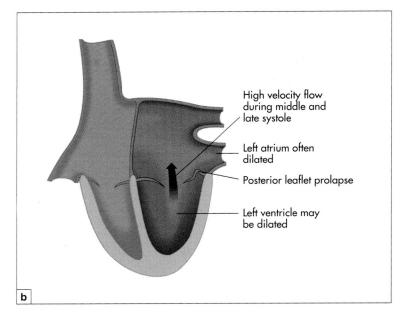

High velocity flow during middle and late systole

Left atrium often dilated

Posterior leaflet prolapse

Left ventricle may be dilated

b

extending into the carotid arteries (Fig 3.43), is characteristic. However, it may be heard widely over the praecordium and extend to the apex. The murmur is loudest with the patient sitting up and in full expiration; associated aortic regurgitation is common; in congenital aortic stenosis where the valve cusps remain mobile and the dome of the valve comes to a sudden halt, an ejection click may precede the murmur—the ejection click is absent if the valve is calcified or if the stenosis is not at the valve level but above or below it.

■ **Signs indicating severe aortic stenosis** (*Good signs guide 3.7*, page 69) (valve area less than 1 cm², or valve gradient greater than 50 mmHg): plateau pulse, carotid pulse reduced in force;

thrill in the aortic area; length of the murmur and lateness of the peak of the systolic murmur, soft or absent A2; left ventricular failure (very late sign); pressure loaded apex beat. These signs are not reliable for distinguishing moderate and severe disease. It is important to remember that the signs of severity of aortic stenosis are less reliable in the elderly.[37]

■ **Causes of aortic stenosis:** (i) degenerative calcific aortic stenosis, particularly in elderly patients; (ii) calcific in younger patients, usually on a congenital bicuspid valve; (iii) rheumatic.

■ **Other types of aortic outflow obstruction are also possible:** (i) supravalvular obstruction; here there is narrowing of the ascending aorta or a fibrous diaphragm just above the aortic

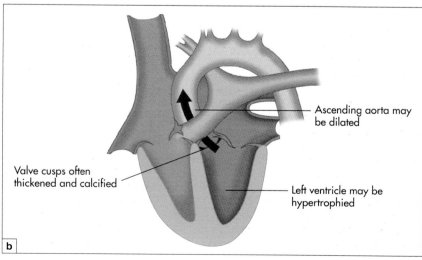

Figure 3.42 Aortic stenosis (AS): (a) murmur, at the aortic area; (b) anatomy

Figure 3.43 Aortic stenosis: listening over the carotid

valve—this is rare and may be associated with a characteristic facies (a broad forehead, widely set eyes and a pointed chin); there is a loud A2 and often a thrill in the area of the sternal notch; (ii) subvalvular obstruction; here there is a membranous diaphragm or fibrous ridge just below the aortic valve; aortic regurgitation is associated and is due to a jet lesion affecting the coronary cusp of the valve; (iii) dynamic left ventricular outflow tract obstruction may occur in hypertrophic cardiomyopathy; here there may be a double apical impulse. Atrial contraction into a stiff left ventricle may be palpable before the left ventricular impulse (only in the presence of sinus rhythm, of course).

Aortic sclerosis presents in the elderly; there are none of the peripheral signs of aortic stenosis. The diagnosis implies the absence of a gradient across the aortic valve despite some thickening and a murmur.

Aortic regurgitation

The incompetent aortic valve allows regurgitation of blood from the aorta to the left ventricle during diastole for as long as the aortic diastolic pressure exceeds the left ventricular diastolic pressure.[38]

- **Symptoms:** occur in the late stages of disease and include exertional dyspnoea, fatigue, palpitations (hyperdynamic circulation) and exertional angina.

- **General signs:** Marfan's syndrome, ankylosing spondylitis or one of the other seronegative arthropathies (page 243) or, rarely, Argyll Robertson pupils (page 301) may be obvious.
- **Pulse and blood pressure:** the pulse is characteristically collapsing, a 'water hammer'[ee] pulse (Table 3.13); there may be a wide pulse pressure. A *bisferiens* pulse (from the Latin, to beat twice) may be a sign of severe aortic regurgitation or of combined aortic regurgitation and aortic stenosis. It is best assessed at the carotid artery, where two beats can be felt in each cardiac cycle. It is probably caused by a Venturi effect in the aorta related to rapid ejection of blood and brief indrawing of the aortic wall, leading to a diminution of the pulse followed by a rebound increase. It was a particular favourite of Galen's.[ff]
- **Neck:** prominent carotid pulsations (Corrigan's sign).
- **Palpation:** the apex beat is characteristically displaced and hyperkinetic. A diastolic thrill may be felt at the left sternal edge when the patient sits up and breathes out.
- **Auscultation** (Figure 3.44 a & b): A2 (the aortic component of the second heart sound) may be soft; a decrescendo high-pitched diastolic murmur beginning immediately after the second heart sound and extending for a variable time into diastole—it is loudest at the third and fourth left intercostal spaces; a systolic ejection murmur is usually present (due to associated aortic stenosis or to torrential flow across a normal diameter aortic valve). Aortic stenosis is distinguished from an aortic flow murmur by the presence of the peripheral signs of significant aortic stenosis, such as a plateau pulse. An *Austin Flint murmur*[gg] should also be listened for. This is a low-pitched rumbling mid-diastolic and

---

ee This Victorian children's toy consisted of a sealed tube half-filled with fluid, with the other half being a vacuum. Inversion of the tube caused the fluid to fall rapidly without air resistance and strike the other end with a noise like a hammer blow. It is not easy to imagine a child today being entertained by this for very long.

ff Claudius Galen (130–200 AD). Born in Pergamum, he worked as a gladiator's surgeon but moved to Rome in 164 AD to become the city's most famous physician. He was the first to describe the cranial nerves. He never performed dissection on human bodies, but his often erroneous anatomical teachings were regarded as infallible for 15 centuries.

gg Austin Flint (1812–1886), New York physician and Professor of Medicine at the New Orleans Medical School, described this murmur in 1862. Author of *The principles and practice of medicine*. He was very much opposed to the naming of signs after people.

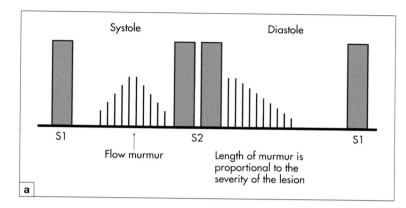

Systole   Diastole

S1   S2   S1

↑
Flow murmur   Length of murmur is
               proportional to the
               severity of the lesion

a

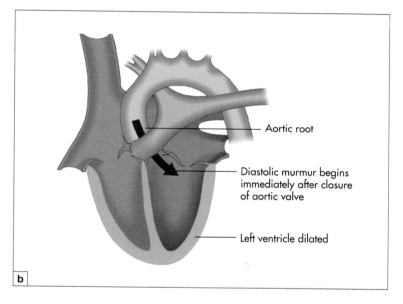

— Aortic root

— Diastolic murmur begins
  immediately after closure
  of aortic valve

— Left ventricle dilated

b

Figure 3.44 Aortic regurgitation: (a) murmur, at the left sternal edge; (b) anatomy

presystolic murmur audible at the apex (the regurgitant jet from the aortic valve causes the anterior mitral valve leaflet to shudder). It can be distinguished from mitral stenosis because S1 (the first heart sound) is not loud and there is no opening snap. Many other signs have been described, but they are interesting rather than helpful (Table 3.13; *Good signs guide 3.8*).

- **Signs indicating severe chronic aortic regurgitation:** collapsing pulse; wide pulse pressure (systolic pressure 80 mmHg more than the diastolic); long decrescendo diastolic murmur; left ventricular S3 (third heart sound); soft A2; Austin Flint murmur; signs of left ventricular failure.
- **Causes of aortic regurgitation:** disease may affect the valvular area or aortic root, and may be acute or chronic.

- **Causes of chronic aortic regurgitation:** (i) valvular—rheumatic (rarely the only murmur in this case), congenital (e.g. bicuspid valve; ventricular septal defect—an associated prolapse of the aortic cusp is not uncommon), seronegative arthropathy, especially ankylosing spondylitis; (ii) aortic root dilatation (murmur may be maximal at the right sternal border)—Marfan's syndrome, aortitis (e.g. seronegative arthropathies, rheumatoid arthritis, tertiary syphilis), dissecting aneurysm.
- **Causes of acute aortic regurgitation** (*Note:* murmur may be soft because of increased left ventricular end-diastolic pressure): (i) valvular—infective endocarditis; (ii) aortic root—Marfan's syndrome, dissecting aneurysm of the aortic root.

GOOD SIGNS GUIDE 3.8 Severity of aortic regurgitation		
Finding	**Positive LR**	**Negative LR**
Typical murmur		
Mild AR or worse	9.9	0.3
Moderate to severe AR	4.3	0.1
Murmur grade 3 or more (moderate to severe AR)	8.2	0.6
Pulse pressure		
>80 mmHg	10.9	–
Other signs— moderate to severe AR		
Sustained or displaced apex	2.4	0.1
Duroziez's sign, pistol shot femorals, water hammer pulse	NS	0.7

NS = not significant.

From McGee S, *Evidence-based physical diagnosis*, Saunders, 2001.

Valve diseases of the right heart

Tricuspid stenosis

This is very rare.

- **The JVP**: raised; giant *a* waves with a slow *y* descent may be seen.
- **Auscultation**: a diastolic murmur audible at the left sternal edge, accentuated by inspiration, very similar to the murmur of mitral stenosis except for the site of maximal intensity and the effect of respiration (louder on inspiration); tricuspid regurgitation and mitral stenosis are often present as well; no signs of pulmonary hypertension.
- **Abdomen**: presystolic pulsation of the liver, caused by forceful atrial systole.
- **Cause of tricuspid stenosis**: rheumatic heart disease.

Table 3.13 Eponymous signs of aortic regurgitation[39]

1 Quincke's sign: capillary pulsation in the nail beds—it is of no value, as this sign occurs normally.
2 Corrigan's sign: prominent carotid pulsations; the Corrigan water hammer pulse sign is present when the patient lies supine with the arms beside the body, the radial pulse is compressed until it disappears, the arm is then lifted perpendicular to the body, the pulse then becomes palpable again even though the same pressure has been maintained on the radial artery.
3 De Musset's sign: head nodding in time with the heart beat.
4 Hill's sign: increased blood pressure (>20 mmHg) in the legs compared with the arms.
5 Mueller's sign: pulsation of the uvula in time with the heart beat.
6 Duroziez's sign: systolic and diastolic murmurs over the femoral artery on gradual compression of the vessel.
7 Traube's sign: a double sound heard over the femoral artery on compressing the vessel distally; this is *not* a 'pistol shot' sound that may be heard over the femoral artery with very severe aortic regurgitation.
8 Mayne's sign: a decrease in diastolic pressure of 15 mmHg when the arm is held above the head compared with that when the arm is at the level of the heart.
9 Rosenbach's liver pulsation sign: liver pulsates in time with the heart beat (in the absence of tricuspid regurgitation).
10 Austin Flint murmur: short rumbling diastolic murmur, thought by Flint to be due to functional mitral stenosis caused by impinging of the AR jet on the anterior mitral valve leaflet.
11 Becker's sign: accentuated retinal artery pulsations.
12 Gerhard's sign: pulsatile spleen.

Note: These signs are amusing, but not often helpful. The signs were named after the following people: Heinrich Quincke (1842–1922), German neurologist; Dominic Corrigan (1802–80), Edinburgh graduate who worked in Dublin and is credited with discovering aortic regurgitation; Alfred de Musset, 19th century French poet who suffered from aortic regurgitation (the sign was noticed by his brother, a physician); Sir Leonard Hill (1866–1952), English physiologist who also described the physiology of the cerebral circulation; Frederick Von Mueller (1858–1941), German physician who also noted an increase in metabolism in exophthalmic goitre; Paul Duroziez (1826–97), French physician; Ludwig Traube (1818–76), Hungarian physician who worked in Germany.

Tricuspid regurgitation (Figure 3.45)

- **The JVP:** large *v* waves; the JVP is elevated if right ventricular failure has occurred.
- **Palpation:** right ventricular heave.
- **Auscultation:** there may be a pansystolic murmur maximal at the lower end of the sternum that increases on inspiration, but the diagnosis can be made on the basis of the peripheral signs alone.
- **Abdomen:** a pulsatile, large and tender liver is usually present and may cause the right nipple to dance in time with the heart beat; ascites, oedema and pleural effusions may also be present.
- **Legs:** dilated, pulsatile veins.
- **Causes of tricuspid regurgitation:**[hh] (i) functional (no disease of the valve leaflets)—right ventricular failure; (ii) rheumatic—only very rarely does rheumatic tricuspid regurgitation occur alone, usually mitral valve disease is also present; (iii) infective endocarditis (right-sided endocarditis in intravenous drug addicts); (iv) tricuspid valve prolapse; (v) right ventricular papillary muscle infarction; (vi) trauma (usually caused by a steering wheel injury to the sternum): (vii) congenital—Ebstein's anomaly.[ii]

Pulmonary stenosis (in adults)

(Figure 3.46)

- **General signs:** peripheral cyanosis, due to a low cardiac output, but only in severe cases.
- **Pulse:** normal or reduced if cardiac output is low.
- **The JVP:** giant *a* waves because of right atrial hypertrophy; the JVP may be elevated.
- **Palpation:** right ventricular heave; thrill over the pulmonary area.
- **Auscultation:** the murmur may be preceded by an ejection click; a harsh and usually loud ejection systolic murmur, heard best in the pulmonary area and with inspiration, is typically present; right ventricular S4 may be present (due to right atrial hypertrophy). It is not well heard over the carotid arteries.
- **Abdomen:** presystolic pulsation of the liver may be present.

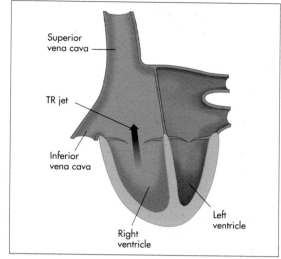

Figure 3.45 Tricuspid regurgitation (TR): anatomy

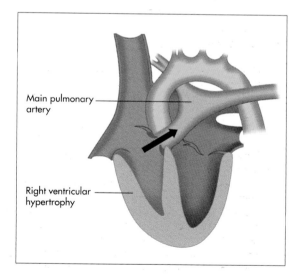

Figure 3.46 Valvar pulmonary stenosis: anatomy

- **Signs of severe pulmonary stenosis:** an ejection systolic murmur peaking late in systole; absence of an ejection click (also absent when the pulmonary stenosis is infundibular—i.e. below the valve level); presence of S4; signs of right ventricular failure.
- **Causes of pulmonary stenosis:** (i) congenital; (ii) carcinoid syndrome (rare).

[hh] Doppler echocardiography has shown that trivial tricuspid regurgitation is very common and is then considered physiological. Christian Doppler (1803–1853) was an Austrian physicist and mathematician.

[ii] Wilhelm Ebstein (1836–1912), Professor of Medicine at Göttingen in Germany, who invented and developed palpation.

Pulmonary regurgitation

This is an uncommon pathological condition; trivial pulmonary regurgitation is often found at echocardiography and is considered physiological.

- **Auscultation:** a decrescendo diastolic murmur which is high pitched and audible at the left sternal edge is characteristic—this typically but not always increases on inspiration (unlike the murmur of aortic regurgitation). It is called the Graham Steell murmur[jj] when it occurs secondary to pulmonary artery dilatation caused by pulmonary hypertension. (*Note:* If there are no signs of pulmonary hypertension a decrescendo diastolic murmur at the left sternal edge is more likely to be due to aortic regurgitation than to pulmonary regurgitation.)
- **Causes of pulmonary regurgitation:** (i) pulmonary hypertension; (ii) infective endocarditis; (iii) following balloon valvotomy for pulmonary stenosis or surgery for pulmonary atresia; (iv) congenital absence of the pulmonary valve.

Prosthetic heart valves

The physical signs with common types of valves are presented in Table 3.14. Mechanical prosthetic valves should have a crisp sound. Muffling of the mechanical sounds may be a sign of thrombotic obstruction of the valve or chronic tissue ingrowth (pannus). After replacement of the aortic valve the presence of audible aortic regurgitation may indicate a *paravalvular leak* often through a stitching hole in the valve sewing ring. As tissue valves age and degenerate they may develop signs of regurgitation or stenosis, or both.

Cardiomyopathy

Hypertrophic cardiomyopathy

(Figure 3.47)

This is abnormal hypertrophy of the muscle in the left ventricular or right ventricular outflow tract, or both. It can obstruct outflow from the left ventricle late in systole when the hypertrophied area contracts. Systolic displacement of the mitral valve apparatus into the left ventricular outflow tract also occurs, causing mitral regurgitation and contributing to the outflow obstruction. Although the outflow tract is narrowed by the hypertrophied septum, the major contribution to the dynamic increase in obstruction comes from the systolic movement of the mitral valve. Variants of

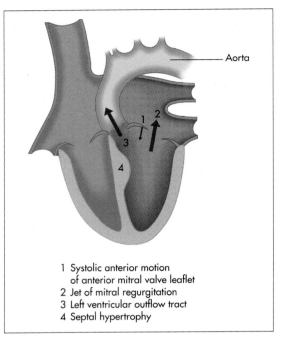

1 Systolic anterior motion of anterior mitral valve leaflet
2 Jet of mitral regurgitation
3 Left ventricular outflow tract
4 Septal hypertrophy

Figure 3.47 Hypertrophic cardiomyopathy: anatomy

hypertrophic cardiomyopathy may involve the mid-ventricle or apex with varying degrees of obstruction.

- **Symptoms:** dyspnoea (increased left ventricular end-diastolic pressure due to abnormal diastolic compliance), angina, syncope or sudden death (secondary to ventricular fibrillation or a sudden increase in outflow obstruction).
- **Pulse:** sharp, rising and jerky. Rapid ejection by the hypertrophied ventricle early in systole is followed by obstruction caused by the displacement of the mitral valve into the outflow tract. This is quite different from the pulse of aortic stenosis.
- **The JVP:** there is usually a prominent *a* wave, due to forceful atrial contraction against a non-compliant right ventricle.
- **Palpation:** double or triple apical impulse, due to presystolic expansion of the ventricle caused by atrial contraction.
- **Auscultation:** late systolic murmur at the lower left sternal edge and apex (due to the obstruction) and a pansystolic murmur at the apex (due to mitral regurgitation); S4.
- **Dynamic manoeuvres:** the outflow murmur is increased by the Valsalva manoeuvre, by standing and by isotonic exercise; it is decreased by squatting and isometric exercise.

[jj] Graham Steell (1851–1942), Manchester physician, described this murmur in 1888.

Table 3.14 Prosthetic heart valves: physical signs

Type	Mitral	Aortic
Ball valve (e.g. Starr-Edwards)*	Sharp mitral opening sound after S2, sharp closing sound at S1 Systolic ejection murmur, no diastolic murmur	Sharp aortic opening sound Systolic ejection murmur (harsh), no diastolic murmur unless a paravalvular leak has occurred, early diastolic murmur indicates AR usually due to a paravalvular leak**
Disc valve (e.g. Bjork-Shiley) †	Sharp closing sound at S1, soft systolic ejection murmur and diastolic rumble (diastolic murmur occasionally)	Sharp closing sound at S2, systolic ejection murmur (soft)
Porcine or bovine pericardial valve‡	Usually sound normal, diastolic rumble mitral opening sound occasionally	Closing sound usually heard, systolic ejection murmur (soft), no diastolic murmur
Bileaflet valve (e.g. St Jude)	—	Aortic valve opening and closing sounds common, soft systolic ejection murmur common
Homograft (human) valve	Normal heart sounds, occasional soft systolic murmur; early diastolic murmur if AR has occurred	

* Modern mechanical valves (e.g. St Jude) make softer opening and closing sounds than older valves. The Starr-Edwards valve is often very noisy and sounds like a ball rattling around in a cage (which is what it is).

† Severe prosthetic dysfunction causes absence of the opening or closing sounds. Ball and cage valves cause more haemolysis than other types and make the most noise, while disc valves are more thrombogenic.

** An aortic regurgitation murmur present after aortic valve replacement suggests regurgitation of the valve ring. It is not uncommon. Less often a mitral regurgitation murmur suggests the same problem with a prosthetic mitral valve.

‡ Bioprosthetic obstruction or patient–prosthetic mismatch cause diastolic rumbling. These valves are used less often in the mitral position because they often have a very limited life there. A degenerated bioprosthetic valve may cause murmurs of regurgitation or stenosis or both.

AR = aortic regurgitation.

(Modified from Smith ND, Raizada V, Abrams J. Auscultation of the normally functioning prosthetic valve. *Ann Intern Med* 1981; 95:594.)

■ **Causes of hypertrophic cardiomyopathy:** (i) autosomal dominant (sarcomeric heavy chain or troponin gene mutation) with variable expressivity; (ii) idiopathic; (iii) Friedreich's ataxia[kk] (page 359).

Dilated cardiomyopathy

This heart muscle abnormality results in a global reduction in cardiac function. Coronary artery disease is excluded as a cause by definition. (Ischaemic cardiomyopathy is a term often used to describe severe myocardial dysfunction secondary to recurrent ischaemic events.) The signs are those of congestive cardiac failure, including those of mitral and tricuspid regurgitation. The heart sounds themselves may be very quiet. Ventricular arrhythmias are common. It is a common indication for cardiac transplantation.

■ **Causes of dilated cardiomyopathy:** (i) idiopathic and familial; (ii) alcohol; (iii) post-viral; (iv) postpartum; (v) drugs (e.g. doxorubicin); (vi) dystrophia myotonica; (vii) haemochromatosis.

[kk] Nikolaus Friedreich (1825–82), German physician, described this disease in 1863. He succeeded Virchow as Professor of Pathological Anatomy at Wurzburg at the age of 31.

Figure 3.48 Ventricular septal defect (VSD): (a) murmur, at the left sternal edge; (b) anatomy

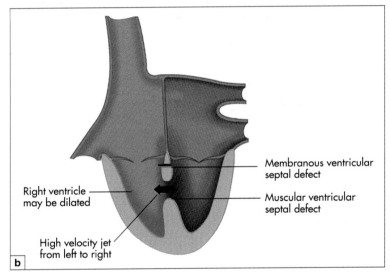

Restrictive cardiomyopathy

This causes similar signs to those caused by constrictive pericarditis (page 63), but Kussmaul's sign is more common and the apex beat is usually easily palpable.

■ **Causes of restrictive cardiomyopathy:** (i) idiopathic; (ii) eosinophilic endomyocardial disease; (iii) endomyocardial fibrosis; (iv) infiltrative disease (e.g. amyloid); (v) granulomas (e.g. sarcoid).

Acyanotic congenital heart disease

Ventricular septal defect

In this condition one or more holes are present in the membranous or muscular ventricular septum.

■ **Palpation:** hyperkinetic displaced apex if the defect is large; and a thrill at the left sternal edge.

■ Auscultation (Figure 3.48 a & b): a harsh pansystolic murmur maximal at, and almost confined to, the lower left sternal edge with a third or fourth heart sound—the murmur is louder on expiration; sometimes a mitral regurgitation murmur is associated. There is often a palpable systolic thrill. The murmur is often louder and harsher when the defect is small.

■ **Causes of ventricular septal defect:** (i) congenital; (ii) acquired—e.g. myocardial infarction involving the septum.

Atrial septal defect

There are two main types: *ostium secundum* (90%), where there is a defect in the part of the septum which does not involve the atrioventricular valves, and *ostium primum*, where the defect does involve the atrioventricular valves.

■ **Palpation:** normal or right ventricular enlargement.

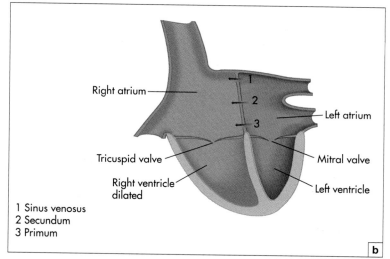

Figure 3.49 Atrial septal defect (ASD): (a) murmur, at the left sternal edge; (b) anatomy

- **Auscultation** (Figure 3.49 a & b): fixed splitting of S2; the defect produces no murmur directly, but increased flow through the right side of the heart can produce a low-pitched diastolic tricuspid flow murmur and more often a pulmonary systolic ejection murmur—these are both louder on inspiration.
- **Signs:** The signs of an ostium primum defect are the same as for an ostium secundum defect, but associated mitral regurgitation, tricuspid regurgitation or a ventricular septal defect may be present. The left ventricular impulse is often impalpable.

Patent ductus arteriosus

(Figure 3.50)

This is a persistent embryonic vessel which connects the pulmonary artery and the aorta. The shunt is from the aorta to the pulmonary artery unless pulmonary hypertension has supervened.

Figure 3.50 Patent ductus arteriosus: anatomy

■ **Pulse and blood pressure:** a collapsing pulse with a sharp upstroke (due to ejection of a large volume of blood into the empty aorta with systole); low diastolic blood pressure (due to rapid decompression of the aorta).

■ **Palpation:** often there is a hyperkinetic apex beat.

■ **Auscultation:** if the shunt is of moderate size a single second heart sound is heard, but if the shunt is of significant size reversed splitting of the second heart sound occurs (due to a delayed A2 because of an increased volume load in the left ventricle); a continuous loud 'machinery' murmur maximal at the first left intercostal space is usually present; flow murmurs through the left side of the heart, including a mitral mid-diastolic murmur, may be heard.

Coarctation of the aorta (Figure 3.51)

This is congenital narrowing of the aorta usually just distal to the origin of the left subclavian artery. It is more common in males. The underlying cause is uncertain but seems related to abnormal placement of tissue involved in the closing of the ductus arteriosus. There is an association with bicuspid aortic valve and Turner's syndrome.

■ **Signs:** the upper body may be better developed than the lower; radiofemoral delay is present, and the femoral pulses are weak; hypertension occurs in the arms but not in the legs; a midsystolic

murmur is usually audible over the praecordium and the back, due to blood flow through collateral chest vessels and across the coarct itself.

Ebstein's anomaly

This is a very rare lesion. The abnormality is a downward displacement of the tricuspid valve apparatus into the right ventricle so that the right atrium becomes very large and consists partly of ventricular muscle, while the right ventricle becomes small. An atrial septal defect is commonly associated. Characteristically, multiple clicks occur due to asynchronous closure of the tricuspid valve. Tricuspid regurgitation is usually present.

Cyanotic congenital heart disease

This is a difficult area. The causes are listed in Table 3.15. The important point to determine is whether or not signs of pulmonary hypertension are present (page 66). Congenital heart disease in which a shunt from the left to the right side of the circulation

Figure 3.51 Coarctation of the aorta: anatomy

Table 3.15 Classification of congenital heart disease
Acyanotic
With left-to-right shunt   Ventricular septal defect   Atrial septal defect   Patent ductus arteriosus
With no shunt   Bicuspid aortic valve, congenital aortic stenosis   Coarctation of aorta   Dextrocardia   Pulmonary stenosis, tricuspid stenosis   Ebstein's anomaly
Cyanotic
Eisenmenger's syndrome (pulmonary hypertension and a right-to-left shunt)   Tetralogy of Fallot   Ebstein's anomaly (if an atrial septal defect and right-to-left shunt are also present)   Truncus arteriosus   Transposition of the great vessels   Tricuspid atresia   Total anomalous pulmonary venous drainage

occurs leads to an increase in pulmonary blood flow. This can cause reactive pulmonary hypertension so that pulmonary pressures eventually exceed systemic pressures. When that happens the systemic to pulmonary (left to right) shunt will reverse. This right-to-left shunt leads to deoxygenated blood being mixed in the systemic circulation, resulting in cyanosis. This is called Eisenmenger's syndrome[ll].

Eisenmenger's syndrome (pulmonary hypertension and a right-to-left shunt)

- **Signs:** central cyanosis; clubbing; polycythaemia; signs of pulmonary hypertension.

It may be possible to decide at what level the shunt occurs by listening to the second heart sound (S2). If there is wide fixed splitting this suggests an atrial septal defect. If a single second heart sound is present, this suggests truncus arteriosus or a ventricular septal defect. A normal or reversed S2 suggests a patent ductus arteriosus.

Tetralogy of Fallot[mm]

There are four features which are due to a single developmental abnormality: (i) ventricular septal defect (VSD); (ii) right ventricular outflow obstruction, which determines the severity of the condition, and can be at the pulmonary valve or infundibular level; (iii) an aorta which overrides the VSD and is responsible for the cyanosis; and (iv) right ventricular hypertrophy secondary to outflow obstruction.

- **Signs:** central cyanosis—this occurs without pulmonary hypertension because venous mixing is possible at the ventricular level, where pressures are balanced. The aorta overrides both ventricles and so receives right and left ventricular blood. Clubbing and polycythaemia are usually present. There may be evidence of right ventricular enlargement—a parasternal impulse at the left sternal edge. A systolic thrill caused by pulmonary valve or right ventricular outflow obstruction may be present. There is no overall cardiomegaly. On auscultation the second heart sound is single and there are no signs of pulmonary hypertension; a pulmonary systolic ejection murmur is present.

[ll] Victor Eisenmenger (1864–1932), German physician. He described this syndrome in 1897.
[mm] Etienne-Louis Fallot (1850–1911), Professor of Hygiene, Marseilles, described this in 1888.

'Grown-up' congenital heart disease

Patients who have been treated for serious congenital cardiac conditions now frequently survive into adult life. Many of the surgical procedures undertaken for these conditions, especially 20 years ago, were palliative rather than curative. The patients present with specific symptoms and signs.

Tetralogy of Fallot

Patients who have had repair of this condition in infancy may present with particular problems. Repair of the right ventricular outflow obstruction and enlargement of the pulmonary valve annulus may leave severe pulmonary regurgitation. This may lead eventually to exertional dyspnoea. The surgery itself has, until recently, required a right ventriculotomy (cutting into the right ventricle). This leaves a scar that can be associated with cardiac rhythm abnormalities in later life. Patients may present with palpitations or syncope.

- **Signs:** may include a median sternotomy scar, a long diastolic murmur of pulmonary regurgitation and signs of right ventricular enlargement (parasternal impulse) and later of tricuspid regurgitation (big *v* waves in the neck and a pulsatile liver).

Transposition of the great arteries

Most adults who have had surgery for this abnormality have had a palliative operation called a Mustard procedure. In this abnormality, the pulmonary artery is connected to the left ventricle and the aorta to the right ventricle. Thus the systemic and pulmonary circulations are in parallel. This is not compatible with life unless some connection between the two circulations is present. Neonates with the condition will have an ASD created soon after birth with a catheter-based balloon (balloon septostomy). This allows mixing of the circulations. Later 'baffles' are created surgically in the atria to direct blood returning from the body into the right atrium across the ASD and into the left atrium, where it is pumped into the pulmonary artery and into the lungs. Blood returning from the lungs into the left atrium is directed across into the right atrium and into the morphological right ventricle and on into the aorta. This means that the morphological right ventricle is working as the systemic ventricle. This arrangement works very well but there are long-term concerns about the ability of the right ventricle to cope with systemic workloads.

- **Symptoms:** symptoms that commonly occur include palpitations caused by supraventricular arrhythmias, dizziness caused by bradycardias and breathlessness related to failure of the systemic ventricle. Occasionally, obstruction of the baffles may occur. The most common problem is with the superior vena caval baffle which leads to facial swelling and flushing.
- **Signs:** include the usual scar, facial flushing and oedema, cyanosis, peripheral oedema from inferior caval baffle obstruction and signs of tricuspid regurgitation. On auscultation there may be a gallop rhythm and the murmurs of mitral and tricuspid regurgitation.

The chest X-ray: a systematic approach

Analysis of the chest X-ray is complementary to the patient's physical examination. It provides much information about the heart and lungs.

The interpretation of the chest X-ray is not easy. It requires knowledge of anatomy and pathology, appreciation of the whole range of normal appearances (Figure 3.52 a & b), and knowledge of the likely X-ray changes occurring with pathological processes. The clinician should feel personally responsible for viewing a patient's radiographs.

Most medical students faced with giving their interpretation of a chest X-ray either opt for a 'spot diagnosis' (usually wrong) or raise their eyes to heaven, hoping for divine inspiration. However, a systematic approach is generally more useful! More is missed by not looking than by not knowing.

Frontal film

Name, date and projection

First, it is important to check the name and date, to be sure that it is the correct patient's film. Checking the left or right marker prevents missing dextrocardia. The film markings will also indicate the projection and patient position. The standard frontal film is taken by a posteroanterior (PA) projection of an erect patient. Anteroposterior and supine films are only second-best. On a supine film there is distension of all the posterior (gravity-dependent) vessels and thus the lung fields appear more plethoric. A small pleural effusion may not be visible if it is lying posteriorly and the heart often appears large on a supine film.

Centring

The medial ends of the clavicles should be equidistant from the midline spinous processes. If the patient is rotated, this will accentuate the hilum that is turned forwards.

Exposure

The quality of the film is important. There should be enough X-ray penetration for the spine to be just seen through the mediastinum, otherwise the film will be too white. With good radiographic technique, the scapulae are projected outside the lung fields.

The film needs to be exposed on full inspiration so that there is no basal crowding of the pulmonary vessels and so that estimation of the cardiothoracic ratio is accurate.

On full inspiration, the diaphragm lies at the level of the tenth or eleventh rib posteriorly or at the level of the sixth costal cartilage anteriorly. The right hemidiaphragm usually lies about 2 cm higher than the left.

Correct orientation

Do not miss dextrocardia—the heart apex will be to the right and the stomach gas to the left. Do not be misled by left or right markers wrongly placed by a radiographer.

Systematic film interpretation

Mediastinum. The trachea should lie in the midline. It may be deviated by a goitre or mediastinal mass. It is normally deviated a little to the left as it passes the aortic knuckle. (The aortic arch becomes wider and unfolded with age because of loss of elasticity.)

The mediastinum, including the trachea, can be deviated by a large pleural effusion, a tension pneumothorax or pulmonary collapse.

Rotation of the patient may make the mediastinum appear distorted.

Hila. The hila are mostly formed by the pulmonary arteries with the upper lobe veins superimposed. The left hilum is higher than the right. The left has a squarish shape whereas the right has a V shape.

A hilum can be more prominent if the patient is rotated. Lymphadenopathy or a large pulmonary artery will cause hilar enlargement.

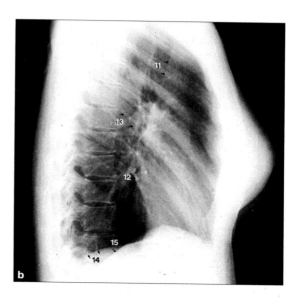

Figure 3.52 Normal chest X-ray

(a) The posteroanterior view shows (1) aortic knuckle; (2) left heart border formed by the lateral border of the left ventricle; (3) left hilum, formed mostly by the left main pulmonary artery and partly by the left upper pulmonary veins; (4) right heart border formed by the right atrium; (5) inferior angle of the scapula; (6) right basal pulmonary artery; (7) medial aspect of the left clavicle; (8) spine of the scapula; (9) right cardiophrenic angle; (10) superimposition of right lateral margins of the superior vena cava and the ascending aorta.

(b) The lateral view shows: (11) anterior border of trachea; (12) pulmonary vein, entering left atrium; (13) oblique fissure; (14) left hemidiaphragm; (15) right hemidiaphragm.

Heart. The heart shape is ovoid with the apex pointing to the left. Characteristically, about two-thirds of the heart projects to the left of the spine.

The right heart border is formed by the outer border of the right atrium, and the left heart border by the left ventricle. The left margin of the right ventricle lies about a thumb's breadth in from the left heart border. (On the surface of the heart, this is marked by the left anterior descending coronary artery.)

The cardiothoracic diameter is a rather approximate way of determining whether the heart is enlarged. If the heart size is more than 50% of the transthoracic diameter, enlargement may be present. Apparent slight cardiac enlargement can occur because of a relatively small AP diameter of the chest. A cardiothoracic ratio at the upper limit of normal should not cause alarm if the patient has no reason to have cardiac failure and no symptoms of it.

Valve calcification, if present, is better seen on the lateral view. On the frontal view, the valve calcification cannot be visualised over the spine.

Diaphragm. The hemidiaphragms visualised on the frontal films are the top of the domes seen tangentially. Much lung in the posterior costophrenic angles is not seen on the frontal film.

If the hemidiaphragms are low and flat, emphysema may be present. A critical look must be made beneath the diaphragm to see if there is free peritoneal gas (Figure 5.23).

Lung fields. On the frontal field, it is convenient to divide the lung fields into zones. It is easy then to compare one zone with another for density differences and the distribution of the vascular 'markings'.

The apices lie above the level of the clavicles. The upper zones include the apices and pass down to the level of the second costal cartilages. The mid-zones lie between the second and fourth costal cartilage levels. The lower zones lie between the fourth and sixth costal cartilages.

The radiolucency of the lung fields is due to the air filling the lung. The 'greyness' is due to blood in the pulmonary vessels.

The upper zones of the lungs are normally less well perfused, resulting in smaller blood vessels. With raised left atrial pressure, there is upper zone blood diversion and the vessels are congested.

An increase in lung radiolucency occurs with pulmonary vessel loss, as also happens with emphysema. Lung radiolucency is lost with an effusion or consolidation.

Terms such as opacity, consolidation and patchy shadowing are used to describe the lung fields. It is usually unwise to attempt to make too precise a diagnosis of the underlying pathology.

The lungs are divided into lobes by reflections of the visceral pleura. The right lung is composed of the upper, middle and lower lobes. On the left, there are only the upper and lower lobes.

The right upper lobe has three segments: anterior, posterior and apical. The right middle lobe has a lateral and medial segment. Apical, medial basal, lateral basal, anterior basal and posterior basal segments compose the lower lobe.

There are three differences in the segmental anatomy of the left lung (Figure 4.8). The left upper lobe has four segments: an apicoposterior, anterior and two lingular segments. The superior and inferior lingular segments are the equivalent of the right middle lobe. The left lower lobe has four segments: it does not contain a medial basal segment.

The fissures are seen as hairline shadows. The horizontal fissure is at the level of the right fourth costal cartilage. The oblique fissures are not seen on the frontal view.

Bones and soft tissue. Nipple shadows are often seen over the lower zones and are about 5 mm in diameter. They can be confused with a 'coin' lesion. In such a case, nipple markers may be helpful.

Look carefully for a missing breast shadow in a female patient. A mastectomy may provide a diagnostic clue to explain bony or pulmonary metastases, or upper zone postradiation fibrosis.

Soft tissue gas may accompany a pneumothorax or be present after a thoracotomy.

Calcified tuberculous glands in the neck should be looked for in patients with lung scarring or calcified hilar lymph nodes.

Check that there are no rib fractures or space occupying lesions. Look for rib notching, due to increased blood flow through intercostal vessels (e.g. coarctation of the aorta). Cervical ribs or a thoracic scoliosis should be noted. Erosions or arthritis around the shoulder joints should be looked for.

Review. Certain parts of the film should be double-checked if the radiograph appears normal.

The retrocardiac region should be looked at again. A collapsed left lower lobe will reveal itself as a triangular opacity behind the heart shadow.

Both apices should be rechecked for lesions, especially Pancoast tumours or tuberculosis.

Has the patient a pneumothorax? There will be a difference between the translucency of the two lungs.

Lateral film

The lateral view is used largely for localisation of an already visible lesion on the frontal film. Examine it just as carefully. Sometimes a lesion is seen only on the lateral view. If there is clinical evidence of heart or lung disease, frontal and lateral views should always be obtained.

- **Points to remember:** (i) the retrosternal and retrocardiac triangles are normally of a similar radiodensity; (ii) the thoracic vertebrae become less opaque lower down the spine, unless there is pulmonary or pleural disease; (iii) the posterior costophrenic angle is sharp unless there is fluid or adjacent consolidation.

The hemidiaphragms are well defined unless there is pleural or pulmonary disease.

The oblique fissure placement is '4 to 4'. It passes from approximately 4 cm behind the anterior costophrenic angle, through the hilum to the T4 vertebral body level.

Heart

The right ventricle forms the anterior heart border on the lateral film. The left atrium forms the upper posterior border.

Mitral valve calcification is seen below an imaginary line drawn from the anterior costophrenic angle to the hilum, whereas aortic valve calcification lies above this line.

Examples of chest X-rays in cardiac disease

The radiological changes seen in pulmonary venous congestion, interstitial pulmonary oedema and alveolar pulmonary oedema are shown in Figures 3.53 to 3.55, respectively. Mitral valve disease is shown in Figure 3.56 a & b, while a ventricular aneurysm is seen in Figure 3.57. The characteristic notching of the inferior aspects of the ribs, due to hypertrophy of the intercostal arteries, appears in Figure 3.58, while the pulmonary plethora that is characteristic of a left-to-right shunt is obvious in Figure 3.59. A prosthetic aortic valve, which was inserted when a regurgitant valve was replaced in a patient with Marfan's syndrome, is illustrated in Figure 3.60.

Figure 3.53 Pulmonary venous congestion

The heart is enlarged due to failure. This failure is not severe enough to cause pulmonary oedema. However, the increased pulmonary venous pressure has caused upper zone blood diversion so the vessels above the hilum appear wider than those below. (The mechanism of the blood diversion is not fully understood.) These changes are seen when the pulmonary venous pressure is about 15 to 20 mmHg.

The cardiothoracic ratio A + B is a useful indicator of cardiac enlargement if it is greater than 50%. The thoracic measurement (T) is the widest diameter above the costophrenic angles, usually at the level of the right hemidiaphragm. The cardiac diameter is the addition of the two widths A and B.

Figure 3.54 Interstitial pulmonary oedema

The heart is moderately enlarged. The interstitial oedema causes fine, diffuse shadowing in the lung fields with blurring of the vessel margins. The escape of fluid into the interstitial tissue occurs when the capillary pressure exceeds the plasma osmotic pressure of 25 mmHg.

The interstitial oedema is characterised by Kerley 'B' lines, which are oedematous interlobular septa. They are best seen peripherally in the right costophrenic angle (arrow), where they lie horizontally, and are about 1 cm long. They contain the engorged lymphatics, which were originally thought by Kerley to be the sole cause of the 'B' lines.

Sternal sutures are present from previous cardiac surgery

Figure 3.55 Alveolar pulmonary oedema

When the pulmonary venous pressure reaches 30 mmHg, oedema fluid will pass into the alveoli. This causes shadowing (patchy to confluent depending on the extent) in the lung fields. This usually occurs first around the hila and gives a bat's wing appearance. These changes are usually superimposed on the interstitial oedema.

A lamellar pleural effusion (arrow) is seen at the right costophrenic angle where Kerley 'B' lines are also evident.

Figure 3.56 Mitral valve disease

The left atrium enlarges because of the pressure and volume load. It bulges posteriorly and to both sides (arrows). The atrial appendage bulges out below the left hilum. The prominent right border of the atrium causes the 'double right heart border' appearance.

To distinguish the valves if calcification is present, draw imaginary lines. On the PA view (a) the line passes from the right cardiophrenic angle to the inferior aspect of the left hilum. The line on the lateral view (b) passes from the antero-inferior angle through the midpoint of the hilum. The aortic valve lies above this line whereas the mitral valve lies below it.

Figure 3.57 Ventricular aneurysm

There is a bulge of the left cardiac border (arrow), which indicates an aneurysm of the left ventricular wall. The most common cause is weakness following myocardial infarction.

Figure 3.58 Aortic coarctation

The classical sign in aortic coarctation is notching of the inferior aspects of the ribs. This is due to hypertrophy of the intercostal arteries in which retrograde flow from the axillary collaterals is taking blood back to the descending aorta.

Because of the increased resistance to the left heart flow, left ventricular hypertrophy and then failure can occur. Failure causing cardiac enlargement has not yet occurred in this patient.

Figure 3.59 Atrial septal defect (ASD)

The most important thing to recognise is that there is pulmonary plethora indicating a left-to-right shunt. Left-to-right shunts occur in ASD, ventricular septal defect (VSD) and patent ductus arteriosus (PDA).

The shunted flow causes enlargement of the main pulmonary artery and its branches. The right hilum is enlarged because of the very dilated right pulmonary artery. The left hilum is hidden by the very dilated main pulmonary artery (arrow).

The ascending aorta is small (in contrast to its enlargement in PDA). The left atrium and ventricle are not enlarged, as they are in VSD and PDA.

Figure 3.60 Marfan's syndrome

The mediastinum is widened by uniform dilatation of the ascending aorta, the aortic arch and the descending aorta. This patient had Marfan's syndrome. Dissecting aneurysms can also occur and have a similar appearance.

There is a prosthetic aortic valve (arrow) from repair of previous regurgitation. Sternal sutures should be noted as well. No left ventricular enlargement is evident at this stage.

Summary
The cardiovascular examination: a suggested method (Figure 3.61)

Position the patient at 45 degrees and make sure his or her chest and neck are fully exposed. Cover the breasts of a female patient with a towel or loose garment.

Inspect while standing back for the appearance of Marfan's, Turner's or Down syndromes. Also look for dyspnoea, cyanosis, jaundice and cachexia.

Pick up the patient's hand. Feel the radial pulse. At the same time inspect the hands for clubbing. Also look for the peripheral stigmata of infective endocarditis: splinter haemorrhages are common (and are also caused by trauma), while Osler's nodes and Janeway lesions are rare. Look quickly, but carefully, at each nail bed, otherwise it is easy to miss these signs. Note any tendon xanthoma (type II hyperlipidaemia).

The pulse at the wrist should be timed for rate and rhythm. Feel for radiofemoral delay (which occurs in coarctation of the aorta) and radio-radial inequality. Pulse character is best assessed at the carotids.

Take the blood pressure (lying and standing or sitting—postural hypotension).

Next inspect the face. Look at the eyes briefly for jaundice (e.g. valve haemolysis) or xanthelasma (type II or type III hyperlipidaemia). You may also notice the classical mitral facies. Then inspect the mouth using a torch for a high arched palate (Marfan's syndrome), petechiae and the state of dentition (endocarditis). Look at the tongue or lips for central cyanosis.

The neck is very important. The jugular venous pressure (JVP) must be assessed for height and character. Use the right internal jugular vein for this assessment. Look for a change with inspiration (Kussmaul's sign).

Now feel each carotid pulse separately. Assess the pulse character.

Proceed to the praecordium. Always begin by inspecting for scars, deformity, site of the apex beat and visible pulsations. Do not forget about pacemaker boxes. Mitral valvotomy scars (usually under the left breast) can be quite lateral and very easily missed.

Palpate for the position of the apex beat. Count down the correct number of interspaces. The normal position is the fifth left intercostal space, one centimetre medial to the midclavicular line. The character of the apex beat is important. There are a number of types. A *pressure-loaded* (hyperdynamic, systolic overloaded) apex beat is a forceful and sustained impulse that is not displaced (e.g. aortic stenosis, hypertension). A *volume-loaded* (hyperkinetic, diastolic overloaded) apex beat is a forceful but unsustained impulse that is displaced down and laterally (e.g. aortic regurgitation, mitral regurgitation). A *dyskinetic* apex beat (cardiac failure) is palpable over a larger area than normal and moves in an uncoordinated way under the examiner's hand. Do not miss the tapping apex beat of mitral stenosis (a palpable first heart sound). The double or triple apical impulse of hypertrophic cardiomyopathy is very important too. Feel also for an apical thrill, and time it.

Then palpate with the heel of your hand for a left parasternal impulse (which indicates right ventricular enlargement or left atrial enlargement) and for thrills. Now feel at the base of the heart for a palpable pulmonary component of the second heart sound (P2) and aortic thrills. Percussion may be helpful if there is uncertainty about cardiac enlargement.

Auscultation begins in the mitral area with both the bell and the diaphragm. Listen for each component of the cardiac cycle separately. Identify the first and second heart sounds and decide if they are of normal intensity and whether the second heart sound is normally split. Now listen for extra heart sounds and for murmurs. Do not be satisfied at having identified one abnormality.

Repeat the approach at the left sternal edge and then the base of the heart (aortic and pulmonary areas). Time each part of the cycle with the carotid pulse. Listen over the carotids.

It is now time to reposition the patient. First put him or her in the left lateral position. Again feel the apex beat for character (particularly tapping) and auscultate. Sit the patient up and palpate for thrills (with the patient in full expiration) at the left sternal edge and base. Then listen in those areas, particularly for aortic regurgitation or a pericardial rub.

Dynamic auscultation should always be done if there is any doubt about the diagnosis. The Valsalva manoeuvre should be performed whenever there is a pure systolic murmur. Hypertrophic cardiomyopathy is easily missed otherwise.

The patient is now sitting up. Percuss the back quickly to exclude a pleural effusion (e.g. due to left ventricular failure), and auscultate for inspiratory crackles (left ventricular failure). If there is a radiofemoral delay, also listen for a coarctation murmur over the back. Feel for sacral oedema and note any back deformity (e.g. ankylosing spondylitis with aortic regurgitation).

Patient lying at 45 degrees

1. **General inspection**
   Marfan's, Turner's, Down syndrome
   Rheumatological disorders, e.g.
      ankylosing spondylitis (aortic
      regurgitation)
   Acromegaly etc
   Dyspnoea

2. **Hands**
   Radial pulses—right and left
   Radiofemoral delay
   Clubbing
   Signs of infective endocarditis—
      splinter haemorrhages etc
   Peripheral cyanosis
   Xanthomata

3. **Blood pressure**

4. **Face**
   Eyes
   • Sclerae—pallor, jaundice
   • Pupils—Argyll Robertson (aortic
      regurgitation)
   • Xanthelasma
   Malar flush (mitral stenosis,
      pulmonary stenosis)
   Mouth
   • Cyanosis
   • Palate (high arched—Marfan's)
   • Dentition

5. **Neck**
   Jugular venous pressure
   • Central venous pressure height
   • Wave form (especially large v
      waves)
   Carotids—pulse character

6. **Praecordium**
   Inspect
   • Scars—whole chest, back
   • Deformity
   • Apex beat—position, character
   • Abnormal pulsations
   Palpate
   • Apex beat—position, character
   • Thrills
   • Abnormal impulses
   NB: Beware of dextrocardia

7. **Auscultate**
   Heart sounds
   Murmurs
   Position patient
   • Left lateral position
   • Sitting forward (forced expiratory
      apnoea)
   NB: Palpate for thrills again after
      positioning
   Dynamic auscultation
   • Respiratory phases
   • Valsalva
   • Exercise (isometric, e.g. hand
      grip)

8. **Back (sitting forward)**
   Scars, deformity
   Sacral oedema
   Pleural effusion (percuss)
   Left ventricular failure (auscultate)

9. **Abdomen** (lying flat—1 pillow
      only)
   Palpate liver (pulsatile etc.),
      spleen, aorta
   Percuss for ascites (right heart
      failure)
   Femoral arteries—palpate,
      auscultate

10. **Legs**
   Peripheral pulses
   Cyanosis, cold limbs, trophic
      changes, ulceration (peripheral
      vascular disease)
   Oedema
   Xanthomata
   Calf tenderness

11. **Other**
   Urine analysis (infective
      endocarditis)
   Fundi (endocarditis)
   Temperature chart (endocarditis)

Figure 3.61 Cardiovascular system

Next lay the patient flat and examine the abdomen properly for hepatomegaly (right ventricular failure) and a pulsatile liver (tricuspid regurgitation). Test for the abdomino-jugular reflux sign if relevant. Feel for splenomegaly (endocarditis) and an aortic aneurysm. Palpate both femoral arteries and auscultate here for bruits. Go on and examine all the peripheral pulses. Look for signs of peripheral vascular disease, peripheral oedema, clubbing of the toes, Achilles tendon xanthomata and stigmata of infective endocarditis.

Finally, examine the fundi (for hypertensive changes, and Roth's spots in endocarditis) and the urine (haematuria in endocarditis). Take the temperature.

References

1. Albert JS. The patient with angina: the importance of careful listening. *J Am Col Cardiol* 1988; 11:27. The history further distinguishes cardiac events even if a coronary angiogram is available.
2. Panju AA, Hemmegan BR, Guyatt GH, Simel DL. Is this patient having a myocardial infarction? *JAMA* 1995; 273:1211–1218. A focused history and examination (and an ECG) can aid subdivision of patients into those highly likely and those highly unlikely to be having a myocardial infarction.
3. Evan AT. Sensitivity and specificity of the history and physical examination for coronary artery disease. *Ann Intern Med* 1994; 120:344–345.
4. Poole-Wilson P. The origin of symptoms in patients with chronic heart failure. *Eur Heart J* 1998; 9 (supplement H):49–53. This article dicusses the lack of correlation between symptoms of heart failure and haemodynamic measurements.
5. Brugada P, Gursoy S, Brugada J, Ardries E. Investigation of palpitations. *Lancet* 1993; 341:1254–1258. Emphasises the role of history taking and examination as well as the ECG in sorting out the patient presenting with palpitations.
6. Calkins H, Shyr Y, Frumin H, Schork A, Morady F. The value of the clinical history in the differentiation of syncope due to ventricular tachycardia, atrioventricular block, and neurocardiogenic syncope. *Am J Med* 1995; 98:365–373. Describes useful historical features in differential diagnosis.
7. Special Writing Group of the Committee on Rheumatic Fever, Endocarditis and Kawasaki Disease of the Council on Cardiovascular Disease in the Young of the American Heart Association. Guidelines for the diagnosis of rheumatic fever. Jones Criteria, 1992 Update. *JAMA* 1992; 268:2069–2073.
8. Myers KA. Does this patient have clubbing? *JAMA* 2001, 286 (3):341–347.
9. Reeves RA. Does this patient have hypertension? *JAMA* 1995; 273:15. An important review of technique and of the errors to avoid.
10. Bellman J, Visintin JM, Salvatore R et al. Osler's manoeuvre: absence of usefulness for the detection of pseudo hypertension in an elderly population. *Am J Med* 1995; 98:42–49. Although it is reproducible, the manoeuvre failed to identify pseudohypertension compared with intra-arterial measurements.
11. Jansen RWMM, Lipsitz LA. Postprandial hypotension: epidemiology, pathophysiology and clinical management. *Ann Intern Med* 1995; 122:186–195. It is important to recognise that blood pressure decreases postprandially and that this can affect interpretation of the blood pressure reading and the management of hypertension.
12. Cook DC. Does this patient have abnormal central venous pressure? *JAMA* 1996; 275:8. A useful review that explains how to examine the veins and conduct the hepatojugular reflux test.
13. Maisel AS, Attwood JE, Goldberger AL. Hepatojugular reflux: useful in the bedside diagnosis of tricuspid regurgitation. *Ann Intern Med* 1984; 101:781–782. This test has excellent sensitivity and specificity.
14. O'Neill TW, Barry M, Smith M, Graham IM. Diagnostic value of the apex beat. *Lancet* 1989; 1:410–411. Palpation of the apex beat beyond the left midclavicular line is specific (59%) for identifying true cardiomegaly.
15. Heckerling PS et al. Accuracy and reproducibility of precordial percussion and palpation for detecting increased left ventricular end-diastolic volume and mass. *JAMA* 1993; 270:16. Percussion has a high sensitivity but low specificity for detecting left ventricular enlargement. Therefore this manoeuvre may have some value despite being previously discredited.
16. Harvey WP. Cardiac pearls. *Disease-a-Month* 1994; 40:41–113. A good review of auscultatory findings that helps demystify the many noises heard when auscultating the heart.
17. Timmis AJ. The third heart sound. *BMJ* 1987; 294:326–327.
18. Folland ED et al. Implications of third heart sounds in patients with valvular heart disease. *N Engl J Med* 1992; 327:458–462. An analysis of patients with valvular regurgitation shows that a third heart sound may occur before cardiac failure has supervened.
19. Benchimol A, Desser KB. The fourth heart sound in patients with demonstrable heart disease. *Am Heart J* 1977; 93:298–301. In 60 out of 100 consecutive patients with normal studies, an S4 was heard. An S4 can be a normal finding although a loud sound is more likely to be pathological.
20. Tyberg TI, Goodyer AVN, Langou RA. Genesis of pericardial knock in constrictive pericarditis. *Am J Cardiol* 1980; 46:570–575. Sudden cessation of ventricular filling generates this sound.
21. Smith ND, Raizada V, Abrams J. Auscultation of the normally functioning prosthetic valve. *Ann Intern Med* 1981; 95:594–598. Provides clear information on auscultatory changes with prosthetic valves.
22. Levine SA. Notes on the gradation of the intensity of cardiac murmurs. *JAMA* 1961; 177:261.
23. Lembo NJ et al. Bedside diagnosis of systolic murmurs. *N Engl J Med* 1988; 318:24. This well-conducted study describes the predictive value of bedside manoeuvres during auscultation.
24. Ewy GA. The abdominojugular test. *Ann Intern Med* 1988; 109:56–60. Note that an abnormal abdominal-jugular test can occur as a result of left heart disease (i.e. elevated pulmonary-capillary wedge pressure).

25. Lederle FA, Walker JM, Reinke DB. Selective screening for abdominal aortic aneurysms with physical examination and ultrasound. *Arch Intern Med* 1988; 148:1753–1756. In fat patients, palpation of aneurysms is unlikely but in thin ones the technique is valuable.

26. Lederle FA, Simel DL. Does this patient have an abdominal aortic aneurysm? *JAMA* 1999; 281:77–82. The only clinical sign of definite value is palpation to detect widening of the aorta. The sensitivity of this sign for aneurysms 5 cm or larger is 76%.

27. Magee TR, Stanley P, Mufti R et al. Should we palpate foot pulses? *Ann Roy Coll Surg Eng* 1992; 74:166–168. Elderly patients who do not have a palpable dorsalis pedis pulse will often have adequate perfusion (unless there is clinical evidence of claudication or foot ulcers). Palpation of the dorsalis pedis is more helpful than the posterior tibial.

28. McGee SR, Boyko EJ. Physical examination and chronic lower-extremity ischemia: a critical review. *Arch Intern Med* 1998; 158:1357–1364. The presence of peripheral arterial disease is positively predicted by abnormal pedal pulses, a unilaterally cool extremity, prolonged venous filling time, and a femoral bruit.

29. O'Keefe ST, Woods BO, Breslin DJ, Tsapatsaris NP. Blue toe syndrome. Causes and management. *Arch Intern Med* 1992; 152:2197–2202. Explains how to identify the cause by clinical methods and directed investigations.

30. Anand SS, Wells PS, Hunt D et al. Does this patient have deep venous thrombosis? *JAMA* 1998; 279:1094–1099. The sensitivity of individual symptoms and signs is 60%–96% and the specificity 20%–72%. Patients can be subdivided into those with a low, intermediate or high pretest probability, based on risk factors and clinical features.

31. Butie A. Clinical examination of varicose veins. *Dermat Surg* 1995; 21:52–56. Techniques are outlined and compared with Doppler ultrasound assessment.

32. Stevenson LW, Perluff JK. The limited reliability of physical signs for estimating hemodynamics in chronic heart failure. *JAMA* 1989; 261:884–888. Physical signs poorly predict haemodynamic changes in heart failure. However, some signs are useful.

33. Khot U, Jia G, Moliterno DJ et al. Prognostic value of physical examination for heart failure in non-ST elevation acute coronary syndromes. *JAMA* 2003; 290: 2174–2181. This analysis of the Killip classification for patients with acute coronary syndromes expands the relevance of the classification from its original use for patients with ST elevation infarction in the pre-thrombolytic era.

34. Klompas M. Does this patient have an acute thoracic dissection? *JAMA*, 2002; 287(17): 2262–2272.

35. Turnbull JM. Is listening for abdominal bruits useful in the evaluation of hypertension? The rational clinical examination. *JAMA* 1995; 274:16. If an abdominal bruit extends into diastole, this has a high predictive value for a clinically important bruit. The pitch and intensity are not helpful.

36. Etchells E, Bell C, Robb K. Does this patient have an abnormal systolic murmur? *JAMA* 1997; 277:564–571. The most useful positive predictive features for aortic stenosis appear to be a slow rate of rise of the carotid pulse, a mid-to-late peak intensity of the murmur and a decreased second heart sound; absence of radiation to the right carotid helps rule it out.

37. Aronow WS. Prevalence and severity of valvular aortic stenosis determined by Doppler echocardiography, and its association with echocardiographic and electrocardiographic left ventricular hypertrophy and physical signs of aortic stenosis in elderly patients. *Am J Cardiol* 1991; 67:776–777. Analysis of the signs of severity of aortic stenosis in elderly patients shows that they are less reliable than in younger patients.

38. Choudhry NK, Etchells EE. Does this patient have aortic regurgitation? *JAMA*, 1999; 281:2231–2238 (Rational Clinical Examination Series).

39. Babu AN, Kymes SM, Carpenter Fryer SM. Eponyms and the diagnosis of aortic regurgitation: What says the evidence? *Ann Intern Med* 2003: 138:736–745.

Suggested reading
Textbooks

Braunwald E, Zipes DP, Libby P. *Heart disease. A textbook of cardiovascular medicine*, 6th edn. Philadelphia: WB Saunders, 2001.

Crawford MH, DiMarco JP, Paulus WJ. *Cardiology*, 2nd edn. London: Mosby, 2004.

chapter 4

The respiratory system and breast examination

A medical chest specialist is long-winded about the short-winded.

Kenneth T Bird (b. 1917)

This chapter deals with common respiratory symptoms, and the examination of the respiratory system and the breasts.

The respiratory history

Presenting symptoms

(Table 4.1)

Cough and sputum

Cough is a common presenting respiratory symptom. It occurs when deep inspiration is followed by explosive expiration. Flow rates of air in the trachea approach the speed of sound during a forceful cough. Coughing enables the airways to be cleared of secretions and foreign bodies. The duration of a cough is important. A cough of recent origin, particularly if associated with fever and other symptoms of respiratory tract infection, may be due to acute bronchitis or pneumonia. A chronic cough associated with wheezing may be due to asthma; sometimes asthma can present with just cough alone. An irritating chronic dry cough can result from oesophageal reflux and acid irritation of the lungs. It may be a feature of late interstitial pulmonary fibrosis. A similar cough is not uncommonly associated with the use of the angiotensin-converting

enzyme (ACE) inhibitors—drugs used in the treatment of hypertension and cardiac failure. Cough that wakes a patient from sleep may be a symptom of cardiac failure or of the reflux of acid from the oesophagus into the lungs that can occur when a person lies down. A chronic cough that is productive of large volumes of purulent sputum may be due to bronchiectasis. A change in the character of a chronic cough may indicate the development of a new and serious underlying problem (e.g. infection or lung cancer).

Patients' descriptions of their cough may be helpful. A cough associated with inflammation of the

Table 4.1 Respiratory history
Major symptoms
Cough
Sputum
Haemoptysis
Dyspnoea (acute, progressive or paroxysmal)
Wheeze
Chest pain
Fever
Hoarseness
Night sweats

epiglottis may have a barking quality. Cough caused by tracheal compression by a tumour may be loud and brassy. Cough associated with recurrent laryngeal nerve palsy has a hollow sound because the vocal cords are unable to close completely; this has been described as a bovine cough. A cough that is worse at night is suggestive of asthma or heart failure, while coughing that comes on immediately after eating or drinking may be due to a tracheo-oesophageal fistula or oesophageal reflux.

It is an important (though perhaps a somewhat unpleasant task) to inquire about the type of sputum produced and then to look at it, if it is available. Be warned that some patients have more interest in their sputum than others and may go into more detail than you really want. A large volume of purulent (yellow or green) sputum suggests the diagnosis of bronchiectasis or lobar pneumonia. Foul-smelling dark-coloured sputum may indicate the presence of a lung abscess with anaerobic organisms. Pink frothy secretions from the trachea, which occur in pulmonary oedema, should not be confused with sputum. Haemoptysis (coughing up of blood) can be a sinister sign of lung disease (Table 4.2) and must always be investigated. It is best to rely on the patient's assessment of the taste of the sputum, which, not unexpectedly, is foul in conditions like bronchiectasis or lung abscess.

Breathlessness (dyspnoea) (Table 4.3)

The awareness that an abnormal amount of work is required for breathing is called dyspnoea. It can be due to respiratory or cardiac disease (page 29). Careful questioning about the timing of onset, severity and pattern of dyspnoea is helpful in making the diagnosis.[1] The patient may be aware of this only on heavy exertion or have much more limited exercise tolerance. Dyspnoea can be graded from I to IV based on the New York Heart Association classification:

- Class I—disease present but no dyspnoea or dyspnoea only on heavy exertion
- Class II—dyspnoea on moderate exertion
- Class III—dyspnoea on minimal exertion
- Class IV—dyspnoea at rest

It is more useful, however, to determine the amount of exertion that actually causes dyspnoea—that is, the distance walked or the number of steps climbed. The association of dyspnoea with wheeze suggests airways disease, which may be due to asthma or chronic obstructive pulmonary disease (chronic airflow limitation). The duration and variability of the dyspnoea are important. Dyspnoea that worsens progressively over a period of weeks, months or years may be due to *pulmonary fibrosis*. Dyspnoea of more rapid onset may be due to an acute respiratory infection (including bronchopneumonia or lobar pneumonia) or to pneumonitis (which may be infective or secondary to a hypersensitivity reaction). Dyspnoea that varies from day to day or even from hour to hour suggests a diagnosis of asthma. Dyspnoea of very rapid onset associated with sharp chest pain suggests a pneumothorax. Dyspnoea that is described by the patient as inability to take a breath big enough to fill the lungs and associated with sighing suggests anxiety. Dyspnoea that occurs on moderate exertion may be due to the combination of obesity and a lack of physical fitness (a not uncommon occurrence).

Wheeze

A number of conditions can cause a continuous whistling noise during breathing. These include asthma or chronic obstructive pulmonary disease, and airways obstruction by a foreign body or tumour. Wheeze is usually maximal during expiration and is accompanied by prolonged expiration.

Table 4.2 Causes of haemoptysis

Respiratory

Bronchitis
Bronchial carcinoma
Bronchiectasis
Pneumonia
(The above four account for about 80% of cases)
Pulmonary infarction
Cystic fibrosis
Lung abscess
Tuberculosis
Foreign body
Goodpasture's* syndrome: pulmonary haemorrhage, glomerulonephritis, antibody to basement membrane antigens
Rupture of a mucosal blood vessel after vigorous coughing

Cardiovascular

Mitral stenosis (severe)
Acute left ventricular failure

Bleeding diatheses

Note: Exclude spurious causes, such as nasal bleeding or haematemesis.
* Ernest W Goodpasture (1886–1960), pathologist at Johns Hopkins, Baltimore. He described this syndrome in 1919.

Table 4.3 Causes of dyspnoea

Respiratory

1 Airways disease	Chronic bronchitis and emphysema (chronic obstructive pulmonary disease)
	Asthma
	Bronchiectasis
	Cystic fibrosis
	Laryngeal or pharyngeal tumour
	Bilateral cord palsy
	Tracheal obstruction or stenosis
	Tracheomalacia
	Cricoarytenoid rheumatoid arthritis
2 Parenchymal disease	Pneumonia
	Allergic alveolitis
	Sarcoidosis
	Pulmonary fibrosis
	Obliterative bronchiolitis
	Diffuse infections
	Acute respiratory distress syndrome (ARDS)
	Infiltrative and metastatic tumour
	Pneumothorax
	Pneumoconiosis
3 Pulmonary circulation	Pulmonary embolism
	Chronic thromboembolic pulmonary hypertension
	Pulmonary arteriovenous malformation
	Pulmonary arteritis
4 Chest wall and pleura	Effusion or massive ascites
	Pleural tumour
	Fractured ribs
	Ankylosing spondylitis
	Kyphoscoliosis
	Neuromuscular diseases
	Bilateral diaphragmatic paralysis

Cardiac

	Left ventricular failure
	Mitral valve disease
	Cardiomyopathy
	Pericardial effusion or constrictive pericarditis
	Intracardiac shunt

Anaemia

Non-cardiorespiratory

	Psychogenic
	Acidosis (compensatory respiratory alkalosis)
	Hypothalamic lesions

Chest pain

Chest pain due to respiratory disease is usually different from that associated with myocardial ischaemia (page 27). The pleura and central airways have pain fibres and may be the source of respiratory pain. Pleural pain is characteristically *pleuritic* in nature: sharp and made worse by deep inspiration and coughing. It is typically localised to one area of the chest. It may be of sudden onset in patients with lobar pneumonia, pulmonary embolism and infarction or pneumothorax, and is often associated with dyspnoea. The sudden onset of pleuritic chest pain and dyspnoea is an urgent diagnostic problem, as all three of these conditions may be life-threatening if not treated promptly.

Other presenting symptoms

Bacterial pneumonia is an acute illness in which prodromal symptoms (fever, malaise and myalgia) occur for a short period (hours) before pleuritic pain and dyspnoea begin. *Viral pneumonia* is often preceded by a longer (days) prodromal illness. Patients may occasionally present with episodes of *fever at night*. Tuberculosis, pneumonia and meso-thelioma should always be considered in these cases. Occasionally patients with tuberculosis present with episodes of *drenching sweating* at night. *Hoarseness* may sometimes be considered a respiratory system symptom. It can be due to transient inflammation of the vocal cords (laryngitis), vocal cord tumour or recurrent laryngeal nerve palsy.

Sleep apnoea is an abnormal increase in the periodic cessation of breathing during sleep. Patients with *obstructive sleep apnoea* (where airflow stops during sleep for periods of at least 10 seconds and sometimes for over 2 minutes, despite persistent respiratory efforts) typically present with daytime somnolence, chronic fatigue, morning headaches and personality disturbances. Very loud snoring may be reported by anyone within earshot. These patients are often obese and hypertensive. Patients with *central sleep apnoea* (where there is cessation of inspiratory muscle activity) may also present with somnolence but do not snore excessively (Table 4.4).

Some patients respond to anxiety by increasing the rate and depth of their breathing. This is called *hyperventilation*. The result is an increase in CO_2 excretion and the development of alkalosis—a rise in the pH of the blood. These patients may complain of variable dyspnoea; they have more difficulty breathing in than out. The alkalosis results in paraesthesiae of the fingers and around the mouth, light-headedness, chest pain and a feeling of impending collapse.

Treatment

It is important to find out what drugs the patient is using, how often they are taken and whether they are inhaled or swallowed. The patient's previous and current medications may give a clue to the current diagnosis. Bronchodilators and inhaled steroids are prescribed for chronic obstructive pulmonary disease, asthma and bronchiectasis. A patient's increased use of bronchodilators suggests poor control of asthma and the need for review of treatment. Chronic respiratory disease, including sarcoidosis, hypersensitivity pneumonias and asthma, may have been treated with oral steroids. Oral steroid use may predispose to tuberculosis. Patients with chronic lung conditions like cystic fibrosis or bronchiectasis will often be very knowledgeable about their treatment and can describe the various forms of physiotherapy that are essential for keeping their airways clear.

Almost every class of drug can produce lung toxicity. Examples include pulmonary embolism from use of the oral contraceptive pill, interstitial lung disease from cytotoxic agents (e.g. methotrexate, cyclophosphamide, bleomycin), bronchospasm from beta-blockers or non-steroidal anti-inflammatory drugs, and cough from ACE inhibitors. Some medications known to cause lung disease may not be mentioned by the patient because they are illegal (e.g. cocaine), are used sporadically (e.g. hydrochlorothiazide), can be obtained over the counter (e.g. tryptophan) or are not taken orally (e.g. timolol; beta-blocker eye drops for glaucoma). The clinician therefore needs to ask about these types of drug specifically.

Past history

One should always ask about previous respiratory illness, including pneumonia, tuberculosis or chronic bronchitis, or abnormalities of the chest X-ray that have previously been reported to the patient. Many previous respiratory investigations may have been memorable, such as bronchoscopy, lung biopsy and video-assisted thoracoscopy. Spirometry, with or without challenge testing for asthma, may have been performed. Many severe asthmatics perform their own regular peak flow testing (page 109). Ask about the results of any of these investigations. Patients with the acquired immunodeficiency syndrome (AIDS) have a high risk of developing *Pneumocystis carinii* pneumonia and indeed other chest infections, including tuberculosis.

Table 4.4 Abnormal patterns of breathing

Type of breathing	Cause(s)
1 Sleep apnoea—cessation of airflow for more than 10 seconds more than 10 times a night during sleep	Obstructive (e.g. obesity with upper airway narrowing, enlarged tonsils, pharyngeal soft tissue changes in acromegaly or hypothyroidism)
2 Cheyne-Stokes* breathing—periods of apnoea (associated with reduced level of consciousness) alternate with periods of hyperpnoea (lasts 30 s on average and is associated with agitation). This is due to a delay in the medullary chemoreceptor response to blood gas changes	Left ventricular failure Brain damage (e.g. trauma, cerebral haemorrhage) High altitude
3 Kussmaul's breathing (air hunger)—deep, rapid respiration due to stimulation of the respiratory centre	Metabolic acidosis (e.g. diabetes mellitus, chronic renal failure)
4 Hyperventilation, which results in alkalosis and tetany	Anxiety
5 Ataxic (Biot†) breathing—irregular in timing and depth	Brainstem damage
6 Apneustic breathing—a post-inspiratory pause in breathing	Brain (pontine) damage
7 Paradoxical respiration—the abdomen sucks inwards with inspiration (it normally pouches outwards due to diaphragmatic descent)	Diaphragmatic paralysis

* John Cheyne (1777–1836), Scottish physician who worked in Dublin, described this in 1818. William Stokes (1804–1878), Irish physician, described it in 1854.
† Camille Biot (b. 1878), French physician.

Occupational history

In no system are the patient's present and previous occupations of more importance.[2] A detailed occupational history is essential. One must ask about exposure to dusts in mining industries and factories (e.g. asbestos, coal, silica, iron oxide, tin oxide, cotton, beryllium, titanium oxide, silver, nitrogen dioxide, anhydrides). Work or household exposure to animals, including birds, is also relevant (e.g. Q fever or psittacosis). Exposure to mouldy hay, humidifiers or air conditioners may also result in lung disease (e.g. allergic alveolitis). The patient may be unaware that his or her occupation involved exposure to dangerous substances; for example, factories making insulating cables and boards very often used asbestos until 25 years ago. Asbestos exposure can result in the development of asbestosis, mesothelioma or carcinoma of the lung up to 30 years later. Relatives of people working with asbestos may be exposed when handling work clothes.

It is most important to find out what the patient actually does when at work, the duration of any exposure, use of protective devices and whether other workers have become ill. An improvement in symptoms over the weekend is a valuable clue to the presence of occupational lung disease, particularly occupational asthma. This can occur as a result of exposure to spray paints or plastic or soldering fumes.

Social history

A smoking history should be routine, as it is the major cause of chronic obstructive pulmonary disease and lung cancer (see Table 1.2, page 6). It also increases the risk of spontaneous pneumothorax and of Goodpasture's syndrome. It is necessary to ask how many packets of cigarettes a day a patient has smoked and how many years the patient has smoked. An estimate should be made of the number of packet years of smoking. Remember that this is based on

20-cigarette packets and that packets of cigarettes are getting larger; curiously, most manufacturers now make packets of 30 or 35. More recently, giant packets of 50 have appeared. These are too large to fit into pockets and must be carried in the hands as a constant reminder to the patient of his or her addiction. Occupation may further affect cigarette smokers; for example, asbestos workers who smoke are at an especially high risk of lung cancer. Passive smoking is now regarded as a significant risk for lung disease and the patient should be asked about exposure to other people's cigarette smoke at home and at work.

Many respiratory conditions are chronic and may interfere with the ability to work. Housing conditions may be inappropriate for a person with a limited exercise tolerance or an infectious disease. An inquiry about the patient's alcohol consumption is important. The drinking of large amounts of alcohol in binges can sometimes result in aspiration pneumonia, and alcoholics are more likely to develop pneumococcal or *Klebsiella* pneumonia. Intravenous drug users are at risk of lung abscess and drug-related pulmonary oedema. Such information may influence the decision about whether to advise treatment at home or in hospital.

Family history

A family history of asthma, cystic fibrosis or emphysema should be sought. Alpha$_1$-antitrypsin deficiency, for example, is an inherited disease, and carriers are extremely susceptible to the development of emphysema. A family history of infection with tuberculosis is also important.

The respiratory examination

Positioning the patient

The patient should be undressed to the waist.[3] If he or she is not acutely ill, the examination is easiest to perform with the patient sitting over the edge of the bed or even on a chair.

General appearance

It is important to look for the following signs before beginning the detailed examination.

Dyspnoea

Watch the patient for signs of dyspnoea at rest. Count the respiratory rate; the normal rate at rest should not exceed 25 breaths per minute (range 16–25). The frequently quoted normal value of 14 breaths per minute is probably too low; normal people can have a respiratory rate of up to 25, and the average is 20 breaths per minute. It is traditional to count the respiratory rate surreptitiously while affecting to count the pulse. The respiratory rate is the only vital sign that is under direct voluntary control. Tachypnoea refers to a rapid respiratory rate of greater than 25. Bradypnoea is defined as a rate below 8, a level associated with sedation and adverse prognosis. In normal relaxed breathing the diaphragm is the only active muscle and is active only in inspiration; expiration is a passive process.

Look to see whether the accessory muscles of respiration are being used. These muscles include the sternomastoids, the platysma and the strap muscles of the neck. Characteristically the accessory muscles cause elevation of the shoulders with inspiration and aid respiration by increasing chest expansion. Contraction of the abdominal muscles may occur in expiration in patients with obstructed airways. In some cases, the pattern of breathing is diagnostically helpful (Table 4.4). Look for pursed lips breathing, which is characteristic of patients with severe chronic obstructive pulmonary disease (COPD). This manoeuvre reduces the patient's breathlessness, possibly by providing continuous positive airways pressure and helping to prevent airways collapse during expiration.

Cyanosis

Central cyanosis is best detected by inspecting the tongue. Examination of the tongue differentiates central from peripheral cyanosis. Lung disease severe enough to result in significant ventilation–perfusion imbalance, such as pneumonia, chronic obstructive pulmonary disease and pulmonary embolism, may cause reduced arterial oxygen saturation and central cyanosis. Cyanosis becomes evident when the absolute concentration of deoxygenated haemoglobin is 5 g/100 mL of capillary blood. Cyanosis is usually obvious when the arterial oxygen saturation falls below 90% in a person with a normal haemoglobin level. Central cyanosis is therefore a relatively late sign of hypoxaemia. In patients with anaemia, cyanosis does not occur until even greater levels of arterial desaturation are reached. The detection of cyanosis is much easier in good (especially fluorescent) lighting

Table 4.5 Some causes of stridor in adults

Sudden onset (minutes)	Anaphylaxis
	Toxic gas inhalation
	Acute epiglottitis
	Inhaled foreign body
Gradual onset (days, weeks)	Laryngeal and pharyngeal tumours
	Cricoarytenoid rheumatoid arthritis
	Bilateral vocal cord palsy
	Tracheal carcinoma
	Paratracheal compression by lymph nodes
	Post-tracheostomy or intubation granulomata

conditions and is said to be more difficult if the patient's bed is surrounded by cheerful pink curtains.

Character of the cough

Coughing is a protective response to irritation of sensory receptors in the submucosa of the upper airways or bronchi. Ask the patient to cough several times. Lack of the usual explosive beginning may indicate vocal cord paralysis (the 'bovine' cough). A muffled, wheezy ineffective cough suggests obstructive pulmonary disease. A very loose productive cough suggests excessive bronchial secretions due to chronic bronchitis, pneumonia or bronchiectasis. A dry, irritating cough may occur with chest infection, asthma or carcinoma of the bronchus and sometimes with left ventricular failure or interstitial lung disease. It is also typical of the cough produced by the ACE inhibitor drugs.

Sputum

Sputum should be inspected. Careful study of the sputum is an essential part of the physical examination. The colour, volume and type (purulent, mucoid or mucopurulent), and the presence or absence of blood, should be recorded.

Stridor

Obstruction of the larynx, trachea or large airways may cause stridor, a rasping or croaking noise loudest on inspiration. This can be due to a foreign body, a tumour, infection (e.g. epiglottitis) or inflammation (Table 4.5). It is a sign that requires urgent attention.

Hoarseness

Listen to the voice for hoarseness, as this may indicate recurrent laryngeal nerve palsy associated with carcinoma of the lung (usually left sided), or laryngeal carcinoma. However, the commonest cause is laryngitis. Non-respiratory causes include hypothyroidism.

The hands

As usual, examination in detail begins with the hands.

Clubbing

Look for clubbing, which is commonly due to respiratory disease (Figure 4.1, Table 3.4). An uncommon but important association with clubbing is *hypertrophic pulmonary osteoarthropathy* (HPO).

Figure 4.1 Finger clubbing

HPO is characterised by the presence of periosteal inflammation at the distal ends of long bones, the wrists, the ankles, the metacarpal and the metatarsal bones. There is swelling and tenderness over the wrists and other involved areas. Rarely HPO may occur without clubbing. The causes of HPO include primary lung carcinoma and pleural mesothelioma. Remember, chronic bronchitis and emphysema do not cause clubbing.

Staining

Look for staining of the fingers (actually caused by tar, as nicotine is colourless), a sign of cigarette smoking. The density of staining does not indicate the number of cigarettes smoked, but depends rather on the way the cigarette is held in the hand.

Wasting and weakness

Compression and infiltration by a peripheral lung tumour of a lower trunk of the brachial plexus results in wasting of the small muscles of the hand and weakness of finger abduction (page 334).

Pulse rate

Tachycardia and pulsus paradoxus are important signs of severe asthma (page 115). Tachycardia is a common side-effect of the treatment of asthma with β-agonist drugs.

Flapping tremor (asterixis)

Ask the patient to dorsiflex the wrists with the arms outstretched and to spread out the fingers. A flapping tremor may occur with severe carbon dioxide retention, usually due to severe chronic obstructive pulmonary disease. However, this is a late and unreliable sign.

The face

Inspect the *eyes* for evidence of Horner's[a] syndrome (a constricted pupil, partial ptosis and loss of sweating), which can be due to an apical lung tumour compressing the sympathetic nerves in the neck (page 320). There may be skin changes on the face that suggest scleroderma or connective tissue disease (page 248).

The *nose* is sited conveniently in the centre of the face. In this position it may readily be inspected

inside and out. Get the patient to tilt the head back. It may be necessary to use a nasal speculum to open the nostrils and a torch. Look for polyps (associated with asthma), engorged turbinates (various allergic conditions) and a deviated septum (nasal obstruction).

As already discussed, look at the *tongue* for central cyanosis. Look in the *mouth* for evidence of an upper respiratory tract infection (a reddened pharynx and tonsillar enlargement, with or without a coating of pus). A broken tooth or a rotten tooth stump may predispose to lung abscess or pneumonia.

Sinusitis is suggested by tenderness over the *sinuses* on palpation. If acute sinusitis is suspected, a torch can be used to transilluminate the frontal and maxillary sinuses.[5] A torch is placed in the patient's mouth and the sinuses examined in a dark room. Normal transillumination generally excludes sinusitis. Complete opacification suggests sinusitis but partial opacification is less helpful. The torch should then be used to look for purulent discharge in the pharynx.

Look at the patient's face for the red, leathery, wrinkled skin of the smoker.[4] There may be facial plethora or cyanosis if superior vena caval obstruction is present (page 116). Some patients with obstructive sleep apnoea will be obese with a receding chin, a small pharynx and a short thick neck.

The trachea

The position of the trachea is most important, and time should be spent establishing it accurately. From in front of the patient the forefinger of the right hand is pushed up and backwards from the suprasternal notch until the trachea is felt (Figure 4.2). If the trachea is displaced to one side, its edge rather than its middle will be felt and a larger space will be present on one side than the other. Slight displacement to the right is fairly common in normal people. This examination is uncomfortable for the patient, so you must be gentle.

Significant displacement of the trachea suggests, but is not specific for, disease of the upper lobes of the lung (Table 4.6).

A tracheal tug is demonstrated when the finger resting on the trachea feels it move inferiorly with each inspiration. This is a sign of gross overexpansion of the chest because of airflow obstruction.

If the patient appears dyspnoeic and use of the accessory muscles of respiration is suspected, the examiner's fingers should be placed in the supraclavicular fossae. When the scalene muscles are

[a] Johann Horner (1831–1886), Professor of Ophthalmology in Zurich, described this syndrome in 1869.

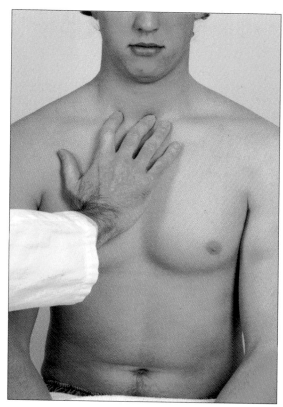

Figure 4.2 Feeling for the position of the trachea—a similar gap should be palpable on each side

Table 4.6 Causes of tracheal displacement

1 Towards the side of the lung lesion
   Upper lobe collapse
   Upper lobe fibrosis
   Pneumonectomy

2 Away from the side of the lung lesion
   (uncommon)
   Massive pleural effusion
   Tension pneumothorax

3 Upper mediastinal masses, such as
   retrosternal goitre

recruited, they can be felt to contract under the fingers. Even more severe dyspnoea will result in use of the sternomastoid muscles. Their contraction is also easily felt with inspiration. Use of these muscles for long periods is exhausting and a sign of impending respiratory failure.

The chest

The chest should be examined anteriorly and posteriorly by inspection, palpation, percussion and auscultation.[3] Compare the right and left sides during each part of the examination.

Inspection

Shape and symmetry of the chest. When the anteroposterior (AP) diameter is increased compared with the lateral diameter, the chest is described as barrel-shaped (Figure 4.3). An increase in the AP diameter compared with the lateral diameter (the thoracic ratio) beyond 0.9 is abnormal and is seen often in patients with severe asthma or emphysema. It is not always a reliable guide to the severity of the underlying lung disease and may be present in normal elderly people.

A **pigeon chest (pectus carinatum)** is a localised prominence (an outward bowing of the sternum and costal cartilages). It may be a manifestation of chronic childhood respiratory illness, in which case

Figure 4.3 Barrel chest

(From FS McDonald, ed., *Mayo Clinic images in internal medicine*, with permission. © Mayo Clinic Scientific Press and CRC Press.)

Figure 4.4 Funnel chest (pectus excavatum)

it is thought to result from repeated strong contractions of the diaphragm while the thorax is still pliable. It also occurs in rickets (page 274).

A **funnel chest (pectus excavatum)** is a developmental defect involving a localised depression of the lower end of the sternum (Figure 4.4). The problem is usually an aesthetic one, but in severe cases lung capacity may be restricted.

Harrison's sulcus[b] is a linear depression of the lower ribs just above the costal margins at the site of attachment of the diaphragm. It can result from severe asthma in childhood, or rickets.

Kyphosis refers to an exaggerated forward curvature of the spine, while scoliosis is lateral bowing. **Kyphoscoliosis** may be idiopathic (80%), secondary to poliomyelitis, or associated with Marfan's syndrome. Severe thoracic kyphoscoliosis may reduce the lung capacity and increase the work of breathing.

Lesions of the chest wall may be obvious. Look for *scars* from previous thoracic operations, or from chest drains for a previous pneumothorax or pleural effusion. Thoracoplasty causes severe chest deformity; this operation was performed for tuberculosis and involved removal of a large number of ribs on one side of the chest to achieve permanent collapse of the affected lung. It is no longer performed because of the availability of effective antituberculous chemotherapy. *Radiotherapy* may cause erythema and thickening of the skin over the irradiated area. There is sharp demarcation between abnormal and normal skin. There may be small tattoo marks indicating the limits of the irradiated area. Signs of radiotherapy usually indicate that the patient has been treated for carcinoma of the lung, breast or, less often, for lymphoma.

Subcutaneous emphysema is a crackling sensation felt on palpating the skin of the chest or neck. On inspection, there is often diffuse swelling of the chest wall and neck. It is caused by air tracking from the lungs and is usually due to a pneumothorax; less commonly it can follow rupture of the oesophagus or a pneumomediastinum (air in the mediastinal space).

Prominent veins may be seen in patients with superior vena caval obstruction. It is important to determine the direction of blood flow (page 147).

Movement of the chest wall should be noted. Look for asymmetry of chest wall movement

[b] Edward Harrison (1766–1838), British general practitioner in Lincolnshire, described this deformity in rickets in 1798. The sign has also been ascribed to Edwin Harrison (1779–1847), a London physician.

Figure 4.5 Inspecting upper lobe expansion: (a) expiration; (b) inspiration—note symmetrical elevation of the clavicles

anteriorly and posteriorly. Assessment of expansion of the upper lobes is best achieved by inspection from behind the patient, looking down at the clavicles during moderate respiration (Figure 4.5). Diminished movement indicates underlying lung disease. The affected side will show delayed or decreased movement. For assessment of lower lobe expansion, the chest should be inspected posteriorly.

Reduced chest wall movement on one side may be due to localised pulmonary fibrosis, consolidation, collapse, pleural effusion or pneumothorax. Bilateral reduction of chest wall movement indicates a diffuse abnormality such as chronic obstructive pulmonary disease or diffuse pulmonary fibrosis.

Look for paradoxical inward motion of the abdomen during inspiration when the patient is supine (indicating diaphragmatic paralysis).

Palpation

Chest expansion. Place the hands firmly on the chest wall with the fingers extending around the sides of the chest. The thumbs should almost meet in the middle line and should be lifted slightly off the chest so that they are free to move with respiration (Figure 4.6). As the patient takes a big breath in, the thumbs should move symmetrically apart at least 5 cm. Reduced expansion on one side indicates a lesion on that side. The causes have been discussed above.

Lower lobe expansion is assessed from the back in this way. Some idea of upper and middle lobe expansion is possible when the manoeuvre is repeated on the front of the chest, but this is better gauged by inspection.

Apex beat. When the patient is lying down, establishing the position of the apex beat may be helpful (page 45), as displacement towards the side of the lesion can be caused by collapse of the lower lobe or by localised pulmonary fibrosis. Movement of the apex beat away from the side of the lung lesion can be caused by pleural effusion or tension pneumothorax. The apex beat is often impalpable in a chest which is hyperexpanded secondary to chronic obstructive pulmonary disease.

Vocal fremitus. Palpate the chest wall with the palm of the hand while the patient repeats 'ninety-nine'. The front and back of the chest are each palpated in two comparable positions, with the palm of one hand on each side of the chest. In this way differences in vibration on the chest wall can be detected. This can be a difficult sign to interpret. It depends on the recognition of changes in vibration conducted to the examiner's hands while the patient speaks. Practice is needed to appreciate the difference between normal and abnormal. Vocal fremitus is more obvious in men because of their lower-pitched voices. It may be absent in normal people (high-pitched voice or thick chest wall). It is only abnormal if different on one side from the other. The causes of change in vocal fremitus are the same as those for vocal resonance (page 108).

Ribs. Gently compress the chest wall antero-posteriorly and laterally. Localised pain suggests a rib fracture, which may be secondary to trauma, or may be spontaneous as a result of tumour deposition, bone disease or sometimes the result of severe and prolonged coughing.

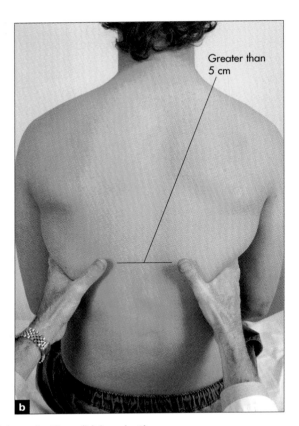

Thumbs not in contact with chest wall

Greater than 5 cm

Figure 4.6 Palpation for lower lobe expansion: (a) expiration; (b) inspiration

Percussion

With the left hand on the chest wall and the fingers slightly separated and aligned with the ribs, the middle finger is pressed firmly against the chest. Then the pad of the right middle finger (the *plexor*) is used to strike firmly the middle phalanx of the middle finger of the left hand (the *pleximeter*) which was often a piece of wood, ivory or a coin in the 19th century but is now always the examiner's finger. The percussing finger (plexor) is quickly removed so that the note generated is not dampened (this may be less important if the pleximeter finger is held firmly on the chest wall, as it should be). The percussing finger must be held partly flexed and a loose swinging movement should come from the wrist and not from the forearm. Medical students will soon learn to keep the right middle fingernail short. Percussion of symmetrical areas of the anterior, posterior and axillary regions is necessary (Figure 4.7). Percussion in the supraclavicular fossa over the apex of the lung should not be omitted.

Percuss the clavicle directly with the percussing finger. On percussion posteriorly, the scapulae should be moved out of the way by asking the patient to move the elbows forward across the front of the chest; this rotates the scapulae anteriorly.

The feel of the percussion note is as important as its sound. The note is affected by the thickness of the chest wall, as well as by underlying structures. Percussion over a solid structure, such as the liver or a consolidated area of lung, produces a dull note. Percussion over a fluid-filled area, such as a pleural effusion, produces an extremely dull (stony dull) note. Percussion over the normal lung produces a resonant note and percussion over hollow structures, such as the bowel or a pneumothorax, produces a hyperresonant note (*Good signs guide 4.1*).

Considerable practice is required before expert percussion can be performed, particularly in front of an audience. The ability to percuss well is usually obvious in clinical examinations and counts in a student's favour, as it indicates a reasonable amount of experience in the wards.

Figure 4.7 Percussion of the chest

(a) Percussing (plexor) finger poised. Inset: plexor finger strikes pleximeter finger. (b) Direct percussion of the clavicle for upper lobe resonance.

GOOD SIGNS GUIDE 4.1
Comparative percussion of the chest

Sign	Positive LR	Negative LR
Dullness—pneumonia	3.0	NS
Hyperresonance—COPD	5.1	NS

NS = not significant.

From McGee S, *Evidence-based physical diagnosis*, Saunders, 2001.

Liver dullness. The upper level of liver dullness is determined by percussing down the anterior chest in the midclavicular line. Normally, the upper level of the liver dullness is the fifth rib in the right midclavicular line. If the chest is resonant below this level, it is a sign of hyperinflation, usually due to emphysema or asthma.

Cardiac dullness. The area of cardiac dullness usually present on the left side of the chest may be decreased in emphysema or asthma.

Auscultation

Breath sounds. Using the diaphragm of the stethoscope, one should listen to the breath sounds in the areas shown in Figure 4.8.[6–8] It is important to compare each side with the other. Remember to listen high up into the axillae and, using the bell of the stethoscope applied above the clavicles, to listen to the lung apices. A number of observations must be made while auscultating and, as with auscultation

of the heart, different parts of the cycle must be considered. Listen for the quality of the breath sounds, the intensity of the breath sounds, and the presence of additional (adventitious) sounds (Figure 4.9).

Quality of breath sounds. *Normal breath sounds* are heard with the stethoscope over nearly all parts of the chest. The patient should be asked to breathe through the mouth so that added sounds from the nasopharynx do not interfere. These sounds are produced in the airways rather than the alveoli. They had once been thought to arise in the alveoli (vesicles) of the lungs and are therefore called vesicular sounds. They have rather fancifully been compared by Laënnec to the sound of wind rustling in leaves. Their intensity is related to total airflow at the mouth and to regional airflow. Normal (vesicular) breath sounds are louder and longer on inspiration than on expiration and there is no gap between the inspiratory and expiratory sounds. They are due to the transmission of air turbulence in the large airways filtered through the normal lung to the chest wall.

With *bronchial breath sounds* turbulence in the large airways is heard without being filtered by the alveoli, producing a different quality. Bronchial breath sounds have a hollow, blowing quality. They are audible throughout expiration and there is often a gap between inspiration and expiration. The expiratory sound has a higher intensity and pitch than the inspiratory sound. Bronchial breath sounds are more easily remembered than described. They are audible in normal people, posteriorly over the right upper chest where the trachea is contiguous with the

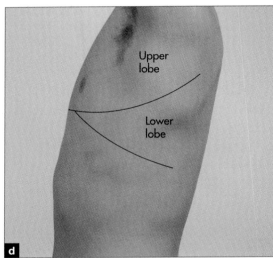

Figure 4.8 Lobes of the lung

(a) Anterior. (b) Posterior. (c) Lobes of the right lung. (d) Lobes of the left lung. Refer to Figure 4.13, page 118, for a list of the segments in each lobe.

right upper bronchus. They are heard over areas of consolidation, as solid lung conducts the sound of turbulence in main airways to peripheral areas without filtering. Causes of bronchial breath sounds are shown in Table 4.7.

Occasionally breath sounds over a large cavity have an exaggerated bronchial quality. This very hollow or *amphoric* sound has been likened to that heard when air passes over the top of a hollow jar (Greek *amphoreus*).

Intensity of the breath sounds. It is better to describe breath sounds as being of normal or reduced intensity than to speak about air entry. The entry of air into parts of the lung cannot be directly gauged from the breath sounds.

Causes of reduced breath sounds include chronic obstructive pulmonary disease (especially emphysema), pleural effusion, pneumothorax, pneumonia, a large neoplasm and pulmonary collapse.

Added (adventitious) sounds. There are two types of added sounds—continuous (wheezes) and interrupted (crackles).

Continuous sounds are called *wheezes*. They are abnormal findings and have a musical quality. The wheezes must be timed in relation to the respiratory cycle. They may be heard in expiration or inspiration,

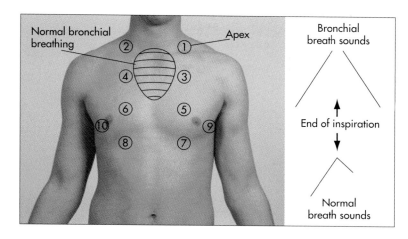

Figure 4.9 Normal and bronchial breath sounds

Auscultate in each area shown (the numbers represent a suggested order). Distinguish normal breath sounds from bronchial breathing.

Table 4.7 Causes of bronchial breath sounds

Common

Lung consolidation (lobar pneumonia)

Uncommon

Localised pulmonary fibrosis
Pleural effusion (above the fluid)
Collapsed lung (e.g. adjacent to a pleural effusion)

Note: The large airways must be patent.

---

or both. Wheezes are due to continuous oscillation of opposing airway walls and imply significant airway narrowing. Wheezes tend to be louder on expiration. This is because the airways normally dilate during inspiration and are narrower during expiration. An inspiratory wheeze implies severe airway narrowing.

The pitch (frequency) of wheezes varies. It is determined only by the velocity of the air jet and is not related to the length of the airway. High-pitched wheezes are produced in the smaller bronchi and have a whistling quality, whereas low-pitched wheezes arise from the larger bronchi.

Wheezes are usually the result of acute or chronic airflow obstruction due to asthma (often high pitched) or chronic obstructive pulmonary disease (often low pitched), secondary to a combination of bronchial muscle spasm, mucosal oedema and excessive secretions. Wheezes are a poor guide to the severity of airflow obstruction. In severe airways obstruction, wheeze can be absent because ventilation is so reduced that the velocity of the air jet is reduced below a critical level necessary to produce the sound.

A fixed bronchial obstruction, usually due to a carcinoma of the lung, tends to cause a localised wheeze, which has a single musical note (mono-phonic) and does not clear with coughing.

Wheezes must be distinguished from stridor (page 99), which sounds very similar to wheeze but is louder over the trachea and is always inspiratory (wheezes usually occur in expiration—the majority—but can occur in both inspiration and expiration).

Interrupted non-musical sounds are best called *crackles*.[9,10] There is a lot of confusion about the naming of these sounds, perhaps as a result of mistranslations of Laënnec. Some authors describe low-pitched crackles as rales and high-pitched ones as crepitations, but others do not make this distinction. The simplest approach is to call all these sounds crackles, but also to describe their timing and pitch.

Crackles are probably the result of loss of stability of peripheral airways that collapse on expiration. With high inspiratory pressures, there is rapid air entry into the distal airways. This causes the abrupt opening of alveoli and of small- or medium-sized bronchi containing secretions in regions of the lung deflated to residual volume. More compliant (distensible) areas open up first, followed by the increasingly stiff areas. Fine and medium-pitched crackles are not caused by air moving through secretions as was once thought but by the opening and closing of small airways.

The timing of crackles is of great importance. *Early inspiratory crackles* (cease before the middle of inspiration) suggest disease of the small airways, and are characteristic of chronic obstructive pulmonary disease.[9] The crackles are heard only in early inspiration and are of medium coarseness. They are different from those heard in left ventricular failure, which occur later in the respiratory cycle.

GOOD SIGNS GUIDE 4.2
Crackles and wheezes

Sign	Positive LR	Negative LR
Crackles		
Pulmonary fibrosis in asbestos workers	5.9	0.2
Pneumonia patients with cough and fever	2.0	0.8
Early inspiratory crackles		
Detecting COPD (patients with crackles)	14.6	NS
Severe disease patients with COPD	20.8	0.1
Unforced (audible during breathing at rest) **wheezing**		
Detecting COPD	6.0	NS

NS = not significant. COPD = chronic obstructive pulmonary disease.
From McGee S, *Evidence-based physical diagnosis*, Saunders, 2001.

Late or *pan-inspiratory crackles* suggest disease confined to the alveoli. They may be fine, medium or coarse in quality. *Fine crackles* have been likened to the sound of hair rubbed between the fingers, or to the sound Velcro makes when pulled apart—they are typically caused by pulmonary fibrosis. Characteristically, more crackles are heard in each inspiration when they are due to fibrosis—up to 14 compared with 1 to 4 for COPD and 4 to 9 for cardiac failure. As fibrosis becomes more severe the crackles extend earlier into inspiration and are heard further up the chest.[c] *Medium crackles* are usually due to left ventricular failure. Here the presence of alveolar fluid disrupts the function of the normally secreted surfactant. *Coarse crackles* are characteristic of pools of retained secretions and have an unpleasant gurgling quality. They tend to change with coughing, which also has an unpleasant gurgling quality. Bronchiectasis is a common cause, but any disease that leads to retention of secretions may produce these features. (See *Good signs guide 4.2*.)

Pleural friction rub: when thickened, roughened pleural surfaces rub together as the lungs expand and contract, a continuous or intermittent grating sound may be audible. A pleural rub indicates pleurisy, which may be secondary to pulmonary infarction or pneumonia. Rarely, malignant involvement of the pleura, a spontaneous pneumothorax or pleurodynia may cause a rub.

Vocal resonance. Auscultation over the chest while a patient speaks gives further information about the lungs' ability to transmit sounds. Over normal lung, the low-pitched components of speech are heard with a booming quality and high-pitched components are attenuated. Consolidated lung, however, tends to transmit high frequencies so that speech heard through the stethoscope takes on a bleating quality (called *aegophony* by Laënnec[11]—from Greek *aix* 'goat', *phone* 'voice'). When a patient with aegophony says 'e' as in 'bee' it sounds like 'a' as in 'bay'.

Ask the patient to say 'ninety-nine' while you listen over each part of the chest. Over consolidated lung the numbers will become clearly audible, while over normal lung the sound is muffled. If vocal resonance is present, bronchial breathing is likely to be heard (Table 4.7). Sometimes vocal resonance is increased to such an extent that whispered speech is distinctly heard; this is called whispering pectoriloquy.

If a very localised abnormality is found at auscultation, try to determine the lobe and approximately which segment or segments are involved (Figure 4.8).

The heart

Lay the patient down at 45 degrees and measure the jugular venous pressure for evidence of right heart failure (page 42). Next examine the praecordium. It is important to pay close attention to the pulmonary component of the second heart sound (P2). This is best heard at the second intercostal space on the left. It should not be louder than the aortic component, best heard at the right second inter-costal space. If the P2 is louder, pulmonary hypertension should be

[c] Expiratory crackles may also occur with lung fibrosis.[10]

strongly suspected. There may be signs of right ventricular failure or hypertension. Pulmonary hypertensive heart disease (cor pulmonale) may be due to chronic obstructive pulmonary disease, pulmonary fibrosis, pulmonary thromboembolism, marked obesity, sleep apnoea or severe kyphoscoliosis.

The abdomen

Palpate the liver for ptosis[d] (page 149), due to emphysema, or for enlargement from secondary deposits of tumour in cases of lung carcinoma.

Other

Pemberton's[e] sign

Ask the patient to lift the arms over the head and wait for one minute.[12] Note the development of facial plethora, cyanosis, inspiratory stridor and non-pulsatile elevation of the jugular venous pressure. This occurs in superior vena caval obstruction (page 261).

Feet

Inspect for swelling (oedema) or cyanosis, which may be clues to cor pulmonale, and look for evidence of deep venous thrombosis.

Respiratory rate on exercise

Patients complaining of dyspnoea should have their respiratory rate measured at rest, at maximal tolerated exertion (e.g. after climbing one or two flights of stairs), and supine. If dyspnoea is not accompanied by tachypnoea when a patient climbs stairs, one should consider the possibility of anxiety or malingering.

Temperature

Fever may occur with any acute or chronic chest infection.

Bedside assessment of lung function

Forced expiratory time

Physical examination should always include an estimate of the forced expiratory time (FET).[13]

Measure the time taken by a patient to exhale forcefully and completely through the open mouth after taking a maximum inspiration. The normal forced expiratory time is 3 seconds or less. Note any audible wheeze or cough. An increased FET indicates airways obstruction. The combination of a significant smoking history and an FET of 9 seconds or more is predictive of chronic obstructive pulmonary disease (positive LR 9.6). A peak flow meter or spirometer, however, will provide a more accurate measurement.

Peak flow meter

A peak flow meter is a simple gauge that is used to measure the maximum flow rate of expired air. Again the patient is asked to take a full breath in, but rather than a prolonged expiration, a rapid forced maximal expiratory puff is made through the mouth. The value obtained (the peak expiratory flow rate, PEFR) depends largely on airways diameter. Normal values for young men are approximately 600 litres a minute and for women 400 litres a minute. The value depends on age, sex and height, so tables of normal values should be consulted. Airways obstruction, such as that caused by asthma or chronic obstructive pulmonary disease, results in a reduced and variable PEFR. It is a simple way of assessing and following patients with airways obstruction, but is rather effort-dependent.

Spirometry (Figure 4.10)

The spirometer records graphically or numerically the forced expiratory volume and the forced vital capacity. The forced expiratory volume (FEV) is the volume of air expelled from the lungs after maximum inspiration using maximum forced effort, and is measured in a given time. Usually this is 1 second (FEV_1). The forced vital capacity (FVC) is the total volume of air expelled from the lungs after maximum inspiratory effort followed by maximum forced expiration. The FVC is often nearly the same as the vital capacity, but in airways obstruction it may be less because of premature airways closure. It is usual to record the best of three attempts and calculate the FEV_1/FVC ratio as a percentage. In healthy youth, the normal value is 80%, but this may decline to as little as 60% in old age. Normal values also vary with sex and race.

Obstructive ventilatory defect. When the FEV_1/FVC ratio is reduced this is referred to as an obstructive defect. Both values tend to be reduced, but the FEV_1 is disproportionately low. The causes are loss of elastic recoil or airways narrowing, as in asthma or chronic obstructive pulmonary disease.

[d] From the Greek word for falling, this was once mostly applied to the eyelid but now seems accepted as a description of the displacement of any organ.
[e] Hugh Pemberton (1891–1956), physician, Liverpool, UK.

Figure 4.10 Spirometry tracings

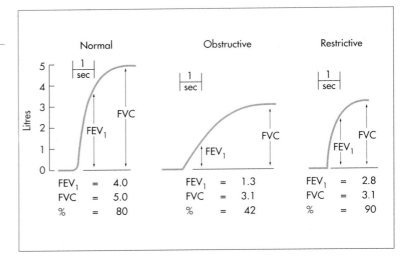

Restrictive ventilatory defect. When the FEV_1/FVC ratio is normal or higher than normal, but both values are reduced, the pattern is described as a restrictive defect. This occurs in parenchymal lung disease, such as pulmonary fibrosis, sarcoidosis, or when lung expansion is reduced by pneumonia or chest wall abnormalities.

Flow volume curve

As an alternative to spirometry, the flow volume curve may be measured using a portable electronic device. This measures expiratory and inspiratory flow as a function of exhaled volume rather than against time. It is a simple and reproducible test easily performed in the respiratory laboratory or at the bedside. The FVC, FEV_1 and various flow measurements (e.g. peak flow) can be calculated from the curve (Figure 4.11 a, b & c).

Correlation of physical signs and respiratory disease (Table 4.8)

Consolidation (lobar pneumonia)

Pneumonia is defined as inflammation of the lung which is characterised by exudation into the alveoli. Pneumonia may be classified on an anatomical basis into lobar, segmental or lobular pneumonia. The signs of lobar pneumonia are characteristic and are referred to clinically as consolidation.[14]

There may be a history of the sudden onset of malaise, chest pain, dyspnoea and fever. Patients may appear very ill and the vital signs, including the temperature, respiratory rate and blood pressure, must be recorded. There may be signs of cyanosis and exhaustion in sick patients.

Signs

- **Expansion:** reduced on the affected side.
- **Vocal fremitus:** increased on the affected side (in other chest disease this sign is of very little use!).
- **Percussion:** dull, but not stony dull.
- **Breath sounds:** bronchial.
- **Additional sounds:** medium, late or pan-inspiratory crackles as the pneumonia resolves.
- **Vocal resonance:** increased.
- **Pleural rub:** may be present.

See also *Good signs guide 4.3*.

Causes

- **Lobar pneumonia:** pneumococcal (90% of cases), *H. influenzae*, staphylococcal.
- **Bronchopneumonia (lobular):** bacteria—*H. influenzae* and *S. pneumoniae* (commonest), viruses such as influenza virus, adenovirus, measles virus, cytomegalovirus. In bronchopneumonia, crackles are often the only chest sign.
- **Primary atypical pneumonia:** *Mycoplasma pneumoniae* (majority), *Chlamydia psittaci*, *Legionella* spp, *Coxiella burnetii* (Q fever).

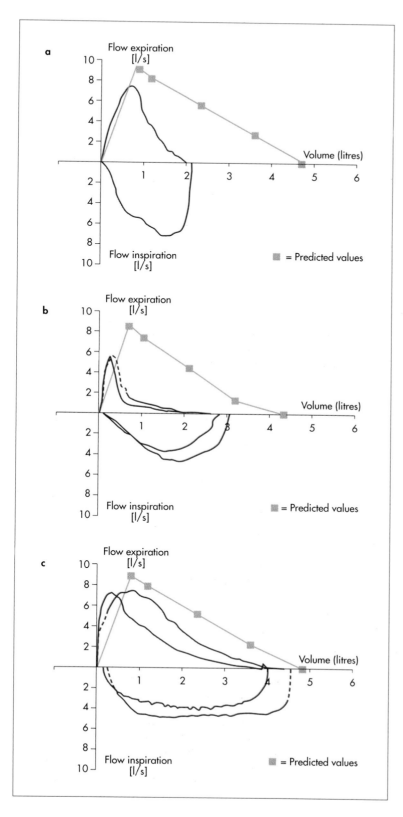

Figure 4.11 Flow volume curve

(a) Restrictive pattern. (b) Obstructive disease with minimal reversibility—chronic obstructive pulmonary disease. (c) Obstructive disease with significant reversibility—asthma.

Table 4.8 Comparison of the chest signs in common respiratory disorders

Disorder	Mediastinal displacement	Chest wall movement	Percussion note	Breath sounds	Added sounds
Consolidation	None	Reduced over affected area	Dull	Bronchial	Crackles
Collapse	Ipsilateral shift	Decreased over affected area	Dull	Absent or reduced	Absent
Pleural effusion	Heart displaced to opposite side (trachea displaced only if massive)	Reduced over affected area	Stony dull	Absent over fluid; may be bronchial at upper border	Absent; pleural rub may be found above effusion
Pneumothorax	Tracheal deviation to opposite side if under tension	Decreased over affected area	Resonant	Absent or greatly reduced	Absent
Bronchial asthma	None	Decreased symmetrically	Normal or decreased	Normal or reduced	Wheeze
Interstitial pulmonary fibrosis	None	Decreased symmetrically (minimal)	Normal unaffected by cough or posture	Normal	Fine, late or pan-inspiratory crackles over affected lobes

Collapse

If a bronchus is obstructed by a tumour mass, retained secretions or a foreign body, the air in the part of the lung supplied by the bronchus is absorbed and the affected part of the lung collapses.

Signs

- **Trachea:** displaced towards the collapsed side.
- **Expansion:** reduced on the affected side with flattening of the chest wall on the same side.
- **Percussion:** dull over the collapsed area.
- **Breath sounds:** reduced, with or without bronchial breathing above the area of collapse.

Note: (i) There may be no signs with complete lobar collapse; (ii) the early changes after the inhalation of a foreign body may be overinflation of the affected side.

Causes

- **Intraluminal:** mucus (e.g. postoperative, asthma, cystic fibrosis), foreign body, aspiration.
- **Mural:** bronchial carcinoma.
- **Extramural:** peribronchial lymphadenopathy, aortic aneurysm.

Pleural effusion

This is a collection of fluid in the pleural space. Note that pleural collections consisting of blood (haemothorax), chyle (chylothorax) or pus (empyema) have specific names, and are not called pleural effusions, although the physical signs are similar.

Signs

- **Trachea and apex beat:** displaced away from a massive effusion.

GOOD SIGNS GUIDE 4.3
Pneumonia

Sign	Positive LR	Negative LR
General appearance		
Cachexia	4.0	NS
Abnormal mental state	2.2	NS
Vital signs		
Temperature >37.8°C	2.2	0.7
Respiratory rate >28/minute	2.2	0.8
Heart rate >100 beats/minute	1.6	0.7
Lung findings		
Percussion dullness	3.0	NS
Reduced breath sounds	2.3	0.8
Bronchial breath sounds	3.3	NS
Aegophony	4.1	NS
Crackles	2.0	0.8
Wheezes	NS	NS

NS = not significant.

From McGee S, *Evidence-based physical diagnosis*, Saunders, 2001.

- **Expansion:** reduced on the affected side.
- **Percussion:** stony dullness over the fluid.
- **Breath sounds:** reduced or absent. There may be an area of bronchial breathing audible above the effusion due to compression of overlying lung.
- **Vocal resonance:** reduced.

Causes

- **Transudate** (less than 30 g of protein per litre of fluid): (i) cardiac failure; (ii) hypoalbuminaemia from the nephrotic syndrome or chronic liver disease; (iii) hypothyroidism; (iv) Meigs syndrome[f] (ovarian fibroma causing pleural effusion and ascites).
- **Exudate** (more than 30 g of protein per litre of fluid): (i) pneumonia; (ii) neoplasm—bronchial carcinoma, metastatic carcinoma, mesothelioma; (iii) tuberculosis; (iv) pulmonary infarction;

(v) subphrenic abscess; (vi) acute pancreatitis; (vii) connective tissue disease such as rheumatoid arthritis, systemic lupus erythematosus; (viii) drugs such as methysergide, cytotoxics; (ix) irradiation; (x) trauma.
- **Haemothorax** (blood in the pleural space): (i) severe trauma to the chest; (ii) rupture of a pleural adhesion containing a blood vessel.
- **Chylothorax** (milky-appearing pleural fluid due to leakage of lymph): (i) trauma or surgery to the thoracic duct; (ii) carcinoma or lymphoma involving the thoracic duct.
- **Empyema** (pus in the pleural space): (i) pneumonia; (ii) lung abscess; (iii) bronchiectasis; (iv) tuberculosis; (v) penetrating chest wound.

Yellow nail syndrome

This is a rare condition which is caused by hypoplasia of the lymphatic system. The nails are thickened and yellow (Figure 4.12) and there is separation of the distal nail plate from the nail bed (onycholysis). It may be associated with a pleural effusion and bronchiectasis, and usually with lymphoedema of the legs.

Pneumothorax

Leakage of air from the lung or a chest wall puncture into the pleural space causes a pneumothorax.

Signs

- **Expansion:** reduced on the affected side.
- **Percussion:** hyperresonance if the pneumothorax is large.
- **Breath sounds:** greatly reduced or absent.
- There may be subcutaneous emphysema.
- There may be no signs if the pneumothorax is small (less than 30%).

Causes

- **'Spontaneous':** (i) subpleural bullae rupture, usually in tall, healthy young males; (ii) emphysema with rupture of bullae, usually in middle-aged or elderly patients with generalised emphysema; (iii) rarely in asthma, lung abscess, bronchial carcinoma, eosinophilic granuloma, end-stage fibrosis or Marfan's syndrome; (iv) iatrogenic (caused by medical intervention), following the insertion of a central venous catheter.
- **Traumatic:** rib fracture, penetrating chest wall injury, or during pleural or pericardial aspiration.

---

[f] Joe Vincent Meigs (1892–1963), Professor of Gynaecology at Harvard, described this in 1937.

Figure 4.12 Yellow nail syndrome: (a) hands; (b) feet

(From FS McDonald, ed., *Mayo Clinic images in internal medicine*, with permission. © Mayo Clinic Scientific Press and CRC Press.)

Tension pneumothorax

This occurs when there is a communication between the lung and the pleural space, with a flap of tissue acting as a valve, allowing air to enter the pleural space during inspiration and preventing it from leaving during expiration. A tension pneumothorax results from air accumulating under increasing pressure in the pleural space; it causes considerable displacement of the mediastinum with obstruction and kinking of the great vessels, and represents a medical emergency.

Signs

- The patient is often tachypnoeic and cyanosed, and may be hypotensive.
- **Trachea and apex beat:** displaced away from the affected side.
- **Expansion:** reduced or absent on affected side.
- **Percussion:** hyperresonant over the affected side.
- **Breath sounds:** absent.
- **Vocal resonance:** absent.

Causes

- Trauma.
- Mechanical ventilation at high pressure.
- Spontaneous (rare cause of tension pneumothorax).

Bronchiectasis

This is a pathological dilatation of the bronchi, resulting in impaired clearance of mucus, and chronic infection. A history of chronic cough and purulent sputum since childhood is virtually diagnostic.

Signs

- **Systemic signs:** fever, cachexia; sinusitis (70%).
- Clubbing and cyanosis (if disease is severe).
- **Sputum:** voluminous, purulent, foul-smelling, sometimes bloodstained.
- Coarse pan-inspiratory or late inspiratory crackles over the affected lobe.
- **Signs of severe bronchiectasis:** very copious sputum and haemoptysis, clubbing, widespread crackles, signs of airways obstruction, signs of respiratory failure and cor pulmonale, signs of secondary amyloidosis (e.g. oedema from proteinuria, cardiac failure, enlarged liver and spleen, carpal tunnel syndrome).

Causes

- **Congenital:** (i) primary ciliary dyskinesia (including the immotile cilia syndrome); (ii) cystic fibrosis; (iii) congenital hypogammaglobulinaemia.
- **Acquired:** (i) infections in childhood, such as whooping cough, pneumonia or measles; (ii) localised disease such as a foreign body, a bronchial adenoma or tuberculosis; (iii) allergic bronchopulmonary aspergillosis—this causes proximal bronchiectasis.

Bronchial asthma

This may be defined as paroxysmal recurrent attacks of wheezing (or in childhood of cough) due to airways narrowing which changes in severity over short periods of time.

Signs

- Wheezing.
- Tachypnoea.
- Dry or productive cough.
- Tachycardia.
- Prolonged expiration.
- Prolonged forced expiratory time (decreased peak flow, decreased FEV_1).
- Use of accessory muscles of respiration.
- Hyperinflated chest (increased anteroposterior diameter with high shoulders and, on percussion, decreased liver dullness).
- Inspiratory and expiratory wheezes.
- **Signs of severe asthma:** appearance of exhaustion and fear, inability to speak because of breathlessness, drowsiness due to hypercapnia (preterminal), cyanosis (a very sinister sign), tachycardia (pulse above 130/minute correlates with significant hypoxaemia), pulsus paradoxus (more than 20 mmHg), reduced breath sounds or a 'silent' chest.

Chronic obstructive pulmonary disease (COPD, chronic airflow limitation)

This represents a spectrum of abnormalities: from predominantly emphysema, where there is pathologically an increase beyond normal in the size of the air spaces distal to the terminal bronchioles, to chronic bronchitis, where there is mucous gland hypertrophy, increased numbers of goblet cells and hypersecretion of mucus in the bronchial tree resulting in a chronic cough and sputum. Chronic obstructive pulmonary disease limitation does not cause clubbing or haemoptysis. Fifty per cent of patients with chronic bronchitis have emphysema, so there is often considerable overlapping of signs.[15]

The diagnosis can often be made on the basis of three findings:

1 A history of heavy smoking (more than 70 packet years).
2 Previous diagnosis of emphysema or COPD.
3 Reduced breath sounds.

If two or three of these are present, the positive LR of COPD is 25.7.

Emphysema

Signs

The patients are usually not cyanosed but are dyspnoeic and are sometimes called 'pink puffers'. The signs result from hyperinflation.

- Barrel-shaped chest with increased anteroposterior diameter.
- Pursed lip breathing (this occurs in emphysema and not in chronic bronchitis): expiration through partly closed lips increases the end-expiratory pressure and keeps airways open, helping to minimise air trapping.
- Use of accessory muscles of respiration and drawing in of the lower intercostal muscles with inspiration.
- **Palpation:** reduced expansion and a hyperinflated chest.
- **Percussion:** hyperresonant with decreased liver dullness.
- **Breath sounds:** decreased, early inspiratory crackles.
- Wheeze is often absent.
- Signs of right heart failure may occur, but only late in the course of the disease, when they usually indicate a preterminal state.

Causes of generalised emphysema

- Usually, smoking.
- Occasionally, alpha$_1$-antitrypsin deficiency.

Chronic bronchitis

This is defined clinically as the daily production of sputum for three months a year for at least two consecutive years.

Signs

The signs are the result of bronchial hypersecretion and airways obstruction.

- Loose cough and sputum (mucoid or mucopurulent).
- **Cyanosis:** these patients are sometimes called 'blue bloaters' because of cyanosis present in the latter stages, and because of associated oedema from right ventricular failure.
- **Palpation:** hyperinflated chest with reduced expansion.
- **Percussion:** increased resonance.
- **Breath sounds:** reduced with end-expiratory high or low-pitched wheezes and early inspiratory crackles.
- Signs of right ventricular failure.

Causes

Smoking is the major cause, but recurrent bronchial infection may cause progression of the disease.

Pulmonary fibrosis

Diffuse fibrosis of the lung parenchyma impairs gas transfer and causes ventilation–perfusion mismatching. It can result from inhalation of mineral dusts (focal fibrosis), replacement of lung tissue following disease which damages the lungs (e.g. tuberculosis) or interstitial disease (e.g. fibrosing alveolitis).

Signs

- **General:** dyspnoea, cyanosis and clubbing may be present.
- **Palpation:** expansion is slightly reduced.
- **Auscultation:** fine (Velcro-like) late inspiratory or pan-inspiratory crackles heard over the affected lobes.
- **Signs of associated connective tissue disease:** rheumatoid arthritis (page 240), systemic lupus erythematosus (page 245), scleroderma (page 247), Sjögren's[g] syndrome (page 217), polymyositis and dermatomyositis (page 355).

Causes

- **Upper lobe:** SCHART—S = silicosis (progressive massive fibrosis), sarcoidosis; C = coal workers' pneumoconiosis (progressive massive fibrosis); H = histiocytosis; A = ankylosing spondylitis, allergic bronchopulmonary aspergillosis; R = radiation; T = tuberculosis.
- **Lower lobe:** RASCO—R = rheumatoid arthritis; A = asbestosis; S = scleroderma; C = cryptogenic fibrosing alveolitis; O = other (drugs, e.g. busulphan, bleomycin, nitrofurantoin, hydralazine, methotrexate, amiodarone).

Tuberculosis

Primary tuberculosis

A Ghon[h] focus with hilar lymphadenopathy occurs usually in children.

Usually no abnormal chest signs are found, but segmental collapse, due to bronchial obstruction by the hilar lymph nodes, occasionally occurs.

Erythema nodosum (page 171) is an important associated sign, but is rare.

Post-primary tuberculosis

Reactivation of a primary lesion or occasionally reinfection are the causes of post-primary or adult tuberculosis. Immune suppression and malnutrition predispose to reactivation of tuberculosis.

There are often no chest signs. The clues to the diagnosis are the classical symptoms of cough, haemoptysis, weight loss, night sweats and malaise.

Miliary tuberculosis

Widespread haematogenous dissemination of tubercle bacilli causes multiple millet-seed tuberculous nodules in various organs—spleen, liver, lymph nodes, kidneys, brain or joints. Miliary tuberculosis may complicate both childhood and adult tuberculosis.

Fever, anaemia and cachexia are the general signs. The patient may also be dyspnoeic, and pleural effusions, lymphadenopathy, hepatosplenomegaly or signs of meningitis may be present.

Mediastinal compression

Mediastinal structures may be compressed by a variety of pathological masses, including carcinoma of the lung (90%), other tumours (lymphoma, thymoma, dermoid cyst), a large retrosternal goitre or rarely an aortic aneurysm.

Signs

- **Superior vena caval obstruction:**[i] the face is plethoric and cyanosed with periorbital oedema; the eyes may show exophthalmos, conjunctival injection, and venous dilatation in the fundi; in the neck the jugular venous pressure is raised but not pulsatile, the thyroid may be enlarged, there may be supraclavicular lymphadenopathy and a positive Pemberton's sign; the chest may show dilated collateral vessels, or signs of lung carcinoma.
- **Tracheal compression:** stridor, usually accompanied by respiratory distress.
- **Recurrent laryngeal nerve involvement:** hoarseness of the voice.
- **Horner's syndrome** (page 320).
- **Paralysis of the phrenic nerve:** dullness to percussion at the affected base, which does not change with deep inspiration (abnormal tidal percussion), and

---

[g] Henrik Samuel Conrad Sjögren (1899–1986), Stockholm ophthalmologist. He described the syndrome in 1933.

[h] Anton Ghon (1866–1936), Austrian pathologist and Professor of Anatomical Pathology in Prague. He described the lesion in 1912.

[i] First described by William Hunter (1718–83; brother of John Hunter) in a patient with a syphilitic aortic aneurysm.

absent breath sounds suggest a paralysed diaphragm due to phrenic nerve involvement.

Carcinoma of the lung

Many patients have no signs.

Respiratory signs

- Haemoptysis.
- Clubbing, sometimes with hypertrophic pulmonary osteoarthropathy (usually not small cell carcinoma).
- Lobar collapse or volume loss.
- Pneumonia.
- Pleural effusion.
- Fixed inspiratory wheeze.
- Tender ribs (secondary deposits of tumour in the ribs).
- Mediastinal compression, including signs of nerve involvement.
- Supraclavicular or axillary lymphadenopathy.

Distant metastases

Brain, liver and bone are the most commonly affected organs.

Non-metastatic extrapulmonary manifestations

- Anorexia, weight loss, cachexia, fever.
- **Endocrine changes:** (i) hypercalcaemia (page 271), due to secretion of parathyroid hormone-like substances, occurs in squamous cell carcinoma; (ii) hyponatraemia—antidiuretic hormone is released by small (oat) cell carcinomas; (iii) ectopic ACTH syndrome (small cell carcinoma); (iv) carcinoid syndrome (small cell carcinoma); (v) gynaecomastia (gonadotrophins—rare; more often squamous cell carcinoma); (vi) hypoglycaemia (insulin-like peptide from squamous cell carcinoma).
- **Neurological manifestations:** Eaton-Lambert[j] syndrome (progressive muscle weakness) and retinal blindness (small cell carcinoma), peripheral neuropathy, subacute cerebellar degeneration, polymyositis, cortical degeneration.
- **Haematological features:** migrating venous thrombophlebitis, disseminated intravascular coagulation, anaemia.
- **Skin:** acanthosis nigricans, dermatomyositis (rare).
- **Renal:** nephrotic syndrome due to membranous glomerulonephritis (rare).

---

[j] ML Eaton, 20th century American physician, and EH Lambert (b. 1915), American neurologist.

Sarcoidosis

This is a systemic disease, characterised by the presence of non-caseating granulomas which commonly affect the lungs, skin, eyes, lymph nodes, liver and spleen, and the nervous system. The aetiology is unknown.

Pulmonary signs

- **Lungs:** no signs usually, although 80% of patients have lung involvement. In severe disease there may be signs of pulmonary fibrosis.

Extrapulmonary signs

- **Skin:** lupus pernio (violaceous patches on the face, especially the nose, fingers or toes), pink nodules and plaques (granulomata) in old scars, erythema nodosum on the shins.
- **Eyes:** ciliary injection, anterior uveitis.
- **Lymph nodes:** generalised lymphadenopathy.
- **Liver and spleen:** enlarged (uncommon).
- **Parotids:** gland enlargement (uncommon) (page 142).
- **Central nervous system:** cranial nerve lesions, peripheral neuropathy (uncommon).
- **Musculoskeletal system:** arthralgia, swollen fingers, bone cysts (rare).
- **Heart:** heart block presenting as syncope, cor pulmonale (both rare).
- Signs of hypercalcaemia (page 272).

Pulmonary embolism

Embolism to the lungs often occurs without symptoms. One should always entertain this diagnosis if there has been sudden and unexplained dyspnoea. Pleuritic chest pain and haemoptysis occur only when there is infarction. Syncope or the sudden onset of severe substernal pain can occur with massive embolism.

- **General signs:** tachycardia, tachypnoea, fever (with infarction).
- **Lungs:** pleural friction rub if infarction has occurred.
- **Massive embolism:** elevated jugular venous pressure, right ventricular gallop, right ventricular heave, tricuspid regurgitation murmur, increased pulmonary component of the second heart sound.
- **Signs of deep venous thrombosis:** fewer than 50% of patients have clinical evidence of a source.

Note: A firm diagnosis cannot be made on the symptoms and signs alone.

The chest X-ray

The radiological appearance of a normal lung, with the lung segments labelled, is shown in Figure 4.13.

The radiological changes of consolidation, pleural effusion, pneumothorax and hydropneumothorax are shown in Figures 4.14 to 4.17.

A pulmonary mass is obvious in Figure 4.18, while multiple metastases are seen in Figure 4.19. Figure 4.20 illustrates the features of emphysema, and primary tuberculosis is shown in Figure 4.21.

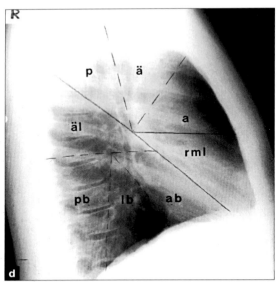

Figure 4.13 Lung segments

(a) Posteroanterior view. (b) CT scan through lung bases. (c) Left lateral view. (d) Right lateral view.

Right upper lobe: ä = apical segment; a = anterior segment, p = posterior segment.

Left upper lobe: ä-p = apico-posterior segment, s = anterior segment, sl = superior lingular segment, il = inferior lingular segment.

Right middle lobe (rml): m = medial segment, l = lateral segment.

Right lower lobe: äl = apical segment, mb = medial basal segment, lb = lateral basal segment, ab = anterior basal segment, pb = posterior basal segment.

Left lower lobe: äl = apical segment, lb = lateral basal segment, ab = anterior basal segment, pb = posterior basal segment.

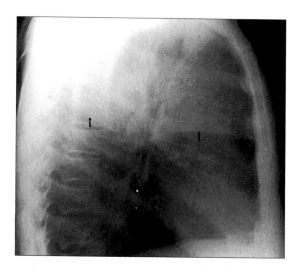

Figure 4.14 Right upper lobe consolidation

The right upper lobe is opacified and is limited inferiorly by the horizontal fissure (arrow). There must be some collapse as well, as the fissure shows some elevation. These changes could be due to a bacterial lobar pneumonia per se, but a central bronchostenotic lesion should be considered. If the pneumonia persists, a bronchoscopy is indicated to search for a central carcinoma.

Figure 4.15
Pleural effusion

The upper margin of the effusion is curved ('meniscus sign'). The left hemidiaphragm is not seen because there is no adjacent aerated lung for contrast. The heart shows some deviation to the right. It is unlikely that this is caused by an effusion of this size. It is probably related to the lower thoracic scoliosis.

Figure 4.16 Pneumothorax

(a) There is a massive right pneumothorax with collapsed lung seen against the hilum (arrow). There is increased translucency because of the absence of vascular shadows. (b) Different patient with a smaller pneumothorax. Small pneumothoraces are easier to see on an expiratory film as the pneumothorax volume remains constant, surrounding the partly deflated lung. The visceral pleural surface is marked (arrow).

Figure 4.18 A pulmonary mass

There is a large solitary mass lesion in the left lower zone. The differential diagnosis is primary or secondary neoplasm, hydatid cyst or large abscess. No air–fluid level is seen within it to indicate cavitation.

Figure 4.17 Hydropneumothorax

An air–fluid level is seen in the upper portion of the right hemithorax. When air and fluid are present in the pleural space, the fluid no longer forms a meniscus at its upper margin. Some aerated lung is seen deep to the fluid.

Figure 4.19 Pulmonary metastases

Multiple rounded opacities are seen in both lung fields, mainly at the left base and around the right hilum. The most likely cause is multiple pulmonary metastases. Other rare possibilities are hydatid cysts, large sarcoid nodules or large rheumatoid nodules. Multiple abscesses are extremely unlikely in the absence of cavitation.

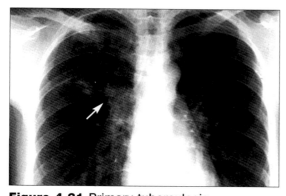

Figure 4.21 Primary tuberculosis

Two small rounded areas of shadowing are seen in the right upper zone (black arrows). The right hilum is enlarged by the enlarged draining lymph nodes (open arrow). This combination of focal shadowing and enlarged lymph nodes is the primary (Ghon) complex of tuberculosis. With healing, calcification may occur in the parenchymal and nodal lesions. In contrast, in tuberculosis reactivation or reinfection, cavitation may occur and there is no lymphadenopathy.

Figure 4.20 Emphysema

The lungs are overinflated with low, flat hemidiaphragms. The level of the hemidiaphragms is well below the anterior aspects of the sixth ribs. The diaphragm normally projects over the sixth rib anteriorly and the tenth intercostal space posteriorly. Count the ribs anteriorly (1–6). There is increased translucency of both upper zones with loss of the vascular markings due to bulla formation (arrow). This increased translucency is not due to overexposure. The hila are prominent because of the enlarged central pulmonary arteries. In contrast, the smaller peripheral pulmonary arteries (the lung markings) are decreased in size and number. This is due to actual destruction, displacement around bullae, and decreased perfusion through emphysematous areas.

Chest X-ray checklist

A – Airway (midline, no obvious deformities, no paratracheal masses).

B – Bones and soft tissue (no fractures, subcutaneous emphysema).

C – Cardiac size, silhouette and retrocardiac density normal.

D – Diaphragms (right above left by 1 cm to 3 cm, costophrenic angles sharp, diaphragmatic contrast with lung sharp).

E – Equal volume (count ribs, look for mediastinal shift).

F – Fine detail (pleura and lung parenchyma).

G – Gastric bubble (above the air bubble one shouldn't see an opacity of any more than 0.5 cm width).

H – Hilum (left normally above right by up to 3 cm, no larger than a thumb), hardware (in the intensive care unit: endotracheal tube, central venous catheters).

Examination of the breasts

Breast examination is a vitally important part of the general physical examination. When it is done properly, the examination takes some time to perform (about 3 minutes per breast). This must obviously be explained to the patient at the start. The examination is only just over 50% sensitive for carcinoma but specificity is as high as 90%. The likelihood ratio of a positive examination is 10.1 and the LR of a negative test is 0.47.[16]

Inspection

Ask the patient to sit up with her chest fully exposed. There is controversy about the value of inspection of the breasts as part of the examination but advanced cancers may be obvious at this stage. Look at the *nipples* for retraction (due to cancer or fibrosis; in some patients retraction may be normal) and Paget's disease of the nipple (where underlying breast cancer causes a unilateral red, bleeding area).

Next inspect the rest of the *skin*. Look for visible veins (which if unilateral suggest a cancer), skin dimpling, and for peau d'orange skin (where advanced breast cancer causes oedematous skin pitted by the sweat glands).

Ask the patient to *raise her arms above her head* and then lower them slowly. Look for tethering of the nipples or skin, a shift in the relative position of the nipples or a fixed mass distorting the breast (Figure 4.22). Also note whether there

Figure 4.22 Carcinoma of the right breast, showing elevation of the breast, dimpling of skin, and retraction of the nipple

are any masses in the axillae. Next ask her to rest her hands on her hips and then press her hands against her hips (the pectoral contraction manoeuvre). This accentuates areas of dimpling or fixation.

Palpation

Examine both the supraclavicular and axillary regions for lymphadenopathy (page 201). Then ask the patient to lie down. The examination can be performed only if the breast tissue is flattened against the chest wall. If the breasts are large, it can be helpful to have the patient place her hand on her forehead for the palpation of the lateral aspect of the breast and bring her elbow up level with the shoulder for the palpation of the medial side of the breast.

Palpation is performed gently with the pulps of the middle three fingers parallel to the contour of the breast. Feel the four quadrants of each breast systematically (Figure 4.23a). The total examination should involve a rectangular area bordered by the clavicle, sternum, mid-axillary line and the bra line. Start in the axilla and palpate in a line down to the bra line inferiorly. The pattern of palpation is like that of mowing a lawn, a series of vertical strips that cover the whole of the rectangle (Figure 4.23b). Each area is palpated three times, using small circular movements and slightly increasing pressure. Palpation is more difficult when a breast implant is present. It is probably best to examine such a patient in a supine position and to keep the ipsilateral arm down at her side.

Next feel behind the nipple for lumps and note if any fluid can be expressed: bright blood (from a duct papilloma, fibroadenosis or carcinoma), yellow serous (fibroadenosis) or serous fluid (early pregnancy), milky (lactation) or green fluid (mammary duct ectasia).

Evaluation of a breast lump

The following points need to be carefully elucidated if a lump is detected.

1   Position—the breast quadrant involved and proximity to the nipple.
2   Size, shape and consistency—a hard, irregular nodule is characteristic of carcinoma.
3   Tenderness—suggests an inflammatory or cystic lesion; breast cancer is usually not tender.
4   Fixation—mobility is determined by taking the breast between the hands and moving it over the chest wall; in advanced carcinoma the lump may be fixed to the chest wall.

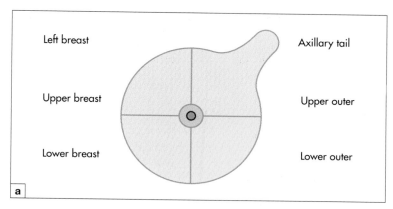

Left breast

Upper breast

Lower breast

Axillary tail

Upper outer

Lower outer

a

b

Figure 4.23 Examination of the breast: (a) quadrants; (b) systematic examination

---

GOOD SIGNS GUIDE 4.4
Breast lump characteristics and likelihood of cancer in a woman of average risk[16]

Sign	Positive LR
Mass	2.1
Fixed	2.4
Hard	1.6
Irregular	1.8
>2 cm diameter	1.9

From McGee S, *Evidence-based physical diagnosis*, Saunders, 2001.

5 Single or multiple lesions present—multiple nodules suggest benign cystic disease or fibro-adenosis.

Remember that many normal breasts have palpable lumps and that although benign lumps tend to be soft, moveable and regular, they can also have the characteristics of malignant lumps (*Good signs guide 4.4*). Causes of a lump in the breast are listed in Table 4.9. In men with true gynaecomastia a disc of breast tissue can be palpated under the areola. This is not present in men who are merely obese. Causes of breast enlargement in men are presented on page 275.

Table 4.9 Causes of a breast lump

Non-tender	Tender
Cyst	Cyst
Carcinoma	Breast abscess
Fibroadenosis (chronic mastitis)	Fibroadenosis
Fibroadenoma (benign highly	Costal cartilage
mobile 'breast mouse')	chondritis
Uncommon causes	Inflammatory breast cancer
• Trauma, fat necrosis	
• Other cysts—e.g. galactocele	
• Other neoplasms—e.g. duct papilloma	
• Chest wall—e.g. lipoma, costal cartilage chondritis	
(causes tenderness but not a lump) (Tietze's* disease)	

* Alexander Tietze (1864–1927), Chief Surgeon, Allerheiligen Hospital, Breslau, Poland. He described the condition in 1921.

Summary

The respiratory examination: a suggested method (Figure 4.24)

Undress the patient to the waist and sit him or her over the side of the bed. While standing back to make your usual inspection, ask if sputum is available for inspection. Purulent sputum always indicates respiratory infection, and a large volume of purulent sputum is an important clue to bronchiectasis. Haemoptysis is also an important sign. Look for dyspnoea at rest and count the respiratory rate. Note any paradoxical inward motion of the abdomen during inspiration (diaphragmatic paralysis). Look for use of the accessory muscles of respiration, and any intercostal indrawing of the lower ribs anteriorly (a sign of emphysema). General cachexia should also be noted.

Pick up the hands. Look for clubbing, peripheral cyanosis, tar staining and anaemia. Note any wasting of the small muscles of the hands and weakness of finger abduction (lung cancer involving the brachial plexus). Palpate the wrists for tenderness (hypertrophic pulmonary osteoarthropathy). While holding the hand, palpate the radial pulse for obvious pulsus paradoxus. Take the blood pressure if indicated.

Go on to the face. Look closely at the eyes for constriction of one of the pupils and for ptosis (Horner's syndrome from an apical lung cancer). Inspect the tongue for central cyanosis.

Palpate the position of the trachea. This is a most important sign, so spend time on it. If the trachea is displaced, you must concentrate on the upper lobes for physical signs. Also note the presence of a tracheal tug, which indicates severe airflow obstruction and feel for the use of the accessory muscles. Now ask the patient to speak (hoarseness) and then cough and note whether this is a loose cough, a dry cough or a bovine cough. Next measure the forced expiratory time (FET). Tell the patient to take a maximal inspiration and blow out as rapidly and forcefully as possible while you listen. Note audible wheeze and prolongation of the time beyond 3 seconds as evidence of chronic obstructive pulmonary disease.

The next step is to examine the chest. You may wish to examine the front first, or go to the back to start. The advantage of the latter is that there are often more signs there, unless the trachea is obviously displaced.

Inspect the back. Look for kyphoscoliosis. Do not miss ankylosing spondylitis, which causes decreased chest expansion and upper lobe fibrosis. Look for thoracotomy scars and prominent veins. Also note any skin changes from radiotherapy.

Palpate first from behind for the cervical nodes. Then examine for expansion—first upper lobe expansion, which is best seen by looking over the patient's shoulders at clavicular movement during moderate respiration. The affected side will show a delay or decreased movement. Then examine lower lobe expansion by palpation. Note asymmetry and reduction of movement.

Now ask the patient to bring his or her elbows together in the front to move the scapulae out of the way. Examine for vocal fremitus, then percuss the back of the chest.

Sitting up (if not acutely ill)

1. **General inspection**
   Sputum mug contents (blood, pus etc)
   Type of cough
   Rate and depth of respiration, and breathing pattern
       at rest
   Accessory muscles of respiration

2. **Hands**
   Clubbing
   Cyanosis (peripheral)
   Nicotine staining
   Wasting, weakness—finger abduction and adduction
       (lung cancer involving the brachial plexus)
   Wrist tenderness (hypertrophic pulmonary
       osteoarthropathy)
   Pulse (tachycardia, pulsus paradoxus)
   Flapping tremor (CO_2 narcosis)

3. **Face**
   Eyes—Horner's syndrome (apical lung cancer), anaemia
   Mouth—central cyanosis
   Voice—hoarseness (recurrent laryngeal nerve palsy)
   Facial plethora—smoker, SVC obstruction

4. **Trachea**

5. **Chest posteriorly**
   Inspect
   • Shape of chest and spine
   • Scars
   • Prominent veins (determine direction of flow)
   Palpate
   • Cervical lymph nodes
   • Expansion
   • Vocal fremitus

   Percuss
   • Supraclavicular region
   • Back
   • Axillae
   • Tidal percussion (diaphragm paralysis)
   Auscultate
   • Breath sounds
   • Adventitious sounds
   • Vocal resonance

6. **Chest anteriorly**
   Inspect
   • Radiotherapy marks, other signs as noted above
   Palpate
   • Supraclavicular nodes
   • Expansion
   • Vocal fremitus
   • Apex beat
   Percuss
   Auscultate
   Pemberton's sign (SVC obstruction)

7. **Cardiovascular system (lying at 45°)**
   Jugular venous pressure (SVC obstruction etc)
   Cor pulmonale

8. **Forced expiratory time**

9. **Other**
   Lower limbs—oedema, cyanosis
   Breasts
   Temperature chart (infection)
   Evidence of malignancy or pleural effusion: examine
       the breasts, abdomen, rectum, lymph nodes etc
   Respiratory rate after exercise

Figure 4.24 Respiratory system
SVC = superior vena cava.

Auscultate the chest. Note breath sounds (whether normal or bronchial) and their intensity (normal or reduced). Listen for adventitious sounds (crackles and wheezes). Finally examine for vocal resonance.

If a localised abnormality is found, try to determine the abnormal lobe and segment.

Return to the front of the chest. Inspect again for chest deformity, distended veins, radiotherapy changes and scars. Palpate the supraclavicular nodes carefully. Then proceed with percussion and auscultation as before. Listen high up in the axillae too. Before leaving the chest feel the axillary nodes and examine the breasts.

Lay the patient down at 45 degrees and measure the jugular venous pressure. Then examine the praecordium and lower limbs for signs of cor pulmonale. Finally examine the liver and take the temperature.

References

1. Schmitt BP, Kushner MS, Wiener SL. The diagnostic usefulness of the history of the patient with dyspnea. *J Gen Intern Med* 1986; 1:386–393. History alone was correct three out of four times when deciding the cause of dyspnoea in defined circumstances.
2. Anonymous. Obtaining an exposure history. Agency for Toxic Substances and Disease Registry. United States Department of Health and Human Services, Public Health Service, Atlanta, Georgia. *Am Fam Phys* 1993; 48:483–491.
3. Mulrow CD, Dolmatch BL, Delong ER et al. Observer variability in the pulmonary examination. *J Gen Intern Med* 1986; 1:364–367. Documents the poor reliability of many respiratory signs.
4. Model D. Smokers face: an underrated clinical sign? *BMJ* 1985; 291:1760–1762. A red face with leathery skin and excessive wrinkling, associated with a gaunt look, may help identify up to half of chronic smokers.
5. Williams JW Jnr, Simel DL, Roberts LR, Samsa GP. Clinical evaluation for sinusitis; making the diagnosis by history and physical examination. *Ann Intern Med* 1992; 117:705–710. The doctor's impression of the likelihood of sinusitis was superior to findings of a purulent nasal discharge, history of maxillary toothache, poor response to nasal decongestants and abnormal transillumination.
6. Kraman SS. Lung sounds for the clinician. *Arch Intern Med* 1986; 146:411–412. Describes the physiological evidence for many auscultatory findings.
7. Earis J. Lung sounds. *Thorax* 1992; 47:671–672.
8. Forgacs P. The functional basis of lung sounds. *Chest* 1978; 73:399–405.
9. Nath AR, Caple LH. Respiratory crackles: early and late. *Thorax* 1974; 29:223–227. Severe airways obstruction causes crackles in the first half of inspiration. In contrast, late crackles are not associated with airways obstruction.
10. Walshaw MJ, Nissa M, Pearson MG et al. Expiratory lung crackles in patients with fibrosing alveolitis. *Chest* 1990; 97:407–409. Inspiratory crackles are usually considered more important, but this report suggests that expiratory crackles occur intermittently in fibrosing alveolitis, usually in mid-expiration.
11. Shapira JD. About egophony. *Chest* 1995; 108:865–867.
12. Wallace C, Siminoski K. The Pemberton sign. *Ann Intern Med* 1996; 125:568–569. Discusses the mechanism of this useful sign, which is present when a large retrosternal goitre compresses the thoracic inlet.
13. Schapira RM, Schapira MM et al. The value of the forced expiratory time in the physical diagnosis of obstructive airways disease. *JAMA* 1993; 270:731–736. In patients with chronic obstructive airways who have a low pretest probability, an appropriate low-end cut-off is required (e.g. 3 seconds).
14. Metlay JP, Kappor WN, Fine MJ. Does this patient have community-acquired pneumonia? Diagnosing pneumonia by history and physical examination. *JAMA* 1997; 278:1440–1445. Normal vital signs and normal chest auscultation substantially reduce the likelihood of pneumonia, but a chest X-ray is required for a firm diagnosis.
15. Holloman DR, Simmel DL, Goldberg JS. Diagnosis of obstructive airways disease from the clinical examination. *J Gen Intern Med* 1993; 8:63–68. A history of smoking, self-reported wheezing and wheezing detected at auscultation combined had a high predictive value for chronic obstructive airways disease. The forced expiratory time added little additional information to these predictors
16. Barton MB, Harris R, Fletcher SW. Does this patient have breast cancer? *JAMA* 1999; 282:1270–1280. The clinical breast examination may have an overall specificity which is high (94%) but the sensitivity is poor (54%). Unfortunately interobserver variation seems to be high.

Suggested reading
Original and review articles

Byrd BF. Close-up: standard breast examination. *CA* 1974; 24:290–293.
Forgacs P. The functional basis of pulmonary sounds. *Chest* 1978; 73:399–405.
Hansen-Flaschen J, Nordberg J. Clubbing and hypertrophic osteoarthropathy. *Clin Chest Med* 1987; 8:287–298.
Kerlikowske K, Smith-Bindman R, Ljung BM et al. Evaluation of abnormal mammography results and palpable breast abnormalities. *Ann Intern Med* 2003; 139:274–284.
Light RW. Pleural effusion. *N Eng J Med* 2002; 346: 1971–1977.

Textbooks

Bourke SJ. *Lecture notes on respiratory disease*, 6th edn. Oxford: Blackwell, 2003.
James DG, Studdy PR. *Color atlas of respiratory diseases*, 2nd edn. Chicago: Mosby-Year Book, 1992.
Seaton A, Haslett C, Leitch AG, Seaton D, eds. *Crofton and Douglas's respiratory diseases*, 5th edn. Oxford: Blackwell, 2000.

chapter 5

The gastrointestinal system

To study the phenomena of disease without books is to sail an uncharted sea, while to study books without patients is not to go to sea at all.

Sir William Osler (1849–1919)

This lord wears his wit in his belly, and his guts in his head.

William Shakespeare, Troilus and Cressida

Gastroenterologists and gastrointestinal surgeons concern themselves with the entire length of the gut, the liver, the exocrine pancreas and the peripheral effects of alimentary disease.

The gastrointestinal history

Presenting symptoms (Table 5.1)

Abdominal pain

There are many causes of abdominal pain, and careful history taking will often lead to the correct diagnosis. The following should be considered.

Frequency and duration. Try to determine whether the pain is acute or chronic, when it began and how often it occurs.

Site and radiation. The site of pain is important. Ask the patient to point to the area affected by pain and to the point of maximum intensity. Parietal peritoneal inflammation that causes pain usually does so in a localised area. Ask about radiation of pain. Pain often radiates through to the back with pancreatic disease or a penetrating peptic ulcer. It may radiate to the shoulder with diaphragmatic irritation or to the neck with oesophageal reflux.

Table 5.1 Gastrointestinal history
Major symptoms
Abdominal pain
Appetite and/or weight change
Postprandial fullness or early satiation, or both
Nausea and/or vomiting
Heartburn and/or acid regurgitation
Waterbrash
Dysphagia
Disturbed defecation (diarrhoea, constipation, faecal incontinence)
Bloating or visible distension, or both
Bleeding (haematemesis, melaena, rectal bleeding)
Jaundice
Dark urine, pale stools
Pruritus
Lethargy
Fever

Character and pattern. The pain may be colicky (coming and going in waves and related to peristaltic movements) or steady. Colicky pain comes from obstruction of the bowel or the ureters. If the pain is chronic, ask about the daily pattern of pain.

Aggravating and relieving factors. Pain due to peptic ulceration may or may not be related to meals. Eating may precipitate ischaemic pain in the gut. Antacids or vomiting may relieve peptic ulcer pain or that of gastro-oesophageal reflux. Defecation or passage of flatus may relieve the pain of colonic disease temporarily. Patients who get some relief by rolling around vigorously are more likely to have a colicky pain, while those who lie perfectly still are more likely to have peritonitis.

Patterns of pain

Peptic ulcer disease. This is classically a dull or burning pain in the epigastrium that is relieved to a degree by food or antacids. It is typically episodic and may occur at night, waking the patient from sleep. This combination of symptoms is suggestive of the diagnosis. The pain is often unrelated to meals, despite classical teaching to the contrary. It is not possible to distinguish duodenal ulceration from gastric ulceration clinically.

Pancreatic pain. This is a steady epigastric pain that may be partly relieved by sitting up and leaning forwards. There is often radiation of the pain to the back, and vomiting is common.

Biliary pain. Although usually called 'biliary colic', this pain is rarely colicky. With cystic duct obstruction there is often epigastric pain. It is usually a severe, constant pain that can last for hours. There may be a history of episodes of similar pain in the past. If cholecystitis develops, the pain typically shifts to the right upper quadrant and becomes more severe.

Renal colic. This is a colicky pain superimposed on a background of constant pain in the renal angle, often with radiation towards the groin. It can be very severe indeed.

Bowel obstruction. This is colicky pain. Periumbilical pain suggests a small bowel origin but colonic pain can occur anywhere in the abdomen. Small bowel obstruction tends to cause more frequent colicky pain (with a cycle every 2 to 3 minutes) than large bowel obstruction (every 10 to 15 minutes). Obstruction is often associated with vomiting, constipation and abdominal distension.

Appetite and weight change

Loss of appetite (anorexia) and weight loss are important gastrointestinal symptoms. The presence of both anorexia and weight loss should make one suspicious of an underlying malignancy, but may also occur with depression and in other diseases (page 257). The combination of weight loss with an increased appetite suggests malabsorption of nutrients or a hypermetabolic state (e.g. thyrotoxicosis). It is important to document when the symptoms began and how much weight loss has occurred over this period. Liver disease can sometimes cause disturbance of taste. This may cause smokers with acute hepatitis and jaundice to give up smoking.

Early satiation and postprandial fullness

Inability to finish a normal meal (early satiation) may be a symptom of gastric diseases, including gastric cancer and peptic ulcer. A feeling of inappropriate fullness after eating can also be a symptom of functional gastrointestinal disease.

Nausea and vomiting

Nausea is the sensation of wanting to vomit. Heaving and retching may occur but there is no expulsion of gastric contents. There are many possible causes for these complaints. Gastrointestinal tract infections (e.g. from food poisoning by *Staphylococcus aureus*) or small bowel obstruction can cause acute symptoms. In patients with chronic symptoms, pregnancy and drugs (e.g. digoxin, opiates, dopamine agonists, chemotherapy) should always be ruled out. In the gastrointestinal tract, peptic ulcer disease with gastric outlet obstruction, motor disorders (e.g. gastroparesis from diabetes mellitus, or after gastric surgery), acute hepatobiliary disease and alcoholism are important causes. Finally, psychogenic vomiting, eating disorders (e.g. bulimia) and, rarely, increased intracranial pressure should be considered in patients with chronic unexplained nausea and vomiting.

The timing of the vomiting can be helpful; vomiting delayed more than 1 hour after the meal is typical of gastric outlet obstruction or gastroparesis, while early morning vomiting before eating is characteristic of pregnancy, alcoholism and raised intracranial pressure. Also ask about the contents of the vomitus (e.g. bile indicates an open connection between the duodenum and stomach, old food suggests gastric outlet obstruction, while blood suggests ulceration).

Heartburn and acid regurgitation

Heartburn refers to the presence of a burning pain or discomfort in the retrosternal area. Typically, this sensation travels up towards the throat and occurs after meals or is aggravated by bending, stooping or lying supine. Antacids usually relieve the pain, at least transiently. This symptom is due to regurgitation of stomach contents into the oesophagus. Usually these contents are acidic, although occasionally alkaline reflux can induce similar problems. Associated with gastro-oesophageal reflux may be *acid regurgitation,* in which the patient experiences a sour or bitter tasting fluid coming up into the mouth. This symptom strongly suggests that reflux is occurring. In patients with gastro-oesophageal reflux disease, the lower oesophageal sphincter muscle relaxes inappropriately. Reflux symptoms may be aggravated by alcohol, chocolate, caffeine, a fatty meal, theophylline, calcium channel blockers and anticholinergic drugs, as these lower the oesophageal sphincter pressure.

Waterbrash refers to excessive secretion of saliva into the mouth and should not be confused with regurgitation; it may occur, uncommonly, in patients with peptic ulcer disease or oesophagitis.

Dysphagia

Dysphagia is difficulty in swallowing. Such difficulty may occur with solids or liquids. The causes of dysphagia are listed in Table 5.2. If a patient complains of difficulty swallowing, it is important to differentiate painful swallowing from actual difficulty.[1] Painful swallowing is termed odynophagia and occurs with any severe inflammatory process involving the oesophagus. Causes include infectious oesophagitis (e.g. *Candida,* herpes simplex), peptic ulceration of the oesophagus, caustic damage to the oesophagus or oesophageal perforation.

If the patient complains of difficulty initiating swallowing, fluid regurgitating into the nose or choking on trying to swallow, this suggests that the cause of the dysphagia is in the pharynx (pharyngeal dysphagia). Causes of pharyngeal dysphagia can include neurological disease (e.g. motor neurone disease, resulting in bulbar or pseudobulbar palsy, see page 317).

If the patient complains of food sticking in the oesophagus, it is important to consider a number of anatomical causes of oesophageal blockage.[1] Ask the patient to point to the site where the solids stick. If there is a mechanical obstruction at the lower end of the oesophagus, most often the patient will localise the dysphagia to the lower retrosternal area. However, obstruction higher in the oesophagus may be felt anywhere in the retrosternal area. If heartburn is also present, for example, this suggests that gastro-oesophageal reflux with or without stricture formation may be the cause of the dysphagia. The actual course of the dysphagia is also a very important part of the history to obtain. If the patient states that the dysphagia is intermittent or is present only with the first few swallows of food, this suggests either a lower oesophageal ring or oesophageal

Table 5.2 Causes of dysphagia

Mechanical obstruction

Intrinsic (within oesophagus)
Reflux oesophagitis with stricture formation
Carcinoma of oesophagus or gastric cardia
Pharyngeal or oesophageal web
Pharyngeal pouch
Schatzki (lower oesophageal) ring
Foreign body

Extrinsic (outside oesophagus)
Goitre with retrosternal extension
Mediastinal tumours, bronchial carcinoma,
  vascular compression (rare)

Neuromuscular motility disorders (hints from the history: solids and liquids equally difficult, symptoms intermittent)

Achalasia
Diffuse oesophageal spasm
Scleroderma

Pharyngeal dysphagia (hints: aspiration, fluid regurgitation into the nose)

Cricopharyngeal dysfunction—Zenker's
  diverticulum
Neurological diseases: bulbar or
  pseudobulbar palsy, myasthenia gravis,
  polymyositis, myotonic dystrophy

spasm. However, if the patient complains of progressive difficulty swallowing, this suggests a stricture, carcinoma or achalasia. If the patient states that both solids and liquids stick, then a motor disorder of the oesophagus is more likely, such as achalasia or diffuse oesophageal spasm.

Diarrhoea

The symptom diarrhoea can be defined in a number of different ways. Patients may complain of frequent stools (more than three per day being abnormal) or they may complain of a change in the consistency of the stools, which have become loose or watery. There are a large number of possible causes of diarrhoea.

Some patients pass small amounts of formed stool more than three times a day because of an increased desire to defecate. The stools are not loose and stool volume is not increased. This is not true diarrhoea. It can occur because of local rectal pathology, incomplete rectal emptying, or because of a psychological disturbance that leads to an increased interest in defecation.

When a history of diarrhoea is obtained, it is also important to determine if this has occurred acutely or whether it is a chronic problem. Acute diarrhoea is more likely to be infectious in nature, while chronic diarrhoea has a large number of causes.

Clinically, diarrhoea can be divided into a number of different groups based on the likely disturbance of physiology.

1 *Secretory diarrhoea* is likely if the diarrhoea is of high volume (commonly more than one litre per day) and persists when the patient fasts; there is no pus or blood, and the stools are not excessively fatty. Secretory diarrhoea occurs when net secretion in the colon or small bowel exceeds absorption; some of the causes include infections (e.g. *E. coli*, *Staphylococcus aureus*, *Vibrio cholerae*), hormonal conditions (e.g. vasoactive intestinal polypeptide-secreting tumour, Zollinger-Ellison[a] syndrome, carcinoid syndrome) and villous adenoma.

2 *Osmotic diarrhoea* is characterised by its disappearance with fasting and by large volume stools related to the ingestion of food. Osmotic diarrhoea occurs due to excessive solute drag; causes include lactose intolerance (disaccharidase deficiency), magnesium antacids or gastric surgery.

3 *Abnormal intestinal motility* (e.g. thyrotoxicosis, the irritable bowel syndrome) can also cause diarrhoea.

4 *Exudative diarrhoea* occurs when there is inflammation in the colon. Typically the stools are of small volume but frequent, and there may be associated blood or mucus (e.g. inflammatory bowel disease, colon cancer).

5 *Malabsorption* of nutrients can result in steatorrhoea. Here the stools are fatty, pale coloured, extremely smelly, float in the toilet bowel and are difficult to flush away. Steatorrhoea is defined as the presence of more than 7 g of fat in a 24-hour stool collection. There are many causes of steatorrhoea (page 170).

Constipation

It is important to determine what patients mean if they say they are constipated. Constipation is a common symptom and can refer to the passage of infrequent stools (fewer than three times per week), hard stools or stools that are difficult to evacuate. This symptom may occur acutely or may be a chronic problem. In many patients, chronic constipation arises because of habitual neglect of the impulse to defecate, leading to the accumulation of large, dry faecal masses. With constant rectal distension from faeces, the patient may grow less aware of rectal fullness, leading to chronic constipation. Constipation may arise from ingestion of drugs (e.g. codeine, antidepressants and aluminium or calcium antacids), and with various metabolic or endocrine diseases (e.g. hypothyroidism, hypercalcaemia, diabetes mellitus, phaeochromocytoma, porphyria, hypokalaemia) and neurological disorders (e.g. aganglionosis, Hirschsprung's[b] disease, autonomic neuropathy, spinal cord injury, multiple sclerosis). Constipation can also arise after partial colonic obstruction from carcinoma; it is, therefore, very important to determine whether there has been a recent change in bowel habit, as this may indicate development of a malignancy. Patients with very severe constipation in the absence of structural disease may be found on a transit study to have slow colonic transit; such slow-transit constipation is most common in young women.

Difficulty with evacuation of faeces may occur with disorders of the pelvic floor muscles or nerves, or anorectal disease (e.g. fissure, or stricture). Patients with this problem may complain of straining, a feeling of anal blockage or even the need to self-digitate.

A chronic but erratic disturbance in defecation (typically alternating constipation and diarrhoea) associated with abdominal pain, in the absence of any structural or biochemical abnormality, is very common; such patients are classified as having the *irritable bowel syndrome*. Patients who report abdominal pain plus two or more of the following symptoms—abdominal pain relieved by defecation, looser or more frequent stools with the onset of abdominal pain, passage of mucus per rectum, a feeling of incomplete emptying of the rectum following defecation and visible abdominal distension—are more likely to have the irritable bowel syndrome than organic disease.

Mucus

The passage of mucus (white slime) may occur because of a solitary rectal ulcer, fistula or villous adenoma, or in the irritable bowel syndrome.

---

[a] Robert Milton Zollinger (b. 1903), American surgeon, and Edwin H Ellison (b. 1918), American physician. This syndrome is characterised by gastric acid hypersecretion, peptic ulceration and in 40% of cases diarrhoea, due to a gastrinoma (gastrin-secreting tumour). It was described in 1955.

[b] Harold Hirschsprung (1830–1916), physician, Queen Louise Hospital for Children, Copenhagen, described this disease in 1888. It had previously been described by Caleb Parry, English physician, in 1825.

Bleeding

Patients may present with the problem of haematemesis (vomiting blood), melaena (passage of jet black stools) or haematochezia (passage of bright red blood per rectum). Sometimes patients may present because routine testing for occult blood in the stools is positive (page 162). It is important to ensure that if vomiting of blood is reported, this is not the result of bleeding from a tooth socket or the nose, or coughing up of blood. Haematemesis indicates that the site of the bleeding is proximal to or at the duodenum. Ask about symptoms of peptic ulceration; haematemesis is commonly due to bleeding chronic peptic ulceration, particularly from a duodenal ulcer. Acute peptic ulcers often bleed without abdominal pain. A Mallory-Weiss tear usually occurs with repeated vomiting; typically the patient reports first the vomiting of clear gastric contents and then the vomiting of blood. Less common causes of upper gastrointestinal bleeding are presented in Table 5.3.

Haemorrhoids and local anorectal diseases such as fissures will commonly present with passing small amounts of bright red blood per rectum. The blood is normally not mixed in the stools but is on the toilet paper, on top of the stools or in the toilet bowl. Melaena usually results from bleeding from the upper gastrointestinal tract, although right-sided colonic and small bowel lesions can occasionally be responsible. Massive rectal bleeding can occur from the distal colon or rectum, or from a major bleeding site higher in the gastrointestinal tract. With substantial lower gastrointestinal tract bleeding, it is important to consider the presence of angiodysplasia or diverticular disease (where bleeding more often occurs from the right rather than the left colon, even though diverticula are more common in the left colon). Less common causes of lower gastrointestinal bleeding are presented in Table 5.3.

Spontaneous bleeding into the skin, or from the nose or mouth, can be a problem for patients with coagulopathy resulting from liver disease.

Jaundice

Usually the relatives notice a yellow discoloration of the sclera or skin before the patient does. Jaundice is due to the presence of excess bilirubin being deposited in the sclera and skin. The causes of jaundice are described on page 164. If there is jaundice, ask about the colour of the urine and stools; pale stools and dark urine occur with obstructive or cholestatic jaundice because urobilinogen is unable to reach the intestine. Also ask about abdominal pain; gallstones, for example, can cause biliary pain and jaundice.[2]

Table 5.3 Causes of acute gastrointestinal bleeding

Upper gastrointestinal tract

More common
1. Chronic peptic ulcer: duodenal ulcer (40%), gastric ulcer
2. Acute peptic ulcer (erosions)

Less common
3. Mallory-Weiss* syndrome (tear at the gastro-oesophageal junction)
4. Oesophageal and/or gastric varices
5. Erosive or ulcerative oesophagitis
6. Gastric carcinoma, polyp, other tumours
7. Dieulafoy's[†] ulcer (single defect that involves an ectatic submucosal artery)
8. Watermelon stomach (antral vascular ectasias)
9. Aortoenteric fistula (usually aortoduodenal and after aortic surgery)
10. Vascular anomalies—angiodysplasia, arteriovenous malformations, blue rubber bleb naevus syndrome, hereditary haemorrhagic telangiectasia, CRST syndrome
11. Pseudoxanthoma elasticum, Ehlers-Danlos[‡] syndrome
12. Amyloidosis
13. Vasculitis
14. Ménétrier's[§] disease
15. Bleeding diathesis
16. Pseudohaematemesis (nasopharyngeal origin)

Lower gastrointestinal tract

More common
1. Angiodysplasia
2. Diverticular disease
3. Colonic carcinoma or polyp
4. Haemorrhoids or anal fissure

Less common
5. Massive upper gastrointestinal bleeding
6. Inflammatory bowel disease
7. Ischaemic colitis
8. Meckel's[#] diverticulum
9. Small bowel disease, e.g. tumour, diverticula, intussusception
10. Haemobilia (bleeding from the gallbladder)
11. Solitary colonic ulcer

---

* George Kenneth Mallory (b. 1900), Professor of Pathology, Boston, and Soma Weiss (1898–1942), Professor of Medicine, Boston City Hospital. They described this syndrome in 1929.
† Georges Dieulafoy (1839–1911), Paris physician.
‡ Edvard Ehlers (1863–1937), German dermatologist, described the syndrome in 1901, and Henri Alexandre Danlos (1844–1912), French dermatologist, described the syndrome in 1908.
§ Pierre Ménétrier (1859–1935), French physician.
# Johann Friedrich Meckel the younger (1781–1833), Professor of Surgery and Anatomy at Halle. His father and grandfather were also professors of anatomy.

CRST = calcinosis, Raynaud's phenomenon, sclerodactyly and telangiectasia.

Figure 5.1 Ehlers-Danlos syndrome: (a) arms; (b) hands

Abnormal elasticity of the skin is typical of the Ehlers-Danlos syndrome. The skin may be greatly stretched and takes much longer than normal to return to its normal position. It is also more fragile than normal. Joint hypermobility occurs in type III Ehlers-Danlos syndrome.

Pruritus

This symptom means itching of the skin and may be either generalised or localised. Cholestatic liver disease can cause pruritus which tends to be worse over the extremities. Other causes of pruritus are discussed on page 388.

Abdominal bloating and swelling

A feeling of swelling (bloating) may be a result of excess gas or a hypersensitive intestinal tract (as occurs in the irritable bowel syndrome). Persistent swelling can be due to ascitic fluid accumulation; this is discussed on page 155. It may be associated with ankle oedema.

Lethargy

Tiredness and easy fatiguability are common symptoms for patients with acute or chronic liver disease, but the mechanism is not known. This can also occur because of anaemia due to gastrointestinal or chronic inflammatory disease. Lethargy is also very common in the general population and is not a specific symptom.

Treatment

The treatment history is very important. Traditional non-steroidal anti-inflammatory drugs (NSAIDs), including aspirin, can induce bleeding from acute or chronic damage to the gastrointestinal tract. As described above, many drugs can result in disturbed defecation. A large number of drugs are also known to affect the liver. For example, acute hepatitis can occur with halothane, phenytoin or chlorothiazide. Cholestasis may occur from a hypersensitivity reaction to chlorpromazine or other phenothiazines, sulphonamides, sulphonylureas, phenylbutazone, rifampicin or nitrofurantoin. Anabolic steroids and the contraceptive pill can cause dose-related cholestasis. Fatty liver can occur with alcohol use, tetracycline, valproic acid or amiodarone. Large blood-filled cavities in the liver called peliosis hepatis can occur with anabolic steroid use or the contraceptive pill. Acute liver cell necrosis can occur if an overdose of paracetamol (acetaminophen) is taken.

Past history

Surgical procedures can result in jaundice from the anaesthesia (e.g. multiple uses of halothane), hypoxaemia of liver cells (hypotension during the operative or postoperative period) or direct damage to the bile duct during abdominal surgery. A history of relapsing and remitting epigastric pain in a patient who presents with severe abdominal pain may indicate that a peptic ulcer has perforated. A past history of inflammatory bowel disease (either ulcerative colitis or Crohn's disease) is important as these are chronic diseases that tend to flare up.

Social history

The patient's occupation may be relevant (e.g. healthcare workers may be exposed to hepatitis). Toxin exposure can also be important in chronic liver disease (e.g. carbon tetrachloride, vinyl chloride). If a patient has symptoms suggestive of liver disease, ask about recent travel to countries where hepatitis is endemic.

The alcohol history is very important, particularly as alcoholics often deny or understate the amount they consume (see Table 1.3).[3] Contact with anybody who has been jaundiced should always be noted. The sexual history should be obtained. A history of any injections (e.g. intravenous drugs, plasma transfusions, dental treatment or tattooing) in a patient who presents with symptoms of liver disease is important, particularly as hepatitis B or C may be transferred in this way.

Family history

A family history of colon cancer or inflammatory bowel disease is important. A positive family history of jaundice, anaemia, splenectomy or cholecystectomy may occur in patients with haemolytic anaemia or congenital or familial hyperbilirubinaemia.

The gastrointestinal examination

Examination of the gastrointestinal system includes a complete examination of the abdomen. It is also important to search for the peripheral signs of gastrointestinal and liver disease. Some signs are more useful than others.[4]

Positioning the patient

For the proper examination of the abdomen it is important that the patient be lying flat with the head resting on a single pillow (Figure 5.2). This relaxes the abdominal muscles and facilitates abdominal palpation. Helping the patient into this position affords the opportunity to make a general inspection.

General appearance

Jaundice

The yellow discoloration of the sclerae (conjunctivae) and the skin that results from hyperbilirubinaemia is best observed in natural daylight (page 164). Whatever the underlying cause, the depth of jaundice can be quite variable.

Weight and wasting

The patient's weight must be recorded. Failure of the gastrointestinal tract to absorb food normally may lead to loss of weight and cachexia. This may also be the result of gastrointestinal malignancy or alcoholic cirrhosis. Folds of loose skin may be visible hanging from the abdomen and limbs. These suggest recent weight loss. Obesity can cause fatty infiltration of the liver (non-alcoholic steatohepatitis) and result in abnormal liver function tests. Anabolic steroid use can induce increase in muscle bulk (sometimes considered desirable) and various liver tumours, including adenomas or hepatocellular carcinomas.

Skin

The gastrointestinal tract and the skin have a common origin from the embryoblast. A number of diseases can present with both skin and gut involvement (Table 5.4, Figures 5.3–5.10).[5]

Pigmentation. Generalised skin pigmentation can result from chronic liver disease, especially in haemochromatosis (due to haemosiderin-stimulating melanocytes, to produce melanin). Malabsorption may result in Addisonian-type pigmentation ('sunkissed' pigmentation) of the nipples, palmar creases, pressure areas and mouth (page 271).

Figure 5.2 Gastrointestinal examination: positioning the patient

Table 5.4 The skin and the gut

Disease	Skin	Gut	Other associations
Gastrointestinal polyposis syndromes			
Peutz–Jeghers syndrome (autosomal dominant)	Pigmented macules on hands, feet, lips	Hamartomatous polyps (rarely adenocarcinoma) in stomach, small bowel, large bowel	
Gardner's* syndrome (autosomal dominant)	Cysts, fibromas, lipomas (multiple)	Polyps, adenocarcinoma in large bowel	Bone osteomata
Cronkhite–Canada syndrome	Alopecia, hyperpigmentation, glossitis, dystrophic nails	Hamartomatous polyps, diarrhoea, exocrine pancreatic insufficiency	
Hormone-secreting tumours			
Carcinoid syndrome	Flushing, telangiectases	Watery diarrhoea, hepatomegaly	Wheeze, right heat murmurs
Systemic mastocytosis (due to mast cell proliferation and histamine release)	Telangiectases, flushing, pigmented papules, pruritus, dermographism, Darier's† sign (rub skin lesion with the blunt end of a pen: a palpable red wheal occurs minutes later)	Peptic ulcer, diarrhoea, malabsorption	Asthma, headache, tachycardia
Glucagonoma (glucagon-secreting tumour)	Migratory necrolytic rash (on flexural and friction areas)	Glossitis, weight loss, diabetes mellitus	
Vascular disorders			
Hereditary haemorrhagic telangiectasia (autosomal dominant)	Telangiectases (especially nail beds, palms, feet)	Gastrointestinal bleeding	Nasopharyngeal bleeding, pulmonary arteriovenous fistulas, high output cardiac failure
Pseudoxanthoma elasticum (autosomal recessive)	Yellow plaques/papules in flexural areas	Bowel bleeding, ischaemia	Angioid streaks in fundus
Blue rubber bleb syndrome	Hemangiomas (e.g. tongue)	Bleeding into bowel or liver	
Degos' disease (malignant atrophic papulosis)	Dome-shaped red papules (early), small porcelain white atrophic scars (late)	Intestinal perforation, infarction (primarily in young men—very rare)	

Table 5.4 (continued)

Disease	Skin	Gut	Other associations
Vascular disorders (continued)			
Acanthosis nigricans	Brown to black skin papillomas (usually axillae)	Carcinoma	Acromegaly, diabetes mellitus
Dermatitis herpetiformis	Pruritic vesicles—typically on knees, elbows, buttocks	Coeliac disease	
Zinc deficiency	Red, scaly, crusting lesions around mouth, eyes, genitalia; white patches on tongue	Diarrhoea (zinc deficiency occurs particularly in setting of Crohn's disease with fistulas, cirrhosis, parenteral nutrition, pancreatitis)	
Porphyria cutanea tarda	Vesicles on exposed skin (e.g. hands)	Alcoholic liver disease	
Inflammatory bowel disease	Pyoderma gangrenosum Erythema nodosum Clubbing Mouth ulcers		
Haemochromatosis (autosomal recessive)	Skin pigmentation (bronze)	Hepatomegaly, signs of chronic liver disease	Diabetes mellitus, heart failure (cardiomyopathy), arthropathy, testicular atrophy
Systemic sclerosis	Skin that is thick and bound down, calcinosis, Raynaud's[‡] phenomenon, sclerodactyly, telangiectases	Gastro-oesophageal reflux, oesophageal dysmotility, small bowel bacterial overgrowth with malabsorption	

* Eldon John Gardner (b. 1909), American geneticist.
† Ferdinand Jean Darier (1856–1938), Paris dermatologist.
‡ Maurice Raynaud (1834–1881), Paris physician.

Figure 5.3 Hyperpigmentation in Cronkhite-Canada syndrome

(From FS McDonald, ed., *Mayo Clinic images in internal medicine*, with permission. © Mayo Clinic Scientific Press and CRC Press.)

Figure 5.5 Glucagonoma: migratory rash involving the groin

(From FS McDonald, ed., *Mayo Clinic images in internal medicine*, with permission. © Mayo Clinic Scientific Press and CRC Press.)

Figure 5.4 Carcinoid syndrome involving the chest and abdomen

(From FS McDonald, ed., *Mayo Clinic images in internal medicine*, with permission. © Mayo Clinic Scientific Press and CRC Press.)

Figure 5.6 Dermatitis herpetiformis

(From FS McDonald, ed., *Mayo Clinic images in internal medicine*, with permission. © Mayo Clinic Scientific Press and CRC Press.)

Figure 5.7 Peutz-Jeghers syndrome, with discrete brown-black lesions of the lips

(Figure 5.7a from Jones DV et al, in Feldman M et al, *Sleisenger & Fordtran's gastrointestinal disease,* 6th edn, Chapter 112. Philadelphia: WB Saunders, 1998, with permission. Figure 5.7b from FS McDonald, ed., *Mayo Clinic images in internal medicine*, with permission. © Mayo Clinic Scientific Press and CRC Press.)

Figure 5.8 Acanthosis nigricans: (a) axilla; (b) chest wall

(From FS McDonald, ed., *Mayo Clinic images in internal medicine*, with permission. © Mayo Clinic Scientific Press and CRC Press.)

Figure 5.9 Hereditary haemorrhagic telangiectasia involving the lips

(From FS McDonald, ed., *Mayo Clinic images in internal medicine*, with permission. © Mayo Clinic Scientific Press and CRC Press.)

Figure 5.10 Porphyria cutanea tarda—scarring from photosensitivity

Peutz-Jeghers[c] syndrome. Freckle-like spots (discrete, brown-black lesions) around the mouth and on the buccal mucosa (Figure 5.7, page 137), and on the fingers and toes, are associated with hamartomas of the small bowel (50%) and colon (30%), which can present with bleeding or intussusception. In this autosomal dominant condition the incidence of gastrointestinal adenocarcinoma is increased.

Acanthosis nigricans. These are brown-to-black velvety elevations of the epidermis due to confluent papillomas and are usually found in the axillae and nape of the neck (Figure 5.8, page 137). Acanthosis nigricans is associated rarely with gastrointestinal carcinoma (particularly stomach) and lymphoma, as well as with acromegaly, diabetes mellitus and other endocrinopathies.

[c] John Peutz (1886–1957), physician at St John's Hospital, The Hague, Holland, first described this condition in 1921. Harold Jeghers (b. 1904), Professor of Medicine, Boston City Hospital, USA, described it in 1949.

Hereditary haemorrhagic telangiectasia

(Rendu–*Osler-Weber syndrome*[d]). Multiple small telangiectasia occur in this disease. They are often present on the lips and tongue (Figure 5.9), but may be found anywhere on the skin. When they are present in the gastrointestinal tract they can cause chronic blood loss or even, occasionally, torrential bleeding. An associated arteriovenous malformation in the liver may be present. This is an autosomal dominant condition and is uncommon.

Porphyria cutanea tarda. Fragile vesicles appear on exposed areas of the skin and heal with scarring (Figure 5.10). The urine is dark in this chronic disorder of porphyrin metabolism associated with alcoholism, liver disease and hepatitis C.

Systemic sclerosis. Tense tethering of the skin in systemic sclerosis is often associated with gastro-oesophageal reflux and gastrointestinal motility disorders (page 247).

Mental state

Assess orientation (pages 287 and 288). The syndrome of hepatic encephalopathy, due to decompensated advanced cirrhosis (chronic liver failure) or fulminant hepatitis (acute liver failure), is an organic neurological disturbance. The features depend on the aetiology and the precipitating factors (page 168). Patients eventually become stuporous and then comatose. The combination of hepatocellular damage and portosystemic shunting due to disturbed hepatic structure (both extrahepatic and intrahepatic) causes this syndrome. It is probably related to the liver's failure to remove toxic metabolites from the portal blood. These toxic metabolites may include ammonia, mercaptans, short-chain fatty acids and amines.

The hands

Even the experienced gastroenterologist must restrain his or her excitement and begin the examination of the gastrointestinal tract with the hands. The signs that may be elicited here give a clue to the presence of chronic liver disease. Whatever its aetiology, permanent diffuse liver damage results in similar peripheral signs. However, none of these signs alone is specific for chronic liver disease.

Figure 5.11 Leuconychia—Terry's nails
(From FS McDonald, ed., *Mayo Clinic images in internal medicine*, with permission. © Mayo Clinic Scientific Press and CRC Press.)

Nails

Leuconychia. When chronic liver or other disease results in hypoalbuminaemia, the nail beds opacify (the abnormality is of the nail bed and not of the nail), often leaving only a rim of pink nail bed at the top of nail (Terry's nails;[e] Figure 5.11). The thumb and index nails are most often involved. The exact mechanism is uncertain. It may be that the explanation is compression of capillary flow by extracellular fluid.

Muehrcke's lines (transverse white lines) can also occur in hypoalbuminaemic states, including cirrhosis. Blue lunulae may be seen in patients with Wilson's disease.

Clubbing. Up to one-third of patients with cirrhosis may have finger clubbing. In at least some cases, this may be related to arteriovenous (AV) shunting in the lungs, resulting in arterial oxygen desaturation. Cyanosis may be associated with severe long-standing chronic liver disease. The cause of this pulmonary AV shunting is unknown. Conditions such as inflammatory bowel disease and coeliac disease, which cause long-standing nutritional depletion, can also cause clubbing.

---

[d] Henri Rendu (1844–1902), French physician. Frederick Weber (1863–1962), English physician. The condition was described in 1907.

[e] These changes were first described by Terry in 1954 in association with cirrhosis. They are also found in patients with cardiac failure and become more common in normal people with age. In a patient under the age of 50, their presence indicates cirrhosis, heart failure or diabetes, with a likelihood ratio of 5.3.

The palms

Palmar erythema ('liver palms'). This is reddening of the palms of the hands affecting the thenar and hypothenar eminences. Often the soles of the feet are also affected. This can be a feature of chronic liver disease. While the finding has been attributed to raised oestrogen levels, it has not been shown to be related to plasma oestradiol levels, so the aetiology remains uncertain. Palmar erythema can also occur with pregnancy, thyrotoxicosis, rheumatoid arthritis, polycythaemia and rarely with chronic febrile diseases or chronic leukaemia. It may also be a normal finding, especially in women and like spider naevi can occur in pregnancy.

Anaemia. Inspect the palmar creases for pallor suggesting anaemia (page 198), which may result from gastrointestinal blood loss, malabsorption (folate, vitamin B_{12}), haemolysis (e.g. hypersplenism) or chronic disease.

Dupuytren's contracture.[f] This is a visible and palpable thickening and contraction of the palmar fascia causing permanent flexion, most often of the ring finger. It is often bilateral and occasionally affects the feet. It is associated with alcoholism (not liver disease), but is also found in some manual workers; it may be familial. The palmar fascia of these patients contains abnormally large amounts of xanthine, and this may be related to the pathogenesis.

Hepatic flap (asterixis[g])

Before leaving the hands one should ask the patient to stretch out the arms in front, separate the fingers and extend the wrists for 15 seconds. Jerky, irregular flexion–extension movement at the wrist and metacarpophalangeal joints, often accompanied by lateral movements of the fingers, constitute the flapping of hepatic encephalopathy (page 168). It is thought to be due to interference with the inflow of joint position sense information to the reticular formation in the brainstem. This results in rhythmical lapses of postural muscle tone. Occasionally the arms, neck, tongue, jaws and eyelids can also be involved. It can be demonstrated if the patient is asked to close the eyes forcefully or to protrude the tongue. The flap is usually bilateral, tends to be absent at rest, and is brought on by sustained posture. The rhythmic movements are not synchronous on each side and the flap is absent when coma supervenes.

Although this flap is a characteristic and early sign of liver failure, it is not diagnostic: it can also occur in cardiac, respiratory and renal failure, as well as in hypoglycaemia, hypokalaemia, hypomagnesaemia or barbiturate intoxication.

An apparent tremor (really a form of choreoathetosis, page 362) may occur in Wilson's disease. A fine resting tremor is common in alcoholism.

The arms

Inspect the upper limbs for *bruising*. Large bruises (ecchymoses) may be due to clotting abnormalities. Hepatocellular damage can interfere with protein synthesis and therefore the production of all the clotting factors (except factor VIII, which is made elsewhere in the reticuloendothelial system). Obstructive jaundice results in a shortage of bile acids in the intestine, and therefore may reduce absorption of vitamin K (a fat-soluble vitamin), which is essential for the production of clotting factors II (prothrombin), VII, IX and X.

Petechiae (pinhead-sized bruises) may also be present (page 199). Chronic excessive alcohol consumption can sometimes result in bone marrow depression, causing thrombocytopenia, which may be responsible for petechiae. In addition, splenomegaly secondary to portal hypertension can cause hypersplenism, with resultant excessive destruction of platelets in the spleen; in severe liver disease (especially acute hepatic necrosis), diffuse intravascular coagulation can occur.

Look for muscle wasting, which is often a late manifestation of malnutrition in alcoholic patients. Alcohol can also cause a proximal myopathy (page 355).

Scratch marks due to severe itch (pruritus) are often prominent in patients with obstructive or cholestatic jaundice. This is commonly the presenting feature of primary biliary cirrhosis[h] before other signs are apparent. The mechanism of pruritus is thought to be retention of an unknown substance normally excreted in the bile, rather than bile salt deposition in the skin as was earlier thought.

Spider naevi (Figure 5.12) consist of a central arteriole from which radiate numerous small vessels which look like spiders' legs. They range in size from just visible to half a centimetre in diameter. Their usual distribution is in the area drained by the

---

[f] Baron Guillaume Dupuytren (1777–1835), Surgeon-in-Chief at the Hotel-Dieu in Paris. A cold, rude, ambitious and arrogant man, he was called 'the Napoleon of surgery'. He saw 10,000 private patients a year.

[g] From Greek *a*, 'not' and *sterixis*, 'fixed position'.

---

[h] Primary biliary cirrhosis (PBC) is an uncommon chronic non-suppurative destructive cholangitis of unknown aetiology; 90% of affected patients are female.

Figure 5.12 A large crop of spider naevi

Figure 5.13 Scleral icterus

superior vena cava, so they are found on the arms, neck and chest wall. They can occasionally bleed profusely. Pressure applied with a pointed object to the central arteriole causes blanching of the whole lesion. Rapid refilling from the centre to the legs occurs on release of the pressure.

The finding of more than two or three spider naevi anywhere on the body is likely to be abnormal. Spider naevi can be caused by cirrhosis, most frequently due to alcohol. They may occur transiently with viral hepatitis. During the second to fifth months of pregnancy, spider naevi frequently appear, only to disappear again within days of delivery. It is not known why they occur only in the upper part of the body. Like palmar erythema they are traditionally attributed to oestrogen excess. Part of the normal hepatic function is the inactivation of oestrogens, which is impaired in chronic liver disease. Oestrogens are known to have a dilating effect on the spiral arterioles of the endometrium, and this has been used to explain the presence of spider naevi, but changes in plasma oestradiol levels have not been found to correlate with the appearance and disappearance of spider naevi.

The differential diagnosis of spider naevi includes *Campbell de Morgan*[i] *spots,* venous stars and hereditary haemorrhagic telangiectasia. Campbell de Morgan spots are flat or slightly elevated red circular lesions that occur on the abdomen or the front of the chest. They do not blanch on pressure and are very common. *Venous stars* are 2 cm to 3 cm lesions that can occur on the dorsum of the feet, legs, back and the lower chest. They are due to elevated venous pressure and are found overlying the main tributary to a large vein. They are not obliterated by pressure.

Figure 5.14 Kayser-Fleischer rings

(From FS McDonald, ed., *Mayo Clinic images in internal medicine*, with permission. © Mayo Clinic Scientific Press and CRC Press.)

The blood flow is from the periphery to the centre of the lesion, which is the opposite of the flow in the spider naevus. Lesions of *hereditary haemorrhagic telangiectasia* (page 201) occasionally resemble spider naevi.

Palpate the axillae for *lymphadenopathy* (page 201). Look in the axillae for acanthosis nigricans.

The face

Eyes

Look first at the sclerae for signs of *jaundice* (Figure 5.13) or *anaemia. Kayser-Fleischer rings*[j] (Figure 5.14) are brownish green rings occurring at

---

[i] Campbell de Morgan (1811–76), London surgeon. He was one of the 300 original Fellows of the Royal College of Surgeons. He described his spots in 1872 and believed them to be a sign of cancer (which they are not).

[j] Bernhard Kayser (1869–1954), German ophthalmologist, described these rings in 1902. Bruno Fleischer (1848–1904), German ophthalmologist, described them in 1903.

Figure 5.15 Amyloidosis causing macroglossia

Note the periorbital purpura that followed a proctoscopic examination, a characteristic (albeit rare) sign. (From FS McDonald, ed., *Mayo Clinic images in internal medicine*, with permission. © Mayo Clinic Scientific Press and CRC Press.)

the periphery of the cornea, affecting the upper pole more than the lower. They are due to deposits of excess copper in Descemet's membrane[k] of the cornea. Slit-lamp examination is often necessary to show them. They are typically found in Wilson's disease[l], a copper storage disease that causes cirrhosis and neurological disturbances. The Kayser-Fleischer rings are usually present by the time neurological signs have appeared. Patients with other cholestatic liver diseases, however, can also have these rings. *Iritis* may be seen in inflammatory bowel disease (page 170).

Xanthelasma are yellowish plaques in the subcutaneous tissues in the periorbital region and are due to deposits of lipids (see Figure 3.12). They may indicate protracted elevation of the serum cholesterol. In patients with cholestasis, an abnormal lipoprotein (lipoprotein X) is found in the plasma and is associated with elevation of the serum cholesterol. Xanthelasma are common in patients with primary biliary cirrhosis (see also Table 3.4).

Periorbital purpura following proctosigmoidoscopy ('black eye syndrome') is a characteristic sign of amyloidosis (perhaps related to factor X deficiency) but is exceedingly rare (Figure 5.15).

Salivary glands

Next inspect and palpate the cheeks over the parotid area for *parotid enlargement* (Table 5.5, Figure 5.16). Ask the patient to clench the teeth so that the mas-

---

Table 5.5 Causes of parotid enlargement
Bilateral
1 Mumps (can be unilateral)
2 Sarcoidosis or lymphoma, which may cause painless bilateral enlargement
3 Mikulicz* syndrome: bilateral painless enlargement of all three salivary glands. This disease is probably an early stage of Sjögren's syndrome
5 Alcohol-associated parotitis
6 Malnutrition
7 Severe dehydration: as occurs in renal failure, terminal carcinomatosis and severe infections
Unilateral
1 Mixed parotid tumour (occasionally bilateral)
2 Tumour infiltration, which usually causes painless unilateral enlargement and may cause facial nerve palsy (page 308)
3 Duct blockage, e.g. salivary calculus
* Johann von Mikulicz-Radecki (1850–1905), Professor of Surgery, Breslau. He described this condition in 1892.

seter muscle is palpable; the normal parotid gland is impalpable but the enlarged gland is best felt behind the masseter muscle and in front of the ear. Parotidomegaly that is bilateral is associated with alcoholism rather than liver disease per se. It is due to fatty infiltration, perhaps secondary to alcohol toxicity with or without malnutrition. A tender, warm, swollen parotid suggests the diagnosis of parotiditis following an acute illness or surgery. A mixed parotid tumour (a pleomorphic adenoma) is the commonest cause of a lump. Parotid carcinoma

---

[k] Jean Descemet (1732–1810), Professor of Surgery and Anatomy, Paris. He described the membrane in 1785.

[l] Samuel Alexander Wilson (1878–1937), London neurologist at Queen Square. His colleagues there included Gowers and Hughlings Jackson. He described his disease in 1912 in his MD thesis. He also described the glabellar tap sign in Parkinson's disease, which is sometimes called Wilson's sign.

Figure 5.16 Parotid gland examination

cases. The presence of fetor hepaticus in a patient with a coma of unknown cause may be a helpful clue to the diagnosis.

Table 5.6 Causes of gum hypertrophy

1 Phenytoin
2 Pregnancy
3 Scurvy (vitamin C deficiency: the gums become spongy, red, bleed easily and are swollen and irregular)
4 Gingivitis, e.g. from smoking, calculus, plaque, Vincent's* angina (fusobacterial membranous tonsillitis)
5 Leukaemia (usually monocytic)

* Jean Hyacinthe Vincent (1862–1950), Professor of Forensic Medicine and French Army bacteriologist, described this in 1898.

Table 5.7 Causes of pigmented lesions in the mouth

1 Heavy metals: lead or bismuth (blue-black line on the gingival margin), iron (haemochromatosis—blue-grey pigmentation of the hard palate)
2 Drugs: antimalarials, the oral contraceptive pill (brown or black areas of pigmentation anywhere in the mouth)
3 Addison's disease (blotches of dark brown pigment anywhere in the mouth)
4 Peutz-Jeghers syndrome (lips, buccal mucosa or palate)
5 Malignant melanoma (raised, painless black lesions anywhere in the mouth)

Table 5.8 Causes of fetor (bad breath)

1 Faulty oral hygiene
2 Fetor hepaticus (a sweet smell)
3 Ketosis (diabetic ketoacidosis results in excretion of ketones in exhaled air, causing a sickly sweet smell)
4 Uraemia (fish breath: an ammoniacal odour)
5 Alcohol (distinctive)
6 Paraldehyde
7 Putrid (due to anaerobic chest infections with large amounts of sputum)
8 Cigarettes

---

may cause a facial nerve palsy (page 308). Feel in the mouth for a parotid calculus, which may be present at the parotid duct orifice (opposite the upper second molar). Mumps also causes acute parotid enlargement which is usually bilateral.

Submandibular gland enlargement is most often due to a calculus. This may be palpable bimanually. The examiner's gloved index finger is placed on the floor of the mouth beside the tongue, feeling between it and fingers placed behind the body of the mandible. It may also be enlarged in chronic liver disease.

The mouth

The teeth and breath. The very beginning of the gastrointestinal tract is, like the very end of the tract, accessible to inspection without elaborate equipment.[6] Look first briefly at the state of the teeth and note whether they are real or false. False teeth will have to be removed for a complete examination of the mouth. Note whether there is gum hypertrophy (Table 5.6) or pigmentation (Table 5.7). Loose-fitting false teeth may be responsible for ulcers and decayed teeth may be responsible for fetor (bad breath).

Other causes of fetor are listed in Table 5.8. These must be distinguished from *fetor hepaticus* which is a rather sweet smell of the breath. It is an indication of severe hepatocellular disease and may be due to methylmercaptans. These substances are known to be exhaled in the breath and may be derived from methionine when this amino acid is not demethylated by a diseased liver. Severe fetor hepaticus that fills the patient's room is a bad sign and indicates a precomatose condition in many

Unless the smell is obvious one should get a patient to exhale through the mouth while one sniffs a little of the exhaled air.

The tongue. Thickened epithelium with bacterial debris and food particles commonly causes a *coating* over the tongue, especially in smokers. It is rarely a sign of disease and is more marked on the posterior part of the tongue where there is less mobility and the papillae desquamate more slowly. It occurs frequently in respiratory tract infections, but is in no way related to constipation or any serious abdominal disorder.

Lingua nigra (black tongue) is due to elongation of papillae over the posterior part of the tongue, which appears dark brown because of the accumulation of keratin. There is no known cause and apart from its aesthetic problems it is symptomless. Bismuth compounds may also cause a black tongue.

Geographical tongue is a term used to describe slowly changing red rings and lines that occur on the surface of the tongue. It is not painful, and the condition tends to come and go. It is not usually of any significance, but can be a sign of riboflavin (vitamin B_2) deficiency.

Leucoplakia is white-coloured thickening of the mucosa of the tongue and mouth; the condition is premalignant. Most of the causes of leucoplakia begin with 'S': sore teeth (poor dental hygiene), smoking, spirits, sepsis or syphilis, but often no cause is apparent. Leucoplakia may also occur on the larynx, anus and vulva.

The term *glossitis* is generally used to describe a smooth appearance of the tongue which may also be erythematous. The appearance is due to atrophy of the papillae, and in later stages there may be shallow ulceration. These changes occur in the tongue often as a result of nutritional deficiencies to which the tongue is sensitive because of the rapid turnover of mucosal cells. Deficiencies of iron, folate and the vitamin B group, especially vitamin B_{12}, are common causes. Glossitis is common in alcoholics and can also occur in the rare carcinoid syndrome. However, many cases, especially those in elderly people, are impossible to explain.

Enlargement of the tongue (*macroglossia*) may occur in congenital conditions such as Down syndrome (page 273) or in endocrine disease, including acromegaly (page 267). Tumour infiltration (e.g. haemangioma or lymphangioma) or infiltration of the tongue with amyloid material in amyloidosis can also be responsible for macroglossia.

Mouth ulcers. This is an important topic because a number of systemic diseases can present with ulcers in the mouth (Table 5.9). *Aphthous ulceration* is the commonest type seen (Figure 5.17). This

Figure 5.17 Aphthous ulceration

(From FS McDonald, ed., *Mayo Clinic images in internal medicine*, with permission. © Mayo Clinic Scientific Press and CRC Press.)

begins as a small painful vesicle on the tongue or mucosal surface of the mouth, which may break down to form a painful, shallow ulcer. These ulcers heal without scarring. The cause is completely unknown. They usually do not indicate any serious underlying systemic disease, but may occur in Crohn's[m] disease or coeliac disease. HIV infection may be associated with a number of mouth lesions (page 403). *Angular stomatitis* refers to cracks at the corners of the mouth; causes include deficiencies in vitamin B_6, vitamin B_{12}, folate and iron.

Candidiasis (moniliasis). Fungal infection with *Candida albicans* (thrush) causes creamy white curd-like patches in the mouth which are removed only with difficulty and leave a bleeding surface. The infection may spread to involve the oesophagus, causing dysphagia or odynophagia. Moniliasis is associated with immunosuppression (steroids, tumour chemotherapy, alcoholism or an underlying immunological abnormality such as HIV infection, or haematological malignancy), where it is due to decreased host resistance. Broad-spectrum antibiotics, which inhibit the normal oral flora, are also a common cause, because fungal overgrowth is permitted. Faulty oral hygiene, iron deficiency and diabetes mellitus can also be responsible. Rarely, chronic mucocutaneous candidiasis, a distinct syndrome comprising recurrent or persistent oral thrush,

---

[m] Burrill Bernard Crohn (1884–1983), American gastroenterologist at Mount Sinai Hospital, New York, described this disease in 1932. It had previously been described by Morgagni (1682–1771) in 1769.

Table 5.9 Causes of mouth ulcers

Common

Aphthous
Drugs (e.g. gold, steroids)
Trauma

Uncommon

Gastrointestinal disease: Crohn's disease,
    ulcerative colitis, coeliac disease
Rheumatological disease: Behçet's* syndrome,
    Reiter's[†] syndrome
Erythema multiforme
Infection: viral—herpes zoster, herpes simplex;
    bacterial—syphilis (primary chancre,
    secondary snail track ulcers, mucous patches),
    tuberculosis
Self-inflicted

* Halusi Behçet (1889–1948), Turkish dermatologist. He
  described the disease in 1937.
[†] Hans Reiter (1881–1969), Berlin bacteriologist, described
  this in 1916.

finger- or toenail bed infection and skin involvement, occurs; in some of these patients, endocrine diseases such as hypoparathyroidism, hypothyroidism or Addison's disease are associated (page 271).

The neck and chest

Palpate the cervical lymph nodes (page 201). It is particularly important to feel for the supraclavicular nodes, especially on the left side. These may be involved with advanced gastric or other gastrointestinal malignancy, or with lung cancer. The presence of a large left supraclavicular node in combination with carcinoma of the stomach is called Troisier's sign.[n] Look for spider naevi.

In males, *gynaecomastia* may be a sign of chronic liver disease. Gynaecomastia may be unilateral or bilateral and the breasts may be tender. This may be a sign of cirrhosis, particularly alcoholic cirrhosis, or of chronic active hepatitis. In chronic liver disease, changes in the oestradiol-to-testosterone ratio may be responsible. In cirrhotic patients, spironolactone, used to treat ascites, is also a common cause. Gynaecomastia may also occur in alcoholics without liver

disease because of damage to the Leydig cells[o] of the testis from alcohol. A number of drugs may rarely cause gynaecomastia (e.g. digoxin, cimetidine).

The abdomen

Self-restraint is no longer required and it is now time to examine the abdomen itself.

Inspection

The patient should lie flat, with one pillow under the head and the abdomen exposed from the nipples to the pubic symphysis (see Figure 5.2). Don't be too eager to begin palpation, as inspection is very often helpful. Inspection begins with a careful look for abdominal *scars,* which may indicate previous surgery or trauma (Figure 5.18). Look in the area around the umbilicus for laparoscopic surgical scars. Older scars are white and recent scars are pink because the tissue remains vascular. Note the presence of stomata (end-colostomy, loop colostomy, ileostomy or ileal conduit) or fistulae.

Generalised abdominal *distension* (Figure 5.19) may be present. All the causes of this sound as if they begin with the letter 'F': fat (gross obesity), fluid (ascites), fetus, flatus (gaseous distension due to bowel obstruction), faeces, 'filthy' big tumour (e.g. ovarian tumour or hydatid cyst) or 'phantom' pregnancy. Look at the shape of the umbilicus, which may give a clue to the underlying cause. An umbilicus buried in fat suggests that the patient eats too much. However, when the peritoneal cavity is filled with large volumes of fluid (ascites) from whatever cause, the abdominal flanks and wall appear tense and the umbilicus is shallow or everted and points downwards. In pregnancy the umbilicus is pushed upwards by the uterus enlarging from the pelvis. This appearance may also result from a huge ovarian cyst.

Local swellings may indicate enlargement of one of the abdominal or pelvic organs. A hernia is a protrusion of an intra-abdominal structure through an abnormal opening; this may occur because of weakening of the abdominal wall by previous surgery (incisional hernia), a congenital abdominal wall defect, or chronically increased intra-abdominal pressure.

Prominent *veins* may be obvious on the abdominal wall. If these are present, the direction of venous flow should be elicited at this stage. A finger is used to occlude the vein and blood is then emptied from the vein below the occluding finger with a second finger. The second finger is removed and, if the vein

[n] Charles Émile Troisier (1844–1919), Professor of Pathology in
  Paris, described this sign in 1886.

[o] Franz von Leydig (1821–1908), Bonn anatomist and zoologist,
  Germany.

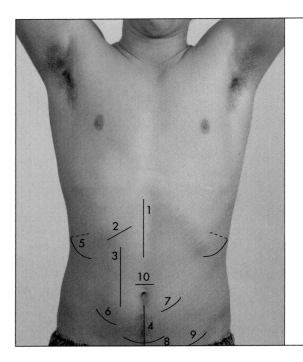

1. Upper midline
2. Right subcostal (Kocher's)
3. Right paramedian
4. Lower midline
5. Nephrectomy
6. Appendicectomy (Gridiron)
7. Transplanted kidney
8. Suprapubic (Pfannensteil)
9. Left inguinal
10. Umbilical port—laparoscopic surgery

Figure 5.18
Abdominal scars

Note: Laparoscopic surgical scars are now common. Most of these procedures include a port about 2 cm in length, just above the umbilicus.

Figure 5.19 Abdomen distended with ascites: umbilicus points downwards, unlike cases of distension due to a pelvic mass

refills, flow is occurring towards the occluding finger (Figure 5.20). Flow should be tested separately in veins above and below the umbilicus. In patients with severe portal hypertension, portal to systemic flow occurs through the umbilical veins, which may, rather rarely, become engorged and distended. The direction of flow then is away from the umbilicus. Because of their engorged appearance they have been likened to the mythical Medusa's hair after Minerva had turned

it into snakes; this sign is called a *caput Medusae* (head of Medusa) but is very rare (Figure 5.21). Usually only one or two veins (often epigastric) are visible. Engorgement can also occur because of inferior vena caval obstruction, usually due to a tumour or thrombosis but sometimes because of tense ascites. In this case the abdominal veins enlarge to provide collateral blood flow from the legs, avoiding the blocked inferior vena cava. The direction of flow is then upwards towards the heart. Therefore, to distinguish caput Medusae from inferior vena caval obstruction, determine the direction of flow *below* the umbilicus; it will be towards the legs in the former and towards the head in the latter. Prominent superficial veins can occasionally be congenital.

Pulsations may be visible. An expanding central pulsation in the epigastrium suggests an abdominal aortic aneurysm. However, the abdominal aorta can often be seen to pulsate in normal thin people.

Visible peristalsis may occur occasionally in very thin normal people; however, it usually suggests intestinal obstruction. Pyloric obstruction due to peptic ulceration or tumour may cause visible peristalsis, seen as a slow wave of movement passing across the upper abdomen from left to right. Obstruction of the distal small bowel can cause similar movements in a ladder pattern in the centre of the abdomen.

Skin lesions should also be noted on the abdominal wall. These include the vesicles of herpes zoster,

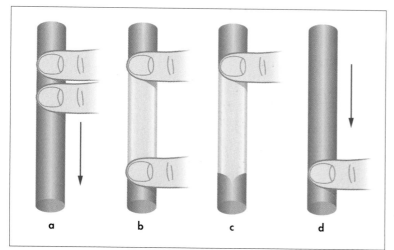

Figure 5.20 Detecting the direction of flow of a vein

(a) Place two fingers firmly on the vein. (b) The second finger is moved along the vein to empty it of blood and keep it occluded. (c) The second finger is removed but the vein does not refill. (d) At repeat testing and removing the first finger, filling occurs, indicating the direction of flow. (Adapted from Swash M, ed. *Hutchison's clinical methods*, 20th edn. Philadelphia: Baillière Tindall, 1995, with permission.)

Figure 5.21 Prominent veins on the abdominal wall

1 = thin veins over the costal margin—not of clinical relevance. 2 = caput Medusae. 3 = inferior vena caval obstruction.
(Based on Swash M, ed. *Hutchison's clinical methods*, 20th edn. Philadelphia: Baillière Tindall, 1995.)

which occur in a radicular pattern (they are localised to only one side of the abdomen in the distribution of a single nerve root). Herpes zoster may be responsible for severe abdominal pain that is of mysterious origin until the rash appears. The Sister Joseph[p] nodule is a metastatic tumour deposit in the umbilicus, the anatomical region where the peritoneum is closest to the skin. Discoloration of the umbilicus where a faintly bluish hue is present is found very rarely, in cases of extensive haemoperitoneum and acute pancreatitis (Cullen's sign[q]—the umbilical 'black eye'). Skin discoloration may also rarely occur in the flanks in severe cases of acute pancreatitis (Grey-Turner's sign[r]).

Stretching of the abdominal wall severe enough to cause rupture of the elastic fibres in the skin produces pink linear marks with a wrinkled appearance, which are called *striae*. When these are wide and purple-coloured, Cushing's syndrome may be the cause (page 269). Ascites, pregnancy or recent weight gain are much more common causes of striae.

Next, squat down beside the bed so that the patient's abdomen is at eye level. Ask him or her to take slow deep breaths through the mouth and watch for evidence of asymmetrical movement, indicating the presence of a mass. In particular a large liver may be seen to move below the right costal margin or a large spleen below the left costal margin.

[p] Sister Joseph of St Mary's Hospital, Rochester, Minnesota, described this sign to Dr William Mayo (1861–1939) of the Mayo Clinic.
[q] Thomas S Cullen (1869–1953), Professor of Gynaecology, Johns Hopkins University, who originally described this sign as an indication of a ruptured ectopic pregnancy.
[r] George Grey-Turner (1877–1951), surgeon, Royal Victoria Infirmary, Newcastle-on-Tyne, England.

Mid-clavicular lines

1. Right hypochondrium
2. Epigastrium
3. Left hypochondrium
4. Right lumbar region
5. Umbilical region
6. Left lumbar region
7. Right iliac fossa
8. Hypogastrium
9. Left iliac fossa

Xiphisternum

Right upper quadrant | Left upper quadrant

Right lower quadrant | Left lower quadrant

Pubic symphysis

Figure 5.22 (a) Regions of the abdomen (b) Quadrants of the abdomen

Palpation

This part of the examination often reveals the most information. Successful palpation requires relaxed abdominal muscles. To this end, reassure the patient that the examination will not be painful and use warm hands. Ask the patient if any particular area is tender and examine this area last. Encourage the patient to breathe gently through the mouth. If necessary, ask the patient to bend the knees to relax the abdominal wall muscles.

For descriptive purposes the abdomen has been divided into nine areas or regions (Figure 5.22). Palpation in each region is performed with the palmar surface of the fingers acting together. For the palpation of the edges of organs or masses, the lateral surface of the forefinger is the most sensitive part of the hand.

Palpation should begin with *light pressure* in each region. All the movements of the hand should occur at the metacarpophalangeal joints and the hand should be moulded to the shape of the abdominal wall. Note the presence of any tenderness or lumps in each region. As the hand moves over each region, the mind should be considering the anatomical structures that underlie it. *Deep palpation* of the abdomen is performed next, though care should be taken to avoid the

Table 5.10 Descriptive features of intra-abdominal masses
For any abdominal mass all the following should be determined:
1 Site: the region involved
2 Tenderness
3 Size (which must be measured) and shape
4 Surface, which may be regular or irregular
5 Edge, which may be regular or irregular
6 Consistency, which may be hard or soft
7 Mobility and movement with inspiration
8 Whether it is pulsatile or not
9 Whether one can get above the mass

tender areas until the end of the examination. Deep palpation is used to detect deeper masses and to define those already discovered. Any mass must be carefully characterised and described (Table 5.10).

Guarding of the abdomen (when resistance to palpation occurs due to contraction of the abdominal muscles) may result from tenderness or anxiety, and may be voluntary or involuntary. The latter suggests

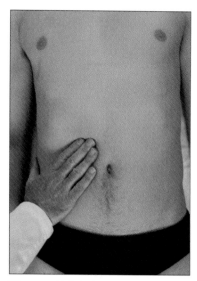

Figure 5.23 Abdominal examination: the liver

peritonitis. *Rigidity* is a constant involuntary contraction of the abdominal muscles always associated with tenderness and indicates peritoneal irritation. *Rebound tenderness* is said to be present when the abdominal wall, having been compressed slowly, is released rapidly and a sudden stab of pain results. This may make the patient wince, so the face should be watched while this manoeuvre is performed. It strongly suggests the presence of peritonitis and should be performed if there is doubt about the presence of localised or generalised peritonitis. Be careful not to surprise your patient by a sudden jabbing and release movement: rebound tenderness should be elicited slowly. If you suspect the patient may be feigning a tender abdomen, test for rebound with your stethoscope after telling the patient to lie still and quiet so that you can hear.

The liver. Feel for hepatomegaly (Figure 5.23).[7] With the examining hand aligned parallel to the right costal margin, and beginning in the right iliac fossa, ask the patient to breathe in and out slowly through the mouth. With each expiration the hand is advanced by 1 or 2 cm closer to the right costal margin. During inspiration the hand is kept still and the lateral margin of the forefinger waits expectantly for the liver edge to strike it.

If the liver edge has been identified, an attempt should be made to feel the surface of the liver. The edge of the liver and the surface itself may be hard or soft, tender or non-tender, regular or irregular,

and pulsatile or non-pulsatile. The normal liver edge may be just palpable below the right costal margin on deep inspiration, especially in thin people. The edge is then felt to be soft and regular with a fairly sharply defined border and the surface of the liver itself is smooth. Sometimes only the left lobe of the liver may be palpable (to the left of the midline) in patients with cirrhosis.

If the liver edge is palpable the total *liver span* can be measured. Remember that the liver span varies with height and is greater in men than women, and that inter-observer error is quite large for this measurement. The normal upper border of the liver is level with the sixth rib in the midclavicular line. At this point the percussion note over the chest changes from resonant to dull (Figure 5.24). To estimate the liver span (Figure 5.24) percuss down along the right midclavicular line until the liver dullness is encountered and measure from here to the palpable liver edge. Careful assessment of the position of the midclavicular line will improve the accuracy of this measurement. The normal span is less than 13 cm. Note that the clinical estimate of the liver span usually underestimates its actual size by 2 to 5 cm.

Other causes of a normal but palpable liver include ptosis due to emphysema, asthma or a sub-diaphragmatic collection, or a Riedel's lobe.[s] The Riedel's lobe is a tongue-like projection of the liver from the right lobe's inferior surface; it can be quite large and rarely extends as far as the right iliac fossa. It can be confused with an enlarged gallbladder or right kidney.

Many diseases cause hepatic enlargement and these are listed in Table 5.11. Detecting the liver edge below the costal margin clinically is highly specific (100%) but insensitive (48%)—positive LR 233.7, negative LR 0.5. Remember, the diseased liver is not always enlarged; a small liver is common in advanced cirrhosis, and the liver shrinks rapidly with acute hepatic necrosis (due to liver cell death and collapse of the reticulin framework).

The gallbladder. The gallbladder is occasionally palpable below the right costal margin where this crosses the lateral border of the rectus muscles. If biliary obstruction or acute cholecystitis is suspected, the examining hand should be oriented perpendicular to the costal margin, feeling from medial to lateral. Unlike the liver edge, the gallbladder, if palpable, will be a bulbous, focal, rounded mass which moves downwards on inspiration. The causes of an enlarged gallbladder are listed in Table 5.12.

[s] Bernhard Riedel (1846–1916), German surgeon, described this in 1888.

Figure 5.24 Percussing the liver span: (a) upper border; (b) lower border

Murphy's sign[t] should be sought if cholecystitis is suspected (*Good signs guide 5.1*). On taking a deep breath, the patient catches his or her breath when an inflamed gallbladder presses on the examiner's hand, which is lying at the costal margin. Other signs are less helpful.

The clinician examining for an enlarged gallbladder must always be mindful of *Courvoisier's law*,[u] which states that, if the gallbladder is enlarged and the patient is jaundiced, the cause is unlikely to be gallstones. Rather, carcinoma of the pancreas or lower biliary tree resulting in obstructive jaundice is likely to be present. This is because the gallbladder with stones is usually chronically fibrosed and therefore incapable of enlargement. Note that if the gallbladder is not palpable, and the patient is jaundiced, some cause other than gallstones is still possible, as at least 50% of dilated gallbladders are impalpable (*Good signs guide 5.2*).

The spleen. The spleen enlarges inferiorly and medially (Figure 5.25). Its edge should be sought below the umbilicus in the midline initially. A two-handed technique is recommended. The left hand is placed posterolaterally over the left lower ribs and the right hand is placed on the abdomen below the umbilicus, parallel to the left costal margin (Figure 5.26a). Don't start palpation too near the costal margin or a large spleen will be missed. As the right hand is advanced closer to the left costal margin, the left hand compresses firmly over the rib cage so as to produce a loose fold of skin (Figure 5.26b); this removes tension from the

---

[t] John Murphy (1857–1916), American surgeon, Professor of Surgery at Rush Medical College, Chicago, described this in 1912.
[u] Ludwig Courvoisier (1843–1918), Professor of Surgery, Switzerland, described this principle in 1890. He was a keen natural historian and wrote 21 papers on entomology.

Table 5.11 Differential diagnosis in liver palpation

Hepatomegaly

1 Massive
- Metastases
- Alcoholic liver disease with fatty infiltration
- Myeloproliferative disease
- Right heart failure
- Hepatocellular cancer

2 Moderate
- The above causes
- Haemochromatosis
- Haematological disease—e.g. chronic leukaemia, lymphoma
- Fatty liver—secondary to e.g. diabetes mellitus, obesity, toxins
- Infiltration—e.g. amyloid

3 Mild
- The above causes
- Hepatitis
- Biliary obstruction
- Hydatid disease
- Human immunodeficiency virus (HIV) infection

Firm and irregular liver

Hepatocellular carcinoma
Metastatic disease
Cirrhosis
Hydatid disease, granuloma (e.g. sarcoid), amyloid, cysts, lipoidoses

Tender liver

Hepatitis
Rapid liver enlargement—e.g. right heart failure, Budd-Chiari* syndrome (hepatic vein thrombosis)
Hepatocellular cancer
Hepatic abscess
Biliary obstruction/cholangitis

Pulsatile liver

Tricuspid regurgitation
Hepatocellular cancer
Vascular abnormalities

* George Budd (1808–1882), Professor of Medicine, King's College Hospital, London, described this in 1845. Hans Chiari (1851–1916), Professor of Pathology, Prague, described it in 1898.

Table 5.12 Gallbladder enlargement

With jaundice

1 Carcinoma of the head of pancreas
2 Carcinoma of the ampulla of Vater*
3 In-situ gallstone formation in the common bile duct
4 Mucocele of the gallbladder due to a stone in Hartmann's† pouch and a stone in the common bile duct (very rare)

Without jaundice

1 Mucocele or empyema of the gallbladder.
2 Carcinoma of the gallbladder (stone hard, irregular swelling)
3 Acute cholecystitis

* Abraham Vater (1684–1751), Wittenberg anatomist and botanist.
† Henri Hartmann (1860–1952), Professor of Surgery, Paris.

GOOD SIGNS GUIDE 5.1
Cholecystitis

Sign	Positive LR	Negative LR
Murphy's sign	2.0	NS
Back tenderness	0.4	2.0
Right upper quadrant mass	NS	NS

NS = not significant.
From McGee S, *Evidence-based physical diagnosis*, Saunders, 2001.

GOOD SIGNS GUIDE 5.2
Gallbladder

Sign	Positive LR	Negative LR
Palpable gallbladder		
Detecting obstructed bile duct in jaundiced patient	26.0	0.7
Malignant obstruction in patient with obstructive jaundice	2.6	0.7

From McGee S, *Evidence-based physical diagnosis*, Saunders, 2001.

Table 5.13 Causes of hepatosplenomegaly

Chronic liver disease with portal hypertension
Haematological disease, e.g. myeloproliferative
   disease, lymphoma, leukaemia, pernicious
   anaemia, sickle cell anaemia
Infection, e.g. acute viral hepatitis, infectious
   mononucleosis, cytomegalovirus
Infiltration, e.g. amyloid, sarcoid
Connective tissue disease, e.g. systemic lupus
   erythematosus
Acromegaly
Thyrotoxicosis

abdominal wall and enables a slightly enlarged soft spleen to be felt as it moves down towards the right iliac fossa at the end of inspiration (Figure 5.26c).

If the spleen is not palpable, the patient must be rolled onto the right side towards the examiner (the right lateral decubitus position) and palpation repeated. Here one begins close to the left costal margin (Figure 5.26d). As a general rule, spleno-megaly becomes just detectable if the spleen is one-and-a-half to two times enlarged. Palpation for splenomegaly is only moderately sensitive but highly specific. The positive LR of splenomegaly when the spleen is palpable is 9.6 and the negative LR of splenomegaly if the spleen is not palpable is 0.6. The

Figure 5.25 Massive splenomegaly: note the splenic notch

causes of splenomegaly are listed in Table 7.6 (page 202). The causes of hepatosplenomegaly are listed in Table 5.13.

The kidneys. The first important differential diag-nosis to consider, if a right or left subcostal mass is palpable, must be a kidney. An attempt to palpate the kidney should be a routine part of the examination. The bimanual method is the best. The patient lies flat on his or her back. To palpate the right kidney, the examiner's left hand slides underneath the back to rest with the heel of the hand under the right loin. The fingers remain free to flex at the metacarpo-phalangeal joints in the area of the renal angle. The flexing fingers can push the contents of the abdomen anteriorly. The examiner's right hand is placed over the right upper quadrant.

First an attempt should be made to capture the kidney between the two hands. It is more often pos-sible to feel a kidney by bimanual palpation (this is traditionally called *ballotting*, although this term should probably be reserved for the palpation of an organ or mass in a fluid medium). In this case the renal angle is pressed sharply by the flexing fingers of the posterior hand. The kidney can be felt to float upwards and strike the anterior hand. The opposite hands are used to palpate the left kidney.

When palpable, the kidney feels like a swelling with a rounded lower pole and a medial dent (the hilum). However, it is unusual for a normal kidney to be felt as clearly as this. The lower pole of the right kidney may be palpable in thin, normal persons. Both kidneys move downwards with inspiration. The causes of kidney enlargement are listed in Table 6.5 (page 186).

It is particularly common to confuse a large left kidney with splenomegaly. The major distinguish-ing features are: (i) the spleen has no palpable upper border—the space between the spleen and the costal margin, which is present in renal enlargement, cannot be felt; (ii) the spleen, unlike the kidney, has a notch that may be palpable; (iii) the spleen moves inferomedially on inspiration while the kidney moves inferiorly; (iv) the spleen is not usually bal-lottable unless gross ascites is present, but the kidney is, again because of its retroperitoneal position; (v) the percussion note is dull over the spleen but is usu-ally resonant over the kidney, as the latter lies posterior to loops of gas-filled bowel; (vi) a friction rub may occasionally be heard over the spleen, but never over the kidney because it is too posterior.

Other abdominal masses. The causes of a mass in the abdomen, excluding the liver, spleen and kid-neys, are summarised in Table 5.14.

Figure 5.26 Palpation of the spleen

(a) Palpation begins in the lower mid-abdomen and finishes up under the left costal margin.
(b) The examiner's hand supports the patient's side...
(c) ...and then rests over the lower costal margin to reduce skin resistance.
(d) If the spleen is not palpable when the patient is flat, he or she should be rolled towards the examiner.

Stomach and duodenum. Although many clinicians palpate the epigastrium to elicit tenderness in patients with suspected peptic ulcer, the presence or absence of tenderness is not helpful in making this diagnosis. With gastric outlet obstruction due to a peptic ulcer or gastric carcinoma (page 173), the 'succussion splash' (the sign of Hippocrates) may occasionally be present. In a case of suspected gastric outlet obstruction, after warning the patient what is to come, grasp one iliac crest with each hand, place your stethoscope close to the epigastrium and shake the patient vigorously from side to side. The listening ears eagerly await a splashing noise due to excessive fluid retained in an obstructed stomach. The test is not useful if the patient has just drunk a large amount of milk or other fluid for his or her ulcer. The clinician must then return 3 hours later, having forbidden the patient to drink anything further.

Pancreas. A pancreatic pseudocyst following acute pancreatitis may, if large, be palpable as a rounded swelling above the umbilicus. It is characteristically tense, does not descend with inspiration and feels fixed. Occasionally a pancreatic carcinoma may be palpable in thin patients.

Aorta. Arterial pulsation from the abdominal aorta may be present, usually in the epigastrium, in thin normal people. The problem is to determine whether such a pulsation represents an aortic aneurysm (usually due to atherosclerosis) or not. Measure the width of the pulsation gently with two fingers by aligning these parallel to the aorta and placing them at the outermost palpable margins. With an aortic aneurysm, the pulsation is expansile (i.e. it enlarges appreciably with systole) (Figure 5.27). If an abdominal aortic aneurysm is larger than 5 cm in diameter, it usually merits surgical repair. The sensitivity of examination for finding an aneurysm of 5 cm or larger is 82%.[8] The sensitivity of the examination for detecting an aneurysm increases *pari passu* with the size of the aneurysm. The overall LR for a significant

Table 5.14 Causes of abdominal masses

Right iliac fossa

Appendiceal abscess or mucocele of the
    appendix
Carcinoma of the caecum or caecal distension
    due to distal obstruction
Crohn's disease (usually when complicated by an
    abscess)
Ovarian tumour or cyst
Carcinoid tumour
Amoebiasis
Psoas abscess
Ileocaecal tuberculosis
Hernia
Transplanted kidney

Left iliac fossa

Faeces (NB: Can often be indented)
Carcinoma of sigmoid or descending colon
Diverticular abscess
Ovarian tumour or cyst
Psoas abscess
Hernia
Transplanted kidney

Upper abdomen

Retroperitoneal lymphadenopathy (e.g.
    lymphoma, teratoma)
Left lobe of the liver
Abdominal aortic aneurysm (expansile)
Carcinoma of the stomach
Pancreatic pseudocyst or tumour
Gastric dilatation (e.g. pyloric stenosis, acute
    dilatation in diabetic ketoacidosis or after
    surgery)
Carcinoma of the transverse colon
Omental mass (e.g. metastatic tumour)
Small bowel obstruction

Pelvis

Bladder
Ovarian tumour or cyst
Uterus (e.g. pregnancy, tumour, fibroids)
Small bowel obstruction

aneurysm when one is suspected on palpation is 2.7, with a negative LR of 0.43 if the examination is normal.

Bowel. Particularly in severely constipated patients with soft abdominal walls and hard faeces, the sigmoid colon is often palpable. Unlike other masses, faeces can usually be indented by the examiner's finger. Rarely, carcinoma of the bowel may be palpable, particularly in the caecum where masses can grow to a large size before they cause obstruction. Such a mass does not move on respiration. In the examination of children or adults with chronic constipation and a megarectum, the enlarged rectum containing impacted stool may be felt above the symphysis pubis, filling a variable part of the pelvis in the midline.

Bladder. An empty bladder is impalpable. If there is urinary retention, the full bladder may be palpable above the pubic symphysis. It forms part of the differential diagnosis of any swelling arising out of the pelvis. It is characteristically impossible to feel the bladder's lower border. The swelling is typically regular, smooth, firm and oval-shaped. The bladder may sometimes reach as high as the umbilicus. It is unwise to make a definite diagnosis concerning a swelling coming out of the pelvis until you are sure the bladder is empty. This may require the insertion of a urinary catheter.

Inguinal lymph nodes. These are described on page 202.

Testes. Palpation of the testes is part of the routine abdominal examination (page 191). Testicular atrophy occurs in chronic liver disease (e.g. alcoholic liver disease, haemochromatosis); its mechanism is believed to be similar to that responsible for gynaecomastia (page 274).

Anterior abdominal wall. The skin and muscles of the anterior abdominal wall are prone to the same sorts of lumps that occur anywhere on the surface of the body (Table 5.15). So to avoid embarrassment it is important not to confuse these with intra-abdominal lumps. To determine whether a mass is in the abdominal wall, ask the patient to fold the arms across the upper chest and sit halfway up. An intra-abdominal mass disappears or decreases in size, but one within the layers of the abdominal wall will remain unchanged.

Pain can arise from the abdominal wall; this can cause confusion with intra-abdominal causes of pain. To test for *abdominal wall pain*, feel for an area of localised tenderness that reproduces the pain while the patient is supine. If this is found, ask the patient to fold the arms across the upper chest and sit halfway up, then palpate again (Carnett's test: described by JB Carnett in 1926). If the tenderness disappears, this suggests that the pain is in the abdominal cavity (as tensed abdominal muscles are protecting the viscera), but if the tenderness persists or is greater, this suggests that the pain is arising from the abdominal wall (e.g. muscle strain, nerve entrapment, myositis).[9,10] However, the Carnett test may occasionally be positive when there is visceral disease with involvement of the parietal peritoneum producing inflammation of the overlying muscle (e.g. appendicitis).

Figure 5.27 Detecting an expansile impulse

A = no impulse; B = transmitted pulsation from a neighbouring artery; C = expansile impulse, the sign of an aneurysm. (Adapted from Clain A, ed. *Hamilton Bailey's physical signs in clinical surgery*, 17th edn. John Wright & Sons, 1986.)

Table 5.15 Some causes of anterior abdominal wall masses

Lipoma
Sebaceous cyst
Dermal fibroma
Malignant deposits—e.g. melanoma, carcinoma
Epigastric hernia
Umbilical or paraumbilical hernia
Incisional hernia
Rectus sheath divarication
Rectus sheath haematoma

Figure 5.28 Percussion of the spleen

Percussion

Percussion is used to define the size and nature of organs and masses, to detect fluid in the peritoneal cavity, and to elicit tenderness in patients with peritonitis.

Liver. The liver borders should be percussed routinely to determine the liver span. If the liver edge is not palpable and there is no ascites, the right side of the abdomen should be percussed in the midclavicular line up to the right costal margin until dullness is encountered. This defines the liver's lower border even when it is not palpable. The upper border of the liver must always be defined by percussing down the midclavicular line (page 104). Loss of normal liver dullness may occur in massive hepatic necrosis, or with free gas in the peritoneal cavity (e.g. perforated bowel).

Spleen. Percussion over the left costal margin may be more sensitive than palpation for detection of enlargement of the spleen. Percuss over the lowest intercostal space in the left anterior axillary line in both inspiration and expiration with the patient supine (Figure 5.28). Splenomegaly should be suspected if the percussion note is dull or becomes *dull on complete expiration*. If the percussion note is dull, palpation should be repeated.

Kidneys. Percussion over a right or left subcostal mass can help distinguish hepatic or splenic from renal masses: in the latter case there will usually be a resonant area because of overlying bowel (be warned, however, that sometimes a very large renal mass may displace overlying bowel).

Bladder. An area of suprapubic dullness may indicate the upper border of an enlarged bladder or pelvic mass.

Ascites. The percussion note over most of the abdomen is resonant, due to air in the intestines.[11] The resonance is detectable out to the flanks. When peritoneal fluid (ascites) collects, the influence of gravity causes this to accumulate first in the flanks in a supine patient. Thus, a relatively early sign of ascites (when at least 2 litres of fluid have accumulated) is a dull percussion note in the flanks (*Good signs guide 5.3*). With gross ascites, the abdomen distends, the flanks bulge, umbilical eversion occurs (see Figure 5.19) and dullness is detectable closer to the midline. However, an area of central resonance will always persist. Routine abdominal examination should include percussion starting in the midline

Figure 5.29 Shifting dullness

(a) Percuss out to the left flank until the percussion note becomes dull. Mark this spot with your finger.

(b) Roll the patient towards you, wait 30 seconds. Shifting dullness is present if the left lateral dull area is now resonant.

with the finger pointing towards the feet; the percussion note is tested out towards the flanks on each side.

If (and only if) dullness is detected in the flanks, the sign of **shifting dullness** should be sought.[11] To detect this sign, while standing on the right side of the bed percuss out to the left flank until dullness is reached (Figure 5.29a). This point should be marked and the patient rolled towards the examiner. Ideally 30 seconds to 1 minute should then pass so that fluid can move inside the abdominal cavity and then percussion is repeated over the marked point (Figure 5.29b).

Shifting dullness is present if the area of dullness has changed to become resonant. This is because peritoneal fluid moves under the influence of gravity to the right side of the abdomen when this is the lowermost point. Very occasionally, fluid and air in dilated small bowel in small intestinal obstruction,

or a massive ovarian cyst filling the whole abdomen, can cause confusion.

To detect a **fluid thrill** (or wave) the clinician asks an assistant (or the patient) to place the medial edges of both palms firmly on the centre of the abdomen with the fingers pointing towards each other. The examiner flicks the side of the abdominal wall, and a pulsation (thrill) is felt by the hand placed on the other abdominal wall. A fluid thrill is of more value when there is massive ascites. Interestingly it may also occur when there is a massive ovarian cyst or a pregnancy with hydramnios.

The presence of dullness or bulging in the flanks has good sensitivity and moderate specificity for the detection of ascites. Shifting dullness has both good sensitivity and specificity. The presence of ankle oedema increases the likelihood of ascites. (See *Good signs guide 5.3*.)

The causes of ascites are listed in Table 5.16.

When significant ascites is present, abdominal masses may be difficult to feel by direct palpation. Here is the opportunity to practise *dipping*. Using the hand placed flat on the abdomen, the fingers are flexed at the metacarpophalangeal joints rapidly so as to displace the underlying fluid. This enables the fingers to reach a mass covered in ascitic fluid. In particular, this should be attempted to palpate an enlarged liver or spleen. The liver and spleen may become ballottable when gross ascites is present.

Auscultation

While some cardiologists believe that the sounds produced in the abdominal cavity are not as varied or as interesting as those one hears in the chest, they have some value.

GOOD SIGNS GUIDE 5.3 Ascites		
Sign	**Positive LR**	**Negative LR**
Inspection		
Bulging flanks	1.9	0.4
Oedema	3.8	0.2
Palpation and percussion		
Flank dullness	NS	0.3
Shifting dullness	2.3	0.4
Fluid wave	5.0	0.5
From McGee S, *Evidence-based physical diagnosis*, Saunders, 2001.		

Table 5.16 Classification of ascites by the serum ascites to albumin concentration gradient

High gradient (>1.1 g/dL)

1 Cirrhosis*
2 Alcoholic hepatitis,
3 Fulminant hepatic failure
4 Congestive heart failure, constrictive pericarditis (cardiac ascites)
5 Budd-Chiari syndrome (hepatic vein thrombosis) or veno-occlusive disease
6 Myxoedema
7 Massive liver metastases

Low gradient (<1.1 g/dL)

1 Peritoneal carcinomatosis
2 Tuberculosis
3 Pancreatic ascites
4 Nephrotic syndrome

* Patients with a high serum-to-ascites albumin concentration gradient most often have portal hypertension.

Bowel sounds. Place the diaphragm of the stethoscope just below the umbilicus. Bowel sounds can be heard over all parts of the abdomen in normal healthy people. They are poorly localised and there is little point in listening for them in more than one place. Most bowel sounds originate in the stomach, some from the large bowel and the rest from the small bowel. They have a soft gurgling character and occur only intermittently. Bowel sounds should be described as either present or absent; the terms 'decreased' or 'increased' are meaningless because the sounds vary, depending on when a meal was last eaten.

Complete absence of any bowel sounds over a 4-minute period indicates paralytic ileus (this is complete absence of peristalsis in a paralysed bowel). As only liquid is present in the gut, the heart sounds may be audible over the abdomen, transmitted by the dilated bowel.

The bowel that is obstructed produces a louder and higher-pitched sound with a tinkling quality due to the presence of air and liquid ('obstructed bowel sounds'). The presence of normal bowel sounds makes obstruction unlikely. Intestinal hurry or rush, which occurs in diarrhoeal states, causes loud gurgling sounds, often audible without the stethoscope. These bowel sounds are called *borborygmi*.

Friction rubs. These indicate an abnormality of the parietal and visceral peritoneum due to inflammation, but are very rare and non-specific. They may be audible over the liver or spleen. A rough creaking or grating noise is heard as the patient breathes. Hepatic causes include a tumour within the liver (hepatocellular cancer or metastases—said to be inaudible in 10% of cases), a liver abscess, a recent liver biopsy, a liver infarct, or gonococcal or chlamydial perihepatitis due to inflammation of the liver capsule (Fitz-Hugh-Curtis syndrome[v]). A splenic rub indicates a splenic infarct.

Venous hums. A venous hum is a continuous, low-pitched, soft murmur that may become louder with inspiration and diminish when more pressure is applied to the stethoscope. Typically it is heard between the xiphisternum and the umbilicus in cases of portal hypertension, but is rare. It may radiate to the chest or over to the liver. Large volumes of blood flowing in the umbilical or para-umbilical veins in the falciform ligament are responsible. These channel blood from the left portal vein to the epigastric or internal mammary veins in the abdominal wall. A venous hum may occasionally be heard over the large vessels such as the inferior mesenteric vein or after portacaval shunting. Sometimes a thrill is detectable over the site of maximum intensity of the hum. The Cruveilhier-Baumgarten[w] syndrome is the association of a venous hum at the umbilicus and dilated abdominal wall veins. It is almost always due to cirrhosis of the liver. It occurs when patients have a patent umbilical vein, which allows portal-to-systemic shunting at this site. The presence of a venous hum or of prominent central abdominal veins suggests that the site of portal obstruction is intrahepatic rather than in the portal vein itself.

Bruits. Uncommonly, an arterial systolic bruit can be heard over the liver. This sound is higher pitched than a venous hum, is not continuous and is well localised. This is usually due to a hepatocellular cancer but may occur in acute alcoholic hepatitis, with an arteriovenous malformation, or transiently after a liver biopsy. Auscultation for renal bruits on either side of the midline above the umbilicus is indicated if renal artery stenosis is suspected (page 187). A bruit in the epigastrium may be heard in patients with chronic intestinal ischaemia from mesenteric arterial stenosis, but may also occur in the absence

---

[v] AH Curtis described hepatic adhesions associated with pelvic inflammatory disease in 1930, while T Fitz-Hugh described right upper abdominal acute gonococcal peritonitis in 1934. However, this syndrome was actually first described by C Stajano in 1920.

[w] Jean Cruveilhier (1791–1874), Professor of Pathological Anatomy, Paris, who had been Dupuytren's registrar, and Paul von Baumgarten (1848–1928), German pathologist.

of pathology. A bruit may occasionally be audible over the spleen when there is a tumour of the body of the pancreas or a splenic arteriovenous fistula.

Hernias

Hernias are of surgical importance and should not be missed during an abdominal examination. They are very frequently the focus of student examinations. This section will be restricted to examination of groin hernias, which comprise inguinal and femoral hernias.

The principal sign of a hernia is that of a lump in the groin region. Naturally, not all lumps in the region are hernias (Table 5.17). A lump that is present on standing or during manoeuvres that raise intra-abdominal pressure (such as coughing or straining), and that disappears on recumbency, is easily identified as a hernia. Some hernias, however, are *irreducible*. Another term used for irreducible is incarcerated, but this term is probably best avoided. Some irreducible hernias contain bowel, which may become *obstructed*, giving rise to symptoms of small bowel obstruction in addition to the irreducible lump. Sometimes the bowel contents' blood supply becomes jeopardised, and these are known as *strangulated* hernias; they are usually painful, red, tense and tender.

Examination technique

A thorough examination for a hernia should be commenced with the patient standing if possible. The patient should be asked to stand with full exposure from the thigh to the upper abdomen.

Inspection is carried out initially. Pay careful attention to scars from previous surgery, which may be difficult to see. Look for obvious lumps and swellings. Before palpation is commenced the patient is asked to turn the head away from the examiner and to cough. The examiner's eyes should be fixed in the region of the pubic tubercle (see below) and note the presence of a visible cough impulse. The patient is then asked to cough again with the examiner inspecting the opposite side.

Of key importance is the position of a hernia in relation to the *pubic tubercle*, which can usually easily be felt *lateral to the symphysis pubis* (2–3 cm from the midline). In the obese individual, it may be difficult to locate the pubic tubercle and in such situations if the thigh is flexed and abducted, the adductor longus muscle can be traced proximally, leading the examiner to the pubic tubercle.

Palpation is commenced with the fingers being placed over the region of the pubic tubercle. Once again the patient is asked to cough and a palpable expansile impulse is sought. If a hernia is present, attempts at reduction should *not* be performed while

Table 5.17 Differential diagnosis of a solitary groin lump
Above the inguinal ligament
Inguinal hernia
Undescended testis
Cyst of the canal of Nuck
Encysted hydrocele or lipoma of the cord
Iliac node
Large femoral hernia (rare)
Below the inguinal ligament
Femoral hernia
Lymph node
Saphena varix (sensation of a 'jet of water' on palpation, disappears when supine)
Femoral aneurysm (pulsatile)
Psoas abscess (associated with fever, flank pain and flexion deformity)

the patient is erect, as it is more difficult and painful than when the patient is placed supine.

The patient is then asked to lie supine on the examination couch. The procedure of inspection and palpation is performed in the same manner again. The exact position of any hernia is usually easier to define with the patient lying supine.

If a lump or cough impulse is present, it must be determined whether this is a hernia and, if so, what sort of hernia. Identify the pubic tubercle. If an inguinal hernia is large, the pubic tubercle may be obscured by the hernia and its position may be less distinct, but an accurate indication can usually be made by comparing the lump with the pubic tubercle on the opposite side.

Inguinal hernias

Inguinal hernias typically bulge above the crease of the groin. They arise from a deficiency *above* the inguinal ligament and this is where they are usually felt (Figure 5.30). The inguinal ligament lies between the anterior superior iliac spine and the pubic tubercle. The pubic tubercle is just above the attachment of the adductor longus tendon to the pubic bone (feel the upper medial aspect of the thigh to palpate the tendon). The internal inguinal ring lies 2 cm above the midpoint of the inguinal ligament.

An *indirect* inguinal hernia protrudes through the deep inguinal ring. The best surface marking for this point is just above the midpoint of the inguinal ligament, which is halfway between the pubic tubercle and the anterior superior iliac spine (it is the

Figure 5.30 Note the elliptical swelling of an indirect inguinal hernia descending into the scrotum on the right side. Also note the globular swelling of a direct inguinal hernia on the left side.

position where the spermatic cord structures enter the inguinal canal). This is lateral to the inferior epigastric vessels. A *direct* hernia, on the other hand, pushes into the inguinal canal posteriorly through a region of weakness known as Hesselbach's triangle.[x] This triangle is bounded inferiorly by the inguinal ligament, laterally by the inferior epigastric vessels and medially by the lateral border of the rectus sheath.

The student may be asked to differentiate between direct and indirect inguinal hernias. However, clinically this is difficult and the true nature of an inguinal hernia can often be determined only at the time of operation. The muscular defect in a direct hernia is usually larger than that of an indirect hernia and as such direct hernias are typically easier to demonstrate, and usually reduce immediately and spontaneously. An indirect hernia may often be felt on palpation to slide along the direction of the inguinal canal under the examining fingers.

A large inguinal hernia may descend through the external ring immediately above the pubic tubercle into the scrotum. Gentle invagination of the scrotum with the tip of the gloved little finger in the external ring may be performed to confirm an indirect hernia in men but this can be difficult to interpret without substantial experience (Figure 5.31). A maldescended testis can be confused with an inguinal hernia; always confirm that there is a testis in each scrotum. A large inguinal hernia may present as a lump in the scrotum. It is important initially in this situation to ascertain whether one can get above the lump. If so, the lump is of primary intrascrotal pathology and is not a hernia.

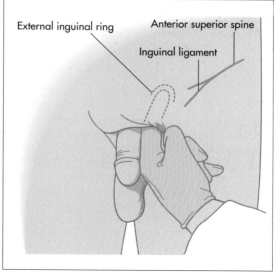

Figure 5.31 To examine the inguinal canal in a male, the scrotum can be invaginated as shown (always wear gloves)

Femoral hernias

Femoral hernias typically bulge into the groin crease at its medial end. Hence they occur lateral to and below the pubic tubercle, just medial to the femoral pulse (about 2 cm away) (Table 5.17). They are less common than inguinal hernias and are not related to the inguinal canal. They are usually smaller and firmer than inguinal hernias and quite commonly do not exhibit a cough impulse. They are frequently irreducible. As such, they are commonly mistaken for an enlarged inguinal lymph

---

[x] Franz Hesselbach (1759–1816), Professor of Surgery, Würzburg, described this triangle bounded by the inguinal ligament, the inferior epigastric artery and the rectus abdominis.

node. A cough impulse in this region needs to be distinguished from the thrill on coughing of a saphena varix.

Remember that hernias are often bilateral and that two different types may occur on the one side. Sometimes there is also a hydrocele (Figure 6.5)—one can get above a hydrocele in the inguinal canal but not a hernia.

Incisional hernias

Any abdominal scar may be the site of a hernia because of abdominal wall weakness. Assess this by asking the patient to cough while you look for abnormal bulges. Next have the patient lift the head and shoulders off the bed while the examiner's hand rests on the forehead and resists this movement. If a bulge is seen, the examiner's other hand should palpate for a fascial layer defect in the muscle.

Rectal examination

The examining physician often hesitates to make the necessary examination because it involves soiling the finger.

William Mayo (1861–1939)

The abdominal examination is not complete without the performance of a rectal examination.[12,13] It should be performed in all patients admitted to hospital who are over the age of 40, unless the examiner has no fingers or acute illness such as myocardial infarction presents a temporary contraindication. Following an explanation as to what is to happen, the patient lies on his or her left side with the knees drawn up and back to the examiner. This is called the left lateral position.

The examiner dons a pair of gloves and begins the inspection of the anus and perianal area by separating the buttocks. The following must be looked for:

1   **Thrombosed external haemorrhoids (piles).** Small (less than 1 cm), tense bluish swellings may be seen on one side of the anal margin. They are painful and are due to rupture of a vein in the external haemorrhoidal plexus. They are also called perianal haematomas.

2   **Skin tags.** These look like tags elsewhere on the body and can be an incidental finding or occur with haemorrhoids or Crohn's disease.

3   **Rectal prolapse.** Circumferential folds of red mucosa are visible protruding from the anus. These may become apparent only when the patient is asked to strain as if to pass stool. A gaping anus suggests loss of internal and external sphincter tone. This may coexist with prolapse.

4   **Anal fissure (fissure-in-ano).** This is a crack in the anal wall which may be painful enough to prevent rectal examination with the finger. Fissures-in-ano usually occur directly posteriorly and in the midline. A tag of skin may be present at the base: this is called a sentinel pile. It indicates that the fissure is chronic. It may be necessary to get the patient to bear down for a fissure to become visible. Multiple or broad-based fissures may be present in patients with inflammatory bowel disease, malignancy or venereal disease.

5   **Fistula-in-ano.** The entrance of this tract may be visible, usually within 4 cm of the anus. The mouth has a red pouting appearance caused by granulation tissue. This may occur with Crohn's disease or perianal abscess (page 170).

6   **Condylomata acuminata (anal warts)** may be confused with skin tags, but are in fact pedunculated papillomas with a white surface and red base. They may surround the anus.

7   **Carcinoma of the anus.** This may be visible as a fungating mass at the anal verge.

8   **Pruritus ani.** The appearance of this irritating anal condition varies from weeping red dermatitis to a thickened white skin.

9   **Excoriation** from diarrhoea.

Next ask the patient to strain: incontinence and leakage of faeces or mucus, abnormal descent of the perineum or the presence of a patulous anus are noted. Internal haemorrhoids can prolapse in the right anterior, right posterior and left lateral positions.

Now the time for action has come. The tip of the gloved right index finger is lubricated and placed over the anus. Ask the patient to breathe in and out quietly through the mouth, as a distraction and to aid relaxation. Slowly increasing pressure is applied with the pulp of the finger until the sphincter is felt to relax slightly. At this stage the finger is advanced into the rectum slowly. During entry, external sphincter tone should be assessed as normal or reduced, but the accuracy has been questioned.[14]

Palpation of the anterior wall of the rectum for the *prostate gland* in the male and for the *cervix* in the female is performed first. The normal prostate is a firm, rubbery bilobed mass with a central furrow. It becomes firmer with age. With prostatic enlargement, the sulcus becomes obliterated and the gland is often asymmetrical. A very hard nodule is apparent when a carcinoma of the prostate is present. The prostate is boggy and tender in prostatitis. A mass above the prostate or cervix may indicate a metastatic deposit on Blumer's shelf.[y]

---

y George Blumer (1858–1940), Professor of Medicine at Yale, in 1909 described cancer in the pouch of Douglas forming a shelf-like structure.

Table 5.18 Causes of a palpable mass in the rectum
Rectal carcinoma
Rectal polyp
Hypertrophied anal papilla
Diverticular phlegmon (recent or old)
Sigmoid colon carcinoma (prolapsing into the pouch of Douglas*)
Metastatic deposits in the pelvis (Blumer's shelf)
Uterine or ovarian malignancy
Prostatic or cervical malignancy (direct extension)
Endometriosis
Pelvic abscess or sarcoma
Amoebic granuloma
Foreign body

Note: Faeces, while palpable, also indent.
* James Douglas (1675–1742), Scottish anatomist and male midwife, Physician to Queen Caroline (wife of George II) in London.

The finger is then rotated clockwise so that the left lateral wall, posterior wall and right lateral wall of the rectum can be palpated in turn. Then the finger is advanced as high as possible into the rectum and slowly withdrawn along the rectal wall. A soft lesion, such as a small rectal carcinoma or polyp, is more likely to be felt this way (Table 5.18).[z] Ask the patient to squeeze your finger with the anal muscles as a further test of anal tone.

Ask the patient to strain and try to expel your finger. If the anal sphincter relaxes, this is normal; if the muscles tighten, this may indicate paradoxical external anal sphincter and puborectalis contraction which, during attempted defecation, blocks stool expulsion (causing constipation) and is termed pelvic floor dyssynergia or pelvic outlet obstruction.

Ask the patient to strain again when the examiner's finger is rotated anteriorly. In this position a *rectocele* (a defect in the anterior wall of the rectum) may be palpable.

After the finger has been withdrawn, the glove is inspected for bright blood or melaena, mucus or pus, and the colour of the faeces is noted. Haemorrhoids are not palpable unless thrombosed. Persistent gaping of the anal canal after withdrawal of the

examining finger may indicate external anal sphincter denervation. The occurrence of significant pain during the examination suggests an anal fissure, an ischiorectal abscess, a recently thrombosed external pile, proctitis or anal ulcers.

Test the *anal wink* (reflex contraction of the anal canal after pinprick testing of the perineum, page 342).

Proctosigmoidoscopy

The examination of the rectum with a sigmoidoscope is an essential part of the physical examination of any patient with symptoms referable to the anorectal region or large bowel. The principal indications include rectal bleeding, chronic diarrhoea, constipation or change in bowel habit. It should also be performed in some patients with abdominal pain, before treatment is begun for any anorectal condition, and before a barium enema is ordered for any reason.

The examination can be performed without anaesthesia, except in patients who have a very painful anal condition.

Procedure

Begin by inspecting the anal area as outlined earlier. Then a digital examination of the rectum is performed.

Explain to the patient what is about to happen. Warn him or her that there will be a feeling of fullness and the desire to defecate, and possibly cramps in the rectal region. The patient is then placed in the left lateral position and asked to relax and breathe quietly through the mouth.

If a rigid sigmoidoscope is to be used, it is warmed slightly and, with the obturator in place, is inserted into the rectum in the direction of the umbilicus until the rectal ampulla is reached (4 to 5 cm). This is the only part of the examination that is performed blind. The obturator is then removed. The tip of the sigmoidoscope is gently swung posteriorly under direct vision to follow the curve of the sacrum. The important landmarks to note during sigmoidoscopy are the anal verge, the dentate line, the anorectal junction, the lowest and middle rectal valves, and finally the rectosigmoid junction. Small amounts of air may be insufflated to assist with this. At about 12 to 15 cm, smooth rectal mucosa gives way to the concentric rugae of the distal sigmoid. It is possible to advance the rigid instrument into the distal sigmoid in the majority of men and in many women. The flexible sigmoidoscope usually can examine the entire left colon in skilled hands. The instrument must *never* be advanced unless the lumen is clearly visible and the patient is not experiencing pain.

[z] It can be useful to perform the rectal examination with the patient supine and the head of the bed elevated; this allows the intra-abdominal contents to descend and a bimanual examination (using the opposite hand to compress the lower abdomen) is possible.

Once the sigmoidoscope has been advanced as far as possible, it should be withdrawn gradually while the circumference of the mucosa is inspected carefully. Look behind for the valves of Houston.[aa] It is possible to sample faeces from areas away from the anal margin, which can be tested for occult blood and subjected to microbiological examination. Mucosal lesions can also be biopsied.

Common abnormalities seen on sigmoidoscopy

1 Blood, seen to be arising from above the highest level examined, indicates that a total examination of the colon by colonoscopy is essential.
2 Erythematous and ulcerated areas indicating inflammation, which may be local or diffuse.
3 Mucosal oedema, where there is loss of the normal vascular pattern of the colon, may be seen in mild inflammatory bowel disease.
4 Polyps, which may be sessile or pedunculated, solitary or multiple.
5 Carcinoma.
6 Strictures, which may be due to carcinoma, Crohn's disease, trauma, ischaemia, radiation or (very rarely) tuberculosis.
7 The orifices of diverticula.
8 Fissures.

If an abnormality of the anal canal is suspected, this is best seen using *anoscopy*, which can be carried out after sigmoidoscopy. Lesions to look for in the anal canal include swellings, masses, fissures, the internal openings of fistulae, squamous metaplasia and haemorrhoids. Haemorrhoids appear as swellings at the site of the normal anal cushions at 3, 7 and 11 o'clock, and they descend on straining. Remember that haemorrhoids are common and may coexist with more sinister bowel disease.

Testing of the stools for blood

Testing of the stools for blood can be helpful, particularly in the assessment of anaemia, iron deficiency, gastrointestinal bleeding or symptoms suggesting colonic cancer. In the guaiac test, stool is placed on a guaiac-impregnated paper; blood results in phenolytic oxidation, causing a blue colour. Newer tests can quantify the amount of blood in the stool. Unfortunately, both false-positive and false-negative results occur with the occult blood tests.

Peroxidase and catalase, present in various foods (e.g. fresh fruit, uncooked vegetables), and haem in red meat can cause false-positive results, as can aspirin, anticoagulants or oral iron. Vitamin C can reduce the sensitivity of guaiac results, and should not be taken before testing.

False-negative results are not uncommon with colorectal neoplasms because they bleed intermittently. Hence, testing for faecal occult blood from the glove after a rectal examination is of little value,[15] and more sensitive and specific testing (e.g. colonoscopy) is required, depending on the clinical setting.

Other

Examine the legs for bruising or oedema, which may be the result of liver disease. Neurological signs of alcoholism (e.g. a coarse tremor) or evidence of thiamine deficiency (peripheral neuropathy or memory loss) may also be present.

Examination of the cardiovascular system may be helpful in patients with hepatomegaly. Cardiac failure is a common cause of liver enlargement and can even cause cirrhosis. Measurement of the patient's temperature is important, especially in an acute abdominal case or if there is any suggestion of infection.

Examine with particular care all lymph node groups, the breasts and chest if there is any evidence of malignant disease such as firm, irregular hepatomegaly (Table 7.7).

Examination of the gastrointestinal contents

Faeces

Never miss an opportunity to inspect a patient's faeces, because considerable information about the gastrointestinal tract can be obtained in this way.

Melaena

Melaena stools are poorly formed, black and have a tarry appearance. They have a very characteristic and offensive smell. The cause is the presence of blood digested by gastric acid and colonic bacteria. Melaena usually indicates bleeding from the oesophagus, stomach or duodenum. The most common cause is acute or chronic peptic ulceration. Less often, right-sided colonic bleeding and

---

[aa] The middle one of three transverse folds of mucous membrane in the rectum, described in 1830 by John Houston (1802–45), Irish surgeon.

(rarely) small-bowel bleeding can cause melaena. The differential diagnosis of dark stools includes ingestion of iron tablets, bismuth, liquorice or charcoal. However, these tend to result in small well-formed non-tarry stools and the offensive smell is absent.

Bright red blood (haematochezia)

This appearance usually results from haemorrhage from the rectum or left colon. Beetroot ingestion can sometimes cause confusion. Blood loss may result from a carcinoma or polyp, an arteriovenous malformation, inflammatory bowel disease or diverticular disease. It can occasionally occur with massive upper gastrointestinal bleeding. The blood is mixed in with the bowel motion if it comes from above the anorectum, but if blood appears on the surface of the motion or only on the toilet paper this suggests, but does not guarantee, that bleeding is from a local rectal cause, such as internal haemorrhoids or a fissure. Dark red jelly-like stools may be seen with ischaemic bowel.

Steatorrhoea

The stools are usually very pale, offensive, smelly and bulky. They float and are difficult to flush away. However, the commonest cause of floating stools is gas and water rather than fat.

Steatorrhoea results from malabsorption of fat. In severe pancreatic disease, oil (triglycerides) may be passed per rectum and this is virtually pathognomonic of pancreatic steatorrhoea (lipase deficiency).

'Toothpaste' stools

Here the faeces are expressed like toothpaste from a tube: the condition is usually due to severe constipation with overflow diarrhoea. It may, however, also occur in the irritable bowel syndrome, with a stricture, or in Hirschsprung's disease.

Rice-water stools

Cholera causes massive excretion of fluid and electrolytes from the bowel, which results in a severe secretory diarrhoea. The pale watery stools are of enormous volume and contain mucous debris.

Vomitus

The clinician who is fortunate enough to have vomitus available for inspection (ill-informed staff may throw out this valuable substance) should not lose the opportunity of a detailed examination. There are a number of interesting types of vomitus.

'Coffee grounds'

An old blood clot in vomitus has the appearance of the dregs of a good cup of coffee. Unfortunately, darker vomitus is often described as having this appearance. This emphasises the need for personal inspection. Iron tablets and red wine, not to mention coffee ingestion, can have the same effect on the vomitus.

Bright red blood (haematemesis)

Look for the presence of fresh clot. It usually indicates fresh bleeding from the upper gastrointestinal tract.

Yellow-green vomitus

This results from the vomiting of bile and upper small bowel contents, often when there is obstruction.

Faeculent vomiting

Here brown offensive material from the small bowel is vomited. It is a late sign of small intestinal obstruction. Recently ingested tea can have the same appearance but lacks the smell.

Brownish-black fluid in large volumes may be vomited in cases of acute dilatation of the stomach. A succussion splash will usually be present. Acute dilatation may occur in association with diabetic ketoacidosis or following abdominal surgery. It represents a medical emergency because of the risk of aspiration; there is a need for urgent placement of a nasogastric tube (Figure 5.39).

Projectile vomiting

This term describes the act of vomiting itself and may indicate pyloric stenosis. It may also occur with raised intracranial pressure.

Urinalysis

Note that testing of the urine can be very helpful in diagnosing liver disease.

Strip colour tests can detect the presence of bilirubin and urobilinogen in the urine. False-positive or false-negative results can occur with vitamin C or even exposure to sunlight.

An understanding of the reasons for the presence of bilirubin or urobilinogen in the urine necessitates an explanation of the metabolism of these substances (Figure 5.32).

Red blood cells are broken down by the reticuloendothelial system, causing the release of haem, which is converted to biliverdin and then *unconjugated bilirubin*, a water-insoluble compound. For

Figure 5.32 Schematic representation of the bilirubin pathway

Increased haemolysis (1) overwhelms the hepatocytes' ability to conjugate bilirubin and excrete the conjugated form, leading to increased serum levels of unconjugated bilirubin. Low levels of glucuronyl transferase (2) (e.g. Gilbert's disease) cause decreased conjugation. Hepatocellular dysfunction (3) causes decreased uptake, conjugation and excretion with increases of unconjugated bilirubin and conjugated bilirubin. Post-hepatic obstruction (4) from stones or tumour prevents passage of bilirubin through the bile ducts into the bowel, leading to increased serum levels of conjugated bilirubin.

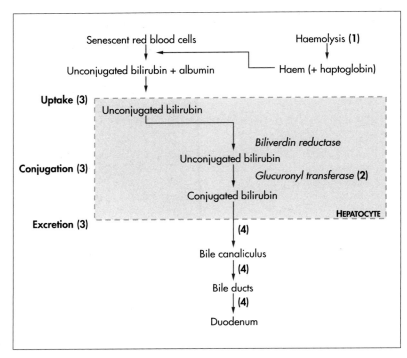

this reason, unconjugated bilirubin released with haemolytic anaemia will not appear in the urine (termed *acholuric jaundice*).

Unconjugated bilirubin is transported in the blood bound largely to albumin but also to other plasma proteins. Unconjugated bilirubin is then taken up by the liver cells and transported to the endoplasmic reticulum, where glucuronyl transferases conjugate bilirubin with glucuronide. This results in the formation of *conjugated bilirubin*, which is water-soluble. Conjugated bilirubin is then concentrated and excreted by the liver cell into the canaliculus.

Conjugated bilirubin is virtually all excreted into the small bowel; it is converted in the terminal ileum and colon to *urobilinogen*, and then to *stercobilin*. Stercobilin is responsible for the normal colour of the stools with other non-bilirubinoid dietary pigments. Up to 20% of urobilinogen is reabsorbed by the bowel, and small amounts are excreted in the urine as urinary urobilinogen. This can often be normally detected by reagent strips.

Total biliary obstruction, from whatever cause, results in absence of urinary urobilinogen, as no conjugated bilirubin reaches the bowel, resulting in pale stools (absence of stercobilin). The conjugated bilirubin, unable to be excreted (the rate-limiting step),

leaks from the hepatocytes into the blood and from there is excreted into the urine (normally there is no bilirubin detected in urine). This results in dark urine (excess conjugated bilirubin). Acute liver damage, as in viral hepatitis, may sometimes initially result in excessive urinary urobilinogen, because the liver is unable to re-excrete the urobilinogen reabsorbed from the bowel. These changes are summarised in Table 5.19.

Examination of the acute abdomen

It is very important to try to determine whether a patient who presents with acute abdominal pain requires an urgent operation or whether careful observation with reassessment is the best course of action.[16] First, take note of the general appearance of the patient. The patient who is obviously distressed with pain or who looks unwell often is, and conversely some reassurance can be gained if a patient does not look sick and appears comfortable.

Assess the patient's vital signs immediately and recheck these at frequent intervals. Signs of reduced circulating blood volume, including tachycardia,

Table 5.19 Changes in urine and faeces with jaundice

Substance and site	Cause of jaundice		
	Haemolysis	Obstruction or cholestasis	Hepatocellular liver disease
Urine			
Bilirubin (conjugated)	Normal*	Raised	Normal or raised
Urobilinogen	Raised	Absent or decreased	Normal or raised
Faeces			
Stercobilinogen	Raised	Absent or decreased	Normal
Causes	Haemolytic anaemia	Extrahepatic biliary obstruction (e.g. gallstones, carcinoma of pancreas or bile duct, strictures of the bile duct), intrahepatic cholestasis (e.g. drugs, recurrent) jaundice of pregnancy)	Hepatitis, cirrhosis, drugs, venous obstruction

* Unconjugated bilirubin levels are elevated in the serum.

postural hypotension, tachypnoea, vasoconstriction and sweating are of great concern. These signs associated with abdominal pain are usually an indication of substantial intra-abdominal blood loss (such as a ruptured aortic aneurism) or of substantial fluid losses (e.g. due to acute pancreatitis), or of septic shock (as with a perforated viscus or abscess).

Inspect the abdomen. Look particularly for lack of movement with respiration, with splinting of the abdominal wall muscles. Note any abdominal distension, visible peristalsis or other lumps and masses, without forgetting the groin region and hernias. Note also any abdominal scars and inquire as to their nature and age.

Palpate very gently. The presence or absence of peritonism is first assessed. Peritonism is an inflammation that causes pain when peritoneal surfaces are moved relative to each other (Table 5.20; see also *Good signs guide 5.4*). Traditionally, rebound tenderness is used to assess whether peritonism is present or not. However, if peritonism is present, this test is far more uncomfortable (and cruel) than eliciting tenderness to light percussion. If the patient is extremely apprehensive, ask him or her first to cough; the reaction will be a guide to the degree of peritonism and also its location. Palpation is then continued slowly,

GOOD SIGNS GUIDE 5.4
Peritonitis

Sign	Positive LR	Negative LR
Abdominal examination		
Guarding	2.6	0.6
Rigidity	5.1	NS
Rebound tenderness	2.1	0.5
Abnormal bowel sounds	NS	0.8
Rectal examination		
Rectal tenderness	NS	NS
Other tests		
Positive abdominal wall tenderness test	0.1	NS

NS = not significant.
From McGee S, *Evidence-based physical diagnosis*, Saunders, 2001.

but more deeply if possible and if masses are sought. Do not forget to palpate for the pulsatile mass of a ruptured aneurysm. This may be quite indistinct.

Then perform light percussion over areas of tenderness. If generalised peritonitis is present, this

Table 5.20 Differential diagnosis of the acute abdomen

Severe abdominal pain with rigidity of the entire abdominal wall and prostration

Perforated peptic ulcer
Perforation of other intra-abdominal organs
Dissecting aneurysm
Severe pancreatitis

Tenderness and rigidity in the right hypochondrium

Acute cholecystitis
Appendicitis in a high appendix
Perforated or penetrating duodenal ulcer
Pleurisy, pneumonitis
Subphrenic abscess
Acute pyelonephritis
Cholangitis
Bleed into an hepatic tumour

Tenderness and rigidity in the left hypochondrium

Pancreatitis
Subphrenic abscess
Diverticulitis
Ruptured spleen
Acute pyelonephritis
Leaking aneurysm of the splenic artery
Acute gastric distension

Tenderness and rigidity in the right iliac fossa

Appendicitis
Perforated or penetrating duodenal ulcer
Crohn's disease or inflamed ileocaecal glands
Inflamed Meckel's diverticulum
Cholecystitis with a low gallbladder

Tenderness and rigidity in the left iliac fossa

Diverticulitis
Colitis
Colonic cancer
Pelvic peritonitis, ruptured ovarian cyst

Periumbilical pain without abdominal signs

Acute mesenteric ischaemia/infarction
Acute appendicitis
Acute small bowel obstruction
Acute pancreatitis

Obstetric and gynaecological causes

Ectopic pregnancy
Torsion of, or haemorrhage into, an ovarian cyst
Acute salpingitis
Ruptured uterus

GOOD SIGNS GUIDE 5.5
Acute bowel obstruction

Sign	Positive LR	Negative LR
Inspection of the abdomen		
Visible peristalsis	18.8	NS
Abdominal distension	9.6	0.4
Palpation		
Guarding	NS	NS
Rigidity	NS	NS
Rebound tenderness	NS	NS
Auscultation		
Increased (obstructed) bowel sounds	5.0	0.6
Abnormal bowel sounds	3.2	0.4
Rectal examination		
Rectal tenderness	NS	NS

NS = not significant.
From McGee S, *Evidence-based physical diagnosis*, Saunders, 2001.

---

almost invariably necessitates a surgical approach, with the notable exception of acute pancreatitis.

Examine for hernias. The presence of a hernia does not necessarily mean that this is the cause of pathology, as they are quite common. However, a tender or irreducible hernia is more likely to be of significance, particularly if this has only very recently been noticed by the patient or has recently become tender.

Auscultation is now performed. In the presence of a bowel obstruction (*Good signs guide 5.5*), bowel sounds will be louder, more frequent and high pitched. In an ileus from any cause, bowel sounds are usually reduced or absent.

Rectal and vaginal examinations are essential; note any tenderness (and its location), masses or blood loss. Per rectal blood should make the examiner think of acute colitis (e.g. Crohn's disease, ulcerative colitis, ischaemic colitis or infectious colitis), or of mesenteric ischaemia. A purulent vaginal discharge suggests salpingitis.

Urinalysis may show glycosuria and ketonuria in diabetic ketoacidosis (which can cause acute abdominal pain), haematuria in renal colic, bilirubinuria in cholangitis or proteinuria in pyelonephritis (page 180).

Examine the *respiratory system* for signs of consolidation, a pleural rub or pleural effusion, and examine the *cardiovascular system* for atrial fibrillation

GOOD SIGNS GUIDE 5.6
Appendicitis

Sign	Positive LR	Negative LR
Vital signs		
Fever	1.8	0.5
Abdominal examination		
Severe right lower quadrant tenderness	NS	0.2
McBurney's point tenderness	3.4	0.4
Rovsing's sign	2.5	0.7
Rectal examination		
Rectal tenderness	NS	NS
Others		
Psoas sign	NS	NS

NS = not significant.
From McGee S, *Evidence-based physical diagnosis*, Saunders, 2001.

(a major cause of embolism to a mesenteric artery) or for signs of a myocardial infarction. Examine the *back* for evidence of spinal disease that may radiate to the abdomen. Remember that herpes zoster may cause abdominal pain before the typical vesicles erupt.

Consider the symptoms and signs of appendicitis. Malaise and fever is usually associated with abdominal pain, which is at first worst in the hypogastrium and then moves to the right iliac fossa. The examination will often reveal tenderness and guarding in the right iliac fossa. The pain and tenderness are usually maximum over *McBurney's point*.[bb] He described this point as $1^{1}/_{2}$ to 2 in (3.8 to 5.0 cm) along a line from the anterior superior iliac spine to the umbilicus. *Rovsing's sign*[cc] is another way of testing rebound tenderness. Press over the patient's left lower quadrant, then release quickly; this causes pain in the right iliac fossa. The *psoas sign* is positive when the patient lies on the left side and the clinician attempts to extend the right hip. If this is painful and resisted, the sign is positive. When the appendix causes pelvic inflammation, rectal examination evokes tenderness on the right side. These signs are of variable usefulness (*Good signs guide 5.6*).

[bb] Charles McBurney (1845-1913). New York surgeon described his sign to the New York Surgical Society in 1889.
[cc] Thorkild Rovsing (1862-1937). Professor of Surgery Copenhagen.

Correlation of physical signs and gastrointestinal disease

Liver disease

Signs

- **Hands:** leuconychia, clubbing, palmar erythema, bruising, asterixis.
- **Face:** jaundice, scratch marks, spider naevi, fetor hepaticus.
- **Chest:** gynaecomastia, loss of body hair, spider naevi, bruising, pectoral muscle wasting.
- **Abdomen:** hepatosplenomegaly, ascites, signs of portal hypertension, testicular atrophy.
- **Legs:** oedema, muscle wasting, bruising.
- **Fever:** may occur in up to one-third of patients with advanced cirrhosis (particularly when this is secondary to alcohol) or if there is infected ascites.

The presence of two or more of the following signs suggests cirrhosis: (i) spider naevi; (ii) palmar erythema; (iii) splenomegaly or ascites; (iv) abnormal collateral veins on the abdomen; (v) ascites. See also *Good signs guide 5.7*.

GOOD SIGNS GUIDE 5.7
Jaundice due to hepatocellular disease

Sign	Positive LR	Negative LR
General appearance		
Weight loss	NS	NS
Skin		
Spider naevi	4.7	0.6
Palmar erythema	9.8	0.5
Distended abdominal veins	17.5	0.6
Abdomen		
Ascites	4.4	0.6
Palpable spleen	2.9	0.7
Palpable gallbladder (Courvoisier's law)	0.04	1.4
Palpable liver	NS	NS
Liver tenderness	NS	NS

NS = not significant.
From McGee S, *Evidence-based physical diagnosis*, Saunders, 2001.

Portal hypertension

Signs

- **Splenomegaly:** correlates poorly with the degree of portal hypertension.
- **Collateral veins:** haematemesis (from oesophageal or gastric varices).
- **Ascites.**

Causes

1 **Cirrhosis** of the liver.
2 **Other causes:**
   (a) *Presinusoidal:* (i) portal vein compression (e.g. lymphoma, carcinoma); (ii) intravascular clotting (e.g. in polycythaemia); (iii) umbilical vein phlebitis.
   (b) *Intrahepatic:* (i) sarcoid, lymphoma or leukaemic infiltrates; (ii) congenital hepatic fibrosis.
   (c) *Postsinusoidal:* (i) hepatic vein outflow obstruction (Budd-Chiari syndrome) may be idiopathic, or caused by myeloproliferative disease, cancer (kidney, pancreas, liver), the contraceptive pill or pregnancy, paroxysmal nocturnal haemoglobinuria (PNH), fibrous membrane, trauma, schistosomiasis; (ii) veno-occlusive disease; (iii) constrictive pericarditis; (iv) chronic cardiac failure.

Hepatic encephalopathy

Grading

Grade 0: normal mental state.
Grade 1: mental changes (lack of awareness, anxiety, euphoria, reduced attention span, impaired ability to add and subtract).
Grade 2: lethargy, disorientation (for time), personality changes, inappropriate behaviour.
Grade 3: stupor, but responsive to stimuli; gross disorientation, confusion.
Grade 4: coma.

Causes

These include:

- Acute liver failure (e.g. postviral hepatitis, alcoholic hepatitis).
- Cirrhosis.
- Chronic portosystemic encephalopathy (e.g. from a portocaval shunt).

Encephalopathy may be precipitated by:

- Diarrhoea, diuretics or vomiting (resulting in hypokalaemia which may increase renal ammonia and other toxin production, or alkalosis which may increase the amount of ammonia and other toxins that cross the blood–brain barrier).
- Gastrointestinal bleeding or a relatively high protein diet (causing an acute increase in nitrogenous contents in the bowel).
- Infection (e.g. urinary tract, chest or spontaneous bacterial peritonitis).
- Acute liver cell decompensation (e.g. from an alcoholic binge or a hepatoma).
- Sedatives.
- Metabolic disturbances such as hypoglycaemia.

Dysphagia

Dysphagia (difficulty in swallowing) and odynophagia (pain on swallowing) are important symptoms of underlying organic disease. It is important to examine such patients carefully for likely causes (see Table 5.2).

Signs

- **General inspection.** Note weight loss, due to decreased food intake or oesophageal cancer per se.
- **The hands.** Inspect the nails for koilonychia (page 198), and the palmar creases for pallor indicative of anaemia. Iron deficiency anaemia can be associated with an upper oesophageal web, which is a thin structure consisting of mucosa and submucosa but not muscle. Iron deficiency anaemia and dysphagia due to an upper oesophageal web is called the Plummer-Vinson[dd] or sometimes the Paterson-Brown-Kelly[ee] syndrome. Also examine the hands for signs of scleroderma (page 248).
- **The mouth.** Inspect the mucosa for ulceration or infection (e.g. candidiasis), which can cause odynophagia; examine the lower cranial nerves for evidence of bulbar or pseudobulbar palsy (page 317).
- **The neck.** Palpate the supraclavicular nodes, which may occasionally be involved with oesophageal cancer (page 201); examine for evidence of retrosternal thyroid enlargement (page 260). A mass on the left side of the neck that is

---

[dd] Henry Plummer (1874–1936), physician at the Mayo Clinic, described the syndrome in 1912; Porter Vinson (1890–1959), physician, Medical College Virginia, described the syndrome in 1919.
[ee] Donald Paterson (1863–1939), Cardiff otolaryngologist, and Adam Brown-Kelly (1865–1941), Glasgow otolaryngologist, described this syndrome in 1919.

accompanied by gurgling sounds may rarely be caused by a Zenker's diverticulum,[ff] an outpouching of the posterior hypopharyngeal wall.

- **The lungs.** Examine for evidence of aspiration into the lungs (due to overflow of retained material, gastro-oesophageal reflux or, rarely, the development of a tracheo-oesophageal reflux from oesophageal cancer).
- **The abdomen.** Feel for hepatomegaly due to secondary deposits from oesophageal cancer and for an epigastric mass from a gastric cancer; perform a rectal examination to exclude melaena (albeit uncommon with oesophageal disease).

Assessment of gastrointestinal bleeding

Haematemesis, melaena or massive rectal bleeding are dramatic signs of gastrointestinal haemorrhage. It is important in such a case to assess the amount of blood loss and attempt to determine the likely site of bleeding. Haematemesis indicates bleeding from a site proximal to, or in, the duodenum.

Assessing degree of blood loss

First take the pulse rate and the blood pressure lying and sitting. As a general rule, loss of 1.5 litres or more of blood volume over a few hours results in a fall in cardiac output, causing hypotension and tachycardia. A pulse rate of more than 100 a minute or a systolic blood pressure of less than 100 mmHg, or a 15 mmHg postural fall in systolic blood pressure, suggests significant recent blood loss. These are indications for blood transfusion. The signs depend to some extent on the state of the patient's cardiovascular system. Those who have pre-existing cardiovascular disease will become shocked much earlier than young fit patients with a normal cardiovascular system.

Once signs of shock are present, massive blood loss has occurred. These signs include peripheral cyanosis with cold extremities, clammy skin, dyspnoea and air hunger; the patients are anxious. The blood pressure is low, with a compensating tachycardia, and the urine output is reduced or absent. These are ominous signs in patients with gastrointestinal haemorrhage. Urgent resuscitative measures must be instituted.

Determining the possible bleeding site

The causes of acute gastrointestinal haemorrhage are listed in Table 5.3.

Examine the patient with *acute upper gastrointestinal bleeding* for signs of chronic liver disease and portal hypertension. Part of the assessment should include inspection of the vomitus and stools (pages 162–163) and a rectal examination. Remember that, of patients with chronic liver disease and upper gastrointestinal bleeding, only about half are bleeding from varices. The others are usually bleeding from peptic ulceration (either acute or chronic). Look for evidence of a bleeding diathesis.

Finally, examine the patient for any evidence of skin lesions that can be associated with vascular anomalies in the gastrointestinal tract, although these are rare (Tables 5.3, 5.4). For example, pseudoxanthoma elasticum is an autosomal recessive disorder of elastic fibres that results in xanthoma-like yellowish nodules, particularly in the axillae or neck. These patients may also have angioid streaks of the optic fundus (page 268) and angiomatous malformations of blood vessels that can bleed into the gastrointestinal tract. Ehlers-Danlos syndrome is a group of connective tissue disorders resulting in fragile and hyperextensible skin. In a number of types, blood vessels are involved. Type IV is characterised by gastrointestinal tract bleeding, spontaneous bowel perforation, minimal skin hyperelasticity and minimal joint hyperextension.

Examine the patient with *acute lower gastrointestinal bleeding* as described above, paying close attention to the abdominal examination and the rectal examination. Inspect the stools and test them for blood. Colonoscopy is a key test for all these patients.

Malabsorption

Numerous diseases can cause maldigestion or malabsorption of food. Fat, protein and/or carbohydrate absorption may be affected.

Signs

- **General:** wasting (protein and fat malabsorption), folds of loose skin (recent weight loss), pallor (anaemia) or pigmentation (e.g. as in Whipple's disease[gg]).

[ff] Friedrich Albert Zenker (1825–1898), Munich pathologist.

[gg] George Hoyt Whipple (1878–1976), Baltimore pathologist, described this rare disease characterised by diarrhoea, arthralgia, central nervous system signs and pigmentation. He shared the 1934 Nobel Prize for work on liver treatment in anaemia and coined the word *thalassaemia*.

- **Stools:** steatorrhoea (pale, bulky and offensive stools).
- **Mouth:** glossitis and angular stomatitis (deficiency in vitamin B_2, vitamin B_6, vitamin B_{12}, folate or niacin), intraoral purpura (vitamin K deficiency) or hyperkeratotic white patches (vitamin A deficiency).
- **Limbs:** bruising (vitamin K deficiency), oedema (protein deficiency), peripheral neuropathy (vitamin B_{12} or thiamine deficiency), bone pain (vitamin D deficiency).
- **Signs suggesting the underlying cause:** in the abdomen these include scars from previous surgery, such as a gastrectomy, operations for Crohn's disease or massive small bowel resection; on the skin dermatitis herpetiformis (itchy red lumps on the extensor surfaces) may be found—this condition is strongly associated with coeliac disease and the histocompatibility antigen HLA-B8; there may be *signs of chronic liver disease*, or *signs of inflammatory bowel disease*.

Causes

Common causes include coeliac disease, chronic pancreatitis and a previous gastrectomy.

Classification of malabsorption

- **Lipolytic phase defects** (pancreatic enzyme deficiency): (i) chronic pancreatitis; (ii) cystic fibrosis.
- **Micellar phase defects** (bile salt deficiency): (i) extrahepatic biliary obstruction; (ii) chronic liver disease; (iii) bacterial overgrowth; (iv) terminal ileal disease, such as Crohn's disease or resection.
- **Mucosal defects** (diseased epithelial lining): (i) coeliac disease; (ii) tropical sprue; (iii) lymphoma; (iv) Whipple's disease; (v) bowel ischaemia or resection; (vi) amyloidosis; (vii) hypogammaglobulinaemia; (viii) HIV infection.
- **Delivery phase defects** (inability to transport fat out of cells to lymphatics): (i) intestinal lymphangiectasia; (ii) abetalipoproteinaemia; (iii) carcinomatous infiltration of lymphatics.

Inflammatory bowel disease

Inflammatory bowel disease refers to two chronic idiopathic diseases of the gastrointestinal tract: ulcerative colitis and Crohn's disease.

Ulcerative colitis

In the gastrointestinal tract only the large bowel is affected. Occasionally the terminal ileum can be secondarily involved (backwash ileitis). The disease almost always involves the rectum and may extend, without skip areas, to involve a variable part of the colon.

- **Abdominal signs:** if there is proctitis only, there are usually no abnormal external findings (except at sigmoidoscopy and biopsy); occasionally, anal fissures are present; with colitis, in the uncomplicated case the abdominal examination may be normal or there may be tenderness and guarding over the affected colon.
- **Signs of complications:** local signs include the following: (i) *toxic dilatation (megacolon)*—one of the most feared complications in which there are signs of distension, generalised guarding and rigidity (peritonism), pyrexia and tachycardia; (ii) *massive bleeding or perforation*; (iii) *carcinoma*—there is an increased incidence of colonic cancer in extensive, long-standing ulcerative colitis.
- **Systemic signs include:** (i) *chronic liver disease*—primary sclerosing cholangitis or cirrhosis; (ii) *anaemia*—due to chronic disease per se, or blood loss, or autoimmune haemolysis; (iii) *arthritis*—there may be a peripheral non-deforming arthropathy affecting particularly the knees, ankles and wrists (10%), and there may be signs of ankylosing spondylitis in 3%; (iv) *skin manifestations:* erythema nodosum (2%) consists of tender red nodules usually on the shins (Figure 5.33); pyoderma gangrenosum (rare) starts as a tender, red raised area which becomes bullous and ulcerates (Figure 5.34)—it may occur anywhere but is often on the anterior aspects of the legs; mouth ulcers are common and are due to aphthous ulceration (5%); finger clubbing may be present; (v) *ocular changes* include conjunctivitis, iritis and episcleritis, which are strongly associated with arthritis and skin rash. (*Conjunctivitis* is an inflammation of the conjunctiva which then appears red and swollen: the eye itself is not tender. *Iritis* is an inflammation of the iris with central scleral injection, which radiates out from the pupil: the eye is tender. *Episcleritis* is a nodule of inflammation on the scleral surface.)

Crohn's disease

The whole of the gastrointestinal tract may be affected from the mouth to the anus. However, most commonly the terminal ileum, with or without the colon, is involved.

- **Abdominal signs:** if the condition affects only the terminal ileum there are often no abnormal

Figure 5.33 Erythema nodosum

(From FS McDonald, ed., *Mayo Clinic images in internal medicine*, with permission. © Mayo Clinic Scientific Press and CRC Press.)

findings, although tenderness, fullness or a mass (either soft or firm) in the right iliac fossa may be present. Occasionally there may be signs of an abdominal abscess: these patients may have a high swinging fever, localised tenderness, a palpable mass and evidence of bowel obstruction (pain, vomiting and constipation with dehydration, abdominal distension and tenderness, and an empty rectum). Anal disease is common, including skin tags, fissures, fistulae and abscesses. Colonic involvement produces the same signs as ulcerative colitis.

- **Signs of complications:** these are similar to those of ulcerative colitis with the following exceptions: (i) *liver disease*—primary sclerosing cholangitis is less common; (ii) *osteomalacia* and *osteoporosis*, which may occur in patients with extensive terminal ileal involvement, results in bone tenderness and fracture; (iii) *signs of malabsorption;* (iv) *finger clubbing* is more common; (v) *signs of gastrointestinal malignancy* (small bowel or colonic carcinoma) are uncommon but the incidence is increased; (vi) the incidence of *gallstones and renal stones* is increased; (vii) *renal disease* due to pyelonephritis, hydronephrosis or very rarely secondary amyloidosis may occur.

The abdominal X-ray: a systematic approach

Interpretation of the plain radiograph requires knowledge of basic anatomy and pathological processes.

The soft tissue density of the abdominal organs is similar to that of water. Therefore they are usually not visible unless outlined by fat or adjacent gas. For example, fluid-filled bowel is not visible, but the bowel walls are outlined by the contained gas.

Because of this intrinsic lack of contrast in the abdomen, radio-opaque contrast media are introduced to show up various organs. Barium meals, barium enemas, intravenous urograms and arteriograms are contrast studies.

Figure 5.34 Pyoderma gangrenosum

(From *Slide atlas of gastroenterology*. London: Gower Medical Publishing, 1985, with permission.)

Radiography

As with the chest X-ray, the name and date should be checked. The left and right sides should be easily distinguished by the stomach gas on the left and the triangular bulky soft tissue of the liver seen in the right hypochondrium.

Review of an abdominal X-ray

- **Boundaries:** diaphragm, psoas muscles, the extraperitoneal fat ('flank lines').
- **Bones:** lower ribs and costal cartilages, lumbar spine, pelvis.
- **Hollow viscera gas:** check gas outlining the stomach, small bowel and large bowel.
- **Solid organs:** size of liver, spleen and kidneys.
- **Pelvic organs:** bladder size.
- **Vascular:** aortic calcification.
- **Abnormalities:** renal or biliary calculi, dilated bowel, free peritoneal gas (Figure 5.35).

Bowel gas pattern

Supine films are taken in most conditions to show the distribution of the bowel gas. In patients with an acute abdomen, a horizontal beam film, usually an erect view, is also taken to show air-fluid levels.

With obstruction, there is an accumulation of fluid and gas proximally.

In inflammatory or ischaemic colitis, the swollen bowel mucosa will be outlined by gas ('thumb-printing').

Bowel dilatation

When an ileus (Figure 5.36) or obstruction (Figures 5.37, 5.38) is present, it is possible to distinguish small- from large-bowel dilatation. The *large-bowel loops* are peripheral, few in number, have diameters greater than 5 cm, contain faeces, and have haustral margins that do not extend across the bowel lumen. In contrast, the *small-bowel loops* are central, multiple, between 3 and 5 cm in diameter, and do not contain faeces. Valvulae conniventes which extend completely across the bowel lumen are seen in the jejunal loops.

With gastric dilatation, the stomach may be massively enlarged and distended with air (Figure 5.39).

Figure 5.35 Free peritoneal gas

The erect chest X-ray is superior to an erect abdominal film for the demonstration of free gas. On the erect chest X-ray, free peritoneal gas is seen below the hemidiaphragm (black arrows). The free gas on the left must be distinguished from gas in the gastric fundus (open arrow). This free gas (black arrow) on the left is crescentic in shape because it outlines the spleen and lies at the apex of the hemidiaphragm. It indicates a perforation of a hollow abdominal viscus unless there has been recent surgery or penetrating trauma.

Figure 5.36 Generalised ileus

The large bowel is filled with gas and is dilated, except in the descending colon. Dilated small bowel is also seen in the right hypochondrium (arrow). As gas is seen around to the rectum (arrow), mechanical obstruction is excluded.

Figure 5.37 Small bowel obstruction

There is gross dilatation of the small bowel. It is recognised as small bowel from its central position and its transverse mucosal bands—the valvulae conniventes (black arrow). Air-fluid levels are seen on the erect view (a). The supine view (b) gives a better view of the distribution of the dilated loops. From the number and position of the displayed dilated loops, the obstruction would be at the level of the mid-small bowel. The round radio-opaque shadow in the left hypochondrium is a tablet (open arrow).

Figure 5.38 Large bowel obstruction

The large bowel is markedly distended around to the sigmoid colon, where it abruptly stops (arrow). The common causes of obstruction are carcinoma or diverticular stricture. The increased peristalsis occurring at the onset of obstruction can remove the gas and faeces distal to the obstruction. Therefore no gas is seen in this patient.

Figure 5.39 Gastric dilatation

The stomach is massively enlarged and distended with air. When this occurs acutely, prompt nasogastric aspiration is necessary. Mechanical obstruction due to a pyloric ulcer or carcinoma needs exclusion. Atonic dilatation is usually a postoperative complication, but may occur with diabetic coma, trauma, pancreatitis or hypokalaemia.

Calcification

Calcification shows up well against the grey, soft tissue densities.

About 90% of renal stones are calcified (Figure 6.1), whereas only 10% of gallstones are calcified. To identify radiolucent gallstones, an ultrasound examination is the test of choice.

Calcification may be seen in the pancreas in chronic pancreatitis (Figure 5.40).

Costal cartilage calcification is commonly seen in elderly patients, projected over the hypochondrial regions.

Calcification in the walls of an abdominal aortic aneurysm may be seen on a lateral abdominal film. Splenic and renal artery aneurysms are also often calcified.

Vascular calcification is often seen in the elderly.

Ascites

With accumulation of peritoneal fluid within the peritoneal cavity, the film looks generally grey and lacks detail. On the supine film the bowel loops float towards the middle of the abdomen.

Figure 5.40 Pancreatic calcification
Stippled calcification is seen in the region of the pancreas (arrow), indicating chronic calcific pancreatitis. The most likely cause is alcohol excess.

Summary

The gastrointestinal examination: a suggested method (Figure 5.41)

Position the patient correctly with one pillow for the head and complete exposure of the abdomen. Look briefly at the general appearance and inspect particularly for signs of chronic liver disease.

Examine the hands. Ask the patient to extend his or her arms and hands and look for the hepatic flap. Look also at the nails for clubbing and for white nails, and note any palmar erythema or Dupuytren's contractures. The arthropathy of haemochromatosis may also be present. Look now at the arms for bruising, scratch marks and spider naevi.

Then go to the face. Note any scleral abnormality (jaundice, anaemia or iritis). Look at the corneas for Kayser-Fleischer rings. Feel for parotid enlargement; then inspect the mouth with a torch and spatula for angular stomatitis, ulceration, telangiectasiae and atrophic glossitis. Smell the breath for fetor hepaticus. Now look at the chest for spider naevi and in men for gynaecomastia and loss of body hair.

Inspect the abdomen from the side, squatting to the patient's level. Large masses may be visible. Ask the patient to take slow deep breaths and look especially for the hepatic, splenic and gallbladder outlines. Now stand up and look for scars, distension, prominent veins, striae, hernia, bruising and pigmentation.

Palpate lightly in each region for masses, having asked first if any area is particularly tender. This will avoid causing the patient pain and may also provide a clue to a site of possible pathology. Next palpate each region more deeply; then feel specifically for hepatomegaly and splenomegaly. If there is hepatomegaly, confirm this with percussion and estimate the span. If no spleen is felt, percuss over the left costal margin in the left anterior axillary line during complete expiration (dullness suggests splenomegaly). Always roll the patient onto the right side and palpate again if the spleen is not felt initially. Attempt now to feel the kidneys bimanually. Remember the important distinguishing features of a spleen as opposed to a kidney.

Percuss routinely for ascites. If the abdomen is resonant right out to the flanks, do not roll the patient over. Otherwise test for shifting dullness. This is performed by percussing away from your side of the bed until you reach a dull note. Then roll the

Lying flat (1 pillow)

1. General inspection
Jaundice (liver disease)
Pigmentation (haemochromatosis, Whipple's disease)
Xanthomata (chronic cholestasis)
Mental state (encephalopathy)

2. Hands

3. Nails
- Clubbing
- Leuconychia

Palmar erythema
Dupuytren's contractures (alcohol)
Arthropathy
Hepatic flap

4. Arms
Spider naevi
Bruising
Wasting
Scratch marks (chronic cholestasis)

5. Face
Eyes
- *Sclera:* jaundice, anaemia, iritis
- *Cornea:* Kayser-Fleischer rings (Wilson's disease)

Parotids (alcohol)
Mouth
- *Breath:* fetor hepaticus
- *Lips:* stomatitis, leucoplakia, ulceration, localised pigmentation (Peutz-Jeghers syndrome), telangiectasia (hereditary haemorrhagic telangiectasia)
- *Gums:* gingivitis, bleeding, hypertrophy, pigmentation, monilia
- *Tongue:* atrophic glossitis, leucoplakia, ulceration

6. Cervical/axillary lymph nodes

7. Chest
Gynaecomastia
Spider naevi
Body hair

8. Abdomen
Inspect
- Scars
- Distension
- Prominent veins—determine direction of flow (caput Medusae; inferior vena cava obstruction)
- Striae
- Bruising
- Pigmentation
- Localised masses
- Visible peristalsis

Palpate
- Superficial palpation—tenderness, rigidity, outline of any mass

Deep palpation—organomegaly (liver, spleen, kidney), abnormal masses

Roll onto right side (spleen)

Percuss
- Liver, spleen
- Ascites—shifting dullness

Auscultate
- Bowel sounds
- Bruits, hums, rubs

9. Groin
Testes
Lymph nodes
Hernial orifices (standing up)

10. Legs
Bruising
Oedema
Neurological signs (alcohol)

11. Other
Rectal examination—inspect (fistulae, tags, blood, mucus), palpate (masses)
Urine analysis (bile)
Cardiovascular system (cardiomyopathy, cardiac failure, constrictive pericarditis)
Temperature chart (infection)

Figure 5.41 Gastrointestinal system

patient towards you and, after waiting a minute or so, begin percussing again for resonance.

By auscultation note the presence of bowel sounds. Next auscultate briefly over the liver, spleen and renal areas, listening for bruits, hums and rubs.

Examine the groins next. Palpate for inguinal lymphadenopathy. Examine for hernias by asking the patient to stand and then cough. The testes must always be palpated. Now look at the legs for oedema and bruising. Neurological examination of the legs may be indicated if there are signs of chronic liver disease.

If the liver is enlarged or cirrhosis is suspected ask the patient to sit up to 45 degrees and estimate the jugular venous pressure. This will avoid missing constrictive pericarditis or chronic cardiac failure as a cause of liver disease, or haemochromatosis, which can cause a dilated cardiomyopathy. While the patient is sitting up, palpate in the supraclavicular fossae for lymph nodes and feel at the back for sacral oedema. If ascites is present, it is necessary to examine the chest for a pleural effusion. If malignant disease is suspected, examine all lymph node groups, the breasts and the lungs.

A rectal examination should always be performed and specimens of the patient's vomitus or faeces should be inspected, if available. Perform a urinalysis (for bilirubin and urobilinogen, and glucose) and check the temperature.

References

1. Hendrix TR. Art and science of history taking in the patient with difficulty swallowing. *Dysphagia* 1993; 8:69–73. A very good review of the key historical features that must be obtained when a patient presents with trouble swallowing.
2. Theodossi A, Knill-Jones RP, Skene A. Interobserver variation of symptoms and signs in jaundice. *Liver* 1981; 1:21–32. The history and examination permitted a correct clinical diagnosis in jaundiced patients two-thirds of the time.
3. Patten A, Saunders JB. The ABC of alcohol; asking the right questions. *BMJ* 1981; 283:1458–1459. Discusses the value of the CAGE screening questions as well as other measures for identifying alcohol abuse.
4. Sibarte V, Shanahan F. Clinical examination of the gastrointestinal system in the 21st century—is the emphasis right? *Am J Gastroenterol* 2004; 99:1874–1875.
5. Walton S, Bennett JR. Skin and gullet. *Gut* 1991; 32:694–697. An excellent review of skin signs in gastroenterology.
6. Beitman RG, Rost SS, Roth JL. Oral manifestations of gastrointestinal disease. *Dig Dis Sci* 1981; 26:741–747. A detailed review.
7. Naylor CD. Physical examination of the liver. (The rational clinical examination.) *JAMA* 1994; 271:1859–1865. A valuable review of technique. Palpation is probably superior to percussion (in part because the midclavicular line is a 'wandering landmark'). Auscultation is usually of minimal value.
8. Fink HA, Lederle FA et al. The accuracy of physical to detect abdominal aortic aneurysm. *Arch Intern Med* 2000;160:833–836.
9. Thomson WH, Francis DM. Abdominal wall tenderness: a useful sign in the acute abdomen. *Lancet* 1977; 2:1053–1054. While abdominal wall pain can be recognised when the patient tenses the abdominal wall muscles, intraperitoneal inflammation can cause a false-positive sign.
10. Srinivasan R, Greenbaum DS. Chronic abdominal wall pain: a frequently overlooked problem. Practical approach to diagnosis and management. *Am J Gastroenterol* 2002; 97:824–830.
11. Williams JW Jr, Simel DL. Does this patient have ascites? How to divine fluid in the abdomen. (The rational clinical examination.) *JAMA* 1992; 267:2645–2648. This review provides information on the discriminant value of signs. Bulging flanks, shifting dullness and a fluid wave are each reasonably sensitive and specific. The presence of ascites is more easily predicted than its absence.
12. Muris JW, Starmans R, Wolfs GG, Pop P, Knottnerus JA. The diagnostic value of rectal examination. *Family Practice* 1993; 10:34–37. A useful procedure in patients with rectal or prostatic symptoms. Based on a literature review but studies in general practice are lacking.
13. Lembo A, Camilleri M. Chronic constipation. *N Engl J Med* 2003; 349:1360–1368.
14. Eckardt VF, Kanzier G. How reliable is digital examination for the evaluation of anal sphincter tone? *Int J Colorectal Dis* 1993; 8:95–97. While this investigation suggests that a rectal examination inadequately assesses the strength of the anal sphincter, these results require confirmation.
15. Longstreth GF. Checking for 'the occult' with a finger: a procedure of little value. *J Clin Gastroenterol* 1988; 10:133–134. A faecal occult blood test from the glove after rectal examination has too many false-positive and false-negative results to be of value.
16. Wagner JM, Mckinney WP, Carpenter JL. Does this patient have appendicitis? *JAMA* 1996; 276:1589–1594. A 'must read' that discusses the key symptoms and signs that help make the correct diagnosis.

Suggested reading

Original and review articles

Chervu A, Clagett GP, Valentine RJ, Myers SI, Rossi PJ. Role of physical examination in detection of abdominal aortic aneurysms. *Surgery* 1995; 117:454–457.

Drossman DA, Talley NJ, Leserman J, Olden KW, Barreiro MA. Sexual and physical abuse and gastrointestinal illness. Review and recommendations. *Ann Intern Med* 1995; 123:782–794.

Editorial. Abdominal wall tenderness test: could Carnett cut costs? *Lancet* 1991; 337:1134.

Murtagh J. Acute abdominal pain: a diagnostic approach. *Aust Fam Phys* 1994; 23:358–361, 364–374.

Sharpstone D, Colin-Jones DG. Chronic, non-visceral abdominal pain. *Gut* 1994; 35:833–836.

Textbooks

Browse NL. *An introduction to the symptoms and signs of surgical disease*, 3rd edn. London: Arnold, 1997.

Ellis H, Calne RY, Watson CJE. *Lecture notes on general surgery*, 10th edn. Oxford: Blackwell, 2003.

Sherlock S, Dooley J. *Diseases of the liver and biliary system*, 11th edn. Oxford: Blackwell, 1997.

Silen W. *Cope's early diagnosis of the acute abdomen*, 20th edn. New York: Oxford University Press, 2000.

Feldman M et al. *Sleisenger & Fordtran's gastrointestinal disease*, 8th edn. Philadelphia: Saunders, 2005.

Talley NJ, Martin CJ, eds. *Clinical gastroenterology. A practical problem-based approach*, 2nd edn. Sydney: Elsevier, 2006.

Yamada T, Alpers DH, Laine L, Owyang C, Powell DW. *Textbook of gastroenterology*, 4th edn. Philadelphia: Lippincott Williams & Wilkins, 2006.

chapter 6

The genitourinary system

You know my method. It is founded upon the observation of trifles.

Sherlock Holmes, created by Sir Arthur Conan Doyle (1859–1930)

The genitourinary history

Presenting symptoms

(Table 6.1)

These may include a change in the appearance of the urine, abnormalities of micturition, suprapubic or flank pain or the systemic symptoms of renal failure. Some patients have no symptoms but are found to be hypertensive or to have abnormalities on routine urinalysis or serum biochemistry. Others may feel unwell without localising symptoms. The major renal syndromes are set out in Table 6.2.

Change in appearance of the urine

Some patients present with discoloured urine. A red discoloration suggests haematuria (blood in the urine).[1] Urethral inflammation or trauma, or prostatic disease, can cause haematuria at the

---

Table 6.1 Genitourinary history

Major symptoms

Change in appearance of urine, e.g. haematuria	Symptoms suggestive of chronic renal failure (uraemia)
Change in urine volume or stream	• Oliguria, nocturia, polyuria
• Polyuria	• Anorexia, a metallic taste, vomiting, fatigue, hiccup, insomnia
• Nocturia	• Itch, bruising, oedema
• Anuria	Menses
• Decrease in stream size	• Age of onset
• Hesitancy	• Regularity
• Dribbling	• Last period (date)
• Urine retention	• Dysmenorrhoea, menorrhagia
• Strangury	Impotence
• Pis-en-deux—double voiding (incomplete bladder emptying)	Loss of libido
• Incontinence of urine	Infertility
Renal colic	Pregnancies: number and any complications
Dysuria (painful micturition), frequency, urgency, incontinence	Urethral or vaginal discharge
Fever, loin pain	Genital rash
Urethral discharge	

Table 6.2 The major renal syndromes

Name	Definition	Example
Nephrotic	Massive proteinuria	Minimal change disease
Nephritic	Haematuria, renal failure	Post-streptococcal glomerulonephritis
Tubulointerstitial nephropathy	Renal failure, mild proteinuria	Analgesic nephropathy
Acute renal failure	Sudden fall in function, rise in creatinine	Acute tubular necrosis
Rapidly progressive renal failure	Fall in renal function, over weeks	Malignant hypertension or 'crescentic' glomerulonephritis
Asymptomatic urinary abnormality	Isolated haematuria, or mild proteinuria	IgA nephropathy

beginning of micturition which then clears, or haematuria only at the end of micturition. Patients with porphyria can have urine that changes colour on standing. Consumption of certain drugs (e.g. rifampicin) or of large amounts of beetroot and, rarely, haemoglobinuria (due to destruction of red blood cells and release of free haemoglobin) can cause red discoloration of the urine (page 190). Patients with severe muscle trauma may have myoglobinuria as a result of muscle breakdown. This can also cause red discoloration. It is worth noting that the colour of the urine is not a reliable guide to its concentration.

Urinary tract infection (UTI)

This condition, which is much more common in women than in men, can be strongly suspected on the basis of the patient's symptoms.[2] These include: dysuria (pain or stinging during urination), frequency (need to pass small amounts of urine frequently), haematuria, and loin or back pain. The presence of these symptoms suggests a urinary tract infection. Physical examination may reveal fevers, rigors, lower abdominal discomfort and loin pain when the renal angle is balloted posteriorly. The latter findings are more suggestive of complicated UTI or pyelonephritis. The presence of a vaginal discharge is against the diagnosis.

Urinary obstruction

Urinary obstruction is a common symptom in elderly men and is most often due to prostatism or bladder outflow obstruction. The patient may have noticed hesitancy (difficulty starting micturition), followed by a decrease in the size of the stream of urine and terminal dribbling of urine. Strangury (recurrently, a small volume is passed with a painful desire to urinate each time) and pis-en-deux/ double voiding (the desire to urinate despite having just done so) may occur.[3] When obstruction is complete, overflow incontinence of urine can occur. Obstruction is associated with an increased risk of urinary infection.

Renal calculi can cause ureteric obstruction (Figure 6.1). The presenting symptom here, however, is usually severe colicky loin pain with radiation of the pain down towards the symphysis pubis or perineum or testis (renal colic). Other causes of urinary obstruction are presented in Table 6.3.

Urinary incontinence

This is the inability to hold urine in the bladder voluntarily. The problem can occur transiently with urinary tract infections, delirium, excess urine output (e.g. from the use of diuretics), immobility (because patients are unable to reach the toilet), atrophic urethritis or vaginitis, or stool impaction.

Common causes of established urinary incontinence include: (i) *stress incontinence* (instantaneous leakage after the stress of coughing or after a sudden rise in intra-abdominal pressure of any cause)—this problem is more common in women; (ii) *overactivity of the detrusor muscle* (characterised by an intense urge to urinate and then leakage of urine in the absence of cough or other stressors)—this occurs in men and women; (iii) *detrusor underactivity*—this is rare and is characterised by urinary frequency, nocturia and the frequent leaking of small amounts of urine; and (iv) *urethral obstruction*—this occurs typically in men with disease of the prostate, and is characterised by dribbling incontinence after incomplete urination—'overflow incontinence'.

Chronic renal failure

The clinical features of chronic renal failure can be deduced in part by considering the normal functions of the kidneys.

Figure 6.1 Renal calculus

Phleboliths (calcifications related to blood vessels) are rounded opacities seen in the pelvis below the level of the ischial spines, whereas ureteric calculi lie above this level, in the line of the ureters. The large staghorn calculus shown here is occupying the calyces of the left renal pelvis. This type of calculus is almost always radio-opaque. An abdominal ultrasound examination (IVPs are almost never performed in this context today) is necessary to check whether there is an obstruction at the pelviureteric junction. In general, 90% of renal calculi are radio-opaque and visible on plain X-ray films. A significant proportion of patients presenting with renal colic due to calcium calculi have hyperparathyroidism.

1   Failure of excretory function leads to accumulation of numerous 'uraemic' toxins, hence the widely used term 'uraemia'. This frequently leads to malaise, lethargy, anorexia, malnutrition and hiccups.
2   Urinary concentrating ability may be lost early, leading to the risk of dehydration; nocturia can be an early symptom.
3   Various factors such as the failure to excrete sodium may lead to hypertension.
4   Damage to the renal tubules may lead to sodium loss and hypotension.
5   Excretion of potassium depends largely on urine volume. Hyperkalaemia usually becomes a problem when a patient is oliguric (passes less than 400 mL urine/day).
6   Failure of acid excretion leads to metabolic acidosis.
7   Failure to hydroxylate vitamin D_3 causes vitamin D deficiency, which in turn leads to compensating (secondary) hyperparathyroidism and therefore a fall in serum calcium and a rise in phosphate. This is responsible for renal bone disease—'renal osteodystrophy'.
8   Failure to secrete erythropoietin leads to normochromic normocytic anaemia.

Adequacy of renal function is defined by the glomerular filtration rate (GFR). This is the volume of blood filtered by the kidneys per unit of time. The normal range is 90–120 mL/min. The GFR is estimated by calculating the clearance of creatinine (a normal breakdown product of muscle) from the blood. The serum creatinine and urea levels also pro-vide a measure of accumulation of uraemic toxins and therefore of renal function.

A uraemic patient may present with anuria (defined as failure to pass more than 50 mL urine daily), oliguria (less than 400 mL urine daily), nocturia (the need to get up during the night to pass urine) or polyuria (the passing of abnormally large volumes of urine) (page 259). Nocturia may be an indication of failure of the kidneys to concentrate urine normally, and polyuria may indicate complete inability to concentrate the urine.

The more general symptoms of renal failure include anorexia, vomiting, fatigue, hiccups and insomnia. Pruritus (a general itchiness of the skin), easy bruising and oedema due to fluid retention may also be present. Other symptoms indicating complications include bone pain, fractures because of renal bone disease, and the symptoms of hypercalcaemia (including anorexia, nausea, vomiting, constipation, increased urination, mental confusion) because of tertiary (or primary) hyperparathyroidism (page 271).[a] Patients may also present with the features of pericarditis (page 29), hypertension (page 31), cardiac failure (page 60), ischaemic heart disease

---

[a]   In secondary hyperparathyroidism, serum calcium is low and phosphate is high. In tertiary hyperparathyroidism, where parathyroid function has become autonomous, serum calcium and phosphate levels are both high.

Table 6.3 Causes of acute renal failure

a. Onset over days

This is defined as a rapid deterioration in renal function severe enough to cause accumulation of waste products, especially nitrogenous wastes, in the body. Usually the urine flow rate is less than 20 mL/hour or 400 mL/day, but occasionally it is normal or increased (high-output renal failure).

Prerenal
Fluid loss: blood, (haemorrhage) plasma or water and electrolytes (diarrhoea and vomiting, dehydration)
Hypotension: myocardial infarction, septicaemic shock, drugs
Renovascular disease: embolus, dissection or atheroma
Increased renal vascular resistance: hepatorenal syndrome

Renal
Acute-on-chronic renal failure (precipitated by infection, dehydration, obstruction or nephrotoxic drugs)— see Table 6.4

Acute renal disease:
• e.g. primary or secondary glomerulonephritis, connective tissue diseases

Acute tubular necrosis secondary to:
• ischaemia (hypovolaemia)
• toxins and drugs (such as aminoglycoside, antibiotics, radiocontrast material, heavy metals)
• rhabdomyolysis, haemoglobinuria

Tubulointerstitial disease:
• e.g. drugs (such as proton pump inhibitors, sulphonamides, cyclosporin A), urate or calcium deposits

Vascular disease:
• e.g. vasculitis, scleroderma

Myeloma
Acute pyelonephritis (rare)

Postrenal (complete urinary tract obstruction)
Urethral obstruction:
• e.g. calculus or blood clot, sloughed papillae, trauma, phimosis or paraphimosis

At the bladder neck:
• e.g. calculus or blood clot, prostatic hypertrophy or cancer

Bilateral ureteric obstruction:
• intraureteric, e.g. blood clot, pyogenic debris, calculi
• extra-ureteric, e.g. retroperitoneal fibrosis (due to radiation, methysergide or idiopathic), retroperitoneal/pelvic tumour or surgery, uterine prolapse

b. Causes of rapidly progressive renal failure (onset over weeks to months)

Urinary tract obstruction
Rapidly progressive glomerulonephritis
Bilateral renal artery stenosis (may be precipitated by angiotensin-converting enzyme inhibitor use)
Multiple myeloma
Scleroderma
Malignant hypertension
Haemolytic uraemic syndrome

Note: Anuria may be due to urinary obstruction, bilateral renal artery occlusion, rapidly progressive (crescentic) glomerulonephritis, renal cortical necrosis or a renal stone in a solitary kidney.

(page 27), neuropathy (page 348) or peptic ulceration (page 128).

Find out whether the patient is undergoing dialysis and whether this is haemodialysis or peritoneal dialysis. There are a number of important questions that must be asked of dialysis patients:

1 What fluid restriction has been recommended?
2 Have phosphate binding drugs been prescribed and when does the patient take these relative to meals?
3 How much weight does the patient gain between each haemodialysis?
4 Does the patient still pass any urine?
5 Is the patient on a renal transplant list?
6 Is the patient compliant with his or her recommended dietary restrictions?

Ask about any complications that have occurred including recurrent peritonitis with peritoneal dialysis or problems with vascular access for haemodialysis.

A common form of treatment for renal failure is renal transplantation. A patient may know how well the graft is functioning, and what the most recent renal function tests have shown. Find out whether the patient knows of rejection episodes, how these were treated, and if there has been more than one renal transplant. It is necessary to ascertain if there have been any problems with recurrent infection, urine leaks or side-effects of treatment. Long-term problems with immunosuppression may have occurred, including the development of cancers, chronic nephrotoxicity (e.g. from cyclosporin or tacrolimus), obesity and hypertension from steroids, or recurrent infections. The patient should be aware of the need to avoid skin exposure to the sun and women should know that they need regular Papanicolaou (Pap) smears for cancer surveillance.

Menstrual and sexual history

A menstrual history should always be obtained. The menarche or date of the first period is important (page 258). The regularity of the periods over the preceding months or years and the date of the last period are both relevant. The patient may complain of dysmenorrhoea (painful menstruation) or menorrhagia (an abnormally heavy period or series of periods).

Vaginal discharge can occur in patients with infections of the genital tract. Sometimes the type of discharge is an indication of the type of infection present (page 194). The history of the number of pregnancies and births is relevant: gravidity refers to the number of times a woman has conceived, while parity refers to the number of babies delivered (live births or stillbirths). One should also ask about any complications that occurred during pregnancy (e.g. hypertension).

The sexual history is also relevant.[4] Ask about contraceptive methods and the possibility of pregnancy.[5] Ask men about erectile dysfunction (impotence).

Treatment

A detailed drug history must be taken. Note all the drugs, including steroids and immunosuppressants and their dosages. In patients with decreased renal function, the dosages of many drugs that are cleared by the kidneys must be adjusted. The patient with chronic renal failure should be well informed about the need for protein, phosphate, potassium, fluid or salt restriction. Patients with urinary tract infections may have had a number of courses of antibiotics. Treatment of hypertension should be documented. Certain drugs should be used with caution. For example, non-steroidal anti-inflammatory drugs can worsen renal function where this is already abnormal.

Past history

Find out whether there have been previous or recurrent urinary tract infections or renal calculi. There may have been operations to remove urinary tract stones, or pelvic surgery may have been performed because of urinary incontinence in women or prostatism in men. The patient may know about the previous detection of proteinuria or microscopic haematuria at a routine examination. Glomerulonephritis will usually have been diagnosed by renal biopsy, a procedure that is often a memorable event. Histories of diabetes mellitus or gout are relevant, as these diseases may lead to renal complications. It is most important to find out about hypertension, because this may not only cause renal impairment but is also a common complication of renal disease. A history of childhood enuresis (bedwetting) beyond the age of three years may be relevant: it can be associated with vesicoureteric reflux and subsequent renal scarring. Renovascular disease is more likely if there is a history of vascular disease elsewhere, such as myocardial ischaemia or cerebrovascular disease. In elderly patients, specific questions relating to ingestion of Bex or Vincent's powders may suggest a diagnosis of analgesic nephropathy. This is particularly important as these patients require surveillance for urothelial malignancy in addition to managing their renal impairment.

Social history

Patients with chronic renal failure may have many social problems. There may be a need for access to equipment at home for dialysis. One must ask detailed questions to find out how the patient is coping with the chronic illness and its complications. Find out how well informed the patient is about the transplant, if this has been the treatment. Also find out what sort of support the patient has obtained from relatives and friends.

Family history

Some forms of renal disease are inherited. Polycystic kidney disease, for example, is an autosomal dominant condition. Ask about diabetes and hypertension in the family. A family history of deafness and renal impairment suggests Alport's syndrome, a hereditary form of nephritis.

The genitourinary examination

A set examination of the genitourinary system is not routinely performed. However, if renal disease is suspected or known to be present then certain signs must be sought. These are mostly the signs of chronic renal failure (uraemia) and its causes (Table 6.4). On the other hand, examination of the male genitalia or female pelvis is part of the routine general examination.

General appearance

The general inspection remains crucial. Look for *hyperventilation*, which may indicate an underlying metabolic acidosis. *Hiccupping* may be present and can be an ominous sign of advanced uraemia. There may be the ammoniacal fish breath (*'uraemic fetor'*) of kidney failure. This musty smell is not easy to describe but once detected is easily remembered. Patients with chronic renal failure commonly have a sallow complexion (a dirty brown appearance or *'uraemic tinge'*). This may be due to impaired excretion of urinary pigments (urochromes) combined with anaemia. The skin colour may be from slate grey to bronze, due to iron deposition in dialysis patients who have received multiple blood transfusions, but these signs are becoming less frequent with the use of exogenous erythropoietin. In terminal renal failure, patients become drowsy and finally sink into a coma due to nitrogen or toxin retention.

Table 6.4 Causes of chronic renal failure

This is defined as a severe reduction in nephron mass over a variable period of time resulting in uraemia.
1 Glomerulonephritis
2 Diabetes mellitus
3 Systemic vascular disease
4 Analgesic nephropathy
5 Reflux nephropathy
6 Hypertensive nephrosclerosis
7 Polycystic kidneys
8 Obstruction
9 Amyloid

Clinical features suggesting that renal failure is chronic rather than acute

Small kidney size (except with polycystic kidneys, diabetes, amyloid and myeloma)
Renal bone disease
Anaemia (with normal red blood cell indices)
Peripheral neuropathy

Twitching due to myoclonic jerks, and tetany and epileptic seizures due to a low serum calcium level and to nitrogen retention, occur late in renal failure. Over-vigorous correction of acidosis (e.g. with bicarbonate infusions) may also precipitate seizures and coma (page 363). There may be subcutaneous nodules due to calcium phosphate deposition.

It is essential to assess the state of hydration in all patients with renal disease (page 21). Severe dehydration can be a cause of acute renal failure and can cause precipitous decompensation in patients with chronic renal failure. Conversely, overhydration can result from intravenous infusions of fluid used in an attempt to correct acute renal failure, resulting in pulmonary oedema (page 29). Patients should be weighed regularly as an objective measure of their fluid status.

The hands

The *nails* should be inspected: look for leuconychia (page 139); Muehrcke's nails[b] refer to paired white transverse lines near the end of the nails; these occur in hypoalbuminaemia (e.g. nephrotic syndrome).[6] A single transverse white band (Mees' lines,[c]

---

[b] RC Meuhrcke reported this sign in the *British Medical Journal* in 1956.
[c] RA Mees reported this sign in 1919.

Figure 6.2 Mees' lines
(From FS McDonald, ed., *Mayo Clinic images in internal medicine*, with permission. © Mayo Clinic Scientific Press and CRC Press.)

Figure 6.2) may occur in arsenic poisoning, as well as in renal failure. Half-and-half nails (distal nail brown or red, proximal nail pink or white) are also seen in chronic renal failure. Non-pigmented indented transverse bands can occur with any cause of a catabolic state (Beau's lines[d]).

Anaemia is common and causes palmar crease pallor. There are a number of causes of anaemia in patients with chronic renal failure, including poor nutrition (especially folate deficiency), blood loss, erythropoietin deficiency, haemolysis, bone marrow depression and the chronic disease state.

Asterixis (page 140) may be present in terminal chronic renal failure.

Inspect the wrist and forearms for scars and palpate for surgically created arteriovenous fistulae or shunts, used for haemodialysis access. There is a longitudinal swelling and a palpable continuous thrill present over the fistula. There may be scars from previous thrombosed shunts or carpal tunnel syndrome surgery present on either side. Look for signs of the carpal tunnel syndrome (page 254).

The arms

Bruising occurs because of nitrogen retention which causes impaired prothrombin consumption, a defect in platelet factor III, and abnormal platelet aggregation in chronic renal failure. *Skin pigmentation* is common, reflecting a failure to excrete urinary pigments. *Scratch marks and excoriations*, due to uraemic pruritus, the precise cause of which is unknown, may be present. This occurs commonly and can be extremely debilitating. *Uraemic frost* is a fine white powder present on the skin where very high concentrations of urea have precipitated out of the sweat in terminal chronic renal failure; it is very rare. Evidence of *vasculitis*, which can cause renal disease, should also be sought (page 246).

Look for signs of *peripheral neuropathy* in the limbs. Sensory impairment is more marked than motor impairment initially (page 348). Myopathy (page 355) and bone tenderness can also occur due to osteomalacia, which results from low 1,25-dihydroxyvitamin D and calcium levels.

The face

The eyes are important; look for signs of *anaemia* and, rarely, *jaundice* (retention of nitrogenous wastes can cause haemolysis). *Band keratopathy* is a calcium deposition beneath the corneal epithelium in line with the interpalpebral fissure—it is due to secondary or tertiary hyperparathyroidism (page 271), or excessive replacement of calcium in patients with chronic renal failure.

The mouth should always be examined. A uraemic *fetor* may be present. This is an ammoniacal, musty odour due to breakdown of urea to ammonia in the saliva. Mucosal *ulcers* can occur as there is a decrease in saliva flow, and patients with chronic renal failure are prone to infection (e.g. thrush), due to decreased acute inflammatory responses as a result of nitrogen retention. Transplant patients treated with calcineurin inhibitors (cyclosporin and tacrolimus) frequently develop *gingival hyperplasia* (thickening of the gums).

The presence of a *rash* or skin tethering may indicate an underlying connective tissue disease such as systemic lupus erythematosus or systemic sclerosis (page 245).

The presence of hearing aids may be consistent with Alport's syndrome (hereditary nephritis often with sensorineural hearing loss and eye disease of the retina or cornea).

The neck

Carefully check the *jugular venous pressure* (page 42) to help assess the intravascular volume status. Auscultate for *carotid artery bruits*; these provide a

---

[d] Joseph Honoré Simon Beau (1806–1865), Paris physician.

clue that there may be generalised atherosclerotic disease (which can cause renal artery stenosis or complicate chronic renal failure). Look for signs of previous *jugular vein puncture* due to previous vascular access insertion ('vascath') for haemodialysis. Surgical scars from previous *parathyroidectomy* performed for management of tertiary hyperparathyroidism may be present.

The chest

Examine the heart and lungs. In chronic renal failure there may be *congestive cardiac failure* due to fluid retention, and *hypertension* as a result of sodium and water retention and excess renin production. Signs of *pulmonary oedema* may also be present due to uraemic lung disease (a type of non-cardiogenic pulmonary oedema), volume overload or uraemic cardiomyopathy.

Pericarditis, which can be fibrinous or haemorrhagic in chronic renal failure, is secondary to retained metabolic toxins and can cause a pericardial effusion; there may be a pericardial rub or signs of cardiac tamponade (page 63). Lung infection is also common due to the immunosuppression present from the chronic renal failure itself or as a result of treatment.

The abdominal examination

Abdominal examination is performed as described on page 174. However, particular attention must be paid to the following.

Inspection

The presence of a Tenckhoff catheter (peritoneal dialysis catheter) should be noted. It is important to look for nephrectomy *scars* (see Figure 5.18). These are often more posterior than one might expect. It may be necessary to roll the patient over and look in the region of the loins. Renal transplant scars are usually found in the right or left iliac fossae. A *transplanted kidney* may be visible as a bulge under the scar, as it is placed in a relatively superficial plane. Peritoneal dialysis results in small scars from catheter placement in the peritoneal cavity; these are situated on the lower abdomen, at or near the midline.

The abdomen may be distended because of large polycystic kidneys or *ascites* (as a result of the nephrotic syndrome, or peritoneal dialysis fluid).

Inspect the scrotum for masses (see page 193) and genital oedema.

Palpation

Particular care is required here so that renal masses (Table 6.5) are not missed. Remember that an enlarged kidney usually bulges forwards, while perinephric

---

Table 6.5 Renal masses

Unilateral palpable kidney

Renal cell carcinoma
Hydronephrosis or pyonephrosis
Xanthogranulomatous pyelonephritis
Polycystic kidneys (with asymmetrical enlargement)
Normal right kidney or solitary kidney
Acute renal vein thrombosis (unilateral)
Acute pyelonephritis
Renal abscess
Compensatory hypertrophy of single functioning kidney

Bilateral palpable kidneys

Polycystic kidneys
Hydronephrosis or pyonephrosis bilaterally
Renal cell carcinoma bilaterally
Diabetic nephropathy (early)
Nephrotic syndrome (Table 6.9)
Infiltrative disease, e.g. amyloid, lymphoma
Acromegaly
Bilateral renal vein thrombosis

---

abscesses or collections tend to bulge backwards. Transplanted kidneys in the right or left iliac fossa may be palpable as well. In polycystic kidney disease, hepatomegaly from hepatic cysts may be found (Table 6.6). Feel for the presence of an enlarged bladder (page 187). Also palpate for an abdominal aortic aneurysm. In the patient with abdominal pain, renal colic should be suspected if there is renal tenderness (LR 3.6) or loin tenderness (LR 27.7).[7]

Balloting

From the French word meaning *to shake about*, balloting is an examination technique for palpating the kidney by attempting to flick it forward. One hand is placed under the renal angle and the examiner's fingers flick upwards while the other hand, placed anteriorly in the right or left upper quadrant, waits to feel the kidney move upwards and then float down again (Figure 6.3).

Percussion

This is necessary to confirm the presence of ascites by examining for shifting dullness. Also percuss for an enlarged bladder. Obesity and ascites make direct percussion of the bladder difficult. This is an opportunity to attempt *auscultatory percussion*.[8] The diaphragm of the stethoscope is placed just above the

Table 6.6 Adult polycystic kidney disease

If you find polycystic kidneys, remember these very important points.

1 Take the blood pressure (75% have hypertension).
2 Examine the urine for haematuria (due to haemorrhage into a cyst) and proteinuria (usually less than 2 g/day).
3 Look for evidence of anaemia (due to chronic renal failure) or polycythaemia (due to high erythropoietin levels). Note that the haemoglobin level is higher than expected for the degree of renal failure.
4 Note the presence of hepatomegaly or splenomegaly (due to cysts). These may cause confusion when one is examining the abdomen.
5 Tenderness on palpation may indicate an infected cyst.

Note: Subarachnoid haemorrhage occurs in 3% of patients with polycystic kidney disease due to rupture of an associated intracranial aneurysm. As polycystic kidney disease is an autosomal dominant condition, all family members should also be assessed.

Fingers flex briskly

Figure 6.3 Balloting the kidneys

border of the symphysis pubis and direct percussion of the abdominal wall performed, starting at the subcostal margin in the middle line. There is a sudden increase in loudness when the upper border of the bladder is reached. It is even possible to estimate the volume of urine in the bladder by this method. An upper border less than 2 cm from the stethoscope suggests a fairly empty bladder, while an upper border more than 8 cm higher corresponds to a urine volume of between 750 mL and a litre.

Auscultation

The important sign here is the presence of a *renal bruit*. Renal bruits are best heard above the umbilicus, about 2 cm to the left or right of the midline. Listen with the diaphragm of the stethoscope over both these areas. Next ask the patient to sit up and listen in both flanks. The presence of a systolic and diastolic bruit is important. A diastolic component makes the bruit more likely to be haemodynamically significant. Its presence suggests renal artery stenosis due to fibromuscular dysplasia or atherosclerosis. Approximately 50% of patients with renal artery stenosis will have a bruit. In a patient with hypertension that is difficult to control, the presence of a systolic/diastolic abdominal bruit has a positive LR for renal artery stenosis of over 40. On the other hand, if only a soft systolic bruit is audible, at least half these patients do not have any significant renal artery stenosis. In such cases the aorta or splenic artery may be the source of the sound. The absence of hypertension makes the diagnosis of renal artery stenosis less likely. The occurrence of unexplained pulmonary oedema of sudden onset ('flash' pulmonary oedema) in patients with renal impairment and hypertension makes a diagnosis of renal artery stenosis more likely.

Rectal and pelvic examination

Here the presence of prostatomegaly[9,10] (page 160) in men and a frozen pelvis from cervical cancer in women is important, as this may be a cause of urinary tract obstruction and secondary renal failure.

The back

Strike the vertebral column gently with the base of the fist to elicit bony tenderness. This may be due to renal osteodystrophy from osteomalacia, secondary hyperparathyroidism or multiple myeloma. Back pain in the context of renal failure should always raise the possibility of an underlying paraproteinaemia.

Gentle use of the clenched fist to strike the patient in the renal angle is known as Murphy's kidney punch (Figure 6.4) and is designed to elicit renal tenderness in patients with renal infection. Similar information may be gained from more gentle balloting of the renal angle when the patient lies supine. Look also for sacral oedema in a patient confined to bed, particularly if the nephrotic syndrome or congestive cardiac failure is suspected.

The legs

The important signs here are oedema, purpura (page 199), livedo reticularis (a red-blue reticular pattern from vasculitis or athero-embolic disease), pigmentation, scratch marks and signs of peripheral vascular disease. Examination for peripheral neuropathy and myopathy is indicated, as in the arms. Gouty tophi or the presence of gouty arthropathy (page 244) may very occasionally provide an

Figure 6.4 Murphy's kidney punch (not too hard)

Table 6.7 Some causes of urine colour changes

Colour	Underlying causes
Very pale or colourless	Dilute urine (e.g. overhydration, recent excessive beer consumption, diabetes insipidus, post-obstructive diuresis)
Yellow-orange	Concentrated urine (e.g. dehydration) Bilirubin Tetracycline, anthracene, sulphasalazine, riboflavin
Brown	Bilirubin Nitrofurantoin, phenothiazines
Pink	Beetroot consumption Phenindione, phenolphthalein (laxatives)
Red	Haematuria, haemoglobinuria, myoglobinuria Porphyrins, rifampicin, pyridium
Green	Methylene blue
Black	Severe haemoglobinuria Methyldopa Melanoma, ochronosis

explanation for the patient's renal failure (although secondary uric acid retention is common with chronic renal failure, it rarely causes clinical gout).

The blood pressure

It is of the utmost importance to take the blood pressure in every patient with renal disease. This is because hypertension can be the cause of renal disease or one of its complications. Test for postural hypotension, as hypovolaemia may precipitate acute renal failure.

The fundi

Examination of the fundi is important. Look especially for Keith-Wegener hypertensive changes (page 64–66) and diabetic changes (page 278). Diabetes can be a cause of chronic renal failure.

The urine

The ghosts of dead patients that haunt us do not ask why we did not employ the latest fad of clinical investigation; they ask why did you not test my urine?

Sir Robert Hutchison (1871–1960)

This valuable fluid must not be discarded in any patient in whom a renal, diabetic, gastrointestinal or other major system disease is suspected.

Colour

Look at the colour of the urine (Table 6.7).

Transparency

Phosphate or urate deposits can occur normally and produce white (phosphate) or pink (urate) cloudiness.

Fainter cloudiness may be due to bacteria. Pus, chyle or blood can cause a more turbid appearance.

Smell

A mild ammoniacal smell is normal. A urinary tract infection causes a fishy smell, and antibiotics can sometimes be smelt in the urine, as can asparagus.

Specific gravity

A urinometer, which is a weighted float with a scale, is used to measure specific gravity. The depth to which the float sinks in the urine indicates the specific gravity, which is read off the scale on the side. The specific gravity can also be estimated by dipstick methods.

Water has a specific gravity of 1, and the presence of solutes (especially heavy solutes such as glucose or an iodine contrast medium) in urine increases the specific gravity. The normal range is 1.002 to 1.025. A consistently low specific gravity suggests chronic renal failure (as there is failure of the kidneys to concentrate the urine) or diabetes insipidus (where there is a deficiency of antidiuretic hormone resulting in passage of a large volume of dilute urine). A high specific gravity suggests dehydration, or diabetes mellitus with the presence of large amounts of glucose in the urine.

There is a rough correlation between the specific gravity of the urine and its osmolarity. For example, a specific gravity of 1.002 corresponds to an osmolarity of 100 mOsm/kg, while a specific gravity of 1.030 corresponds to 1200 mOsm/kg.

Chemical analysis

A chemical reagent colour strip allows simultaneous multiple analyses of pH, protein, glucose, ketones, blood, nitrite, specific gravity, presence of leucocytes, bile and urobilinogen. The strip is dipped in the urine and colour changes are measured after a set period. The colours are compared with a chart provided.

pH

Normal urine is acid, except after meals when for a short time it becomes alkaline (the alkaline tide). Measuring the pH of urine is helpful in a number of critical circumstances. Sometimes the urine has to be made alkaline for therapeutic purposes, such as treating myoglobinuria or recurrent urinary calculi due to uric acid or cystine. Distal renal tubular acidosis should be suspected if the early morning urine is consistently alkaline and cannot be acidified. Urinary tract infections with urea-splitting organisms, such as *Proteus mirabilis*, can also cause an alkaline urine which, in turn, favours renal calcium stone formation.

Protein

The colours are compared with a chart provided. The strip tests give only a semi-quantitative measure of urinary protein (+ to ++++) and, if positive, must be confirmed by other tests. One-third of measured urinary protein is albumin and two-thirds is globulin. A reading of + of proteinuria may be normal, as up to 150 mg of protein a day is lost in the urine. Causes of abnormal amounts of protein in the urine are listed in Tables 6.8 and 6.9. Chemical dipsticks

---

Table 6.8 Causes of proteinuria

Persistent proteinuria

1. Renal disease
Almost any renal disease may cause a trace of proteinuria. Moderate or large amounts tend to occur with glomerular disease (Table 6.9).

2. No renal disease (functional)
Exercise
Fever
Hypertension (severe)
Congestive cardiac failure
Burns
Blood transfusion
Postoperative
Acute alcohol abuse

Orthostatic proteinuria
Proteinuria that occurs when a patient is standing but not when recumbent is called orthostatic proteinuria. In the absence of abnormalities of the urine sediment, diabetes mellitus, hypertension or reduced renal function, this entity probably has a benign prognosis.

---

do not detect the presence of Bence-Jones proteinuria[e] (immunoglobulin light chains).

If proteinuria is detected on dipstick testing, this should be quantified with a 24-hour urinary collection, and careful urine (phase-contrast) microscopy should be carried out to look for evidence of active renal disease.

Glucose and ketones

A semi-quantitative measurement of glucose and ketones is available. Glycosuria usually indicates diabetes mellitus, but can occur with other diseases (Table 6.10). False-positive or false-negative results can occur with vitamin C (large doses), tetracyclines or levodopa ingestion.

Ketones in the urine of patients with diabetes mellitus are an important indication of the presence of diabetic ketoacidosis (Table 6.10). The three ketone bodies are acetone, beta-hydroxybutyric acid and acetoacetic acid. Lack of glucose (starvation) or lack of glucose availability for the cells (diabetes mellitus) causes activation of carnitine acetyltransferase, which

---

[e] Henry Bence-Jones (1818–73), physician at St George's Hospital, London, described this in 1848.

Table 6.9 Nephrotic syndrome

Definition

1 Proteinuria (>3.5 g per 24 hours) (*Note:* the other features can all be explained by loss of protein.)
2 Hypoalbuminaemia (serum albumin <30 g/L, due to proteinuria)
3 Oedema (due to hypoalbuminaemia)
4 Hyperlipidaemia (due to increased LDL and cholesterol, possibly from loss of plasma factors that regulate lipoprotein synthesis)

Causes

Primary renal pathology
1 Membranous glomerulonephritis
2 Minimal change glomerulonephritis
3 Focal and segmental hyalinosis and sclerosis
4 Mesangiocapillary (membranoproliferative) glomerulonephritis
5 Crescentic glomerulonephritis

Secondary renal pathology
1 Drugs: e.g. penicillamine, probenecid, gold, captopril, heroin, non-steroidal anti-inflammatory drugs
2 Systemic disease: e.g. SLE, diabetes mellitus, amyloid
3 Malignancy: e.g. carcinoma, lymphoma, multiple myeloma
4 Infections: e.g. hepatitis B, infective endocarditis, malaria, HIV
5 Allergy: e.g. vaccines, bee sting

LDL = low density lipoprotein.
SLE = systemic lupus erythematosus.
HIV = human immunodeficiency virus.

Table 6.10 Causes of glycosuria and ketonuria

Glycosuria

Diabetes mellitus
Other reducing substances (false-positives): metabolites of salicylates, ascorbic acid, galactose, fructose
Impaired renal tubular ability to absorb glucose (renal glycosuria)
• e.g. Fanconi syndrome* (proximal renal tubular disease)

Ketonuria

Diabetic ketoacidosis
Starvation

* Guido Fanconi (1892–1972), Zürich paediatrician, described this in 1936. It had previously been described by Guido De-Toni in 1933 and is sometimes called the De-Toni-Fanconi syndrome.

---

accelerates fatty acid oxidation in the liver. However, the pathway for the conversion of fatty acids becomes saturated, leading to ketone body formation. The strip colour tests react only to acetoacetic acid.

Blood

Blood in the urine (haematuria) is abnormal and can be seen with the naked eye if 0.5 mL is present per litre of urine (Table 6.11). A positive dipstick test is abnormal and suggests haematuria, haemoglobinuria (uncommon) or myoglobinuria (also uncommon). The presence of more than a trace of protein in the urine in addition suggests that the blood is of renal origin. False-positive or false-negative results can occur if vitamin C is being taken.

Nitrite

If positive, this usually indicates infection with bacteria that produce nitrite. False-positive or false-negative results occur with vitamin C ingestion. More specific dipstick tests for white cells are now available; a positive test has an LR of 4.2 for a urinary infection and a negative test has an LR of 0.3.

The urine sediment

Every patient with suspected renal disease should have a midstream urine sample examined. Centrifuge 10 mL of the urine at 2000 rpm for four minutes. Remove the supernatant, leaving 0.5 mL; shake well to re-suspend, then place one drop on a slide with a coverslip. Look at the slide using a low-power microscope, and at specific formed elements under the high-power field (hpf) for identification. There is a significant false-negative rate when there are low numbers of formed elements in the urine.

Look for red blood cells, white blood cells and casts.

Red blood cells (RBCs)

These appear as small circular objects without a nucleus. Usually none are seen, although up to 5 RBCs/low-power field (lpf) may be normal in very concentrated urine. If their numbers are increased,

Table 6.11 Causes of positive dipstick test for blood in the urine

Haematuria

Renal
Glomerulonephritis
Polycystic renal disease
Pyelonephritis
Renal cell carcinoma
Analgesic nephropathy
Malignant hypertension
Renal infarction, e.g. infective endocarditis, vasculitis
Bleeding disorders

Renal tract
Cystitis
Calculi
Bladder or ureteric tumour
Prostatic disease, e.g. cancer, benign prostatic hypertrophy
Urethritis

Haemoglobinuria

Intravascular haemolysis, e.g. microangiopathic haemolytic anaemia, march haemoglobulinuria, prosthetic heart valve, paroxysmal nocturnal haemoglobinuria, chronic cold agglutinin disease

Myoglobinuria

This is due to rhabdomyolysis (muscle destruction):
• Muscle infarction, e.g. trauma
• Excessive muscle contraction, e.g. convulsions, hyperthermia, marathon running
• Viral myositis, e.g. influenza, Legionnaires' disease
• Drugs or toxins, e.g. alcohol, snake venom, statins
• Idiopathic

try to determine whether the RBCs originate from the glomeruli (more than 80% of the RBCs are dysmorphic—irregular in size and shape) or the renal tract (the RBCs are typically uniform).

White blood cells (WBCs)

These cells have lobulated nuclei. Usually fewer than 6 WBCs/hpf are present, although up to 10 may be normal in very concentrated urine. Tubular epithelial cells have a compact nucleus and are larger. Pyuria

indicates urinary tract inflammation. Bacteria may also be seen if there is infection, but bacterial contamination is more likely if squamous epithelial cells (which are larger and have single nuclei) are prominent. Urine culture is essential, as pyuria is an insensitive guide to infection. Sterile pyuria is characteristic of renal tuberculosis but may also occur in acute or chronic tubulo-interstitial disease.

Casts

Casts are cylindrical moulds formed in the lumen of the renal tubules or collecting ducts. They are signs of a damaged glomerular basement membrane or damaged tubules. The size of a cast is determined by the dimension of the lumen of the nephron in which it forms.

Hyaline casts are long cylindrical structures. One or two RBCs or WBCs may be present in the cast. Normally there are fewer than 1 per low-power field. They consist largely of Tamm-Horsfall mucoprotein secreted by the renal tubules.

Granular casts are abnormal cylindrical granular structures that arise from the tubules, usually in patients with proteinuria. They consist of hyaline material containing fragments of serum proteins.

Red cell casts are always abnormal and indicate primary glomerular disease (haematuria of glomerular origin or vasculitis). They contain 10 to 50 red cells, which are well defined.

With **white cell casts** many WBCs adhere to or inside the cast. These are abnormal, indicating bacterial pyelonephritis or, less commonly, glomerulonephritis, kidney infarction or vasculitis.

Fatty casts (i.e. the presence of fat in casts) are suggestive of the nephrotic syndrome.

Male genitalia

Inspect the genitals for evidence of mucosal ulceration. This can occur in a number of systemic diseases, including Reiter's syndrome (page 243) and the rare Behçet's syndrome (page 251). If necessary, retract the foreskin to expose the glans penis. For aesthetic and protective reasons, it is essential to wear gloves for this examination. This mucosal surface is prone to inflammation or ulceration in both infective and connective tissue diseases (Table 6.12). Look also for urethral discharge. If there is a history of discharge, attempt to express fluid by compressing or 'milking' the shaft. Any fluid obtained must be sent for microscopic examination and culture.

Inspect the scrotum with the patient standing. Usually the left testis hangs lower than the right.

Table 6.12 Causes of genital lesions

Ulcerative

Herpes simplex (vesicles followed by ulcers: tender)

Syphilis (non-tender)

Malignancy (squamous cell carcinoma: non-tender)

Chancroid (*Haemophilus ducreyi* infection: tender)

Behçet's syndrome

Non-ulcerative

Balanitis, due to Reiter's syndrome or poor hygiene

Venereal warts

Primary skin disease, e.g. psoriasis

Note: Always consider AIDS.

This is the only part of the body that consistently does not appear bilaterally symmetrical on inspection. Torsion of the testis may cause the involved testis to appear higher and to lie more transversely than normal. Inspect for oedema of the skin, sebaceous cysts, tinea cruris or scabies. Scrotal oedema is common in severe cardiac failure and may occur with the nephrotic syndrome and ascites.

Palpate each testis gently using the fingers and thumb of the right hand.[11] The testes are normally equal in size, smooth and relatively firm. Absence of one or both testes may be due to previous excision, failure of the testis to descend, or a retractile testis. In children the testis may retract as examination of the scrotum begins because of a marked cremasteric reflex (page 342). A maldescended testis (one that lies permanently in the inguinal canal or higher) has a high chance of developing malignancy. An exquisitely tender, indurated testis suggests orchitis.[12] This is often due to mumps in postpubertal patients and occurs about 5 days after the parotitis. An undescended testis may be palpable in the inguinal canal, usually at or above the external inguinal ring. The presence of small firm testes suggests an endocrine disease (hypogonadism) or testicular atrophy due to alcohol or drug ingestion.

Feel posteriorly for the epididymis and then upwards for the vas deferens and the spermatic cord. It should be possible to differentiate the vas from the testis.

A varicocele feels like a bag of worms in the scrotum. The testis on the side of the varicocele often lies horizontally. It is unclear whether this is a cause or effect of the varicocele. A left varicocele is sometimes found when there is underlying left renal tumour or left renal vein thrombosis. The significance of the rarer right varicocele is disputed.[13]

Differential diagnosis of a scrotal mass (Figure 6.5)

If a mass is palpable in the scrotum, decide first whether it is possible to get above it. Have the patient stand up. If no upper border is palpable, it must be descending down the inguinal canal from the abdomen and is therefore an inguino-scrotal hernia (page 159).

If it is possible to get above the mass, it is necessary to decide whether it is separate from or part of the testis, and to test for translucency. This is performed using a transilluminoscope (a torch). With the patient in a darkened room, a small torch is applied to the posterior part of the swelling by invaginating the scrotal wall. A cystic mass will light up while a solid mass remains dark.

A mass that is part of the testis and that is solid (non-translucent) is likely to be a tumour, or rarely a syphilitic gumma. The testes may be enlarged and hard in men with leukaemia. A mass that is cystic (translucent) with the testis within it is a hydrocele (a collection of fluid in the tunica vaginalis of the testis). A mass that appears separate from the testis and transilluminates is probably a cyst of the epididymis, while a similar mass that fails to transilluminate is probably the result of chronic epididymitis. By feeling along the testicular–epididymal groove it is usually possible to separate an epididymal mass from the testis itself.

Pelvic examination

The pelvic examination should be performed as the final part of any complete physical examination.[14] The patient should have first emptied her bladder. She should be on her back with her legs apart and her knees bent (the lithotomy position). The left lateral position (page 160) is used when the woman cannot assume the lithotomy position or when a view of the anterior vaginal wall is required: for example, when a urinary fistula is suspected.

The perineum should be brightly illuminated by a lamp. Put a glove on each hand. Inspect first the external genitalia. Note any rash (e.g. sclerotic white areas of leucoplakia, or redness, swelling and excoriation from thrush or trichomoniasis), ulceration, warts, scars, sinus openings or other lesions. Separate the labia with the thumb and forefinger of the

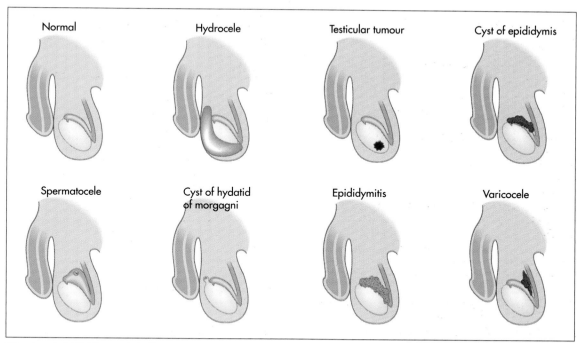

Figure 6.5 Differential diagnosis of a scrotal mass

(Adapted from Dunphy JE, Botsford TW. *Physical examination of the surgical patient. An introduction to clinical surgery*, 4th edn. Philadelphia: WB Saunders, 1975.)

right hand. A Bartholin[f] cyst or abscess is palpated between the thumb and index finger in the posterior part of the labia major; the normal gland is impalpable. Note the size and shape of the clitoris, and the presence or absence of a discharge from the urethral orifice and vaginal outlet. A bloody vaginal discharge suggests menstruation, a miscarriage, cancer or a cervical polyp or erosion. A purulent discharge suggests vaginitis, cervicitis or endometritis (e.g. gonorrhoea) or a retained tampon. *Trichomonas vaginalis* causes a frothy, watery, pale, yellow-white discharge, while thrush (*Candida albicans*) causes a thick cheesy discharge associated with excoriations and pruritus.

Ask the patient to bear down; a cystocele (descent of the bladder through the anterior vaginal wall) or rectocele (descent of the rectum through the posterior vaginal wall) or uterine prolapse may become apparent. Then ask the patient to cough; this may demonstrate stress incontinence. Note the presence of vaginal atrophy in older women.

Next insert the lubricated index and middle finger into the vagina. Locate the cervix first: it normally points towards the posterior vaginal wall. Note the position, size, shape, consistency, tenderness and mobility. Next palpate the anterior, posterior and lateral fornices. Usually the ovaries are not palpable. If a mass is palpable, its characteristics and location should be noted.

Bimanual palpation of the uterus is now performed; the fingers in the vagina are kept high up while the left hand presses downwards and backwards above the pubic symphysis. Note whether the uterus is anterior (anteverted) or posterior (retroverted). Also note its size, shape and consistency and feel for tenderness and mobility. A large nodular mobile uterus suggests fibroids, while smooth enlargement of the uterus suggests pregnancy, adenomyosis or submucous fibroids.

A speculum examination of the vagina and cervix is made by introducing a well-lubricated warm bivalve speculum in an upwards direction and with the blades closed, while the other hand separates the labia. The blades are opened once the speculum is fully introduced, and the vagina and cervix are inspected. A smear for cervical cytology

---

[f] Caspar Bartholin Secundus (1655–1738), Professor of Philosophy at Copenhagen at the age of 19, then Professor of Medicine, Anatomy and Physics. He described the glands in 1677.

1. **General inspection**
   Mental state
   Hyperventilation (acidosis), hiccups
   Sallow complexion ('uraemic tinge')
   Hydration
   Subcutaneous nodules (calcium phosphate deposits)

2. **Hands**
   Nails—leuconychia; white lines; distal brown arc
   Arterio-venous fistulae
   Asterixis
   Neuropathy

3. **Arms**
   Bruising
   Pigmentation
   Scratch marks/excoriations
   Myopathy

4. **Face**
   Eyes—anaemia, jaundice, band keratopathy
   Mouth—dryness, ulcers, fetor, gingival hypertrophy
   Rash (lupus, vasculitis etc)

5. **Neck**
   Jugular venous pressure
   Carotid bruits
   Scars from previous vascath insertion
   Parathyroidectomy scars

6. **Abdomen**
   Tenckhoff catheter
   Scars—dialysis, operations
   Kidneys—transplant kidney
   Bladder
   Liver
   Lymph nodes
   Ascites
   Bruits
   Rectal examination (prostatomegaly, frozen pelvis, bleeding)

7. **Back**
   Nephrectomy scar
   Tenderness
   Oedema

8. **Chest**
   Heart—heaving apex, pericarditis, failure
   Lungs—infection, pulmonary oedema

9. **Legs**
   Oedema—nephrotic syndrome, cardiac failure
   Bruising
   Pigmentation
   Scratch marks/excoriation
   Neuropathy
   Vascular access

10. **Urine analysis**
    Specific gravity, pH
    Glucose—diabetes mellitus
    Blood—'nephritis', infection, stone
    Protein—'nephritis' etc

11. **Other**
    Blood pressure—lying and standing
    Fundoscopy—hypertensive and diabetic changes etc
    Rash, livedo reticularis

Figure 6.6 Chronic renal failure

(Papanicolaou[g] or 'Pap' smear) can be taken to detect cervical dysplasia or cancer. This is done using a spatula that is placed firmly against the cervical os and rotated through 360 degrees. The test is more accurate if some endocervical cells are also obtained. This can be done with a separate brush designed to fit into the os. A smear of vaginal wall cells for hormonal assessment can be taken with the other end of the spatula. The samples are smeared thinly on microscopic slides and placed immediately in fixative. Wet slides can also be prepared for *Trichomonas* or thrush, and cultures obtained for gonorrhoea if indicated.

---

[g] George N Papanicolaou (1884–1962), New York physician.

Summary

Examination of a patient with chronic renal failure: a suggested method (Figure 6.6)

Lay the patient flat in bed while performing the usual general inspection. Note particularly the patient's mental state and the presence of a sallow complexion, whether the patient appears properly hydrated and whether there is any hyperventilation or hiccupping.

The detailed examination begins with the hands and the examination of the nails, which may reveal leuconychia, white transverse lines (Muehrcke's nails), a single white band (Mees' lines), or a distal brown arc (half-and-half nails). Examine the wrists and arms for vascular access. Get the patient to hold out the hands and look for asterixis. Then inspect the arms for bruising, subcutaneous nodules (calcium phosphate deposits), pigmentation, scratch marks and gouty tophi.

Go on now to the face and begin by examining the eyes for anaemia, jaundice or band keratopathy. Examine the mouth for dryness, ulcers or fetor, and note the presence of any vasculitic rash on the face.

The patient should be lying flat while the abdomen is examined for scars indicating peritoneal dialysis or operations, including renal transplants. Palpate for the kidneys, including transplanted kidneys, then examine the liver and spleen. Feel for an abdominal aortic aneurysm. Percuss over the bladder, determine if there is ascites, and listen for renal bruits. Rectal examination is indicated to detect prostatomegaly or bleeding.

Sit the patient up and palpate the back for tenderness and sacral oedema.

Look at the jugular venous pressure with the patient at 45 degrees. Examine the heart for signs of pericarditis or cardiac failure and the lungs for pulmonary oedema.

Lay the patient down again. Look at the legs for oedema (due to the nephrotic syndrome or cardiac failure), bruising, pigmentation, scratch marks or the presence of gout. Examine for peripheral neuropathy (decreased sensation, loss of the more distal reflexes).

Examination ends with measurement of the blood pressure, lying and standing (for orthostatic hypotension), and fundoscopy to look for hypertensive and diabetic changes. Finally urinalysis is performed, testing for specific gravity, pH, glucose, blood, protein or leucocytes.

References

1. Marazzi P, Gabriel R. The haematuria clinic. *BMJ* 1994; 308:356.
2. Bent S, Nallamothu BK, Simel DL et al. Does this woman have an acute uncomplicated urinary tract infection? *JAMA* 2002, 287; 20:2701–2710. Dysuria, frequency, haematuria, back pain and costovertebral tenderness increase the likelihood of urinary tract infection (positive LRs between 1.5 and 2.0). No vaginal discharge or irritation decreased the likelihood.
3. Dawson C, Whitfield H. Urological evaluation (ABC of urology). *BMJ* 1996; 312:695–698. This article provides useful definitions and interpretation of symptoms.
4. Dean J. ABC of sexual health: examination of patient with sexual problems. *BMJ* 1998; 317:1641–1643.
5. Bastian LA, Pistcitelli JT. Is this patient pregnant? Can you reliably rule in or rule out early pregnancy by clinical examination? *JAMA* 1997; 278:586–591. Clinical features (amenorrhoea, morning sickness, tender breasts, enlarged uterus after 8 weeks with a soft cervix) cannot reliably diagnose early pregnancy—a pregnancy test, however, can
6. Muehrcke RC. The fingernails in chronic hypoalbuminaemia: a new physical sign. *BMJ* 1956; 1:1327–1328. The classic description of this sign.
7. McGee S. *Evidence-based physical diagnosis*. Philadelphia: WB Saunders, 2001, 627.
8. Guarino JR. Auscultatory percussion of the urinary bladder. *Arch Intern Med* 1985; 145:1823–1825. This careful study makes a convincing case for the use of this technique, especially in obese patients or those with ascites.
9. Guinan P, Bush I, Ray V et al. The accuracy of the rectal examination in the diagnosis of prostate carcinoma. *N Engl J Med* 1980; 303:499–503. Suggests that rectal examination is an excellent technique for distinguishing benign prostatic hyperplasia and cancer, but this has subsequently been questioned.
10. Schroder FH. Detection of prostate cancer. *BMJ* 1995; 310:140–141.
11. Zornow DH, Landes RR. Scrotal palpation. *Am Fam Physician* 1981; 23:150–154. Describes standard examination techniques.
12. Rabinowitz R, Hulbert WC Jr. Acute scrotal swelling. *Urol Clin Nth Am* 1995; 22:101–105.
13. Roy CR, Wilson T, Raife M, Horne D. Varicocele as the presenting sign of an abdominal mass. *J Urol* 1989; 141:597–599. A sign of late-stage renal cell carcinoma, due to testicular vein compression, but can be on the left or right side!
14. Deneke M, Wheeler L, Wagner G, Ling FW, Buxton BH. An approach to relearning the pelvic examination. *J Fam Pract* 1982; 14:782–783. Provides some useful hints.

Suggested reading

Textbooks

Davison AM et al (ed). *Oxford textbook of clinical nephrology*. Oxford: Oxford University Press, 2005.

chapter 7

The haematological system

[T]he blood is the generative part, the fountain of life, the first to live, the last to die and the primary seat to the soul.

William Harvey (1578–1657)

The haematological history

Presenting symptoms

(Table 7.1)

Patients with anaemia may present with weakness, tiredness, dyspnoea, fatigue or postural dizziness. Anaemia due to iron deficiency is often the result of gastrointestinal blood loss, or sometimes recurrent heavy menstrual blood loss, and so these symptoms should be sought. Disorders of platelet function or blood clotting may present with easy bruising or bleeding problems. Recurrent infection may be the first symptom of a disorder of the immune system, including leukaemia or HIV infection. The patient may have noticed lymph node enlargement, which can occur with lymphoma or leukaemia.

Treatment

Anaemia may have been treated with iron supplements or B_{12} injections. Anti-inflammatory drugs or anticoagulants may be the cause of bleeding. Treatment for leukaemia or lymphoma may have involved chemotherapy, radiotherapy or both.

Past history

A history of gastric surgery or malabsorption may give a clue regarding the underlying cause of an anaemia. Anaemia in patients with systemic disease such as rheumatoid arthritis or uraemia can be multifactorial. Previous blood transfusions may have been required to treat the anaemia. On the other hand, patients with polycythaemia may have had many venesections (page 209).

Table 7.1 Haematological history

Major symptoms

Symptoms of anaemia: weakness, tiredness, dyspnoea, fatigue, postural dizziness

Bleeding (menstrual, gastrointestinal)

Easy bruising, purpura, thrombotic tendency

Infection, fever or jaundice

Lymph gland enlargement

Bone pain

Paraesthesiae (e.g. B_{12} deficiency)

Skin rash

Weight loss

Table 7.2 Causes of ecchymoses

Thrombocytopenia or platelet dysfunction (Table 7.3)

Coagulation disorders

Acquired
Vitamin K deficiency (leading to factor II, VII, IX and X deficiency)
Liver disease (impaired synthesis of clotting factors)
Anticoagulants, e.g. heparin, warfarin, proteins with anticoagulant activity
Disseminated intravascular coagulation

Congenital (rarely cause ecchymoses and usually present with haemorrhage)
Haemophilia A (factor VIII deficiency)
Haemophilia B (factor IX deficiency, Christmas disease)
Von Willebrand's disease (an inherited abnormality of the von Willebrand protein, which is part of the factor VIII complex and causes a defect in platelet adhesion)

Senile ecchymoses (due to loss of skin elasticity)

Social history

A patient's racial origin is relevant. Thalassaemia is common in people of Mediterranean or southern Asian origin. Rarely, very strict vegetarian diets can result in vitamin B_{12} deficiency.

Family history

There may be a history of thalassaemia or sickle cell anaemia in the family. Haemophilia is a sex-linked recessive disease while von Willebrand's disease[a] is autosomal dominant with incomplete penetrance (Table 7.2).

The haematological examination

Haematological assessment does not depend only on the microscopic examination of the blood constituents. Physical signs, followed by examination of

Figure 7.1 Digital infarction

the blood film, can give vital clues about underlying disease. Haematological disease can affect the red blood cells, the white cells, the platelets and other haemostatic mechanisms as well as the mononuclear-phagocyte (reticuloendothelial) system.

General appearance

Position the patient as for the gastrointestinal examination—lying on the bed with one pillow. Note the patient's *racial* origin (e.g. thalassaemia). *Pallor* should be looked for as it may indicate anaemia.[1–3] If there is any *bruising*, look at its distribution and extent. *Jaundice* may be present and can indicate haemolytic anaemia. *Scratch marks* (following pruritus, which sometimes occurs with lymphoma and myeloproliferative disease) should be noted.

The hands

The detailed examination begins in the usual way with assessment of the hands. Look at the nails for *koilonychia*—these are dry, brittle, ridged, spoon-shaped nails, which are rarely seen today. They can be due to severe iron deficiency anaemia, although the mechanism is unknown. Occasionally koilonychia may be due to fungal infection. They may also be seen in Raynaud's phenomenon (page 217). Digital infarction (Figure 7.1) may be a sign of abnormal globulins (e.g. cryoglobulinaemia). Pallor of the nail beds may occur in anaemia but is an unreliable sign. Pallor of the *palmar creases* suggests that the haemoglobin level is less than 70 g/L, but this is also a rather unreliable sign.[1]

Note any changes of rheumatoid or gouty *arthritis*, or connective tissue disease (Chapter 8). Rheumatoid arthritis, when associated with splenomegaly and neutropenia, is called Felty's

[a] EA von Willebrand (1870–1949), Swedish physician, described this in 1926.

Figure 7.2 Thrombocytopenic purpura

syndrome[b]: the mechanism of the neutropenia is unknown, but it can result in severe infection. Felty's syndrome can also be associated with thrombocytopenia (Figure 7.2), haemolytic anaemia, skin pigmentation and leg ulceration. Gouty tophi and arthropathy may be present in the hands. Gout may be a manifestation of a myeloproliferative disease. Connective tissue diseases can cause anaemia because of the associated chronic inflammation.

Now take the *pulse*. A tachycardia may be present. Anaemic patients have an increased cardiac output and compensating tachycardia because of the reduced oxygen-carrying capacity of their blood.

Look for *purpura* (Figure 7.2), which is really any sort of bruising, due to haemorrhage into the skin. The lesions can vary in size from pinheads called *petechiae* (from Latin *petechia* 'a spot') (Table 7.3) to large bruises called *ecchymoses* (Table 7.2).

If the petechiae are raised (*palpable purpura*), this suggests an underlying systemic vasculitis, where the lesions are painful, or bacteraemia.

The forearms

If thrombocytopenia or capillary fragility is suspected, the Hess test[c] may be indicated. A blood pressure cuff, placed over the upper arm, is inflated to a point 10 mmHg above the diastolic blood pressure. Wait for 5 minutes, then deflate the cuff and wait for another 5 minutes before inspecting the arm. Look for petechiae, which are usually most prominent in the cubital fossa and near the wrist, where the skin is most lax. Fewer than 5 petechiae per cm^2 is normal, while more than 20 is definitely abnormal,

---

[b] Augustus Roi Felty (1895–1963), physician, Hartford Hospital, Connecticut, described this in 1924.
[c] Alfred Hess (1875–1933), Professor of Paediatrics, New York, described this in 1914.

Table 7.3 Causes of petechiae

Thrombocytopenia
Platelet count <100 x10^9/L

Increased destruction
Immunological:
- immune thrombocytopenic purpura (ITP)
- systemic lupus erythematosus
- drugs, e.g. quinine, sulphonamides, methyldopa

Non-immunological:
- damage, e.g. prosthetic heart valve
- consumption, e.g. disseminated intravascular coagulation (DIC)
- loss, e.g. haemorrhage

Reduced production
Marrow aplasia, e.g. drugs, chemicals, radiation
Marrow invasion, e.g. carcinoma, myeloma, leukaemia, fibrosis

Sequestration
Hypersplenism

Platelet dysfunction
Congenital or familial
Acquired:
- myeloproliferative disease
- dysproteinaemia
- chronic renal failure, chronic liver disease
- drugs, e.g. aspirin

Bleeding due to small vessel disease
Infection:
- infective endocarditis
- septicaemia (e.g. meningococcal)
- viral exanthemata (e.g. measles)

Drugs, e.g. steroids
Scurvy (vitamin C deficiency)—classically perifollicular purpura on the lower limbs, which is almost diagnostic of this condition
Cushing's syndrome
Vasculitis:
- polyarteritis nodosa
- Henoch-Schönlein purpura*

Fat embolism
Dysproteinaemia

---

* Eduard Henoch (1820–1910), Professor of Paediatrics, Berlin, described this in 1865, and Johannes Schönlein (1793–1864), Berlin physician, described it in 1868.

Figure 7.3 Feeling for the epitrochlear lymph node

suggesting thrombocytopenia, abnormal platelet function or capillary fragility. This test is not commonly performed these days.

Epitrochlear nodes

These must always be palpated. The best method is to place the palm of the right hand under the patient's left elbow (Figure 7.3). The examiner's thumb can then be placed over the appropriate area, which is proximal and slightly anterior to the medial epicondyle. This is repeated with the left hand for the other side. An enlarged epitrochlear node is usually pathological. It occurs with local infection, non-Hodgkin's lymphoma[d] or rarely syphilis. Note the features listed in Table 7.4.

Axillary nodes

To palpate these the examiner raises the patient's arm and, using the left hand for the right side, pushes his or her fingers as high as possible into the axilla. The patient's arm is then brought down to rest on the examiner's forearm. The opposite is done for the other side (Figure 7.4).

There are five main groups of axillary nodes: (i) central; (ii) lateral (above and lateral); (iii) pectoral (medial); (iv) infraclavicular; and (v) subscapular (most inferior) (Figure 7.5). An effort should be made to feel for nodes in each of these areas of the axilla.

---

[d] Thomas Hodgkin (1798–1866), famous student at Guy's Hospital, London, described his disease in 1832. The first case he described was a patient of Richard Bright's. Hodgkin was one of the first to use the stethoscope in England. On failing to be appointed a physician, he gave up medicine and became a missionary.

Table 7.4 Characteristics of lymph nodes

During the palpation of lymph nodes the following features must be considered:
Site
Palpable nodes may be localised to one region (e.g. local infection, early lymphoma) or generalised (e.g. late lymphoma). The palpable lymph node areas are: • epitrochlear • axillary • cervical and occipital • supraclavicular • para-aortic (rarely palpable) • inguinal • popliteal
Size
Large nodes are usually abnormal (greater than 1 cm)
Consistency
Hard nodes suggest carcinoma deposits, soft nodes may be normal, and rubbery nodes may be due to lymphoma.
Tenderness
This implies infection or acute inflammation.
Fixation
Nodes that are fixed to underlying structures are more likely to be infiltrated by carcinoma than mobile nodes.
Overlying skin
Inflammation of the overlying skin suggests infection, and tethering to the overlying skin suggests carcinoma.

The face

The *eyes* should be examined for the presence of scleral jaundice, haemorrhage or injection (due to increased prominence of scleral blood vessels, as in polycythaemia). Conjunctival pallor suggests anaemia and is more reliable than examination of the nail beds or palmar creases.[3] In northern Europeans the combination of prematurely grey hair and blue eyes may indicate a predisposition to the auto-immune disease *pernicious anaemia*, where there is

Patient's arm rests on the examiner's to relax shoulder

Figure 7.4 Feeling for the axillary lymph nodes

Figure 7.6 Cervical and supraclavicular lymph nodes

1 = submental; 2 = submandibular; 3 = jugular chain;
4 = supraclavicular; 5 = posterior triangle;
6 = postauricular; 7 = preauricular; 8 = occipital.

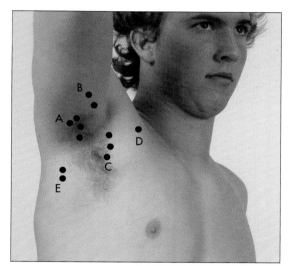

Figure 7.5 The main groups of axillary lymph nodes

A = central; B = lateral; C = pectoral; D = infraclavicular;
E = subscapular.

Look to see if the tonsils are enlarged. *Waldeyer's ring*[e] is a circle of lymphatic tissue in the posterior part of the oropharynx and nasopharynx, and includes the tonsils and adenoids. Sometimes non-Hodgkin's lymphoma will involve Waldeyer's tonsillar ring, but Hodgkin's disease rarely does.

Cervical and supraclavicular nodes

Sit the patient up and examine the cervical nodes from behind. There are eight groups. Attempt to identify each of the groups of nodes with your fingers (Figure 7.6). First palpate the submental node, which lies directly under the chin, and then the submandibular nodes, which are below the angle of the jaw. Next palpate the jugular chain, which lies anterior to the sternomastoid muscle, and then the posterior triangle nodes, which are posterior to the sternomastoid muscle. Palpate the occipital region for occipital nodes and then move to the postauricular node behind the ear and the preauricular node in front of the ear. Finally from the front, with the patient's shoulders slightly shrugged, feel in the supraclavicular fossa and at the base of

a vitamin B_{12} deficiency due to lack of intrinsic factor secretion by an atrophic gastric mucosa.

The *mouth* should be examined for hypertrophy of the gums, which may occur with infiltration by leukaemic cells, especially in acute monocytic leukaemia, or with swelling in scurvy (see Table 5.6). Gum bleeding must also be looked for, and ulceration, infection and haemorrhage of the buccal and pharyngeal mucosa noted. Atrophic glossitis occurs with megaloblastic anaemia or iron deficiency anaemia.

[e] Heinrich Wilhelm Gottfried von Waldeyer-Hartz (1836–1921), Berlin anatomist.

Table 7.5 Causes of lymphadenopathy

Generalised lymphadenopathy

Lymphoma (rubbery and firm)
Leukaemia (e.g. chronic lymphocytic leukaemia,
    acute lymphocytic leukaemia)
Infections: viral (e.g. infectious mononucleosis,
    cytomegalovirus, HIV), bacterial (e.g.
    tuberculosis, brucellosis, syphilis), protozoal
    (e.g. toxoplasmosis)
Connective tissue diseases: e.g. rheumatoid
    arthritis, systemic lupus erythematosus
Infiltration: e.g. sarcoid
Drugs: e.g. phenytoin (pseudolymphoma)

Localised lymphadenopathy

Local acute or chronic infection
Metastases from carcinoma or other solid
    tumour
Lymphoma, especially Hodgkin's disease

Table 7.6 Causes of splenomegaly

Massive

Common
Chronic myeloid leukaemia
Myelofibrosis

Rare
Malaria
Kala azar
Primary lymphoma of spleen

Moderate

The above causes
Portal hypertension
Lymphoma
Leukaemia (acute or chronic)
Thalassaemia
Storage diseases, e.g. Gaucher's disease*

Small

The above causes
Other myeloproliferative disorders:
• polycythaemia rubra vera
• essential thrombocythaemia
Haemolytic anaemia
Megaloblastic anaemia (rarely)
Infection:
• viral (e.g. infectious mononucleosis, hepatitis)
• bacterial (e.g. infective endocarditis)
• protozoal (e.g. malaria)
Connective tissue diseases:
• rheumatoid arthritis
• systemic lupus erythematosus
• polyarteritis nodosa
Infiltrations:
• e.g. amyloid, sarcoid
Splenomegaly may be found in 3–12% of the
    normal population.

Note: Secondary carcinomatosis is a *rare* cause of
splenomegaly.
* Phillipe Charles Ernest Gaucher (1854–1918), who
    described this in 1882, was physician and dermatologist
    at the Hôpital St-Louis, Paris.

the sternomastoid muscle for the supraclavicular nodes. Causes of lymphadenopathy, localised and generalised, are given in Table 7.5. Note that small cervical nodes are often palpable in normal young people.[4,5]

Bone tenderness

While the patient is sitting up, tap over the spine with the fist for bony tenderness. This may be caused by an enlarging marrow due to infiltration by myeloma, lymphoma or carcinoma, or due to malignant disease of the bony skeleton. Also gently press the sternum and both clavicles with the heel of the hand and then test both shoulders by pushing them towards each other with your hands.

The abdominal examination

Lay the patient flat again. Examine the abdomen carefully (page 145), especially for splenomegaly[6] (Table 7.6), hepatomegaly, para-aortic nodes, inguinal nodes and testicular masses. Remember that a central deep abdominal mass may occasionally be due to enlarged para-aortic nodes. Para-aortic adenopathy strongly suggests lymphoma or lymphatic leukaemia. The rectal examination may reveal evidence of bleeding or a carcinoma.

Assessment of the patient with suspected malignancy is presented in Table 7.7.[7]

Inguinal nodes

There are two groups—one along the inguinal ligament and the other along the femoral vessels. Small, firm mobile nodes are commonly found in otherwise normal subjects.

Table 7.7 Assessing the patient with suspected malignancy

1 Palpate all draining lymph nodes.
2 Examine all remaining lymph node groups.
3 Examine the abdomen, particularly for hepatomegaly and ascites.
4 Feel the testes.
5 Perform a rectal examination and pelvic examination.
6 Examine the lungs.
7 Examine the breasts.
8 Examine all the skin and nails for melanoma.

The legs

Inspect for any bruising, pigmentation or scratch marks. Palpable purpura over the buttocks and legs are present in Henoch-Schönlein purpura[f] (Figure 7.7). Leg ulcers may occur above the medial or lateral malleolus in association with haemolytic anaemia (including sickle cell anaemia and hereditary spherocytosis), probably as a result of tissue infarction due to abnormal blood viscosity. Leg ulcers can also occur with thalassaemia, macroglobulinaemia, thrombotic thrombocytopenic purpura and polycythaemia, as well as in Felty's syndrome.

Very occasionally, popliteal nodes may be felt in the popliteal fossa.

The legs should also be examined for evidence of the neurological abnormalities caused by vitamin B_{12} deficiency: peripheral neuropathy and subacute combined degeneration of the spinal cord (page 353). Vitamin B_{12} is an essential cofactor in the conversion of homocysteine to methionine; in B_{12} deficiency, the lack of methionine impairs methylation of myelin basic protein. Deficiency of vitamin B_{12} can also result in optic atrophy and mental changes. Lead poisoning causes anaemia and foot (or wrist) drop.

The fundi

Examine the fundi. An increase in blood viscosity, which occurs in diseases such as macroglobulinaemia, myeloproliferative disease or chronic granulocytic leukaemia, can cause engorged retinal vessels and later papilloedema (page 298). Haemorrhages may occur because of a haemostatic disorder. Retinal lesions (multiple yellow-white patches) may

---

[f] Henoch-Schönlein purpura is also characterised by glomerulonephritis (manifested by haematuria and proteinuria), arthralgias and abdominal pain.

Figure 7.7 Henoch-Schönlein purpura
(From FS McDonald, ed., *Mayo Clinic images in internal medicine*, with permission. © Mayo Clinic Scientific Press and CRC Press.)

be present in toxoplasmosis (see Figure 13.5) and cytomegalovirus infections (see Figure 13.6).

Examination of the peripheral blood film

This is a simple and useful clinical investigation.

A properly made peripheral blood film is one of the simplest, least invasive and most readily accessible forms of 'tissue biopsy', and can be a very useful diagnostic tool in clinical medicine. An examination of the patient's blood film can (i) assess whether the morphology of red cells, white cells and platelets is normal; (ii) help to characterise the type of anaemia; (iii) detect the presence of abnormal cells and provide clues about quantitative changes in plasma proteins—e.g. paraproteinaemia; (iv) help to make the diagnosis of an underlying infection, malignant infiltration of the bone marrow or primary proliferative haematological disorder. The following pages present illustrated examples of some clinical problems diagnosed by examination of the blood film (Figures 7.8 to 7.20).

Figure 7.8 Iron deficiency anaemia

Red cells show varying shape and size and are generally hypochromic.

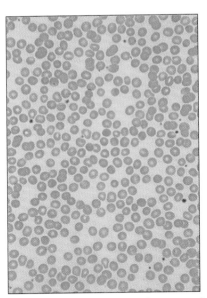

Figure 7.10 Spherocytic anaemia

Hereditary spherocytosis or autoimmune haemolytic anaemia. The numerous red blood cells which are small, round and lack central pallor are spherocytes (the big red blood cells are probably reticulocytes).

Figure 7.9 Megaloblastic anaemia

Red cells are macrocytic with many oval forms and the neutrophil is hypersegmented.

Figure 7.11 Autoagglutination

Cold haemagglutinin disease. Film shows clumping of red cells (low power).

Figure 7.12 Microangiopathic haemolysis (e.g. disseminated intravascular coagulation)

Frequent fragmented (bitten) red cells.

Figure 7.14 Leucoerythroblastic film

Film indicative of bone marrow infiltration. Shows circulating nucleated red blood cells and immature white cells.

Figure 7.13 Sickle cell anaemia

Film shows several sickle-shaped cells with target cells probably secondary to the 'autosplenectomy' that occurs in this disease.

Figure 7.15 Myelofibrosis

Film shows a dysplastic nucleated red blood cell, frequent tear-drop poikilocytes and a primitive granulocyte.

Figure 7.16 Postsplenectomy picture

Film shows several Howell-Jolly bodies, target cells and crenated cells.

Figure 7.18 Viral illness (e.g. infectious mononucleosis)

Film shows two atypical or 'switched-on' lymphocytes.

Figure 7.17 Malaria

The two red cells in the centre show the trophozoite.

Figure 7.19 Bacterial infection (e.g. pneumonia, infective endocarditis)

The white cell in the centre is a band form with prominent 'toxic' granules.

Figure 7.20 Acute leukaemia
The film shows two very primitive white cells with prominent nucleoli.

Correlation of physical signs and haematological disease

Anaemia

Anaemia is a reduction in the concentration of haemoglobin below 135 g/L in an adult man and 115 g/L in an adult woman. Anaemia is not a disease itself but results from an underlying pathological process (Table 7.8). It can be classified according to the blood film. Red blood cells with a low mean cell volume (MCV) appear small (microcytic) and pale (hypochromic). Those with a high MCV appear large and round or oval-shaped (macrocytic). Alternatively, the red blood cells may be normal in shape and size (normochromic, normocytic) but reduced in number.

Signs of a severe anaemia of any cause include pallor, tachycardia, wide pulse pressure, systolic ejection murmurs due to a compensatory rise in cardiac output, and cardiac failure if myocardial reserve is reduced. There may be signs of the underlying cause.

Pancytopenia

Signs

There may be clinical evidence of anaemia, leucopenia (reduced numbers of white blood cells resulting in susceptibility to infection) and thrombocytopenia (petechiae and bleeding)—a deficiency in all three bone marrow cell lines. If confirmed on a blood count, this condition is called pancytopenia.

Causes

- **Aplastic anaemia:** severe hypoplasia of the erythroid, myeloid and platelet precursor cell lines in the bone marrow, resulting in a bone marrow that is fatty and empty of cells. The causes are listed in Table 7.8; 50% have no cause identified.
- **Marrow infiltration** by leukaemia, lymphoma, carcinoma, myeloma, myelofibrosis or granulomata.
- **Other:** acute leukaemia (subleukaemic phase), pernicious anaemia, hypersplenism, systemic lupus erythematosus, folate deficiency.

Acute leukaemia

Leukaemia is a neoplastic proliferation of one of the blood-forming cells. Acute leukaemia presents with marrow failure from progressive infiltration of the marrow with immature cells. The course is rapidly fatal without treatment. Acute leukaemias can be divided into two main types: acute lymphoblastic leukaemia and acute myeloid leukaemia.

General signs of acute leukaemia

Pallor (anaemia), fever (which usually indicates infection secondary to neutropenia) and petechiae (thrombocytopenia) are all due to bone marrow failure. Weight loss, muscle wasting (hypercatabolic state) and localised infections (e.g. of the tonsils or perirectal region, due to leucopenia) also occur.

Signs of infiltration of the haemopoietic system

These include: (i) bony tenderness, due to infiltration or infarction; (ii) lymphadenopathy (slight to moderate, especially in acute lymphoblastic leukaemia); (iii) splenomegaly (slight to moderate, occurs especially in acute lymphoblastic leukaemia; the spleen may be tender due to splenic infarction); and (iv) hepatomegaly (slight to moderate).

Table 7.8 Causes of anaemia

Microcytic anaemia

Iron deficiency anaemia (iron is essential for haem production)
- chronic bleeding (commonest cause, usually from gastrointestinal or menstrual loss)
- malabsorption, e.g. gastrectomy, coeliac disease
- hookworm (blood loss)
- pregnancy (increased demand)
  Note: Dietary inadequacy alone is rarely the sole cause.

Thalassaemia minor (an abnormal haemoglobin)
Sideroblastic anaemia (iron incorporation into haem is abnormal)
Long-standing anaemia of chronic disease

Macrocytic anaemia

Megaloblastic bone marrow (oval macrocytes on the blood film)
- vitamin B_{12} deficiency due to:
  pernicious anaemia
  gastrectomy
  tropical sprue or bacterial overgrowth
  ileal disease, e.g. Crohn's disease, ileal resection (>60 cm)
  fish tapeworm (*Diphyllobothrium latum*) in Scandinavia especially
  poor diet (vegans, very rare)
- folate deficiency due to:
  dietary deficiency, especially alcoholics
  malabsorption, especially coeliac disease
  increased cell turnover, e.g. pregnancy, leukaemia, chronic haemolysis, chronic inflammation
  antifolate drugs, e.g. phenytoin, methotrexate, sulphasalazine

Non-megaloblastic bone marrow (round macrocytes on the blood film)
- alcohol
- cirrhosis of the liver
- reticulocytosis, e.g. haemolysis, haemorrhage
- hypothyroidism
- marrow infiltration
- myelodysplastic syndrome
- myeloproliferative disease

Normocytic anaemia

Bone marrow failure:
- aplastic anaemia (bone marrow fatty or empty), e.g. drugs (such as chloramphenicol, indomethacin, phenytoin, gold, sulphonamides, antineoplastics), radiation, systemic lupus erythematosus, viral hepatitis, pregnancy, Fanconi syndrome, idiopathic
- ineffective haematopoiesis (normal or increased bone marrow cellularity), e.g. myelodysplastic syndrome, paroxysmal nocturnal haemoglobinuria
- infiltration, e.g. leukaemia, lymphoma, myeloma, granuloma, myelofibrosis

Anaemia of chronic disease:
- chronic inflammation, e.g. infection (abscess, tuberculosis), connective tissue disease
- malignancy
- endocrine deficiencies, e.g. hypothyroidism, hypopituitarism, Addison's disease
- liver disease
- chronic renal failure
- malnutrition

Haemolytic anaemia:
- intracorpuscular defects, e.g. hereditary spherocytosis, elliptocytosis; haemoglobinopathies—sickle cell anaemia, thalassaemia; paroxysmal nocturnal haemoglobinuria (PNH)
- extracorpuscular defects: e.g. immune–autoimmune (warm or cold antibody) incompatible blood transfusion; hypersplenism; trauma (marathon runners, prosthetic heart valves); microangiopathic—disseminated intravascular coagulation); toxic—malaria.

Signs of infiltration of other areas

There may be: (i) tonsillar enlargement (especially in acute lymphoblastic leukaemia); (ii) swelling or bleeding of the gums, especially in monocytic leukaemia; (iii) pleural effusions; (iv) nerve palsies, involving the spinal nerve roots or the cranial nerves; or (v) meningism (page 363) due to infiltration of the meninges, especially in acute lymphoblastic leukaemia.

Chronic leukaemia

This is a haematological malignancy in which the leukaemic cell is at first well differentiated. These have a better prognosis untreated than acute leukaemia. There are two main types: chronic myeloid leukaemia and chronic lymphocytic leukaemia.

Signs of chronic myeloid leukaemia

This is one of the myeloproliferative disorders. There is an expanded granulocytic mass in the bone marrow, liver and spleen.

General signs may include pallor (anaemia due to bone marrow infiltration) and secondary gout (common).

Haemopoietic system signs include massive splenomegaly and moderate hepatomegaly. (Note: Lymphadenopathy is usually a sign of blast transformation.)

Signs of chronic lymphocytic leukaemia

There may be tiredness and pallor. Recurrent acute infections occur.

Haemopoietic system signs include marked or moderate lymphadenopathy and moderate hepatosplenomegaly.

Other abnormalities may include a Coombs'[g] test – positive haemolytic anaemia, herpes zoster skin infections and nodular infiltrates.

Myeloproliferative disease

This is a group of disorders of the stem cell. These include polycythaemia rubra vera, myelofibrosis, chronic myeloid leukaemia and essential thrombo-

cythaemia. Overlapping clinical and pathological features occur in these disorders. Therefore, patients may have signs of one or more of the conditions. Any of them may progress to acute myeloid leukaemia.

Polycythaemia

This is an elevated haemoglobin concentration and can result from an increased red blood cell mass or a decreased plasma volume. Polycythaemia rubra vera results from an autonomous increase in the red blood cell production. Patients with polycythaemia often have a striking ruddy, plethoric appearance. To examine a patient with suspected polycythaemia, assess for both the manifestations of polycythaemia rubra vera and for other possible underlying causes of polycythaemia (Table 7.9).

Look at the patient and estimate the state of hydration (dehydration alone can cause an elevated haemoglobin due to haemoconcentration). Note if there is a Cushingoid (page 269) or virilised (page 274) appearance. Cyanosis may be present because of an underlying condition such as cyanotic congenital heart disease or chronic lung disease. All these diseases can result in secondary polycythaemia.

The arms should be inspected for scratch marks; pruritus occurs in polycythaemia rubra vera, possibly due to basophil histamine release. Take the blood pressure: very rarely a phaeochromocytoma will cause secondary polycythaemia and hypertension.

Examine the eyes. Look for injected conjunctivae. Fundal hyperviscosity changes, including engorged, dilated retinal veins and haemorrhages, may be present. Inspect the tongue for central cyanosis.

Examine the cardiovascular system for signs of cyanotic congenital heart disease and the respiratory system for signs of chronic lung disease. The abdomen must be carefully assessed for splenomegaly, which occurs in 80% of cases of polycythaemia rubra vera but does not usually occur with the other causes of polycythaemia. There may be evidence of chronic liver disease or hepatocellular carcinoma, which may cause secondary polycythaemia. Palpate for the kidneys and perform a urinalysis. In women palpate the uterus. Polycystic kidney disease, hydronephrosis, renal carcinoma and uterine fibromata can all rarely cause secondary polycythaemia.

The legs must be inspected for scratch marks, gouty tophi and arthropathy, as well as for signs of

[g] Robin Coombs (b. 1921), Quick Professor of Biology, Cambridge.

Table 7.9 Polycythaemia

Signs of polycythaemia rubra vera

Plethoric appearance including engorged
    conjunctival and retinal vessels (not specific)
Scratch marks (generalised pruritus)
Splenomegaly (80%)
Bleeding tendency (platelet dysfunction)
Peripheral vascular and ischaemic heart disease
    (thrombosis, slow circulation)
Gout
Mild hypertension

Causes of polycythaemia

Absolute polycythaemia (increased red cell
    mass)
Idiopathic: polycythaemia rubra vera
Secondary polycythaemia
• Increased erythropoietin:
        renal disease—polycystic disease,
            hydronephrosis, tumour
        hepatocellular carcinoma
        cerebellar haemangioblastoma
        uterine fibroma
        virilising syndromes
        Cushing's syndrome
        phaeochromocytoma
• Hypoxic states (erythropoietin secondarily
    increased)
        chronic lung disease
        sleep apnoea
        cyanotic congenital heart disease
        abnormal haemoglobins
        carbon monoxide poisoning

Relative polycythaemia (decreased plasma
    volume)
Dehydration
Stress polycythaemia: Gaisböck's* disease

* Felix Gaisböck (1868–1955), German physician, described
    this in 1905.

peripheral vascular disease. In polycythaemia rubra vera, secondary gout occurs due to the increased cellular turnover resulting in hyperuricaemia. Peripheral vascular disease occurs in polycythaemia rubra vera because of thrombosis (as there is increased platelet adhesiveness and accelerated atherosclerosis) and slowed circulation due to hyperviscosity.

Look for cerebellar signs (page 327), which may be due to the presence of a cerebellar haemangio-blastoma, a very rare cause of secondary polycythaemia. Examine the central nervous system for signs of a stroke due to thrombosis (page 347).

Myelofibrosis

This is a clonal haemopoietic stem cell disorder with fibrosis as a secondary phenomenon. Gradual replacement of the marrow by fibrosis and progressive splenomegaly characterise the disease.

- **General signs** include pallor (anaemia occurs in most patients eventually) and petechiae (in 20% of patients, due to thrombocytopenia).
- **Haemopoietic system signs** include splenomegaly (in almost all cases, and often to a massive degree—there may also be a splenic rub due to splenic infarction), hepatomegaly (occurs in 50% and can be massive) and lymphadenopathy (very uncommon).
- **Other signs** are bony tenderness (uncommon) and gout (occurs in 5%).

Chronic myeloid leukaemia

(See page 209.)

Essential thrombocythaemia

This is a sustained elevation of the platelet count above normal without any primary cause.

- **General signs** include spontaneous bleeding and thrombosis.
- **Haemopoietic system signs** include splenomegaly.
- **Causes of thrombocytosis** (platelet count more than 400×10^9/L) include: (i) following haemorrhage or surgery; (ii) postsplenectomy; (iii) iron deficiency; (iv) chronic inflammatory disease; (v) malignancy.
- **Causes of thrombocytosis** (platelet count more than 800×10^9/L) include: (i) myeloproliferative disease; (ii) secondary to recent splenectomy or malignancy occasionally.

Lymphoma

This is a malignant disease of the lymphoid system. There are two main clinicopathological types: Hodgkin's disease (with the characteristic Reed-Sternberg cell[h]) and non-Hodgkin's lymphoma. Signs of lymphoma depend on the stages of the disease (Table 7.10).

[h] Dorothy Reed (1874–1964), pathologist at Johns Hopkins Hospital, Baltimore, described these cells in 1906 and Karl Sternberg (1872–1935), pathologist, described giant cells in 1898.

Table 7.10 Staging of lymphoma: Ann Arbor classification

Stage I

Disease confined to a single lymph node region or a single extralymphatic site (IE)

Stage II

Disease confined to two or more lymph node regions on one side of the diaphragm

Stage III

Disease confined to lymph nodes on both sides of the diaphragm with or without localised involvement of the spleen (IIIS), other extralymphatic organ or site (IIIE), or both (IIIES)

Stage IV

Diffuse disease of one or more extralymphatic organs (with or without lymph node disease)

For any stage: a = no symptoms; b = fever, weight loss greater than 10% in 6 months, night sweats.

Hodgkin's disease often presents in stage I or II, while non-Hodgkin's lymphoma usually presents in stage III or IV.

Signs of Hodgkin's disease

1 Lymph node enlargement: discrete, rubbery, painless, large and superficial nodes, often confined to one side and one lymph node group.
2 Weight loss and fever with or without infection (reduced cell-mediated immunity) suggest a poor prognosis.
3 Splenomegaly and hepatomegaly. Splenomegaly does not always indicate extensive disease.
4 Organ infiltration occurs with late disease. Look especially for signs of: (i) lung disease, such as a pleural effusion; (ii) bone pain or pathological fractures (rare); (iii) spinal cord or nerve compression (rare); and (iv) nodular skin infiltrates (rare).

Signs of non-Hodgkin's lymphoma

1 Lymph node enlargement: often more than one site is involved and Waldeyer's ring is more commonly affected.
2 Hepatosplenomegaly is common.
3 Systemic signs (for example weight loss or fever) are less common.

4 Signs of extranodal spread are more common.
5 The disease may sometimes arise at an extranodal site (e.g. the gastrointestinal tract).

Multiple myeloma

This is a disseminated malignant disease of plasma cells.

General signs

There may be signs of anaemia (due to bone marrow infiltration or as a result of renal failure), purpura (due to bone marrow infiltration and thrombocytopenia) or infection (particularly pneumonia).

Bony tenderness and pathological fractures may be present. Weight loss may be a feature. Skin changes include hypertrichosis, erythema annulare, yellow skin and secondary amyloid deposits. There may be signs of spinal cord compression, or mental changes (due to hypercalcaemia).

Look for signs of chronic renal failure, which may be due to tubular damage from filtered light chains, uric acid nephropathy, hypercalcaemia, urinary tract infection, secondary amyloidosis or plasma cell infiltration.

Summary
The haematological examination: a suggested method (Figure 7.21)

Position the patient as for a gastrointestinal examination. Make sure he or she is fully undressed. Look for bruising, pigmentation, cyanosis, jaundice and scratch marks (due to myeloproliferative disease or lymphoma). Also note the presence of frontal bossing and the racial origin of the patient.

Pick up the patient's hands. Look at the nails for koilonychia (spoon-shaped nails, which are rarely seen today and indicate iron deficiency) and the changes of vasculitis. Pale palmar creases may indicate anaemia (typically the haemoglobin level has to be lower than 70 g/L). Evidence of arthropathy may be important (e.g. rheumatoid arthritis and Felty's syndrome, recurrent haemarthroses in bleeding disorders, secondary gout in myeloproliferative disorders).

Examine the epitrochlear nodes. Note any bruising. Remember, petechiae are pinhead haemorrhages, while ecchymoses are larger bruises.

Go to the axillae and palpate the axillary nodes. There are five main areas: central, lateral (above

Lying flat (1 pillow)

1. General inspection
Bruising (thrombocytopenia,
  scurvy etc)
- Petechiae (pinhead bleeding)
- Ecchymoses (large bruises)
Pigmentation (lymphoma)
Rashes and infiltrative lesions
  (lymphoma)
Ulceration (neutropenia)
Cyanosis (polycythaemia)
Plethora (polycythaemia)
Jaundice (haemolysis)
Scratch marks (myeloproliferative
  diseases, lymphoma)
Racial origin

2. Hands
Nails—koilonychia, pallor
Palmar crease pallor (anaemia)
Arthropathy (haemophilia,
  secondary gout, drug treat-
  ment etc)
Pulse

3. Epitrochlear and axillary nodes

4. Face
Sclera—jaundice, pallor,
  conjunctival suffusion
  (polycythaemia)
Mouth—gum hypertrophy
  (monocytic leukaemia etc.),
  ulceration, infection,
  haemorrhage (marrow aplasia
  etc.); atrophic glossitis, angular
  stomatitis (iron, vitamin
  deficiencies)

5. Cervical nodes (sitting up)
Palpate from behind

6. Bony tenderness
Spine
Sternum
Clavicles
Shoulders

**7. Abdomen (lying flat) and
genitalia**
Detailed examination

8. Legs
Vasculitis (Henoch-Schönlein
  purpura—buttocks, thighs)
Bruising
Pigmentation
Ulceration (e.g.
  haemoglobinopathies)
Neurological signs (subacute
  combined degeneration,
  peripheral neuropathy)

9. Other
Fundi (haemorrhages,
  infection etc)
Temperature chart (infection)
Urine analysis (haematuria,
  bile etc)
Rectal and pelvic examination
  (blood loss)

Figure 7.21 Haematological system

and lateral), pectoral (most medial), infraclavicular and subscapular (most inferior).

Look at the face. Inspecting the eyes, note jaundice, pallor or haemorrhage of the sclerae, and the injected sclerae of polycythaemia. Examine the mouth. Note gum hypertrophy (e.g. from acute monocytic leukaemia or scurvy), ulceration, infection, haemorrhage, atrophic glossitis (e.g. from iron deficiency, or vitamin B_{12} or folate deficiency) and

angular stomatitis. Look for tonsillar and adenoid enlargement (Waldeyer's ring).

Sit the patient up. Examine the cervical nodes from behind. There are eight groups: submental, submandibular, jugular chain, supraclavicular, posterior triangle, postauricular, preauricular and occipital. Then feel the supraclavicular area from the front. Tap the spine with your fist for bony tenderness (caused by an enlarging marrow—e.g. in myeloma or carcinoma). Also gently press the sternum, clavicles and shoulders for bony tenderness.

Lay the patient flat again. Examine the abdomen. Focus on the liver and spleen. Feel for para-aortic nodes. Don't forget to feel the testes, and to perform a rectal and pelvic examination (for tumour or bleeding). Spring the hips for pelvic tenderness. Palpate the inguinal nodes. There are two groups— along the inguinal ligament and along the femoral vessels.

Examine the legs. Note particularly leg ulcers. Examine the legs from a neurological aspect, for evidence of vitamin B_{12} deficiency or peripheral neuropathy from other causes. Remember, hypothyroidism can cause anaemia and neurological disease.

Finally, examine the fundi, look at the temperature chart, and test the urine.

References

1. Strobach RS, Anderson SK, Doll DC, Ringenberg QS. The value of the physical examination in the diagnosis of anaemia: correlation of the physical findings and the haemoglobin concentrations. *Arch Intern Med* 1988; 148:831–832. Palmar crease pallor can occur above a haemoglobin of 70 g/L.
2. Nardone DA, Roth KM, Mazur DJ, McAfee JH. Usefulness of physical examination in detecting the presence or absence of anemia. *Arch Intern Med* 1990; 150:201–204.
3. Sheth TN, Choudray NK, Bowes M, Detsky AS. The relation of conjunctival pallor to the presence of anemia. *J Gen Intern Med* 1997; 12:102–106. The presence of conjunctival pallor is a useful indicator of anaemia, but its absence is unhelpful. It is also a reliable sign.
4. Linet OI, Metzler C. Practical ENT: incidence of palpable cervical nodes in adults. *Postgrad Med* 1977; 62:210–211, 213. In young adults without chronic disease, palpable cervical lymph nodes are often detected but are not clinically important. Remember, posterior cervical nodes are almost never normal.
5. Robertson TI. Clinical diagnosis in patients with lymphadenopathy. *Med J Aust* 1979; 2:73–76.
6. Grover SA, Barkun AN, Sackett DL. Does this patient have splenomegaly? *JAMA* 1993; 270:2218–2221. A valuable guide to assessment of splenomegaly, although the recommendations are controversial. A combination of percussion and palpation may best identify splenomegaly, but in contrast to hepatomegaly, percussion may be modestly more sensitive, according to the few available studies. Our conclusion is that this needs to be better established; in practice splenomegaly is often missed by percussion alone.
7. Anonymous. Cancer detection in adults by physical examination. US Public Health Service. *Am Fam Phys* 1995; 51:871–874, 877–880, 883–885.

Suggested reading

Textbooks

Hoffbrand AV, Moss P, Pettit JE. *Essential haematology*, 4th edn. London: Blackwell, 2001.

Provan D, ed. *ABC of clinical haematology*, 2nd edn. London: BMJ Publishing Group, 2003.

chapter 8

The rheumatological system

The rheumatism is a common name for many aches and pains which have yet got no peculiar appellation, though owing to very different causes.

William Heberden (1710–1801)

Rheumatology is 'the study of the Rheumatic Diseases including arthritis, rheumatic fever, fibrositis, neuralgia, myositis, bursitis, gout and other conditions producing somatic pain, stiffness and soreness' (*Oxford English Dictionary*, 2nd edn, 1989). The rheumatological system therefore includes diseases of the joints, tendons and muscles.

The rheumatological history

Presenting symptoms

(Table 8.1)

Peripheral joints

Pain and swelling. The underlying aetiology of joint pain can often be determined by establishing the distribution and duration of joint involvement. Remember, *arthralgia* is the presence of joint pain without swelling, while with *arthritis* there is usually pain and swelling. Determine whether one or many joints are involved.

It is often useful to ask the patient to point to the painful place or area. For example, pain said to affect the knee may be in the popliteal fossa, the knee joint itself or in the supra- or infrapatellar bursa. Remember also that pain in the knee or lower thigh may be referred from the hip.

Table 8.1 Rheumatological history—major symptoms

Joints
Pain
Swelling
Morning stiffness
Loss of function
Deformity
Weakness
Instability
Changes in sensation

Eyes
Dry eyes and mouth
Red eyes

Systemic
Raynaud's phenomenon
Rash, fever, fatigue, weight loss, diarrhoea, mucosal ulcers

Find out if the symptoms are of an acute or chronic nature and whether they are getting better or worse. The effect of rest and exercise on the joint pain should be determined. Patients with rheumatoid arthritis have joint symptoms which are worse after rest, while those with osteoarthritis have pain

Table 8.2 Causes of monoarthritis

A single hot red swollen joint (acute monoarthritis)

Septic arthritis
- Haematogenous—e.g. staphylococcal or gonococcal (latter may be polyarticular)
- Secondary to penetrating injury

Traumatic
Gout, pseudogout, or hydroxyapatite arthropathy
Haemarthrosis—e.g. haemophilia
Seronegative spondyloarthritis (occasionally)

A single chronic inflamed joint (chronic monoarthritis)

Chronic infection—e.g. tuberculosis
Seronegative spondyloarthritis
Pigmented villonodular synovitis

Table 8.3 Causes of polyarthritis

Acute polyarthritis

Infection—viral, bacterial
Onset of chronic polyarthritis

Chronic polyarthritis

Rheumatoid arthritis
Seronegative spondyloarthritis
Primary osteoarthritis
Gout, pseudogout, or hydroxyapatite arthropathy
Connective tissue disease, e.g. systemic lupus erythematosus
Infection, e.g. Lyme arthritis, spirochaetal infection (rare)

Table 8.4 Patterns of polyarthropathy

Rheumatoid arthritis

This is usually a symmetrical arthritis.
Hands: proximal interphalangeal, metacarpophalangeal and wrist joints
Elbows
Small joints of the upper cervical spine
Knees
Feet: tarsal and metatarsophalangeal joints

Seronegative spondyloarthritis

This is commonly an asymmetrical arthritis.

Ankylosing spondylitis
Sacroiliac joints and spine
Hips, knees and shoulders

Psoriatic arthritis
Terminal interphalangeal joints
Sacroiliac joints
Rheumatoid pattern

Reiter's syndrome
Sacroiliac joints and spine
Hips
Knees
Ankles and most of the joints of the feet

Primary osteoarthritis

This is usually symmetrical and can affect many joints.
Fingers: distal (Heberden's nodes) and proximal (Bouchard's nodes) interphalangeal joints, and metacarpophalangeal joints of the thumbs
Acromioclavicular joints
Small joints of the spine (lower cervical and lumbar)
Knees
Metatarsophalangeal joints of the great toes

Secondary osteoarthritis

This is asymmetrical and affects previously injured, inflamed or infected weightbearing joints
Hip
Knee
Intervertebral disc

which is worse after exercise. Ask about the sequence of onset of joint involvement. Precipitating factors such as trauma should be noted. The causes of monoarthritis (single joint) and polyarthritis (more than one joint), and the patterns of polyarthritis in various diseases, are presented in Tables 8.2, 8.3 and 8.4.

Morning stiffness. Ask about the presence of early morning stiffness and the length of time that this stiffness lasts. Morning stiffness classically occurs in rheumatoid arthritis and other inflammatory arthropathies, and the duration of stiffness is a guide to its severity.

Deformity. The patient may have noticed deformity of a joint or bone. If there has been progressive change in the shape of the area this is more likely to be significant.

Instability. Joint instability may be described by the patient as a 'giving way', or occasionally 'coming

Table 8.5	Functional assessment in rheumatoid arthritis
Class	**Assessment**
Class 1	Normal functional ability
Class 2	Ability to carry out normal activities, despite discomfort or limited mobility of one or more joints
Class 3	Ability to perform only a few of the tasks of the normal occupation or of self-care
Class 4	Complete or almost complete incapacity with the patient confined to wheelchair or to bed

out', of the joint in certain conditions. This may be due to true dislocation (for example, with the shoulder or the patella) or alternatively to muscle weakness or ligamentous problems.

Change in sensation: Change in sensation may occur as a result of nerve entrapment or injury, and sometimes as a result of ischaemia. Ask about numbness or paraesthesiae. The distribution of the change of sensation should help to distinguish nerve damage or entrapment (a specific distribution) from ischaemia.

Back pain

This is a very common symptom. It is most often a consequence of local musculoskeletal disease. Ask where the pain is situated, whether it began suddenly or gradually, whether it is localised or diffuse, whether it radiates to the limbs or elsewhere and whether the pain is aggravated by movement, coughing or straining. Musculoskeletal pain is characteristically well localised and is aggravated by movement. If there is a spinal cord lesion there may be pain that occurs in a dermatomal distribution. This helps to localise the level of the lesion (page 330). Diseases such as osteoporosis (with crush fractures), osteomalacia or infiltration of carcinoma, leukaemia or myeloma may cause progressive and unremitting back pain. The pain may be of sudden onset but is usually self-limiting if it results from the crush fracture of a vertebral body. In ankylosing spondylitis the pain is usually situated over the sacroiliac joints and lumbar spine.[1,2] Pain from diseases of the abdomen and chest can also be referred to the back.

Limb pain

This can occur from disease of the musculoskeletal system, the skin, the vascular system or the nervous system.

Musculoskeletal pain may be due to trauma. Muscle disease such as *polymyositis* can present with an aching pain in the proximal muscles around the shoulders and hips associated with weakness. Pain and stiffness in the shoulders and hips in patients over the age of 50 years may be due to *polymyalgia rheumatica*. Bone disease such as osteomyelitis, osteomalacia, osteoporosis or tumours can cause limb pain. Inflammation of tendons (*tenosynovitis*) can produce local pain over the affected area.

Vascular disease may also produce pain in the limbs. Acute arterial occlusion causes severe pain of sudden onset (page 57). Chronic peripheral vascular disease can result in calf pain on exercise that is relieved by rest. This is called intermittent claudication (page 31). Venous thrombosis can also cause diffuse aching pain in the legs associated with swelling (page 58).

Nerve entrapment and neuropathy can both cause limb pain (page 343). Injury to peripheral nerves can result in vasomotor changes and severe limb pain. This is called *causalgia*. Even following amputation of a limb, phantom limb pain may develop and persist as a chronic problem.

Raynaud's phenomenon

Raynaud's phenomenon[a] is an abnormal response of the fingers and toes to cold. The fingers first turn white, then blue and finally red after exposure to cold. It is during the red phase that the pain is most severe. Patients with Raynaud's disease have Raynaud's phenomenon without an obvious underlying cause. However, it tends to be familial and females are more likely to be affected. In connective tissue diseases, Raynaud's phenomenon can occur and may lead to the formation of digital ulcers (Table 8.6).

Dry eyes and mouth

Dry eyes and dry mouth are characteristic of Sjögren's syndrome (Table 8.7). This syndrome may occur in isolation (primary Sjögren's) or in association with rheumatoid arthritis and other connective tissue disease. Mucus-secreting glands become infiltrated with lymphocytes and plasma cells, which cause atrophy and fibrosis. The dry eyes

---

[a] Maurice Raynaud (1834–1881) described this in his first work, published in Paris in 1862.

Table 8.6 Causes of Raynaud's phenomenon (white-blue-red fingers and toes in response to cold)

Reflex

Raynaud's disease (idiopathic)
Vibrating machinery injury
Cervical spondylosis

Connective tissue disease

Scleroderma, CRST syndrome, mixed
    connective tissue disease
Systemic lupus erythematosus
Polyarteritis nodosa
Rheumatoid arthritis
Polymyositis

Arterial disease

Embolism or thrombosis
Buerger's disease (thromboangiitis obliterans)
Trauma

Haematological

Polycythaemia
Leukaemia
Dysproteinaemia
Cold agglutinin disease

Poisons

Drugs: beta-blockers, ergotamine
Vinyl chloride

CRST = calcinosis, Raynaud's, sclerodactyly and telangiectasiae.

Table 8.7 Clinical features of Sjögren's syndrome

In this syndrome mucus-secreting glands are infiltrated by lymphocytes and plasma cells, which cause atrophy and fibrosis of glandular tissue.
1 Dry eyes: conjunctivitis, keratitis, corneal ulcers (rarely vascularisation of the cornea)
2 Dry mouth
3 Chest: infection secondary to reduced mucus secretion or interstitial pneumonitis
4 Kidneys: renal tubular acidosis or nephrogenic diabetes insipidus
5 Genital tract: atrophic vaginitis
6 Pseudolymphoma: lymphadenopathy and splenomegaly, which may rarely progress to a true (usually non-Hodgkin's) lymphoma

Note: This syndrome occurs in rheumatoid arthritis and with the connective tissue diseases.

can result in conjunctivitis, keratitis and corneal ulcers. Sjögren's syndrome can also have an effect on other organs such as the lungs or kidneys.

Red eyes

The seronegative spondyloarthropathies and Behçet's[b] syndrome (page 251) but not rheumatoid arthritis may be complicated by iritis (central scleral injection (a 'red eye') radiating out from the pupil) (see Figure 8.35).

Systemic symptoms

A number of other symptoms may occur with specific rheumatological diseases. *Fatigue* is common with connective tissue disease. *Weight loss* and *diarrhoea* may occur with scleroderma, because of small

bowel bacterial overgrowth. Mucosal ulcers are common in some connective tissue diseases such as systemic lupus erythematosus (SLE). Specific rashes can also occur. *Generalised stiffness* can be due to rheumatoid arthritis or scleroderma, but other causes include systemic infection (e.g. influenza), excessive exercise, polymyalgia rheumatica, neuromuscular disease (e.g. extrapyramidal disease, tetanus, myotonia, dermatomyositis) and hypothyroidism. Finally, *fever* may be associated with the connective tissue diseases.

Treatment history

Document current and previous anti-arthritic medications (e.g. aspirin, other non-steroidal anti-inflammatory drugs, gold, methotrexate, penicillamine, chloroquine, steroids, anti-tumour necrosis factor α therapy). Any side-effects of these drugs (e.g. gastric ulceration or haemorrhage, from aspirin) also need to be identified. Ask about physiotherapy and joint or tendon surgery in the past.

Past history

It is important to inquire about any history of trauma or surgery in the past. Similarly, a history of recent infection, including hepatitis, streptococcal pharyngitis, rubella, dysentery, gonorrhoea and tuberculosis, may be relevant to the onset of arthralgia or arthritis. A history of tick bite may indicate that the patient has Lyme disease. Inflammatory bowel disease can result in arthritis, as described on

[b] Halushi Behçet (1889–1948), Turkish dermatologist.

page 170. A history of psoriasis may indicate that the arthritis is due to psoriatic arthropathy. It is also important to inquire about any history of arthritis in childhood.

Social history

Determine the patient's domestic set-up and occupation. This is particularly relevant if a chronic disabling arthritis has developed. Any history of sexually transmitted disease in the past is important, but non-specific urethritis and gonorrhoea are especially relevant.

Family history

Some diseases associated with chronic arthritis run in families. These including rheumatoid arthritis, gout and primary osteoarthritis, haemochromatosis, the seronegative spondyloarthropathies and inflammatory bowel disease. A family history of bleeding disorder may explain an acutely swollen tender joint in a boy (haemophilia).

The rheumatological examination

There are certain established ways of examining the joints and related structures[3] and it is important to be aware of the numerous systemic complications of rheumatological diseases. The actual system of examination depends on the patient's history and sometimes on the examiner noticing an abnormality on general inspection. Formal examination of all the joints is rarely part of the routine physical examination, but students should learn how to handle each joint properly. Diseases of the extra-articular soft tissues are particularly common.

General inspection

This is important for two reasons: first, it gives an indication of the patient's functional disability, which is essential in all rheumatological assessments; and second, certain conditions can be diagnosed by careful inspection. Look at the patient as he or she walks into the room. Does walking appear to be painful and difficult? What posture is taken, does the patient require assistance such as a stick, is there obvious deformity and what joints does it involve? Note the pattern of joint involvement, which gives a clue about the likely underlying disease (Tables 8.2 to 8.4).

For a more detailed examination the patient should be undressed as far as practical, usually to the underclothes. Depending on the patient's condition and the parts of the body to be examined, the examination may be best begun with the patient in bed, sitting over the side of the bed or in a chair, or standing. The opportunity of watching the patient remove the clothes should not be lost because arthritis can interfere with this essential daily task.

Principles of joint examination

Certain general rules apply to the examination of all the joints and they can be summarised as: *look, feel, move, measure,* and *compare with the opposite side.*

Look

The first principle is always to compare right with left. Remember that joints are three-dimensional structures and need to be inspected from the front, the back and the sides. The skin is inspected for *erythema* indicating underlying inflammation and suggesting active arthritis or infection, *atrophy* suggesting chronic underlying disease, *scars* indicating previous operations such as tendon repairs or joint replacements, and *rashes.* For example, psoriasis is associated with a rash and polyarthritis (inflammation of more than one joint). The psoriatic rash consists of scaling erythematous plaques on extensor surfaces. The nails are often also affected (page 262). Also look for a vasculitic skin rash (inflammation of the blood vessels of the skin), which can range in appearance from palpable purpura or livedo reticularis (bluish-purple streaks in a net-like pattern) to skin necrosis.

Note any *swelling* over the joint. There are a number of possible causes: these include effusion into the joint space, hypertrophy and inflammation of the synovium (e.g. rheumatoid arthritis) or bony overgrowths at the joint margins (e.g. osteoarthritis). It may also occur when tissues around the joints become involved, as with the tendonitis or bursitis of rheumatoid arthritis.

Deformity is the sign of a chronic, usually destructive arthritis, and ranges from mild ulnar deviation of the metacarpophalangeal joints in early rheumatoid arthritis to the gross destruction and disorganisation of a denervated (Charcot's[c]) joint (rare) (Figure 9.16). Deviation of the part of the body away from the midline is called *valgus* deformity and towards the midline, *varus* deformity. For example,

---

[c] Jean Martin Charcot (1825–1893), Parisian physician and neurologist. He became Professor of Nervous Diseases, holding the first Chair of Neurology in the world. His pupils included Babinski, Marie and Freud.

genu valgum means knock-kneed and *genu varum*, bow-legged.

Look for abnormal bone alignment. *Subluxation* is said to be present when displaced parts of the joint surfaces remain partly in contact. *Dislocation* is used to describe displacement where there is loss of contact between the joint surfaces.

Muscle wasting results from a combination of disuse of the joint, inflammation of the surrounding tissues and sometimes nerve entrapment. It tends to affect muscle groups adjacent to the diseased joint (e.g. quadriceps wasting with active arthritis of the knee) and is a sign of chronicity.

Feel

Palpate for skin *warmth*. This is done traditionally with the backs of the fingers where temperature appreciation is said to be better. A cool joint is unlikely to be involved in an acute inflammatory process. A swollen and warm joint may be affected by active synovitis (see below), infection (e.g. *Staphylococcus*) or crystal arthritis (e.g. gout).

Tenderness is a guide to the acuteness of the inflammation. The patient must be told to let the examiner know if the examination is becoming uncomfortable. Tenderness can be graded as follows:
Grade I: patient complains of pain
Grade II: patient complains of pain and winces
Grade III: patient complains of pain, winces, and withdraws the joint
Grade IV: patient does not allow palpation

This may result from joint inflammation or from lesions outside the joints (periarticular tissues). Infected joints are extremely tender and patients will often not let the examiner move the joint at all. Palpation of a joint or area for tenderness must be performed gently and the patient's face rather than the joint itself should be watched for signs that the examination is uncomfortable.

Palpate the joint deliberately now, if possible, for evidence of *synovitis*, which is a soft and spongy (boggy) swelling. This must be distinguished from an *effusion*, which tends to affect large joints but can occur in any joint. Here the swelling is fluctuant and can be made to shift within the joint (page 237). *Bony swelling* feels hard and immobile, and suggests osteophyte formation or subchondral bone thickening.

Move

Much information about many joints is gained by testing the range of *passive* movement. (Passive movement is obviously contraindicated in cases of recent injury to the limb or joint, such as a suspected fracture.) The patient is asked to relax and let the examiner move the joint. This must be attempted gently and will be limited if the joint is painful (secondary to muscle spasm), if a tense effusion is present or if there is a fixed deformity. The joints may have limited extension (called fixed flexion deformity) or limited flexion (fixed extension deformity). Passive movement of the spine is not a practical manoeuvre (unless the examiner is very strong) and active movement is tested here. *Active* movement is more helpful in assessing integrated joint function. Hand function (page 226) and gait are usually applied as tests of *function*.

Stability of the joint is important and depends largely on the surrounding ligaments. This is tested by attempting to move the joint gently in abnormal directions.

Joint crepitus, which is a grating sensation or noise from the joint, indicates irregularity of the articular surfaces. Its presence suggests chronicity.

Measure

Accurate measurement of the range of movement of a joint is possible with a goniometer, which is a hinged rod with a protractor in the centre. The jaws are opened and lined up with the joint. Measurement of joint movements is performed from the zero starting position. For most joints this is the anatomical position in extension—e.g. the straightened knee. Movement is then recorded as the number of degrees of flexion from this position. A knee with a fixed flexion deformity may be recorded as 30 to 60 degrees, which indicates that there is 30 degrees of fixed flexion deformity and that flexion is limited to 60 degrees. At some joints both flexion and extension from the anatomical position can be measured, as at the wrists. The goniometer is not routinely used by non-rheumatologists and there is a wide range of normal values for joint movement. Most clinicians estimate the approximate joint angles.

A tape measure is useful for measuring and following serially the quadriceps muscle bulk and in examination of spinal movements (page 233).

Assessment of individual joints

The hands and wrists (Figure 8.1)

History. *Pain* may be present in some or all of the joints. It is more likely to be vague or diffuse if it has radiated from the shoulder or neck or is due to carpal tunnel syndrome, and to be localised if it is

Sitting up (hands on a pillow)

1. General inspection
Cushingoid
Weight
Iritis, scleritis etc
Obvious other joint disease

2. Look
Dorsal aspect
• Wrists
   Skin—scars, redness, atrophy,
      rash
   Swelling—distribution
   Deformity
   Muscle wasting
• Metacarpophalangeal joints
   Skin
   Swelling—distribution
   Deformity—ulnar deviation, volar
      subluxation etc
• Proximal and distal
      interphalangeal joints
   Skin
   Swelling—distribution
   Deformity—swan necking,
      boutonnière, Z etc

• Nails
   Psoriatic changes—pitting,
      ridging, onycholysis,
      hyperkeratosis, discoloration

3. Feel and move passively
Wrists
• Synovitis
• Effusions
• Range of movement
• Crepitus
• Ulnar styloid tenderness
Metacarpophalangeal joints
• Synovitis
• Effusions
• Range of movement
• Crepitus
• Subluxation
Proximal and distal interphalangeal
   joints
• As above

Palmar tendon crepitus
Carpal tunnel syndrome tests
Palmar aspect
• Skin—scars, palmar erythema,
   palmar creases (anaemia)
• Muscle wasting

4. Hand function
Grip strength
Key grip
Opposition strength
Practical ability

5. Other
Elbows—subcutaneous nodules—
   psoriatic rash
Other joints
Signs of systemic disease

Figure 8.1 Examination of the hands and wrists

due to arthritis. *Stiffness* is typically worse in the mornings in rheumatoid arthritis. *Swelling* of the wrist may indicate arthritis or tendon sheath inflammation. Swelling of individual joints suggests arthritis. *Deformity* of the fingers and hand due to rheumatoid arthritis or of the fingers as a result of arthritis or gouty tophi may be the presenting complaint. The sudden onset of deformity suggests tendon rupture. *Locking or snapping* of a finger (trigger finger) is typical of inflammation of a flexor tendon sheath (tenovaginitis). *Loss of function* is a serious problem when it involves the numerous functions of the hand and wrist. The history should include an assessment of the difficulties the patient has in using the hands and wrists. *Neurological symptoms* as a result of nerve compression may cause paraesthesiae or limitation of complicated hand functions.

Figure 8.2 The hands in rheumatoid arthritis

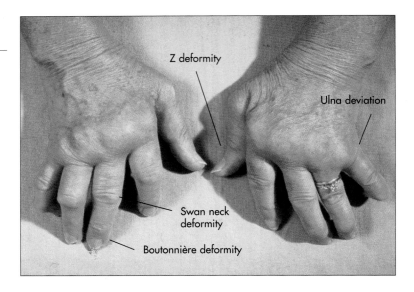

Examination. First sit the patient over the side of the bed and place the hands on the pillow with palms down. Often examination of the hands alone will give enough information for the examiner to make a diagnosis. As a result this is quite a popular test in viva voce examinations.

Look. Start the examination at the *wrists and forearms*. Inspect the skin for erythema, atrophy, scars and rashes. Look for swelling and its distribution. Next look at the wrist for swelling, deformity, ulnar and styloid prominence. Then look for muscle wasting of the intrinsic muscles of the hand. This results in the appearance of hollow ridges between the metacarpal bones. It is especially obvious on the dorsum of the hand.

Go on to the *metacarpophalangeal joints*. Again note any skin abnormalities, swelling or deformity. Look especially for ulnar deviation and volar (palmar) subluxation of the fingers. Ulnar deviation is deviation of the phalanges at the metacarpophalangeal joints towards the medial (ulnar) side of the hand. It is usually associated with anterior subluxation of the fingers (Figure 8.2). These deformities are characteristic but not pathognomonic of rheumatoid arthritis (Table 8.8).

Next inspect the *proximal interphalangeal* and *distal interphalangeal* joints. Again note any skin changes and joint swelling. Look for the characteristic deformities of *rheumatoid arthritis*. These include *swan neck* and *boutonnière* deformity of the fingers and *Z deformity* of the thumb (Figure 8.2).

They are due to joint destruction and tendon dysfunction. The swan neck deformity is hyperextension at the proximal interphalangeal joint and fixed flexion deformity at the distal interphalangeal joint. It is due to subluxation at the proximal interphalangeal joint and tendon shortening at the distal interphalangeal joint. The boutonnière (buttonhole) deformity consists of fixed flexion of the proximal interphalangeal joint and extension of the distal interphalangeal joints. This is due to protrusion of the proximal interphalangeal joint through its ruptured extensor tendon. The Z deformity of the thumb consists of hyperextension of the interphalangeal joint and fixed flexion and subluxation of the metacarpophalangeal joint.

Now look for the characteristic changes of *osteoarthritis* (Figure 8.3). Here the distal interphalangeal and first carpometacarpal joints are usually

Table 8.8 Differential diagnosis of a deforming polyarthropathy

Rheumatoid arthritis
Seronegative spondyloarthropathy, particularly psoriatic arthritis, ankylosing spondylitis or Reiter's disease
Chronic tophaceous gout (rarely symmetrical)
Primary generalised osteoarthritis
Infection, e.g. Lyme arthritis

Figure 8.3 The hands (a) and the feet (b) of a patient with osteoarthritis

Showing Heberden's nodes (distal interphalangeal joints), Bouchard's nodes (proximal interphalangeal joints) and bunions.

involved. *Heberden's nodes*[d] are a common deformity caused by marginal osteophytes that lie at the base of the distal phalanx. Less commonly, the proximal interphalangeal joints may be involved and osteophytes here are called *Bouchard's*[e] nodes.

Look also to see if the phalanges appear *sausage-shaped*. This is characteristic of psoriatic arthropathy, but can also occur in patients with ankylosing spondylitis and Reiter's disease. It is due to interphalangeal arthritis and flexor tendon sheath oedema. Finger shortening due to severe destructive arthritis also occurs in psoriatic disease and is called *arthritis mutilans*. The hand may take up a *main en lorgnette* ('hand holding long-handled opera glasses') appearance due to a combination of shortening and telescoping of the digits.

Now examine the *nails*. Characteristic *psoriatic* nail changes may be visible: these include pitting (small depressions in the nail), onycholysis (Figure 8.4) and, less commonly, hyperkeratosis (thickening of the nail), ridging and discoloration. The presence of *vasculitic* changes around the nailfolds implies active disease. These consist of black to brown 1 to 2 mm lesions due to skin infarction and occur typically in rheumatoid arthritis (Figure 8.5). Splinter haemorrhages may be present in patients with systemic lupus erythematosus (and infective endocarditis) and are due to vasculitis. Unlike nailfold infarcts they are located under the nails in the nail beds. Periungual telangiectasiae occur in systemic lupus erythematosus, scleroderma or dermatomyositis.

Figure 8.4 Psoriatic nails

Showing onycholysis and discoloration, with typical pitting and ridging.

The hands should now be turned over and the *palmar surfaces* revealed. Look at the palms for scars (from tendon repairs or transfers), palmar erythema, and muscle wasting of the thenar or hypothenar eminences (due to disuse, vasculitis or peripheral nerve entrapment).

Feel and move. Turn the hands back again to the palm-down position. Palpate the *wrists* with both thumbs placed on the dorsal surface by the wrists supported underneath by the index fingers (Figure 8.6). Feel gently for synovitis (boggy swelling) and effusions. The wrist should be gently dorsiflexed (normally possible to 75 degrees) and palmar flexed (also possible to 75 degrees) with the examiner's thumbs. Then radial and ulnar deviation (20 degrees) is tested (Figure 8.7). Note any tenderness or limitation of movement or joint crepitus.

---

[d] William Heberden (1710–1801), London physician, and doctor to George III and Samuel Johnson, described these in 1802. He was the first person to describe angina.
[e] Charles Jacques Bouchard (1837–1915), Parisian physician.

Figure 8.5 Rheumatoid vasculitis (arrows)

Figure 8.6 Palpating the wrist joint —approved method

Palpate the ulnar styloid for tenderness, which can occur in rheumatoid arthritis.

Test for tenderness at the tip of the radial styloid. This suggests de Quervain's[f] tenosynovitis (page 255).

Feel for tenderness in the anatomical snuff box if scaphoid injury is suspected (Figure 8.7). Test for tenderness distal to the head of the ulna for extensor carpi ulnaris tendonitis.

Go on now to the *metacarpophalangeal joints*, which are palpated in a similar way with the two thumbs. Again passive movement is tested. Volar subluxation can be demonstrated by flexing the metacarpophalangeal joint with the proximal phalanx held between the thumb and forefinger. The metacarpophalangeal joint is then rocked backwards and forwards (Figure 8.8). Very little movement occurs with this manoeuvre at a normal joint. Considerable movement may be present when ligamentous laxity or subluxation is present.

Palpate the *proximal* and *distal interphalangeal* joints for tenderness, swelling and osteophytes.

Next test for *palmar tendon crepitus*. The palmar aspects of the examiner's fingers are placed against the palm of the patient's hand while he or she flexes and extends the metacarpophalangeal joints. Inflamed palmar tendons can be felt creaking in their thickened sheaths and nodules can be palpated. This indicates tenosynovitis.

A *trigger finger* may also be detected by this manoeuvre. Here the thickening of a section of digital flexor tendon is such that it tends to jam when passing through a narrowed part of its tendon sheath. Rheumatoid arthritis is an important cause. Typically, flexion of the finger occurs freely up to a certain point where it sticks and cannot be extended (as flexors are more powerful than extensors). The application of greater force overcomes the resistance with a snap.

If the carpal tunnel syndrome is suspected, ask the patient to flex both wrists for 30 seconds—paraesthesiae will often be precipitated in the affected hand if the syndrome is present (*Phalen's*[g] *wrist flexion test*). The paraesthesiae (pins and needles) are in the distribution of the median nerve (page 331), when thickening of the flexor retinaculum has entrapped the nerve in the carpal tunnel (Table 8.9). This test is more reliable than *Tinel's*

[f] Fritz de Quervain (1868–1940), Professor of Surgery in Berne, Switzerland.

[g] George Phalen, orthopaedic surgeon, the Cleveland Clinic.

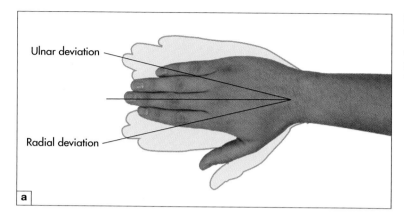

Figure 8.7 Movements of the wrist

(a) Ulnar and radial deviation.
(b) Dorsal and palmar flexion.

Ulnar deviation

Radial deviation

a

Dorsal flexion

Neutral

Palmar flexion

b

Figure 8.8 Examination for volar subluxation at the metacarpophalangeal joints

Table 8.9 Causes of carpal tunnel syndrome

Occupation-related:	Pregnancy
working with	Gout
wrists and	Obesity
hands flexed	Amyloid
Rheumatoid arthritis	Diabetes mellitus
Hypothyroidism	Idiopathic
Acromegaly	Carpal bone
	osteomyelitis

sign[h], in which tapping over the flexor retinaculum which lies at the proximal part of the palm may cause similar paraesthesiae.[4]

Now test active movements. First assess *wrist flexion and extension* as shown in Figure 8.9 (a and b). Compare the two sides. Now go on to *thumb movements* (Figure 8.10a, b, c and d). The patient holds the hand flat, palm upwards and the examiner's hand holds the patient's fingers. Test *extension* by asking the patient to stretch the thumb outwards, *abduction* by asking for the thumb to be pointed straight upwards, *adduction* by asking him or her to squeeze the examiner's finger, and *opposition* by getting the patient to touch the little finger with the thumb. Look for limitation of these movements and discomfort caused by them. Next test *metacarpophalangeal and interphalangeal movements*. As a

---

[h] Jules Tinel (1879–1952), physician and neurologist in Paris. In 1915 he described tingling in the distribution of a nerve that had been severed and was regrowing when it was percussed.

Figure 8.9 (a) Active wrist extension and (b) active wrist flexion

Figure 8.10 Thumb movements

(a) Extension. (b) Abduction.
(c) Adduction. (d) Opposition.

Figure 8.11 Screening metacarpophalangeal and interphalangeal movements

(a) Flexion. (b) Extension.

Figure 8.12 Testing the superficial and profundus flexor tendons

(a) Flexor profundus. (b) Flexor superficialis.

Figure 8.13 The key grip

Figure 8.14 Testing opposition strength

screening test, ask the patient to make a fist then to straighten out the fingers (Figure 8.11a and b). Then test the fingers individually. If active flexion of one or more fingers is reduced, test the superficial and profundus flexor tendons (Figure 8.12a and b). Hold the proximal finger joint extended and instruct the patient to bend it (Figure 8.12a); the distal finger-tip will flex if the flexor profundus is intact. Then hold the other fingers extended (to inactivate the profundus) and check finger flexion (inability indi-cates the superficialis is unable to work). The most common tendon ruptures are of the extensors of the fourth and fifth fingers.

Function. It is important to test the function of the hand. *Grip strength* is tested by getting the patient to squeeze two of the examiner's fingers. Even an angry patient will rarely cause pain if given only two fingers. Serial measurements of grip strength can be made by asking the patient to squeeze a partly inflated sphygmomanometer cuff and noting the

pressure reached. *Key grip* (Figure 8.13) is the grip with which a key is held between the pulps of the thumb and forefinger. Ask the patient to hold this grip tightly and try to open up his or her fingers. *Opposition strength* (Figure 8.14) is where the patient opposes the thumb and individual fingers. The difficulty with which these can be forced apart is assessed. Finally, *a practical test*, such as asking the patient to undo a button or write with a pen, should be performed.

Tests of hand function should be completed by formally assessing for neurological changes (page 331).

Examination of the hands is not complete with-out feeling for the *subcutaneous nodules* of rheumatoid arthritis near the elbows (Figure 8.15). These are 0.5 to 3 cm firm, shotty, non-tender lumps which occur typically over the olecranon. They may be attached to bone. They are found in rheumatoid factor-positive rheumatoid arthritis. Rheumatoid

Figure 8.15 Subcutaneous nodules in rheumatoid arthritis

Table 8.10 Causes of arthritis plus nodules*

Rheumatoid arthritis
Systemic lupus erythematosus (rare)
Rheumatic fever (Jaccoud's[†] arthritis) (very rare)
Granulomas—e.g. sarcoid (very rare)

* Gouty tophi and xanthomata from hyperlipidaemia may cause confusion.
† François Jaccoud (1830–1913), Professor of Medicine, Geneva.

---

nodules are areas of fibrinoid necrosis with a characteristic histological appearance and are probably initiated by a small vessel vasculitis. They are localised by trauma but can occur elsewhere, especially attached to tendons, over pressure areas in the hands or feet, in the lung, pleura, myocardium or vocal cords. The combination of arthritis and nodules suggests the diagnostic possibilities listed in Table 8.10.

The elbows

History. *Pain* from the elbow is usually diffuse and may radiate down the forearm. It may occur over the lateral or medial epicondyle if the patient has tendonitis (tennis or golfer's elbow). The patient may have noticed some swelling as a result of inflammation. *Swelling* over the back suggests olecranon bursitis. *Stiffness* may interfere with elbow movements and the patient may complain of difficulty combing the hair. When supination and pronation are affected the patient may complain of difficulty with carrying and holding. If the patient is aware of the elbow moving abnormally this suggests *instability* of the joint and may be a result of rheumatoid arthritis or trauma. Ulnar nerve trauma at the elbow may lead to a complaint of *numbness* or *paraesthesiae* in the distribution of that nerve.

Examination. *Watch* as the patient undresses, for difficulty disentangling the arms from clothing. The upper arms should be exposed completely. Note any deformity or difference in the normal 5 to 10 degree valgus position (carrying angle) as the patient stands with the palms facing forward.

Look for a joint effusion, which appears as a swelling on either side of the olecranon. Discrete swellings over the olecranon or over the proximal subcutaneous border of the ulna may be due to rheumatoid nodules, gouty tophi, an enlarged olecranon bursa or rarely to other types of nodules (Table 8.10).

Feel for tenderness, particularly over the lateral and medial epicondyles, which may indicate tennis or golfer's elbow (page 252), respectively. Palpate any discrete swellings. Rheumatoid nodules are quite hard, may be tender and are attached to underlying structures. Gouty tophi have a firm feeling and often appear yellow under the skin, but are sometimes difficult to distinguish from rheumatoid nodules. A fluid collection in the olecranon bursa is softly fluctuant and may be tender if inflammation is present. These collections are associated with rheumatoid arthritis and gout, but often occur independently of these diseases.

Move the elbow joints passively. The elbow is a hinge joint. The zero position is when the arm is fully extended (0 degrees). Normal flexion is possible to 150 degrees. Limitation of extension is an early sign of synovitis.

If lateral epicondylitis is suspected, ask the patient to extend the wrist actively against resistance (see Figure 8.50). Test the range of active movements by standing in front of the patient and demonstrating. If there is any deformity or complaint of numbness, a neurological examination of the hand and arm are indicated for ulnar nerve entrapment.

The shoulders

Movements of the shoulder are a result of a combination of ball and socket articulation at the glenohumeral joint and motion between the scapula and the thorax. The shoulder joint is most frequently affected by a number of non-arthritic conditions involving its bursa and surrounding tendons—e.g. 'frozen (stiff) shoulder', tendonitis, bursitis. All of these disorders affect movement of the shoulder.

History. *Pain* is the most common symptom of patient with shoulder problems.[5] Typically it is felt over the front and lateral part of the joint. It may radiate to the insertion of the deltoid or even further. Pain felt over the top of the shoulder is more likely to come from the acromioclavicular joint or from the neck. *Deformity* has to be severe before it becomes obvious. *Stiffness* may severely limit shoulder movement. *Instability* may cause the alarming feeling that the shoulder is jumping out of its socket. This is most likely to occur during abduction and external rotation (e.g. while attempting to serve a tennis ball). *Loss of function* may result in difficulty using the arms at above shoulder height or reaching around to the back.

Examination. *Watch* the patient undressing and note forward, backward and upward movements of the shoulders and whether these seem limited or cause the patient pain. Stand back and compare the two sides. The arms should be held at the same level and the outlines of the acromioclavicular joints should be the same. There may be wasting of one of the deltoid muscles that will not be obvious unless the two are compared.

Look at the joint. A swelling may be visible anteriorly, but unless effusions are large these are difficult to detect. Look for asymmetry and for scars as a result of injury or previous surgery.

Feel for tenderness and swelling. Stand beside the patient, rest one hand on the shoulder and move the arm into different positions (see below). As the shoulder moves, feel the acromioclavicular joint and then move the hand along the clavicle to the sternoclavicular joint.

Move the joint. The zero position is with the arm hanging by the side of the body so that the palm faces forwards (Figure 8.16). *Abduction* tests glenohumeral abduction, which is normally possible to 90 degrees. For the right shoulder the examiner stands behind the patient resting the left hand on the patient's shoulder, while the right hand abducts the elbow from the shoulder. *Elevation* is usually possible to 180 degrees when it is performed actively, as movement of the scapula is then included. *Adduction* is possible to 50 degrees. The arm is carried forwards across the front of the chest. *External rotation* is possible to

65 degrees. With the elbow bent to 90 degrees the arm is turned laterally as far as possible. *Internal rotation* is usually possible to 90 degrees. It is tested actively by asking the patient to place his or her hand behind the back and then to try to scratch the back as high up as possible with the thumb. Patients with rotator cuff problems complain of pain when they perform this manoeuvre. *Flexion* is possible to 180 degrees, of which the glenohumeral joint contributes about 90 degrees. *Extension* is possible to 65 degrees (Figure 8.17). The arm is swung backwards as in marching. During all these manoeuvres, limitation with or without pain and joint crepitus are assessed.

Rapid assessment of shoulder movement is possible using the three-step 'Apley[i] scratch test' (Figure 8.18). Stand behind and ask the patient to scratch an imaginary itch over the opposite scapula, first by reaching over the opposite shoulder, next by reaching behind the neck and finally by reaching behind the back.

The anterior stability of the shoulder joint is best assessed by the 'apprehension' test. Stand behind the patient, abduct, extend and externally rotate the shoulder (Figure 8.17c) while pushing the head of the humerus forwards with the thumb. The patient will strongly resist this manoeuvre if there is impending dislocation. There will be a similar response if the arm is adducted and internally rotated and posterior dislocation is about to occur.

This is also the time to test biceps function. The patient flexes the elbow against resistance. A ruptured biceps tendon causes the biceps muscle to roll up into a ball.

As a general rule, intra-articular disease produces *painful* limitation of movement in *all* directions, while tendonitis produces painful limitation of movement in *one* plane only, and tendon rupture or neurological lesions produce *painless* weakness. For example, if the abnormal sign is limited shoulder abduction in the middle range (45 to 135 degrees), this suggests 'rotator cuff' problems (i.e. the supraspinatus, infraspinatus, subscapularis and teres minor muscles) rather than arthritis (page 229).

In bicipital tendonitis there is localised tenderness on palpating over the groove. The supraspinatus tendon is a little higher, just under the anterior surface of the acromion. Supraspinatus tendonitis is common. Testing for it involves placing a finger

---

[i] Alan Apley, orthopaedic surgeon, St Thomas's Hospital, London.

Figure 8.16 Movements of the shoulder joint

(a) Abduction using the glenohumeral joint. (b) Abduction using the glenohumeral joint and the scapula. (c) Extension. (d) Adduction.

over the head of the tendon while the shoulder is in extension. As this pushes the tendon forwards against the examiner's finger, the movement is painful. When the shoulder is then flexed the tendon moves away and the pain disappears.

Don't forget that arthritis affecting the acromio-clavicular joint can be confused with glenohumeral disorders. Also remember to examine the neck and axillae in patients with shoulder pain.

**Figure 8.17
Examining the
shoulder joint**

(a) Extension.
(b) Flexion.
(c) Apprehension
test.
(d) Internal
rotation and
abduction.

Figure 8.18 Apley scratch test to assess shoulder movements

Figure 8.19 Examining the temporomandibular joints

Figure 8.20 Rheumatoid arthritis

Note the head tilt due to right atlantoaxial subluxation, the rheumatoid hands and the subcutaneous rheumatoid nodules.

The temporomandibular joints

History. The usual symptoms of temporomandibular joint dysfunction include clicking and pain on opening the mouth. The jaw may sometimes lock in the open position.

Examination. *Look* in front of the ear for swelling. *Feel* by placing a finger just in front of the ear while the patient opens and shuts the mouth (Figure 8.19). The head of the mandible is palpable as it slides forwards when the jaw is opened. Clicking and grating may be felt. This is sometimes associated with tenderness if the joint is involved in an inflammatory arthritis. Rheumatoid arthritis may affect the temporomandibular joint.

The neck

History. *Pain* is the most common neck symptom. There may be a history of trauma. The pain may have begun suddenly, suggesting a disc prolapse, or more gradually due to disc degeneration. Postural tendon and muscle strains are common causes of temporary neck pain. *Deformity* may occur as a result of muscle spasm or sometimes following disc prolapse. *Stiffness*

is a common problem often associated with pain and muscle spasm. *Neurological symptoms* suggest nerve root irritation or compression. Ask about paraesthesiae and weakness in the arms and hands.

Examination. The patient should be undressed so as to expose the neck, shoulders and arms.

Look at the cervical spine while the patient is sitting up and note particularly his or her posture (Figure 8.20). *Movement* should be tested actively. Flexion is tested by asking the patient to try to touch his or her chest with the chin (normal flexion is possible to 45 degrees). Extension (Fig 8.21a) is tested by asking the patient to look up and back (normally possible to 45 degrees). Lateral bending (Fig 8.21b) is tested by getting the patient to touch his or her shoulder with the ear; lateral bending is normally possible to 45 degrees. Rotation is tested by getting the patient to look over the shoulder to the right and then to the left. This is normally possible to 70 degrees.

Figure 8.21 Movements of the neck

(a) Extension—'Look up and back'.
(b) Lateral bending—'Now touch your right ear onto your shoulder' (45 degrees); rotation—'Now look over your shoulder to the right and then to the left' (70 degrees).

Figure 8.22 Examining the spinous processes

Feel the posterior spinous processes. This is often easiest to do when the patient lies prone with the chest supported by a pillow and the neck slightly flexed. The examiner should feel for tenderness and uneven spacing of the spinous processes. Tenderness of the facet joints will be elicited by feeling a finger's breadth lateral to the middle line on each side (Figure 8.22).

Neurological examination of the upper limbs, including testing of shoulder abduction (C5, C6) and the serratus anterior muscle (C5, C6, C7), is part of the assessment of the neck (page 323).

The thoracolumbar spine and sacroiliac joints

History. Lower back pain is a very common symptom. The discomfort is usually worst in the lumbosacral area. Ask whether the onset was sudden and associated with lifting or straining or whether it was gradual.[1,2] Stiffness and pain in the lower back that is worse in the morning is characteristic of an inflammatory spondyloarthropathy. Pain that shoots from the back into the buttock and thigh along the sciatic nerve distribution is called '*sciatica*'. In sciatic nerve compression at a lumbosacral nerve root, the pain is often aggravated by coughing or straining. 'Lumbago' however is often due to referred pain (e.g. from the vertebral joints). There may be other *neurological symptoms* in the legs due to nerve compression or irritation. The distribution of the paraesthesiae or weakness may indicate the level of spinal cord or nerve root abnormality. One should also ask about urinary incontinence and retention, which can be a result of cauda equina involvement.

Examination. To start the examination, have the patient standing and clothed only in underpants. *Look* for deformity, inspecting from both the back and side. Note especially loss of the normal thoracic kyphosis and lumbar lordosis, which is typical of ankylosing spondylitis. Also note any evidence of scoliosis, a lateral curvature of the spine which may be simple ('C' shaped) or compound ('S' shaped) and which can result from trauma, developmental abnormalities, vertebral body disease (e.g. rickets, tuberculosis) or muscle abnormality (e.g. polio).

Feel each vertebral body for tenderness and palpate for muscle spasm.[1]

Movement is assessed actively. Bending movements largely take place at the lumbar spine, while rotational movements occur at the thoracic spine. Range of movement is tested by observation and the use of Schober's test (see below) (Figure 8.23).

Flexion is tested by asking the patient to touch the toes with the knees straight. The normal range of flexion is very wide. Many people can reach only halfway down the shins when the knees are kept straight. As the patient bends look at the spine, there is normally a gentle curve along the back from the shoulders to the pelvis. Patients with advanced ankylosing spondylitis have a flat ankylosed spine and all the bending occurs at the hips. Test *extension* by asking the patient to lean backwards. Patients with back pain usually find this less uncomfortable than bending forwards. *Lateral bending* is assessed by getting the patient to slide the right hand down the right leg as far as possible without bending forwards, and then the same for the left side. This movement tends to be restricted early in ankylosing spondylitis. *Rotation* is tested with the patient sitting on a stool (to fix the pelvis) and asking him or her to rotate the head and shoulders as far as possible to each side. This is best viewed from above.

Measure the lumbar flexion with *Schober's test*. A mark is made at the level of the posterior iliac spine on the vertebral column (approximately at L5). One finger is placed 5 cm below and another 10 cm above this mark. The patient is then asked to touch the toes. An increase of less than 5 cm in the distance between the two fingers indicates limitation of lumbar flexion. The finger-to-floor distance at full flexion can be measured serially to give an objective indication of disease progression.

Assess *straight leg raising* (Lasègue's[j] test includes passive ankle dorsiflexion). With the patient lying down, lift the straightened leg if sciatica is suspected

---

Figure 8.23 Movements of the thoracolumbar spine

(a) Flexion. (b) Extension. (c) Lateral bending. (d) Rotation.

Left

Right

(normal 80 to 90 degrees). This will be limited by pain in lumbar disc prolapse (less than 60 degrees).

Now get the patient to lie in bed on the stomach. Look for gluteal wasting. The sacroiliac joints lie underneath the dimples of Venus[k]. By tradition, firm palpation with both palms overlying each other is used to elicit tenderness in patients with sacroiliitis. Test each side separately.

The complete examination of the back also requires neurological assessment of the lower limbs (page 335).[6]

The hips

History. The patient with hip problems will often have *pain* that is felt anteriorly in the groin or may radiate to the knee. Athletes with 'groin strain' often have adductor tendonitis or osteitis pubis caused by trauma. A *limp* may be noticed by the patient. When associated with pain it is a compensating mechanism but, when painless, may be due to differing limb length or instability of the joint. Patients are sometimes aware of *clicking* or *snapping* coming from the region of the hip. This may be due to a psoas bursitis or to slipping of the tendon of the gluteus maximus over the edge of the greater trochanter. *Functional impairment* usually results in difficulty walking and climbing stairs. Sitting down and standing up can become progressively more uncomfortable because of stiffness and pain.

Examination. *Watch* the patient walking into the room and note the use of a walking stick, a slow obviously uncomfortable gait or a limp.

Get the patient to lie down, first on the back.

---

[k] Roman goddess of love—her ancient Greek equivalent was Aphrodite.

Looking at the hip joint itself is not possible because so much muscle overlies it. However, the examiner must inspect for scars and deformity. The patient may adopt a position with one leg rotated because of pain.

Feel just distal to the mid-point of the inguinal ligament for joint tenderness. Now feel for the positions of the greater trochanters. The examiner's thumbs are placed on the anterior superior iliac spines on each side while the fore and middle fingers move posteriorly to find the tips of the greater trochanters. These should be at the same level. If one side is higher than the other, the higher side is likely to be the abnormal one.

Move the hip joint passively (Figure 8.24). *Flexion* is tested by flexing the patient's knee and moving the thigh towards the chest. The examiner keeps the pelvis on the bed by holding the other leg down. A fixed flexion deformity (inability to extend a joint normally) may be masked by the patient's arching the back and tilting the pelvis forward and increasing lumbar lordosis unless *Thomas's test*[l] is applied. The legs are fully flexed to straighten the pelvis. One leg is then extended. A fixed flexion deformity (e.g. as result of osteoarthritis) will prevent straightening. *Rotation* is tested with the knee and hip flexed. One hand holds the knee, the other the foot. The foot is then moved medially (*external rotation of the hip*, normally possible to 45 degrees), then laterally (*internal rotation of the hip*, normal to 45 degrees). *Abduction* is tested by standing on the same side of the bed as the leg to be tested. The right hand grasps the heel of the right leg while the left hand is placed over the anterior superior iliac spine to steady the pelvis. The leg is then moved outwards as far as possible. This is normally possible to 50 degrees. *Adduction* is the opposite. The leg is carried immediately in front of the other limb and this is normally possible to 45 degrees.

Ask the patient to roll over onto the stomach. *Extension* is then tested by placing one hand over the sacroiliac joint while the other elevates each leg. This is normally possible to about 30 degrees. Ask the patient to stand now and perform the Trendelenburg[m] test. The patient stands first on one leg and then on the other. Normally the non-weightbearing hip rises, but with proximal myopathy (page 355) or hip joint disease the non-weightbearing side sags.

Finally, the true *leg length* (from the anterior superior iliac spine to the medial malleolus) and apparent leg length (from the umbilicus to the same lower point) for each leg should be measured. A difference in true leg length indicates hip disease on the shorter side, while apparent leg length differences are due to tilting of the pelvis.

In patients with osteoarthritis of the joint, internal rotation, abduction and extension are usually restricted.[7]

The knees

History. *Pain* is a common knee problem. If there has been an injury or it is due to a mechanical abnormality, it is often localised. Inflammatory diseases more often cause diffuse pain. *Stiffness* is usually of gradual onset and is typical of osteoarthritis. It tends to be worse after inactivity. *Locking* of the knee usually means there is a sudden inability to reach full extension. Unlocking may occur just as suddenly. The cause is mechanical: a loose body or torn meniscus has become wedged between the articular surfaces of the joint. *Swelling* may occur suddenly after an injury, suggesting it is due to haemarthrosis from a fracture or ligamentous tear, or after a few hours when a torn meniscus is more likely to be the cause. Arthritis and synovitis cause a chronic swelling. Patients sometimes notice *deformity*, which in later life is usually due to arthritis. Sometimes the patient may complain that the knee is *unstable* or *gives way*. Patellar instability and ruptured ligaments may present this way. One should always ask about *loss of function*. There is often a reduced ability to walk distances, climb stairs and get into and out of chairs.

Examination. This is performed with the patient in a number of positions and, of course, walking.[8,9] Even more than with the other joints, it is important to examine the more normal or uninjured knee first. This will help with the interpretation of changes in the other knee and give the patient more confidence that the examination will not be painful.

Look first with the patient lying down on the back with both knees and thighs fully exposed. The affected knee will often be flexed, the most comfortable position. Note any quadriceps wasting. This begins quite soon after knee abnormalities lead to disuse of the muscle. Examine the knees themselves for skin changes, scars, swelling and deformity. Compare each side with the other. Localised swellings may move about as the knee flexes and extends. They are often cartilaginous loose bodies. Fixed lumps in the line of the joint may be meniscal cysts.

Swelling of the synovium is usually seen medial to the patella and in the joint's suprapatellar extension. Loss of the peripatellar grooves may be an

---

l   Hugh Thomas (1834–91), 'the father of orthopaedic surgery', worked in Liverpool as a bone setter but did not have a hospital appointment.

m   Friedrich Trendelenburg (1844–1924), Professor of Surgery at Rostock, Bonn and Leipzig.

Figure 8.24 Movements of the hip

(a) Flexion. (b) Extension. (c) Flexion, knee bent.
(d) Internal rotation. (e) External rotation. (f) Abduction.

Figure 8.25 Testing for patellar effusion

(a) The patellar tap. (b) The bulge sign: compressing the suprapatellar pouch.

early sign of an effusion. Assess fixed flexion deformity by squatting down and looking at each knee from the side. A space under the knee will be visible if there is permanent flexion deformity arthritis.

Varus and valgus deformity may be obvious here but are more easily seen when the patient stands. Varus deformity is often related to osteoarthritis and valgus deformity to rheumatoid arthritis.

Now watch as the patient flexes and straightens each knee in turn. As the knee extends the patella glides upwards and remains centred over the femoral condyles. If there is patellar subluxation it will slip laterally during knee flexion and return to the middle line during knee extension.

Feel the quadriceps for wasting. Palpate over the knees for warmth and synovial swelling.

Test carefully for a joint effusion. The *patellar tap* is used to confirm the presence of large effusions (Figure 8.25). One hand rests over the lower part of the quadriceps muscle and compresses the suprapatellar bursa. The other hand pushes the patella downwards. The sign is positive if the patella is felt to sink and then comes to rest with a tap as it touches the underlying femur. The *bulge sign* is used to detect small effusions. Here the left hand compresses the suprapatellar pouch while the fingers of the right hand are run along the groove beside the patella on one side and then the other. A bulging along the groove due to a fluid wave, on the side not being compressed, is a sign of a small effusion.

Examine for patellofemoral lesions by sliding the patella sideways across the underlying femoral condyles.

Move the joint passively. Test *flexion* (normally possible to 135 degrees) and *extension* (normal to 5 degrees) by resting one hand on the knee cap while the other moves the leg up and down (Figure 8.26a). The range of movements and the presence of crepitus are noted. While holding the knee flexed, feel for and attempt to localise tenderness. Feel gently for tenderness along the joint line at the patellar ligament and at the sites of attachment of the collateral ligaments.

Test the *ligaments* next. The lateral and medial *collateral ligaments* are assessed by having the knee slightly flexed while holding the leg, with the examiner's forearm resting along the length of the tibia; lateral and medial movements of the leg on the knee joint are tested (Figure 8. 26b). Meanwhile the thigh is steadied with the other hand. Movements of more than 5 to 10 degrees are abnormal. The *cruciate ligaments* (Figure 8.26c) are tested next. The examiner steadies the patient's foot with an elbow or by sitting on it. The patient's knee is flexed to 90 degrees. The examiner's hands grasp the tibia and attempt anterior and posterior movements of the leg on the knee joint. Movement may be detected by the examiner's thumbs positioned at the joint margins. Again, movement of more than 5 to 10 degrees is abnormal. Increased anterior movement suggests anterior cruciate ligamentous laxity and increased posterior movement suggests posterior cruciate ligamentous laxity. The Lachman test may be more accurate (positive LR 42.0, negative LR 0.1).[8] Here the knee is flexed 20 to 30 degrees while the patient is lying supine. Grasp the femur (place your hand above the knee) to steady it, then grab the lower leg below the knee and give it a quick forward tug. It is abnormal when there is exaggerated anterior tibial movement or the knee fails to stop with a thud.

When recurrent dislocation or subluxation of the patella is suspected, the *patellar apprehension test* should be performed. Push the patella firmly in a lateral direction while slowly flexing the knee. The patient's face should be studied for the anxious look that suggests impending dislocation (it is then time to suspend the test).

Figure 8.26 Knee examination

(a) Testing knee flexion. (b) Testing the collateral ligaments. (c) Testing the cruciate ligaments.

Figure 8.27 Baker's cyst of the right knee, viewed from behind

Figure 8.28 Apley's grinding test (push hard)

Ask the patient to roll into the prone position. Look and feel in the popliteal fossa for a Baker's cyst[n]. This is a pressure diverticulum of the synovial membrane that occurs through a hiatus in the knee capsule (Figure 8.27). It is best seen with the knee extended. Rupture of this into the calf muscle

produces signs that may mimic a deep venous thrombosis (page 58). It must be distinguished from an aneurysm of the popliteal artery, which will be pulsatile, and a bony tumour (very hard).

This is also the position in which Apley's[o] *grinding test* may be performed (Figure 8.28). This is a test of meniscal damage. The patient's leg is flexed to 90 degrees, the examiner stabilises the thigh by kneeling lightly on it and while pressing on the foot rotates the leg backwards and forwards. Pain or clicking make the test positive. The *distraction test* is the opposite. Here the patient's leg is pulled upwards

[n] William Baker (1839–1896), surgeon at St Bartholomew's Hospital, London, described this in 1877.

[o] Alan Apley, orthopaedic surgeon, St Thomas's Hospital, London.

so as to take the strain off the menisci and stretch the ligaments. If the patient finds the test painful, a ligamentous abnormality may be the cause.

McMurray's[p] test (Figure 8.29) is another way of detecting a meniscal tear. The patient lies on the back, the examiner stands on the opposite side to be tested and holds the ankle. The examiner's other hand sits on the medial side of the knee and pushes to apply valgus force. The patient's leg is then extended from the flexed position while being internally and then externally rotated. The test is positive if there is a popping sensation, which may be followed by inability to extend the knee. The likelihood ratios of both these tests are not high. McMurray's has a positive LR of 1.3 and a negative LR of 0.8 for meniscal tear.[8]

Stand the patient up. Look particularly for varus (bow-leg) and valgus (knock-knee) deformity.

Finish with a test of function. Get the patient to walk to and fro. Study the gait and the movement of the knees, particularly for a sideways wobble.

The ankles and feet

History. The usual symptom is pain. If this is present only when the patient wears shoes, the shoes rather than the feet may be the problem. There may be a specific area that is painful and the patient should be asked to point to this. Very severe pain involving the first metatarsophalangeal joint is usually due to gout. Pain right over one of the metatarsals that comes on after unusually vigorous exercise may be due to a stress fracture. *Metatarsalgia* is a non-localised ache that spreads across the forefoot. It can occur in normal feet after prolonged standing but also occurs in a number of other foot conditions.

There may be deformity involving the ankle or toes. Patients find this especially troublesome if it makes it difficult to put on shoes. The patient may have noticed swelling; ask if this is painful or not and whether it involves one or both feet. Bilateral swelling is more likely due to inflammation. Swelling over the medial aspect of the first metatarsal head (a bunion) occurs commonly as people get older, but may be associated with rheumatoid arthritis.

Paraesthesiae in the feet may have been noticed. Try to find out the distribution of the abnormal sensation which may be a result of peripheral nerve injury or peripheral neuropathy. Coldness of the feet is very common but cyanosis and ulceration are more worrying problems. Chronic foot ulcers mean diabetes must be excluded.

Figure 8.29 McMurray's test of the knee

Figure 8.30 Sausage-shaped first and second toes in psoriatic arthritis

Examination. This examination includes the ankles, feet and toes.

Look at the skin. Note any swelling, scars, deformity or muscle wasting. Deformities affecting the forefoot include hallux valgus (fixed lateral deviation of the main axis of the big toe), clawing (fixed flexion deformity) and crowding of the toes, as occurs in rheumatoid arthritis. Sausage deformities of the toes occur with psoriatic arthropathy, ankylosing spondylitis and Reiter's[q] disease (Figure 8.30). Look for the nail changes that suggest psoriasis. Inspect the transverse arch of the foot, which runs underneath the metatarsophalangeal joints, and the longitudinal arch, which runs from the first metatarsophalangeal joint to the heel. These arches, which bear the weight of the body, may be flattened in arthritic conditions of the foot like rheumatoid arthritis. Calluses over the metatarsal

[p] Thomas McMurray (1888-1949), the first professor of orthopaedic surgery in Liverpool.

[q] Hans Reiter (1881–1969), Professor of Hygiene in Berlin, described the syndrome in 1916.

Figure 8.31 Rheumatoid feet showing bilateral hallux valgus and calluses over the metatarsal heads

Figure 8.32 Rheumatoid nodule of the Achilles tendon

heads on the plantar surface of the foot occur with subluxation of these joints (Figure 8.31).

Feel, starting with the ankle, for swelling around the lateral and medial malleoli. This should not be confused with pitting oedema (page 57). *Move* the *talar (ankle) joint*, grasping the midfoot with one hand. *Dorsiflexion* is tested by raising the foot towards the knee—normally possible to 20 degrees—and *plantar flexion* by performing the opposite manoeuvre, which is normally possible to 50 degrees.

With the subtalar joint, only *inversion* and *eversion* of the foot on the ankle are tested. Tenderness on movement is more important than range at this joint. The midtarsal (midfoot) joint allows rotation of the forefoot when the hindfoot is fixed. This is done by steadying the ankle with one hand and rotating (twisting) the forefoot. Again, tenderness rather than range of movement is noted.

Squeeze the *metatarsophalangeal joints* by compressing the first and fifth metatarsals between your thumb and forefinger. Tenderness suggests inflammation, common in early rheumatoid arthritis. Press upwards from the sole of the foot just proximal to the proximal metatarsophalangeal joints of the third and fourth toes. Pain here suggests *Morton's*[r] metatarsalgia. This is due to entrapment and swelling of the digital nerve between the toes. It is associated with pain and numbness of the sides of these toes.

Each *individual interphalangeal joint* is then assessed by feeling and moving. These are typically affected in the seronegative spondyloarthropathies. Extremely tender involvement of the first metatarso-

phalangeal joint is characteristic of acute gout. In this case the joint also looks red and swollen.

Palpate the *Achilles tendon* for rheumatoid nodules (Figure 8.32) and tenderness due to Achilles tendonitis. An old Achilles tendon rupture may be detected by squeezing the calf: normally the foot plantar flexes unless the tendon has previously ruptured (Simmond's[s] test). Also palpate the inferior aspect of the *heel* for tenderness; this may indicate plantar fasciitis, which occurs in the seronegative spondyloarthropathies and sometimes for no apparent reason.

Correlation of physical signs and rheumatological disease

Rheumatoid arthritis

(Figures 8.20 and 8.33)

This is a chronic systemic inflammatory disease of unknown aetiology which characteristically involves the joints. In the majority of cases, patients with rheumatoid arthritis have rheumatoid factor

---

[r] Thomas Morton (1835–1903), general and eye surgeon, Philadelphia Hospital, performed one of the first appendicectomies.

[s] Franklin Simmonds, orthopaedic surgeon, Rowley Bristow Hospital, Surrey, UK; he is now retired.

1. **General inspection**
   Cushingoid appearance
   Weight

2. **Hands**

3. **Arms**
   Entrapment neuropathy (e.g. carpal tunnel)
   Subcutaneous nodules
   Elbow joint
   Shoulder joint
   Axillary nodes

4. **Face**
   Eyes—dry eyes (Sjögren's), scleritis, episcleritis,
      scleromalacia perforans, anaemia, cataracts
      (steroids, chloroquine)
   Fundi—hyperviscosity
   Face—parotids (Sjögren's)
   Mouth—dryness, ulcers, dental caries
   Temporomandibular joint (crepitus)

5. **Neck**
   Cervical spine
   Cervical nodes

6. **Chest**
   Heart—pericarditis, valve lesions
   Lungs—effusion, fibrosis, infarction, infection,
      nodules (and Caplan's syndrome)

7. **Abdomen**
   Splenomegaly (e.g. Felty's syndrome)
   Inguinal nodes

8. **Hips**

9. **Knees**

10. **Lower limbs**
    Ulceration (vasculitis)
    Calf swelling (ruptured synovial cyst)
    Peripheral neuropathy
    Mononeuritis multiplex
    Cord compression

11. **Feet**

12. **Other**
    Urine: protein, blood (drugs, vasculitis, amyloidosis)
    Rectal examination (blood)

Figure 8.33 Rheumatoid arthritis

present in the serum (seropositive disease). These are heterogeneous antibodies directed against the Fc portion of altered immunoglobulin (IgG), but are not specific for rheumatoid arthritis.

To examine the patient with suspected rheumatoid arthritis sit him or her up in bed or on a chair.

General inspection

Look to see whether the patient has a Cushingoid appearance due to steroid treatment (page 267), or whether there are signs of weight loss that may indicate active disease.

The hands

Put the hands on a pillow. Look especially for symmetrical small joint polyarthritis (the distal interphalangeal joints are usually spared). The other common abnormalities are ulnar deviation, volar subluxation of the metacarpophalangeal joints, and Z deformity of the thumb with swan neck and boutonnière deformity of the fingers. Examine the fingernails for vasculitic changes and look for wasting of the small muscles of the hand. Look at the palms for palmar erythema. Feel the palms for palmar tendon crepitus while the patient extends and flexes the fingers. Look for signs of an ulnar nerve palsy (from ulnar nerve entrapment at the elbow) and a median nerve palsy (carpal tunnel).

The wrists

Look for synovial thickening and perform Phalen's sign (carpal tunnel).

Figure 8.34 Nodular scleritis involving the sclera lateral to the iris

The elbows

Look around the elbows for rheumatoid nodules, which suggest seropositive disease, and examine the elbow joint. Flexion contractures are common.

The shoulders and axillae

Here look for tenderness and limitation of movement. Also palpate the axillary nodes because enlarged nodes may indicate active disease of joints in the area that they drain.

The eyes

Look at the eyes for redness and dryness (Sjögren's syndrome) (Table 8.7), which occurs in 10% to 15% of cases. Note also scleritis (an elevated white or purple-red lesion, which is pathologically a rheumatoid nodule and usually appears surrounded by the intense redness of the injected sclera) (Figure 8.34). These nodules occur especially in the superior parts of the sclera and are often bilateral, but affect only 1% of patients. Iritis does *not* occur.

With severe scleritis, scleral thinning may occur, exposing the underlying choroid. This is called scleromalacia. Look for cataracts due to steroid treatment. Conjunctival pallor may be present, indicating anaemia due to iron deficiency. This can be a result of blood loss from non-steroidal anti-inflammatory drug use, folate deficiency from a poor diet, hypersplenism or chronic inflammation, or some combination of these.

The parotids

Look for enlargement of the parotid glands, as occurs with Sjögren's syndrome.

The mouth

Look for dryness of the mouth and dental caries (Sjögren's syndrome), and ulcers related to drug treatment (e.g. gold).

The temporomandibular joints

Feel the temporomandibular joints for crepitus as the patient opens and shuts the mouth.

The neck

Go on to examine the cervical spine for tenderness, muscle spasm and reduction of rotational movement. Examine for cervical lymphadenopathy.

The chest

Now examine the lungs for signs of pleural effusions or pulmonary fibrosis. Caplan's syndrome[t] is the presence of rheumatoid lung nodules in combination with pneumoconiosis.

The heart

Listen to the heart for a pericardial rub (relatively common) and for murmurs indicating valvular regurgitation (especially the aortic valve), which may occur due to nodular involvement of a heart valve.

The abdomen

Feel the abdomen for splenomegaly (this occurs in up to 10% of patients and suggests the possibility of Felty's syndrome (page 202)) and hepatomegaly (e.g. drug induced by methotrexate). Feel the inguinal lymph nodes.

The lower limbs

Examine the hips for limitation of joint movement, although this occurs only uncommonly. The knees, however, are more often affected and here one must note any quadriceps wasting, synovial effusions and flexion contractures. Valgus deformity and ligamentous instability may occur as late complications. Look in the popliteal fossae for Baker's cysts. Go on to look at the lower parts of the legs for ulceration; this can occur as a vasculitic complication of Felty's syndrome. Examine for a stocking distribution peripheral neuropathy and for mononeuritis multiplex of the nerves of the lower limbs. There may also be signs of spinal cord compression due to anterior dislocation of the first cervical vertebra or vertical subluxation of the odontoid process.

[t] Anthony Caplan, Welsh physician, described this in 1953.

The ankles and feet (Figures 8.31, 8.32)

Now look for foot drop (peroneal nerve entrapment or vasculitis) and examine the ankle joint for limitation of movement. Look at the metatarsophalangeal joints for swelling and subluxation. There may also be lateral deviation and clawing of the toes. Remember that the interphalangeal joints are very rarely involved. Finally, feel the Achilles tendon for nodules—a sign of seropositive disease.

Seronegative spondyloarthropathies

Four conditions are generally accepted as belonging to this group: ankylosing spondylitis, psoriatic arthritis, Reiter's disease and enteropathic arthritis. These are called the seronegative spondyloarthropathies because they were originally distinguished from rheumatoid arthritis by the absence of rheumatoid factor in the serum. However, up to 30% of patients with otherwise classical rheumatoid arthritis are rheumatoid factor negative. The seronegative spondyloarthropathies overlap clinically and pathologically, and have an association with HLA-B27.

Ankylosing spondylitis

The following areas should be examined.

The back and sacroiliac joints: may show loss of lumbar lordosis and thoracic kyphosis; severe flexion deformity of the lumbar spine (rare); tenderness of the lumbar vertebrae; reduction of movement of the lumbar spine in all directions; and tenderness of the sacroiliac joints.

The legs: Achilles tendonitis; plantar fasciitis; signs of cauda equina compression (rare)—lower limb weakness, loss of sphincter control, saddle sensory loss.

The lungs: decreased chest expansion (less than 5 cm); signs of apical fibrosis.

The heart: signs of aortic regurgitation.

The eyes: acute iritis (tends to recur)—painful red eye (10%–15%) (Figure 8.35).

Rectal and stool examination: signs of inflammatory bowel disease (either ulcerative colitis or Crohn's disease). *Note:* Signs of secondary amyloidosis—for example, hepatosplenomegaly, renal enlargement, proteinuria—may be present, although this is a very rare complication.

Reiter's syndrome

Classically this disease follows urethritis or diarrhoea, with conjunctivitis and arthritis (usually asymmetrical) of the large weightbearing joints such

Figure 8.35 Iritis of the right eye

Figure 8.36 Circinate balanitis

as the hip, knee or ankle. The following areas should be examined.

The genital region: urethral discharge; circinate balanitis—scaly, superficial reddened erosions with well-demarcated borders on the glans penis (Figure 8.36).

The prostate: prostatitis.

The eyes: conjunctivitis; iritis (rare).

The mouth: painless ulcers.

The back: sacroiliac joints (may be unilaterally involved).

The lower limbs (more commonly affected): knees, ankles; metatarsophalangeal joints; plantar fasciitis, Achilles tendonitis; keratoderma blennorrhagica on the sole (non-tender reddish-brown macules, which become scaling papules: Figure 8.37)—this is indistinguishable from pustular psoriasis; nails thickened, opaque and brittle.

The hands (less commonly involved): wrists; metacarpophalangeal joints, proximal interphalangeal joints, distal interphalangeal joints; keratoderma blennorrhagica on the palms; nail changes.

Cardiovascular system: aortic regurgitation (rare).

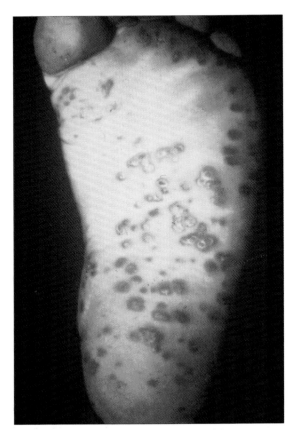

Figure 8.37 Reiter's syndrome with keratoderma blennorrhagica

(From FS McDonald, ed., *Mayo Clinic images in internal medicine*, with permission. © Mayo Clinic Scientific Press and CRC Press.)

Figure 8.38 Gouty tophi of the fingers

Figure 8.39 Gouty tophus of the ear

Psoriatic arthritis

Five per cent of patients with psoriasis (page 390) have arthritis.

Examine as for rheumatoid arthritis, but include the sacroiliac joints. There are five distinct groups of psoriatic arthritis.

1 Monoarticular and oligoarticular arthritis of the hands and feet (note sausage-shaped digits in Figure 8.30). Most psoriatic arthritis is of this type.
2 Similar to rheumatoid arthritis (but seronegative).
3 Distal interphalangeal joint involvement with psoriatic nail changes (Figure 8.4).
4 Arthritis mutilans (destructive polyarthritis).
5 Sacroiliitis with or without peripheral joint involvement.

Enteropathic arthritis

There are two patterns of involvement of the joints with ulcerative colitis and Crohn's disease.

1 **Peripheral joint disease.** This is an asymmetrical oligoarthropathy, usually affecting the lower limbs, especially the knees and ankles. It rarely causes deformity.
2 **Sacroiliitis.** This is indistinguishable clinically from ankylosing spondylitis.

Gouty arthritis

Begin with the feet, as acute gouty arthritis affects the metatarsophalangeal joint of the great toe in 75% of cases. Next examine the ankles and knees, which tend to be involved after recurrent attacks. The fingers, wrists and elbows are affected late (Figure 8.38). Palpate for gouty tophi (these are

1. General inspection
Cushingoid
Weight
Mental state
2. Hands
Vasculitis
Rash
Arthropathy
3. Arms
Livedo reticularis
Purpura
Proximal myopathy (active disease or steroids)

4. Head
Alopecia, lupus hairs
Eyes—scleritis, cytoid lesions etc
Mouth—ulcers, infection
Rash—butterfly
Cranial nerve lesions
Cervical adenopathy
5. Chest
Cardiovascular system—pericarditis
Respiratory system—pleural effusion, pleurisy,
pulmonary fibrosis, collapse or infection
6. Abdomen
Hepatosplenomegaly
Tenderness
7. Hips
Aseptic necrosis
8. Legs
Feet—red soles, small joint synovitis
Rash
Ulcers over the malleoli e.g. antiphospholipid
syndrome
Proximal myopathy
Neuropathy
Mononeuritis multiplex
Cerebellar ataxia
Hemiplegia
9. Other
Urine analysis (proteinuria)
Blood pressure (hypertension)
Temperature chart

Figure 8.40 Systemic lupus erythematosus

urate deposits with inflammatory cells surrounding them) (Latin *tophus,* 'chalk stone'). The presence of tophi indicates chronic recurrent gout. They tend to occur over the joint synovia, the olecranon bursa, the extensor surface of the forearm, the helix of the ear (Figure 8.39), and in the infrapatellar and Achilles tendons.

Finally, examine for signs of the causes of secondary gout: increased purine turnover due to myeloproliferative disease (page 209), lymphoma (page 210) or leukaemia; and decreased renal urate excretion due to renal disease or hypothyroidism. Hypertension, diabetes mellitus and ischaemic heart disease are more common among sufferers of gout.

Calcium pyrophosphate arthropathy (pseudogout)

This may present a similar picture to that described above for true gout, but usually large joints (especially the knees) are involved. In a minority of patients there will be signs of hyperparathyroidism (page 271), haemochromatosis or true gout.

Calcium hydroxyapatite arthropathy

This causes large joint arthritis (especially knee and shoulder) and is more common in elderly patients.

Systemic lupus erythematosus (SLE)

This is a multisystemic chronic inflammatory disease of unknown origin, named because the erosive nature of the condition was likened to the damage caused by a hungry wolf (Latin *lupus*[u] 'wolf') (Figure 8.40).

---

[u] Lupus has been used as a name for any erosive disease of the skin; for example, lupus vulgaris is tuberculosis of the skin.

General inspection

Look for weight loss (due to chronic inflammation) or a Cushingoid appearance (steroid treatment). While taking the history note any abnormal mental state—psychosis may occur due to the lupus itself or to steroid therapy.

Hands

Note any vasculitis around the nail bed, particularly telangiectasia and erythema of the skin of the nail base. A rash may occur—photosensitivity is common.

Raynaud's phenomenon may occur if the examiner is lucky and the weather cold (Table 8.6). Characteristically the affected fingers become white, then cyanosed and finally become red and tender due to reactive hyperaemia (i.e. white–blue–red).

Examine for arthropathy: synovitis of the proximal and metacarpophalangeal joints, which is not destructive (non-erosive), may occur in SLE.

Forearms

Livedo reticularis may occur here; in Latin this describes skin discoloration in the form of a small net. This is formed by connected bluish-purple streaks without discrete borders. They occur usually on the limbs and are associated with various connective tissue diseases.[10] Look for purpura (due to vasculitis[11] or autoimmune thrombocytopenia). Examine for a proximal myopathy (due to the disease itself or to steroid treatment). Subcutaneous nodules very rarely occur in SLE. The axillary nodes may be enlarged but will not be tender.

The head and neck

Alopecia (hair loss) is an important diagnostic clue that occurs in about two-thirds of patients. Look especially for lupus hairs, which are short, broken hairs above the forehead. The hair as a whole may be coarse and dry as in hypothyroidism.

Examine the eyes for scleritis and episcleritis (see Figure 8.34). The eyes may be red and dry (Sjögren's syndrome). Pallor of the conjunctivae occurs with anaemia, usually due to chronic disease. Occasionally jaundice due to autoimmune haemolytic anaemia may be found. Perform a fundoscopy for cytoid bodies, which are hard exudates (white spots) due to aggregates of swollen nerve fibres and are secondary to vasculitis.

A facial rash may be diagnostic (Figure 8.41). The classical rash is an erythematous 'butterfly rash' over the cheeks and bridge of the nose. Mouth ulcers on the soft or hard palate may occur and the mouth may be dry (Sjögren's syndrome).

Discoid lupus may be found in the same area or affect different parts of the body. Lesions begin as

Figure 8.41 Butterfly rash of systemic lupus erythematosus

spreading red plaques which have a central area of hyperkeratosis and follicular plugging. An active lesion has an oedematous edge. The appearance may suggest psoriasis. A healed lesion may have marginal hyperpigmentation with central atrophy and depigmentation. The scalp, external ear and face are most commonly affected, but in some patients lesions may occur all over the arms and chest.

After examining the face, feel for cervical lymphadenopathy, which is usually non-tender.

The chest

Signs of a pericardial rub (from pericarditis) may be found. In the respiratory examination a pleural rub (pleuritis), a pleural effusion, pulmonary fibrosis, pulmonary collapse or pulmonary hypertension may be detected. Chest disease is probably most often secondary to an interstitial pneumonitis rather than to vasculitis of the lungs.

The abdomen

Splenomegaly, usually mild, can be detected in 10% of cases. Hepatomegaly (mild) may occur in uncomplicated cases. Chronic liver disease due to chronic hepatitis ('lupoid hepatitis') is a separate disease rather than a variant of SLE.

The hips

Examine the hip joint movements: in aseptic (avascular) necrosis there is tenderness on movement, with preservation of hip extension but loss of the other movements. This is due to ischaemia of the femoral head and may be related to steroid use or to the SLE itself.

The legs

Examine for proximal myopathy and peripheral neuropathy (mainly sensory) (page 348).

Rarely there may be signs of hemiplegia, cerebellar ataxia or chorea.

Leg ulceration over the malleoli, due to vasculitis or the antiphospholipid syndrome,[10] is important. Very occasionally the toes may be gangrenous. There may be ankle oedema from the nephrotic syndrome or fluid retention from steroids.

Urine and blood pressure

Perform a urine analysis (for proteinuria and haematuria) and take the blood pressure (for hypertension). Renal disease is a common complication of SLE.

Temperature

Take the temperature, as fever is common in SLE, either from secondary infection or from the disease per se.

Scleroderma (progressive systemic sclerosis)

This is a disorder of connective tissue with prominent cutaneous fibrosis. There may be occlusion of the microvasculature of the fingers, gut, lungs, heart and kidneys. The CREST syndrome (calcinosis, Raynaud's phenomenon, oesophageal motility disturbance, sclerodactyly and telangiectasia) is a more localised form of scleroderma with a better prognosis.

General inspection (Figure 8.42)

Look for cachexia due to dysphagia (from an oesophageal motility disturbance) or malabsorption (due to bacterial overgrowth).

1. **General appearance**
   'Bird-like' facies
   Weight-loss (malabsorption)

2. **Hands**
   CRST—calcinosis, atrophy distal tissue pulp (Raynaud's), sclerodactyly, telangiectasia
   Dilated capillary loops (nailfolds)
   Small joint arthropathy and tendon crepitus
   Fixed flexion deformity
   Hand function

3. **Arms**
   Oedema (early), or skin thickening and tightening
   Pigmentation
   Vitiligo
   Hair loss
   Proximal myopathy

4. **Head**
   Alopecia
   Eyes—loss of eyebrows, anaemia, difficulty with closing
   Mouth—puckered, difficulty with opening
   Pigmentation

   Telangiectasia
   Neck muscles—wasting and weakness

5. **Dysphagia**

6. **Chest**
   Tight skin ('Roman breastplate')
   Heart—cor pulmonale, pericarditis, failure
   Lungs—fibrosis, reflux pneumonitis, chest infections

7. **Legs**
   Skin lesions
   Vasculitis

8. **Other**
   Blood pressure (hypertension with renal involvement)
   Urine analysis (proteinuria)
   Temperature chart (infection)
   Stool examination (steatorrhoea)

Figure 8.42 Scleroderma

Skin changes in scleroderma vary. There may be an early oedematous phase with non-tender pitting oedema of the hands which appear tightly swollen. In patients with progressive disease the oedematous skin is replaced by indurated skin which appears thickened, hard and tight. This phase usually begins in the fingers (Table 8.11).

The hands

Examine the hands. Note particularly *calcinosis* (palpable nodules due to calcific deposits in the subcutaneous tissue of the fingers), *Raynaud's phenomenon* sometimes causing atrophy of the finger pulps (due to ischaemia) (Figure 8.43), *sclerodactyly* (tightening of the skin of the fingers leading to tapering), and multiple large *telangiectasia* on the fingers (Figure 8.44).

Look for *contraction deformity of the fingers*, which is relatively common (Figure 8.45), and for synovitis, although this is uncommon. The nails can be affected by Raynaud's (page 217). It can be

Figure 8.43 Digital infarcts

Figure 8.44 Telangiectasia of the hands in the CREST syndrome

---

Table 8.11 Differential diagnosis of thickened tethered skin

CREST syndrome
Systemic sclerosis (scleroderma)
Mixed connective tissue disease (an overlap syndrome including features of systemic sclerosis, systemic lupus erythematosus and polymyositis)
Eosinophilic fasciitis—widespread skin thickening due to inflammation of the fascia often following excessive muscle exercise; occurs in association with eosinophilia and hypergammaglobulinaemia
Localised morphea—heterogeneous group of disorders where there are small areas of sclerosis: most common type is morphea, which begins with large plaques of red or purple skin that evolve into sclerotic areas and may regress spontaneously over years
Chemically induced: vinyl chloride, pentazocine, bleomycin
Pseudoscleroderma: porphyria cutanea tarda, acromegaly, carcinoid syndrome
Scleroedema: thickened skin over the shoulders and upper back in diabetes mellitus
Graft versus host disease
Silicosis
Eosinophilic myalgia syndrome (L-tryptophan)
Toxic oil syndrome

---

useful to inspect the nailfolds using a hand-held magnifying glass: in scleroderma you may see dilated capillary loops but this is not diagnostic. These are best viewed on the fourth digit. Assessing hand function is important in this disease.

The arms

Determine the extent of skin tethering in the arms. If the skin thickening extends above the wrists to the arms, legs or trunk, the diagnosis is *diffuse scleroderma* rather than *CREST*. If the skin thickening extends only to the elbows and face this is called *limited scleroderma*. Assess for proximal myopathy due to myositis.

The face

The skin of the face is involved in progressive disease. There is loss of normal wrinkles and skinfolds as well as of the eyebrows. The face appears pinched and expressionless ('bird-like' facies). Inspect for malar telangiectasia and look for salt-and-pepper pigmentation. Ask the patient to close the eyes—skin

Figure 8.45 Systemic sclerosis: signs in the hands

Sclerodactyly, tethered smooth skin, calcinosis and ulceration, atrophy of finger pulps due to Raynaud's phenomenon, and fixed flexion deformities of the fingers.

tethering may make this incomplete. The eyes may be dry (Sjögren's syndrome), though this is uncommon, and the conjunctivae pale (there are a number of reasons for anaemia, including the presence of chronic disease, bleeding from oesophagitis, and microangiopathic haemolytic anaemia).

Ask the patient to open the mouth fully. It may appear puckered and narrow. Inability to open the mouth so that there is more than 3 cm of clearance between the incisors indicates abnormal restriction.

The chest

Inspect the skin of the chest wall, which may have acquired a tight, thickened appearance, like ancient Roman breastplate armour.

Examine the lungs for pulmonary fibrosis, evidence of reflux pneumonitis, or (rarely) a pleural effusion or alveolar cell carcinoma.

Examine the heart for cor pulmonale secondary to pulmonary fibrosis or for pericarditis. Left ventricular failure may also occur due to myocardial involvement.

The legs

Look for signs of vasculitis, ulceration and skin involvement. Peripheral neuropathy is rare.

Urinalysis and blood pressure

These are very important because renal involvement is common in scleroderma and is often associated with severe hypertension. Renal disease is one of the most common causes of death.

The stool

Look for evidence of steatorrhoea (due to malabsorption from bacterial overgrowth). A summary of the physical signs that can be found in scleroderma is presented in Figure 8.42.

Rheumatic fever

This is an inflammatory disease which is a delayed sequel to infection with group A beta-haemolytic *Streptococcus*. It is uncommon in Western nations today. It is diagnosed by finding two major or one major and two minor criteria, plus evidence of recent streptococcal infection.

Major criteria: (i) carditis (causing tachycardia, murmurs, cardiac failure, pericarditis); (ii) polyarthritis; (iii) chorea (page 362); (iv) erythema marginatum (see below); (v) subcutaneous nodules (painless mobile swellings).

Minor criteria: (i) fever; (ii) arthralgia; (iii) previous rheumatic fever; (iv) acute phase proteins; (v) prolonged PR interval on the electrocardiogram.

Examining the patient with suspected rheumatic fever

First examine the large joints of the limbs for effusions and synovitis. Two or more joints must be involved (classically there is a transient migratory polyarthritis). Feel for subcutaneous nodules over bony prominences. Look for a rash. Erythema marginatum is a slightly raised pink or red rash that blanches with pressure. The red rings have a clear centre and round margins, and occur on the trunk and proximal limbs; the rash is not found on the face. Look for choreiform movements. Their onset is usually delayed until about 3 months after the throat infection.

Now examine the cardiovascular system for any signs of pancarditis: (i) a pericardial rub due to

Table 8.12 The vasculitides

Clinical syndrome	Major vessels inflamed or involved	Important clinical features*
1 Hypersensitivity vasculitis Causes: • Connective tissue diseases—e.g. rheumatoid arthritis, SLE • Infection—e.g. hepatitis B • Drugs—(the Ps) e.g. penicillin, phenothiazines, phenylbutazone propylthiouracil (and many others) • Haematological diseases —e.g. essential cryoglobulinaemia, paraproteinaemia • Idiopathic	Capillaries and venules (leucocytoclastic vasculitis)	Very variable: • Urticaria • Palpable purpura, livedo reticularis • Henoch-Schönlein purpura • Digital infarcts • Features of underlying disease
2 Allergic granulomatosis (NB: Blood eosinophilia common) Cause: unknown	Small arteries and veins	• Signs of asthma, eosinophilia • Similar to PAN (see below)
3 Wegener's† granulomatosis Cause: unknown	Arteries, capillaries and venules	• Upper respiratory tract: sinusitis, saddle nose deformity • Lungs: pneumonitis • Renal: hypertension, signs of renal failure, haematuria • Eyes: conjunctivitis, uveitis • Skin: similar to hypersensitivity vasculitis
4 Polyarteritis nodosa (PAN) Cause: unknown Associated with hepatitis B (20%)	Medium and small arteries (fibrinoid necrosis)	• Digital gangrene, ulceration • Renal: hypertension, signs of renal failure, haematuria • GIT: haematemesis, melaena • Lung: signs of pneumonitis, effusion • CNS: mononeuritis multiplex, retinal vasculitis • Skin: similar to hypersensitivity vasculitis

GIT = gastrointestinal tract. SLE = systemic lupus erythematosus. PAN = polyarteritis nodosa. CNS = central nervous system.
* Common general findings include fatigue, fever, weight loss, anaemia and hypoalbuminaemia.
† Friedrich Wegener, German pathologist.

Table 8.12 The vasculitides (continued)

Clinical syndrome	Major vessels inflamed or involved	Important clinical features*
5 Behçet's syndrome Cause: unknown	Medium to small arteries and veins	• Oral and genital ulcers • Eyes: uveitis • Asymmetrical large joint polyarthropathy • Thrombophlebitis • Rash • CNS: cranial or spinal cord lesions
6 Giant cell arteritis (NB: Polymyalgia rheumatica, a related disease) Cause: unknown	Large and medium arteries	• Tender extracranial arteries particularly the temporal • Visual disturbance, sudden blindness • Jaw claudication
7 Aortic arch (Takayasu's)‡ arteritis Cause: unknown	Aorta and its branches	• Hypertension • Loss of upper limb pulses Signs have been termed 'reverse coarctation'

GIT = gastrointestinal tract. SLE = systemic lupus erythematosus. PAN = polyarteritis nodosa. CNS = central nervous system.
‡ Mikito Takayasu (1860–1938), Japanese Professor of Ophthalmology

pericarditis; (ii) congestive cardiac failure due to myocarditis; (iii) mitral or aortic regurgitation due to acute endocarditis.

Finally, take the temperature.

The vasculitides

This is a heterogeneous group of disorders characterised by inflammation and damage to blood vessels.[11] The clinical features and major vessels involved are shown in Table 8.12.

Soft tissue rheumatism

This includes a number of common, painful conditions that arise in soft tissue, often around a joint. The problem may be general—for example, fibromyalgia; or restricted to a single anatomical region—for example, tendon, tenosynovium, enthesis or bursa. There are a large number of these conditions; the more common ones are described here.

Fibromyalgia syndrome

This syndrome is a common, frequently overlooked condition that mostly affects women in their 40s and 50s. It presents with a variable group of symptoms including widespread musculoskeletal aches and pains, and severe and easy fatiguability. The musculoskeletal pain is mostly axial (neck and back) and diffuse. It is made worse by stress or cold. Pain may be felt 'all over' and is unresponsive to anti-inflammatory drug treatment. The combination of pain and fatigue may cause the patient severe disability. There is usually a poor sleep pattern. The patient wakes up not feeling refreshed, and more tired in the morning than later in the day. Note that no abnormal pathology has been found in the joints, muscles or tendons of these patients.

Examination. Look for the characteristic multiple hyperalgesic tender points (Figure 8.46). These areas are tender to finger pressure in normal people but in affected patients there is marked tenderness and a definite withdrawal response. This response should be obtained in at least 10 sites in the upper and lower limbs and on both sides (i.e. it is widespread and symmetrical). Next examine for hyperalgesia at control sites such as the forehead or distal forearm, where it should be absent.

The diagnosis is based on the presence of typical symptoms and multiple hyperalgesic tender sites (with negative control sites). Inflammatory and endocrine disease must be excluded.

Shoulder syndromes

Soft tissue disorders of the shoulder are common and have certain particular clinical features.

Rotator cuff syndrome

Supraspinatus tendonitis is the commonest form of rotator cuff syndrome. It is associated with degeneration and subsequent inflammation in the supraspinatus tendon as it is compressed between the acromion and humeral head when the arm is raised. It mostly affects 40–50-year-olds. Symptoms may begin following unaccustomed physical activities such as gardening.

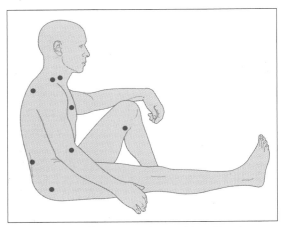

Figure 8.46 Frequent sites of localised tenderness in the fibromyalgia syndrome

Examination. Examine the shoulder joint. Note pain on abduction of the arm (Figure 8.47), with a painful arc of movement between 60 and 120 degrees of abduction. Involvement of other rotator cuff tendons causes similar painful movement.

Frozen shoulder

Capsulitis of the shoulder, or frozen shoulder, is associated with limitation of active and passive arm movements in all directions. It may follow immobilisation of the arm after a stroke. There is typically a sudden onset of shoulder pain, which is worse at night and radiates to the base of the neck and down the arm. Pain is made worse by shoulder movement and may be bilateral. Pain and stiffness usually subside over a period of months. Complete movement may not be regained.

Examination. Examine the shoulders. There is global restriction of movement of the shoulder—that is, it is frozen.

Elbow epicondylitis (tennis and golfer's elbow)

Many contact and non-contact sports can cause physical injury, although serious injuries are rather uncommon with certain sports (e.g. synchronised swimming). There may be pain over the epicondyles of the elbow. The *lateral epicondyle* is the most often affected and is called 'tennis elbow'. Pain arises from the site of insertion of the extensor muscle tendons into the lateral epicondyle (enthesis). Involvement of the medial epicondyle at the site of insertion of the flexor tendons of the forearm causes medial

Figure 8.47 Inflammation of the rotator cuff tendons may cause a 'painful arc' during abduction of the arm

The initial movement (a) is painless but the next 90 degrees of movement (b) causes pain. When the arm reaches full abduction (c) the pain eases as the pressure is taken off the rotator cuff apparatus.

Figure 8.48 Examination of the elbow

Looking for signs of lateral epicondylitis. Palpation over the forearm extensor muscle origin elicits pain. Straining the muscles by resisted extension of the wrist exacerbates the symptoms.

Figure 8.50 Testing for lateral epicondylitis

Figure 8.49 Examination to elicit signs of medial epicondylitis

Local pressure over the medial epicondyle elicits pain. Symptoms are exacerbated by resisted flexion of the wrist and fingers.

epicondylitis—'golfer's elbow'. These conditions are also common in manual workers such as painters.

Examination. Examine for local tenderness over the lateral (Figure 8.48) or medial epicondyle (Figure 8.49). Ask the patient to extend the fingers against resistance (Figure 8.50). This will make the pain of lateral epicondylitis worse. Ask the patient to flex the fingers against resistance. This will exacerbate the pain of medial epicondylitis.

Tenosynovitis of the wrist

Inflammation of the synovial tubes in which tendons run can occur in patients with rheumatoid arthritis but also in otherwise healthy people. The cause is often unaccustomed repetitive movement. A common site for tenosynovitis is at the wrist, where it involves the long extensor and abductor tendons of the thumb (De Quervain's tenosynovitis) (Figure 8.51).

Examination. This reveals tenderness and swelling on the radial side of the wrist (radial styloid). There is pain on active or passive movement of the thumb. Confirm the diagnosis by performing Finkelstein's test.[v] Hold the patient's hand with the thumb tucked into the palm and then quickly turn the wrist into full ulnar deviation (Figure 8.52). An alternative approach that is reported to produce fewer false positives involves gripping the patient's thumb rather than tucking the thumb into the palm.[12] Sharp pain will occur in the tendon sheath when the test is positive. Examine also the other common sites of tendon involvement—the flexor tendons of the fingers and the Achilles tendon.

Bursitis

Bursae are found in areas exposed to mechanical strain or trauma, either at the site where muscle or tendon glides over bone or muscle, or superficially where bony prominences are exposed to mechanical stress. Bursitis usually occurs as a local soft-tissue inflammatory reaction to unusual mechanical pressure. It may be associated with rheumatoid arthritis, gout or sepsis. Common sites include the prepatellar area (housemaid's knee) (Figure 8.53), over the olecranon (olecranon bursitis) and over the greater trochanter (trochanteric bursitis).

[v] Harry Finkelstein (1865–1939), surgeon, Hospital for Joint Diseases, New York.

Figure 8.51 A patient with de Quervain's tenosynovitis

There is characteristic swelling of the tendon sheath of the abductor pollicis brevis over the styloid process of the radius.

Figure 8.52 Finkelstein's test

Nerve entrapment syndromes

These are caused by compression of peripheral nerves at vulnerable sites and are associated with pain, paraesthesiae and numbness in a particular nerve distribution.

Carpal tunnel syndrome

Compression of the median nerve at the wrist is the most frequent form. This seems hardly surprising when one remembers that the carpal tunnel, sandwiched between the carpal bones and the carpal ligament, contains 9 flexor tendons as well as the median nerve. These patients complain of numbness and paraesthesiae in the median nerve distribution (the 3 median fingers and the medial side of the ring finger. Symptoms often wake patients from sleep and may radiate up the forearm ($^1/_3$ of cases). The commonest cause is an overuse tenosynovitis of the flexor tendon sheaths at the wrist. Fluid retention during pregnancy or from use of the oral contraceptive pill can also produce carpal tunnel symptoms. In addition, median nerve compression can occur in rheumatoid arthritis, hypothyroidism, acromegaly and amyloidosis.

Examination. Symptoms can be reproduced by gentle percussion over the carpal tunnel while the wrist is held in extension (Tinel's sign). This sign is negative in up to 30% of patients with electrophysiologically proven median nerve compression. Prolonged (60 seconds) passive wrist flexion (Phalen's test) has a lower false-negative rate (positive LR 1.3, negative LR 0.7). Look for wasting in the median nerve distribution, and loss of motor (thenar muscle strength: weak thumb abduction) and sensory function. These signs occur only in advanced cases.

Meralgia[w] paraesthetica

Compression of the lateral cutaneous nerve of the thigh causes paraesthesiae and sensory loss over the lateral side of the thigh (page 342). This entirely sensory nerve passes through the lateral part of the inguinal ligament only just medial to the anterior superior iliac spine. Here it is subject to compression in patients who are obese, wear tight or heavy belts or spend long periods sitting. Diabetes, pregnancy and trauma can also be causes of problems with the nerve.

---

[w] The Greek word *meros* means thigh and *algia* means painful.

Figure 8.53 A red, swollen and painful prepatellar bursa

(a) Anterior view. (b) Lateral view.

Tarsal tunnel syndrome

This may be caused by compression of the posterior tibial nerve in its fibro-osseous canal formed by the flexor retinaculum and the tarsal bones. Symptoms include burning pain and paraesthesiae in toe, sole and heel. Patients are often woken with pain at night and as with the carpal tunnel syndrome, this may radiate upwards. Walking may improve the symptoms. Causes include diabetes, synovitis from rheumatoid arthritis, bony deformity and flexor tenosynovitis. Hypertrophy of the abductor hallucis muscle, which occurs in intemperate runners, is an occasional cause.

Examination There is usually tenderness over the nerve posterior to the medial malleolus. There may be a positive Tinel's sign over the tarsal tunnel. Motor findings include weakness of toe flexion and of the intrinsic muscles of the foot.

Morton's metatarsalgia

This is caused by compression of the interdigital plantar nerves by the transverse metatarsal ligament. Patients complain of a burning pain or ache that extends distally from the affected web space to the toes (most often the third and fourth).

Examination. There is often tenderness over the involved metatarsal head and a painful nodule may be palpable.

References

1. Van den Hoogen HMM, Koes BW, Van Eijk JTM, Bouter LM. On the accuracy of history, physical, and the erythrocyte sedimentation rate in diagnosing low back pain in general practice: a criteria based review of the literature. *Spine* 1995; 20:318–327. Unfortunately, distinguishing mechanical from non-mechanical causes of low back pain such as ankylosing spondylitis is clinically difficult. However, tenderness to pressure over the anterior superior iliac spines and over the lower sacrum may, based on other studies, be somewhat helpful for the positive diagnosis of ankylosing spondylitis.

2. Deyo RA, Rainville J, Kent DL. What can the history and physical examination tell us about low back pain? *JAMA* 1992; 268:760–765.

3. Fuchs HA. Joint counts and physical measures. *Rheum Dis Clin Nth Am* 1995; 21:429–444. Describes useful quantitative methods to evaluate tenderness, pain on motion, swelling, deformity and limitation of movement.

4. Katz JN, Larson ME, Sabra A et al. The carpal syndrome: diagnostic utility of the history and physical examination findings. *Ann Intern Med* 1990; 112:321–327. This study compares the neurophysiological assessment of the carpal tunnel syndrome with the information obtained by examination and history. No single symptom or sign is sufficiently predictive.

5. Glockner SM. Shoulder pain: a diagnostic dilemma. *Am Fam Phys* 1995; 51:1677–1687, 1690–1692. Reviews the utility of symptoms and signs in differential diagnosis.

6. Katz JN, Dalgas M, Stucki G et al. Degenerative lumbar spinal stenosis. Diagnostic value of the history and physical examination. *Arth Rheum* 1995; 38:1236–1241. Describes symptoms (severe lower limb pain which is absent when the patient is seated) and signs (including a wide-based gait, positive Romberg's sign, thigh pain with lumbar extension) that help predict this rare condition in older patients.

7. Murtagh J. Diagnosis of early osteoarthritis of the hip joint: the four-step stress test. *Aust Fam Phys* 1990; 19:389. Discusses the diagnosis of osteoarthritis of the hip in a systematic way, suggesting a four-step approach.

8. Solomon DH, Simel DL, Bates DW et al. Does this patient have a torn meniscus or ligament of the knee? *JAMA* 2001; 286: 1610–1620.

9. Scholten RJ, Opstetten W, vander Plas CG et al. Accuracy of physical diagnostic tests for assessing ruptures of the anterior cruciate ligament: a meta-analysis. *J Fam Pract* 2003; 52:689–694.

10. Grob JJ, Bonerandi JJ. Cutaneous manifestations associated with the presence of the lupus-anticoagulant. *J Am Acad Dermatol* 1986; 15:211–219. Antiphospholipid antibody syndrome can be associated with leg ulcers (that resemble pyoderma gangrenosum), livedo reticularis and fingertip ischaemia.

11. Stevens GL, Adelman HM, Wallach PM. Palpable purpura: an algorithmic approach. *Am Fam Phys* 1995; 52:1355–1362.

12. Elliott BG. Finkelstein's test: a descriptive error that can produce a false-positive. *J Hand Surg Br* 1992; 17:481–482. Careful explanation of the performance of this test (which is often misunderstood) appears in this article. Movement with the thumb folded into the hand can produce a false-positive result.

Suggested reading
Original and review articles

Deyo RA, Weinstein JN. Low back pain. *N Engl J Med* 2001; 344:363–370.

Kataria PK, Brent LH. Spondyloarthropathies. *Am Fam Physician* 2004; 69: 2853–2860.

Textbooks

Apley AG, Solomon L. *Physical examination in orthopaedics*. Oxford: Butterworth-Heinemann, 1997.

Hochberg M, Silman AJ, Smolen JS, Weinblatt ME, Weisman MH. *Rheumatology*, 3rd edn. St Louis: Mosby, 2003.

Shipley M. *A color atlas of rheumatology*, 3rd edn. St Louis: Mosby-Yearbook, Europe Limited, 1998.

Snaith ML. *ABC of rheumatology*, 3rd edn. London: BMJ Publishing Group, 2004.

Solomon L, Nayagam D, Warwiak D. *Apley's system of orthopaedics and fractures*, 8th edn. London: Butterworth-Heineman, 2001.

chapter 9

The endocrine system

A physician is obligated to consider more than a diseased organ,
more even than the whole man—he must view the man in his world.

Harvey Cushing (1869–1939)

The endocrine history

Presenting symptoms

(Table 9.1)

Hormones control so many aspects of body function that the manifestations of endocrine disease are protean. Symptoms can include changes in body weight, appetite, bowel habit, hair distribution, pigmentation, sweating, height and menstruation, galactorrhoea (unexpected breast-milk production—in men and women), as well as polydipsia, polyuria, lethargy, headaches and loss of libido and erectile dysfunction. Many of these symptoms have other causes as well and must be carefully evaluated. On the other hand, the patient may know which endocrine organ or group of endocrine organs has been causing a problem. In particular, there may be a history of a thyroid condition or diabetes mellitus. A list of common symptoms associated with various endocrine diseases is presented in Table 9.1. In this section some of the important symptoms associated with endocrine disease will be discussed.

Changes in appetite and weight

An increased appetite associated with weight loss classically occurs in thyrotoxicosis or uncontrolled diabetes mellitus. An increased appetite with weight gain may occur in Cushing's syndrome, hypoglycaemia or in hypothalamic disease. A loss of appetite with weight loss can occur with adrenal insufficiency but is also seen in anorexia nervosa and with gastrointestinal disease (particularly malignancy). A loss of appetite with weight gain can occur in hypothyroidism.

Changes in bowel habit

Diarrhoea is associated with hyperthyroidism and adrenal insufficiency, while constipation may occur in hypothyroidism and hypercalcaemia.

Changes in sweating

Increased sweating is characteristic of hyperthyroidism, phaeochromocytoma, hypoglycaemia and acromegaly, but may also occur in anxiety states and at the menopause (page 392).

Changes in hair distribution

Hirsutism refers to an increased growth of body hair in women. The clinical evaluation and differential diagnosis are presented on page 274. The absence of facial hair in a man suggests hypogonadism, while temporal recession of the scalp hair in women occurs with androgen excess. The decrease in adrenal androgen production that occurs as a result of hypogonadism or adrenal insufficiency can cause loss of axillary and pubic hair in both sexes.

Lethargy

This common symptom can be due to a number of different diseases. Patients with hypothyroidism, Addison's disease and diabetes mellitus can present with this problem. Anaemia, connective tissue diseases, chronic infection (e.g. HIV, infective endocarditis), drugs (e.g. sedatives, diuretics causing electrolyte disturbances), chronic liver disease, renal failure and occult malignancy may also result in lethargy. Importantly, depression is a common cause of this symptom (page 371).

Table 9.1 Endocrine history

Major symptoms
Appetite and weight changes
Disturbed defecation
Sweating
Hair distribution
Lethargy
Skin changes
Pigmentation
Stature
Loss of libido, erectile dysfunction
Menstruation
Polyuria
Lump in the neck (goitre)

Syndromes
Thyrotoxicosis: preference for cooler weather, weight loss, increased appetite (polyphagia), palpitations, increased sweating, nervousness, irritability, diarrhoea, amenorrhoea, muscle weakness, exertional dyspnoea
Hypothyroidism (myxoedema): preference for warmer weather, lethargy, swelling of eyelids (oedema), hoarse voice, constipation, coarse skin, hypercarotenaemia
Diabetes mellitus: polyuria, polydipsia, thirst, blurred vision, weakness, infections, groin itch, rash (pruritus vulvae, balanitis), weight loss, tiredness, lethargy, disturbance of conscious state
Hypoglycaemia: morning headaches, weight gain, seizures, sweating
Primary adrenal insufficiency: pigmentation, tiredness, loss of weight, anorexia, nausea, diarrhoea, nocturia, mental changes, seizures (hypotension, hypoglycaemia)
Acromegaly: fatigue, weakness, increased sweating, heat intolerance, weight gain, enlarging hands and feet, enlarged and coarsened facial features, headaches, decreased vision, voice change, decreased libido, erectile dysfunction (impotence)

Changes in the skin

The skin becomes coarse, pale and dry in hypothyroidism, and dry and scaly in hypoparathyroidism. Soft tissue overgrowth occurs in acromegaly. Flushing of the skin of the face and neck occurs in the carcinoid syndrome (due to the release of vasoactive peptides from the tumour). Soft tissue overgrowth occurs in acromegaly and skin tags may appear in the axillae. These are called molluscum fibrinosum.

Acanthosis nigricans can also occur in acromegaly and in insulin-resistant states including Cushing's syndrome and polycystic ovarian syndrome. Xanthelasma can be present in patients with diabetes or hypothyroidism.

Changes in pigmentation

Increased pigmentation may be reported in primary adrenal insufficiency, Cushing's syndrome or acromegaly. Decreased pigmentation occurs in hypopituitarism. Localised depigmentation is characteristic of vitiligo, which may be associated with certain endocrine diseases such as Hashimoto's[a] disease with hypothyroidism and Addison's disease with adrenal insufficiency.

Changes in stature

Tallness may occur in children for constitutional reasons (tall parents) or, rarely, may reflect growth hormone excess (leading to gigantism), gonadotrophin deficiency, Klinefelter's syndrome[b], Marfan's syndrome or generalised lipodystrophy. Short stature can also result from endocrine disease, as discussed on page 272.

Erectile dysfunction (impotence)

A persistent inability to attain or sustain penile erections may occasionally be due to primary hypogonadism or to secondary hypogonadism due to hyperprolactinaemia. More often, it is related to emotional disorders; vascular disease, autonomic neuropathy (e.g. in diabetes mellitus or alcoholism), spinal cord disease or testicular atrophy can also cause this problem.

Galactorrhoea

Hyperprolactinaemia (usually the result of pituitary adenoma) can also cause galactorrhoea in up to 80% of women and 30% of men. Galactorrhoea in men occurs from a normal-appearing male breast.

Menstruation

Failure to menstruate is termed *amenorrhoea*. *Primary amenorrhoea* is defined as a failure to start menstruating by 17 years of age. True primary amenorrhoea may result from ovarian failure (e.g. X chromosomal abnormalities such as Turner's syndrome) or from pituitary or hypothalamic disease (e.g. tumour, trauma or idiopathic disease). Excess androgen production or systemic disease (e.g. malabsorption, chronic renal failure, obesity) can also result in primary amenorrhoea.

[a] Hakaru Hashimoto (1881–1934), Japanese surgeon.
[b] Harry Fitch Klinefelter (b. 1912), Baltimore physician, described the condition when he was a medical student.

Apparent primary amenorrhoea can also occur if menstrual flow cannot escape: for example, if there is an imperforate hymen. *Secondary amenorrhoea* is defined as the cessation of menstruation for 6 months or more. Pregnancy and menopause are common causes. The polycystic ovarian syndrome, hyperprolactinaemia, virilising syndromes or hypothalamic or pituitary disease can also result in this problem, as can use of the contraceptive pill or psychiatric disease.

Polyuria

Polyuria is defined as a urine volume of more than 3 litres/day. Patients who report urinary frequency may find it difficult to tell if large volumes of urine are being passed. Causes include diabetes mellitus (due to excessive filtration of glucose, a poorly resorbed solute); diabetes insipidus (due to inadequate renal water conservation from a central deficiency of antidiuretic hormone, or a lack of renal responsiveness to this hormone); primary polydipsia, where a patient drinks excessive water (due to psychogenic or hypothalamic disease or drugs such as chlorpromazine or thioridazine); hypercalcaemia; and tubulointerstitial or cystic renal disease.

Past history

A previous history of any endocrine condition must be uncovered. This includes surgery on the neck for a goitre. A partial thyroidectomy or radio-iodine (^{131}I) treatment in the past can lead to eventual hypothyroidism. The same may apply to radiation of the thyroid for carcinoma. A woman may have been diagnosed with diabetes mellitus after the birth of a large baby. There may be a past history of hypertension, which is occasionally due to an endocrine condition (e.g. phaeochromocytoma, Cushing's syndrome or Conn's syndrome). Previous thyroid surgery can be associated with hypoparathyroidism because of surgical damage to the parathyroid glands.

Previous treatment of a patient's thyroid problems may have included the use of antithyroid drugs, thyroid hormone or radioactive iodine. Surgery on the adrenals or pituitary may have been performed and this may leave the patient with decreased adrenal or pituitary function.

Patients with diabetes mellitus have an important chronic condition. Treatment may be with diet, insulin or oral hypoglycaemic agents. One must determine how well the patient understands the condition and whether he or she understands the principles of the diabetic diet and adheres to it. Find out how the blood sugar levels are monitored and whether or not the patient adjusts the insulin dose. Most patients should now be able to monitor their own blood sugar levels at home using a glucometer. There is now good evidence that tight control of blood sugar levels reduces the incidence of diabetic complications. The patient should be aware of the need for attention to the feet and eyes to help prevent complications.

Patients with hypopituitarism or hypoadrenalism may be on steroid replacement; some of these people also require mineralocorticoid replacement. Details of the patient's dosage schedule should be obtained.

Social history

Many of these conditions are chronic and their complications serious. How well the patient copes with various problems and the conditions at home and work will have an important effect on the success of treatment.

Family history

There may be a history in the family of thyroid conditions or diabetes mellitus. Occasionally a family history of a multiple endocrine neoplasia (MEN) syndrome may be obtained. These are rare autosomal dominant conditions. They include pituitary tumours, medullary carcinoma of the thyroid, hyperparathyroidism, phaeochromocytoma and pancreatic tumours.

The endocrine examination

A formal examination of the whole endocrine system is rarely performed (page 280); it is more usual to examine for signs of specific endocrine diseases. Usually there will be some clue from the history and general inspection to indicate what approach should be pursued.

The thyroid

The thyroid gland[c]

The examiner of the thyroid gland is fortunate that this gland has been placed conveniently in the front of the neck (Table 9.2).[1,2]

---

[c] The first person to distinguish an enlarged thyroid from cervical lymphadenopathy was the Roman medical writer, Aulus Aurelius Cornelius Celsus (53 BC—7 AD). He is more famous for describing the four cardinal signs of inflammation: redness, swelling, heat and tenderness.

Inspection. The normal thyroid may be just visible in a thin young person below the cricoid cartilage. Usually only the isthmus is visible as a diffuse central swelling. Enlargement of the gland, called a goitre (Latin *guttur*, 'throat'), should be apparent on inspection (see *Good signs guide 9.1*) especially if the patient extends the neck. Look at the front and sides of the neck and decide whether there is localised or general swelling of the gland. In normal people the line between the cricoid cartilage and the suprasternal notch should be straight. An outward bulge suggests the presence of a goitre. Remember that 80% of people with a goitre are biochemically euthyroid, 10% are hypothyroid and 10% are hyperthyroid.

Table 9.2 Causes of neck swellings

Midline

Goitre (moves up on swallowing)
Thyroglossal cyst (moves on poking out the tongue with the jaw stationary)
Submental lymph nodes
Parathyroid gland (very rare)

Lateral

Lymph nodes
Salivary glands (e.g. stone, tumour)
• Submandibular gland
• Parotid gland (lower pole)
Skin: sebaceous cyst or lipoma
Lymphatics: cystic hygroma (translucent)
Carotid artery: aneurysm or rarely tumour (pulsatile)
Pharynx: pharyngeal pouch, or brachial arch remnant (brachial cyst)

GOOD SIGNS GUIDE 9.1
Detection of a goitre
(compared with ultrasound findings)

Sign	Positive LR
No goitre on inspection or palpation	0.4
Goitre palpated and visible only on neck extension	NS
Goitre palpated and visible with neck in normal position	26.3

NS = not significant.
From McGee S, *Evidence-based physical diagnosis*, Saunders, 2001.

The temptation to begin touching a swelling as soon as it has been detected should be resisted until a glass of water has been procured. The patient takes sips from this repeatedly so that swallowing is possible without discomfort. Ask the patient to swallow and watch the neck swelling carefully. Only a goitre or a thyroglossal cyst, because of attachment to the larynx, will rise during swallowing. A thyroid gland fixed by neoplastic infiltration may not do so, but this is rare. Swallowing also allows the shape of the gland to be seen better. It should be noted whether an inferior border is visible as the gland rises. The thyroglossal cyst is a midline mass that can present at any age. It is an embryological remnant of the thyroglossal duct. Characteristically it rises when the patient protrudes the tongue.

Inspect the skin of the neck for scars. A thyroidectomy scar forms a ring around the base of the neck in the position of a high necklace. Also look for prominent veins. Dilated veins over the upper part of the chest wall, often accompanied by filling of the external jugular vein, suggest retrosternal extension of the goitre (thoracic inlet obstruction). Rarely, redness of the skin over the gland occurs in cases of suppurative thyroiditis.

Palpation. Palpation is best begun from *behind* (Figure 9.1). Both hands are placed with the pulps of the fingers over the gland. The patient's neck should be slightly flexed so as to relax the sternomastoid muscles. Feel systematically both lobes of the gland and its isthmus.

Figure 9.1 Palpating the thyroid from behind while the patient swallows sips of water

Figure 9.2 Goitre: (a) large; (b) massive.

Consider the following:

- **Size:** only an approximate estimation is possible (Figure 9.2). Feel particularly carefully for a lower border, because its absence suggests retrosternal extension.
- **Shape:** note whether the gland is uniformly enlarged or irregular and whether the isthmus is affected. If a *nodule* that feels distinct from the remaining thyroid tissue is palpable, determine its location, size, consistency, tenderness and mobility. Also decide whether the whole gland feels nodular (multinodular goitre).
- **Consistency:** may vary in different parts of the gland. Soft is normal; the gland is often firm in simple goitre and typically rubbery hard in Hashimoto's thyroiditis. A stony, hard node suggests carcinoma, calcification in a cyst, fibrosis or Riedel's thyroiditis.
- **Tenderness:** a feature of thyroiditis (subacute or rarely suppurative), or less often of a bleed into a cyst or carcinoma.
- **Mobility:** carcinoma may tether the gland.

Repeat the assessment while the patient swallows.

Decide if a thrill is palpable over the gland, as occurs when the gland is unusually metabolically active as in thyrotoxicosis.

Palpate the cervical lymph nodes (page 201). These may be involved in carcinoma of the thyroid. Feel each carotid artery—absence of its pulsation may very occasionally indicate malignant infiltration by thyroid carcinoma.

Move to the *front*. Palpate again. Localised swellings may be more easily defined here. Note the position of the trachea, which may be displaced by a retrosternal gland.

Percussion. The upper part of the manubrium can be percussed from one side to the other. A change from resonant to dull indicates a possible retrosternal goitre, but this is not a very reliable sign.

Auscultation. Listen over each lobe for a bruit. This is a sign of increased blood supply which may occur in hyperthyroidism, or occasionally from the use of antithyroid drugs. The differential diagnosis also includes a carotid bruit (louder over the carotid itself) or a venous hum (obliterated by gentle pressure over the base of the neck). If there is a goitre, apply mild compression to the lateral lobes and listen again for stridor.

Pemberton's sign. Get the patient to lift both arms as high as possible. Wait a few moments, then search the face eagerly for signs of congestion (plethora) and cyanosis. Associated respiratory distress and inspiratory stridor may occur. Look at the neck veins for distension (venous congestion). Ask the patient to take a deep breath in through the mouth and listen for stridor. This is a test for thoracic inlet obstruction due to a retrosternal goitre or any retrosternal mass.[3]

Examination of the thyroid should be part of every routine physical examination. Causes of a goitre are listed in Table 9.3.

Hyperthyroidism (thyrotoxicosis)

This is a disease caused by excessive concentrations of thyroid hormones. Many of the clinical features of thyrotoxicosis are characterised by signs of sympathetic overactivity such as tremor, tachycardia and sweating. The explanation is not entirely clear. Catecholamine secretion is usually normal in hyperthyroidism; however, thyroid hormone potentiates the effects of

Table 9.3 Goitre

Causes of a diffuse goitre
(patient often euthyroid)
Idiopathic (majority)
Puberty or pregnancy
Thyroiditis
- Hashimoto's
- Subacute (gland usually tender)
Simple goitre (iodine deficiency)
Goitrogens—iodine excess, drugs (e.g. lithium, phenylbutazone)
Inborn errors of thyroid hormone synthesis—e.g. Pendred's* syndrome (an autosomal recessive condition associated with nerve deafness)

Causes of a solitary thyroid nodule

Benign:
- Dominant nodule in a multinodular goitre
- Degeneration or haemorrhage into a colloid cyst or nodule
- Follicular adenoma
- Simple cyst (rare)
Malignant:
- Carcinoma—primary or secondary (e.g. renal cell carcinoma)
- Lymphoma (rare)

* Vaughan Pendred (b. 1869), London physician.

GOOD SIGNS GUIDE 9.2
Thyrotoxicosis

Sign	Positive LR	Negative LR
Pulse		
≥90/min	4.4	0.2
Skin		
Moist and warm	6.7	0.7
Thyroid		
Enlarged	2.3	0.1
Eyes		
Eyelid retraction	31.5	0.7
Lid lag	17.6	0.8
Neurological		
Fine tremor	11.4	0.3

From McGee S, *Evidence-based physical diagnosis*, Saunders, 2001.

Figure 9.3 Onycholysis (Plummer's nails)

catecholamines, possibly by increasing the number of adrenergic receptors in the tissues.

The commonest cause of thyrotoxicosis in young people is Graves' disease,[d] an autoimmune disease where circulating immunoglobulins stimulate thyroid stimulating hormone (TSH) receptors on the surface of the thyroid follicular cells.

Examine a suspected case of thyrotoxicosis as follows (see *Good signs guide 9.2*).

General inspection. Look for signs of weight loss, anxiety and the frightened facies of thyrotoxicosis.

The hands. Ask the patient to put out the arms and look for a fine tremor (due to sympathetic overactivity). Laying a sheet of paper over the patient's fingers may more clearly demonstrate this tremor, to the amazement of less-experienced colleagues.

Look at the nails for *onycholysis* (Plummer's[e] nails) (Figure 9.3). Onycholysis (where there is sep-

aration of the nail from its bed) is said to occur particularly on the ring finger, but can occur on all the fingernails, and is apparently due to sympathetic overactivity. It is rarely seen in association with Graves' disease. Inspect now for thyroid acropathy (acropathy is another term for clubbing) seen rarely in Graves' disease but not with other causes of thyrotoxicosis.

Inspect for palmar erythema and feel the palms for warmth and sweatiness (sympathetic overactivity).

Take the pulse. Note the presence of sinus tachycardia (sympathetic overdrive) or atrial fibrillation (due to a shortened refractory period of atrial cells

[d] Robert Graves (1796–1853), Dublin physician.
[e] Henry Plummer (1874–1936), physician at the Mayo Clinic, USA.

Figure 9.4 Thyrotoxicosis: thyroid stare and exophthalmos

Table 9.4 Causes of exophthalmos

Bilateral

Graves' disease

Unilateral

Tumours of the orbit: e.g. dermoid, optic nerve
    glioma, neurofibroma, granuloma
Cavernous sinus thrombosis
Graves' disease
Pseudotumours of the orbit

related to sympathetic drive and hormone-induced changes). The pulse may also have a collapsing character due to a high cardiac output.

Test for proximal myopathy and tap the arm reflexes for abnormal briskness, especially in the relaxation phase (page 325).

The eyes. Examine the eyes for exophthalmos, which is protrusion of the eyeball from the orbit (Figure 9.4, Table 9.4). This may be very obvious, but if not, look carefully at the sclerae, which in exophthalmos are not covered by the lower eyelid. Next look from behind over the patient's forehead for exophthalmos, where the eye will be visible anterior to the superior orbital margin. Now examine for the complications of proptosis, which include: (i) chemosis (oedema of the conjunctiva and injection of the sclera, particularly over the insertion of the lateral rectus); (ii) conjunctivitis; (iii) corneal ulceration (due to inability to close the eyelids); (iv) optic atrophy (rare and possibly due to optic nerve stretching); and (v) ophthalmoplegia (the inferior rectus muscle power tends to be lost first, and later convergence is weakened).

The mechanism of exophthalmos is uncertain. It occurs only in Graves' disease. It may precede the onset of thyrotoxicosis, or may persist after the patient has become euthyroid. It is characterised by an inflammatory infiltrate of the orbital contents, but not of the globe itself. The orbital muscles are particularly affected and an increase in their size accounts for most of the increased volume of the orbital contents and therefore for protrusion of the globe. It is probably due to an autoimmune abnormality.

Next examine for the components of thyroid ophthalmopathy, which are related to sympathetic overactivity and are not specific for Graves' disease. Look for the thyroid stare (a frightened expression) and lid retraction (where there is sclera visible above the iris). Test for lid lag (von Graefe's sign[f]) by asking the patient to follow your finger as it descends at a moderate rate from the upper to the lower part of the visual field. Descent of the upper lid lags behind descent of the eyeball.

If ptosis is present, one should rule out myasthenia gravis, which can be associated with autoimmune disease.

The neck. Examine for thyroid enlargement, which is usually detectable (60–90% of patients). In Graves' disease the gland is classically diffusely enlarged and is smooth and firm. An associated thrill may be present. Absence of thyroid enlargement makes Graves' disease unlikely, but does not exclude it. Possible thyroid abnormalities in patients who are thyrotoxic but do not have Graves' disease include a toxic multinodular goitre, a solitary nodule (toxic adenoma), or subacute thyroiditis (de Quervain's[g] thyroiditis). In de Quervain's thyroiditis there is typically a moderately enlarged firm and tender gland. Thyrotoxicosis may occur without any goitre, particularly in elderly patients. Alternatively, in hyperthyroidism due to an abnormality of trophoblastic tissue (a hydatidiform mole or choriocarcinoma of the testis or uterus), or excessive thyroid hormone replacement, the thyroid gland will not usually be palpable. These causes are rare.

If a thyroidectomy scar is present, assess for hypoparathyroidism (Chvostek's[h] or Trousseau's[i] signs (page 272)). These signs are most often present in the first few days after operation.

The arms. Ask the patient to raise the arms above the head and so test for proximal myopathy.

---

f Friedrich von Graefe (1828–70), Professor of Ophthalmology in Berlin, described this in 1864. He was one of the most famous ophthalmologists of the 19th century. Horner was one of his pupils. He died of tuberculosis at the age of 42.
g Fritz de Quervain (1868–1940), Professor of Surgery, Berne, Switzerland.
h Franz Chvostek (1835–84), Viennese physician.
i Armand Trousseau (1801–1867), Parisian physician.

Table 9.5 Thyrotoxicosis and hypothyroidism

Causes of thyrotoxicosis

Primary
Graves' disease
Toxic multinodular goitre
Toxic uninodular goitre: usually a toxic adenoma
Hashimoto's thyroiditis (early in its course; later it produces hypothyroidism)
Subacute thyroiditis (transient)
Postpartum thyroiditis (non-tender)
Iodine-induced ('Jod-Basedow phenomenon'* — iodine given after a previously deficient diet)

Secondary
Pituitary (very rare): TSH hypersecretion
Hydatidiform moles or choriocarcinomas: HCG secretion (rare)
Struma ovarii (rare)
Drugs, e.g. excess thyroid hormone ingestion, amiodarone

Causes of hypothyroidism

Primary
Without a goitre (decreased or absent thyroid tissue):
• Idiopathic atrophy
• Treatment of thyrotoxicosis—e.g. ^{131}I, surgery
• Agenesis or a lingual thyroid
• Unresponsiveness to TSH
With a goitre (decreased thyroid hormone synthesis):
• Chronic autoimmune diseases—e.g. Hashimoto's thyroiditis
• Drugs, e.g. lithium, amiodarone
• Inborn errors (enzyme deficiency)
• Endemic iodine deficiency or iodine-induced hypothyroidism

Secondary
Pituitary lesions (Table 9.7)

Tertiary
Hypothalamic lesions

Transient
Thyroid hormone treatment withdrawn
Subacute thyroiditis
Postpartum thyroiditis

* Carl von Basedow (1799–1854), German general practitioner, described this in 1840 (*Jod* = iodine in German).
TSH = thyroid stimulating hormone. HCG = human chorionic gonadotrophin.

The chest. Gynaecomastia (page 274) occurs occasionally. Examine the heart for systolic flow murmurs (due to increased cardiac output) and signs of congestive cardiac failure, which may be precipitated by thyrotoxicosis in older people.

The legs. Look first for pretibial myxoedema. This takes the form of bilateral firm, elevated dermal nodules and plaques, which can be pink, brown or skin-coloured. They are caused by mucopolysaccharide accumulation. Despite the name, this occurs only in Graves' disease and not in hypothyroidism. Test now for proximal myopathy and hyperreflexia in the legs.

Hypothyroidism (myxoedema)

Hypothyroidism (deficiency of thyroid hormone) is due to primary disease of the thyroid or, less commonly, is secondary to pituitary or hypothalamic failure (Table 9.5). Myxoedema implies a more severe form of hypothyroidism. In myxoedema, for unknown reasons, hydrophilic mucopolysaccharides accumulate in the ground substance of tissues including the skin. This results in excessive interstitial fluid, which is relatively immobile, causing skin thickening and a doughy induration.

Examine the patient with suspected hypothyroidism as follows (see *Good signs guide 9.3*):

General inspection. Look for signs of obvious mental and physical sluggishness, or evidence of the very rare 'myxoedema madness'. Hypothyroid speech is a feature in about a third of patients. This is characteristically slow, nasal and deep in pitch. Obesity is no more common than in euthyroid people.

The hands. Note peripheral cyanosis (due to reduced cardiac output) and swelling of the skin, which may appear cool and dry. The yellow discoloration of hypercarotenaemia (there is slowing down of hepatic metabolism of carotene) may be seen on the palms. Look for palmar crease pallor—anaemia may be due to: (i) chronic disease; (ii) folate deficiency secondary to bacterial overgrowth, or vitamin B_{12} deficiency due to associated pernicious anaemia; or (iii) iron deficiency due to menorrhagia.

Take the pulse, which may be of small volume and slow. Test for sensory loss, as the carpal tunnel is thickened in myxoedema (page 331).

The arms. Test for proximal myopathy (rare) and a 'hung-up' biceps reflex (see below).

The face. Inspect the face (Figure 9.5). The skin, but not the sclera, may appear yellow due to hypercarotenaemia. The skin may be generally thickened,

GOOD SIGNS GUIDE 9.3 Hypothyroidism		
Sign	**Positive LR**	**Negative LR**
Skin		
Coarse	5.6	0.7
Cool and dry	4.7	0.9
Cold palms	NS	NS
Dry palms	NS	NS
Periorbital puffiness	2.8	0.6
Puffiness of wrists	2.9	0.7
Loss of eyebrow hair	1.9	NS
Speech		
Hypothyroid speech	5.4	0.7
Thyroid gland		
Goitre	2.8	0.6
Pulse		
<70/min	4.1	0.8

NS = not significant.

From McGee S, *Evidence-based physical diagnosis*, Saunders, 2001.

Figure 9.5 Myxoedema

Table 9.6 Neurological associations of hypothyroidism

Common

Entrapment: carpal tunnel, tarsal tunnel
Delayed ankle jerks
Muscle cramps

Uncommon

Peripheral neuropathy
Proximal myopathy
Hypokalaemic periodic paralysis
Cerebellar syndrome
Psychosis
Coma
Unmasking of myasthenia gravis
Cerebrovascular disease
High cerebrovascular fluid protein
Nerve deafness

and alopecia may be present, as may vitiligo (an associated autoimmune disease).

Inspect the eyes for periorbital oedema. Loss or thinning of the outer third of the eyebrows can occur in myxoedema but is also common in healthy persons. Look for xanthelasma (due to associated hypercholesterolaemia) (page 40, 41). Palpate for coolness and dryness of the skin and hair. There may be thinning of the scalp hair.

Look at the tongue for swelling. Ask the patient to speak and listen for coarse, croaking, slow speech. Bilateral nerve deafness may occur with endemic or congenital hypothyroidism.

The thyroid gland. A primary decrease in thyroid hormone results in a compensatory oversecretion of TSH. A goitre will result if there is viable thyroid tissue.

Many cases of hypothyroidism are not associated with an enlarged gland as there is little thyroid tissue. The exceptions include severe iodine deficiency, enzyme deficiency (inborn errors of metabolism), late Hashimoto's disease or treated thyrotoxicosis (Table 9.5).

The chest. Examine the heart for a pericardial effusion and the lungs for pleural effusions.

The legs. There may be non-pitting oedema. Ask the patient to kneel on a chair with the ankles exposed. Tap the Achilles tendon with a reflex hammer. There is normal contraction followed by delayed relaxation of the foot in hypothyroidism (the 'hung-up' reflex) (page 268). Examine for signs of peripheral neuropathy and for other uncommon neurological abnormalities associated with hypothyroidism (Table 9.6).

The pituitary

Pituitary tumours can present in two ways: as a result of (i) local effects such as headaches, visual field loss and loss of acuity; and (ii) changes in pituitary hormone secretion. These changes include: (i) excess growth hormone, causing acromegaly; (ii) excess adrenocorticotrophic hormone (ACTH), causing Cushing's syndrome; and (iii) excess prolactin, causing secondary amenorrhoea or male infertility or deficiency (hypopituitarism).

Table 9.7 Causes of hypopituitarism

Space-occupying lesion
- Pituitary tumour (non-secretory or secretory)
- Other tumours: craniopharyngioma, metastatic carcinoma, sarcoma
- Granulomata: e.g. sarcoid, tuberculosis
Iatrogenic: e.g. surgery or irradiation
Head injury
Sheehan's syndrome* (postpartum pituitary haemorrhage resulting in necrosis of the gland)
Infarction or pituitary apoplexy
Idiopathic

* Harold Sheehan (b. 1900), Professor of Pathology, Liverpool, England, described the syndrome in 1937.

Panhypopituitarism

This is a deficiency of most or all of the pituitary hormones and is usually due to a space-occupying lesion or destruction of the pituitary gland (Table 9.7). Hormone production is often lost in the following order: (i) growth hormone (dwarfism in children, insulin sensitivity in adults); (ii) prolactin (failure of lactation after delivery); (iii) gonadotrophins (loss of secondary sexual characteristics, secondary amenorrhoea in women, loss of libido and infertility in men); (iv) TSH (hypothyroidism): and (v) ACTH (hypoadrenalism and hyperpigmentation), with loss of secondary sexual hair due to decreased adrenal androgen production.

However, isolated single hormonal deficiencies or multiple deficiencies may occur in any combination.

General inspection. The patient may be of short stature (failure of growth hormone secretion before growth is complete). Look for pallor of the skin (due to anaemia or occasionally ACTH deficiency because of the loss of its melanocyte-stimulating activity), fine-wrinkled skin and lack of body hair (due to gonadotrophin deficiency). There may be complete absence of the secondary sexual characteristics (Table 9.8) if gonadotrophin failure occurred before puberty.

The face. Look at the face more closely. Multiple skin wrinkles around the eyes are characteristic of

---

Table 9.8 Secondary sexual development (Tanner stages)

This occurs at puberty in response to pituitary gonadotrophins

Males

1 Preadolescent
2 Enlargement of testes and scrotum
3 Lengthening of penis
4 Increase in penis breadth, glans development and scrotal darkening
5 Adult: above, plus public hair spread to medial surface of the thighs

Females

Breasts	*Pubic hair*
1 Preadolescent	1 No pubic hair
2 Breast bud (elevation of breasts and papilla)	2 Sparse growth, mainly over the labia
3 Enlargement of breast and areola (no separation of contours)	3 Darker, coarser, more curled hairs but sparse over the junction of the pubes
4 Areola and papilla project above breast level (secondary mound)	4 Adult type but no hair spread to medial surface of thighs
5 Adult: areola is recessed and papilla projects	5 Adult: horizontal pattern and hair spread to medial thighs

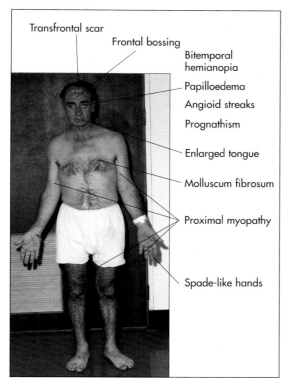

Transfrontal scar
Frontal bossing
Bitemporal hemianopia
Papilloedema
Angioid streaks
Prognathism
Enlarged tongue
Molluscum fibrosum
Proximal myopathy
Spade-like hands

Figure 9.6 Acromegaly

gonadotrophin deficiency. Inspect the forehead carefully for hypophysectomy scars—transfrontal scars will be apparent (Figure 9.6) but not transsphenoidal ones, as this operation is performed through the base of the nose, via an incision under the upper lip.

Examine the eyes (page 297). The visual fields must be assessed for any defects, especially bitemporal hemianopia (an enlarging pituitary tumour may compress the optic chiasm) and the fundi examined for optic atrophy (optic nerve compression from a pituitary tumour). Assess the third, fourth, sixth and first division of the fifth cranial nerves, as these may be affected by extrapituitary tumour expansion into the cavernous sinus (Figure 9.7).

Feel the facial hair over the bearded area in men for normal beard growth (which is lost with gonadotrophin deficiency).

The chest. Go on to the chest. Look for skin pallor and for a decrease in nipple pigmentation. In men, decreased body hair (axillary and chest) may be present. In women, secondary breast atrophy may be found.

The genital region. Loss of pubic hair occurs in both sexes. In men, testicular atrophy may be present. Atrophied testes are characteristically small and firm. The normal-sized testis is about 15 to 25 mL in volume.

The ankle reflexes. Test for 'hung-up' jerks (Figure 9.8). These are an important sign of pituitary hypothyroidism. Occasionally, pituitary hypothyroid patients may be slightly overweight, but the classical myxoedematous appearance is usually absent.

Acromegaly[j]

This is excessive secretion of growth hormone, typically due to an eosinophilic pituitary adenoma. Growth hormone stimulates the liver and other tissues to produce somatomedins which in turn promote growth. Growth hormone is also a protein anabolic hormone exerting its effects at the ribosomal level, and it is diabetogenic as it exerts an anti-insulin effect in muscle and increases hepatic glucose release.

Gigantism is the result of growth hormone hypersecretion occurring before puberty and fusion of the epiphyses. It results in massive skeletal as well as soft-tissue growth. Acromegaly occurs when the growth plates have fused, so that only soft tissue and flat bone enlargement are possible.

General inspection. The face and body habitus may be characteristic (Figure 9.6).

The hands. Sit the patient on the side of the bed and look at the hands. Notice a wide spade-like shape (due to soft tissue and bony enlargement). Increased sweating and warmth of the palms may be noted. This is due to an increased metabolic rate. The skin may appear thickened. Changes of osteoarthritis in the hands are common and are due to skeletal overgrowth. Examine for median nerve entrapment, which can occur because of soft-tissue overgrowth in the carpal tunnel area.

The arms. Proximal myopathy may be present (page 355). Palpate behind the medial epicondyle (the 'funny bone') for ulnar nerve thickening.

The axillae. Carefully inspect the axillae for skin tags (called molluscum fibrosum, which are nontender skin-coloured protrusions). Summon up courage and feel for greasy skin. Look for acanthosis nigricans.

The face. Look for a large supraorbital ridge, which causes frontal bossing (this may also occur

---

[j] The acral parts are the hands and feet.

Figure 9.7 The cavernous sinus and its relationship with the cranial nerves and pituitary gland

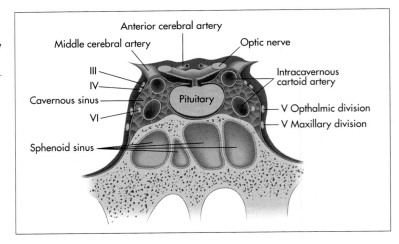

Figure 9.8 Testing ankle jerks (second method—see also page 339)

This method best demonstrates the 'hang-up' reflexes of hypothyroidism. Look for rapid dorsiflexion followed by slow plantar flexion as the tendon is tapped.

occasionally in Paget's disease, rickets, achondroplasia or hydrocephalus). The lips may be thickened.

Examine the eyes for visual field defects: classically there may be bitemporal hemianopia if the pituitary tumour is large. Look in the fundi for optic atrophy (due to nerve compression) and papilloedema (due to raised intracranial pressure with an extensive tumour). The presence of angioid streaks (red, brown or grey streaks that are three to five times the diameter of a retinal vein and appear to emanate from the optic disc) should also be sought: these are due to degeneration and fibrosis of Bruch's membrane. One should also note hypertensive changes or diabetic changes in the fundus. Ocular palsies may occur with an extensive pituitary tumour.

Look in the mouth for an enlarged tongue that may not fit neatly between the teeth. The teeth themselves may be splayed and separated, with malocclusion as the jaw enlarges. The lower jaw may look square and firm (as it does on some American actors). When the jaw protrudes it is called prognathism (Greek *pro* 'forwards', *gnathos* 'jaw').

The neck. The thyroid may be diffusely enlarged or multinodular (all the internal organs may enlarge under the influence of growth hormone). Listen to the voice for hoarseness.

The chest. Look for coarse body hair and gynaecomastia. Examine the heart for signs of arrhythmias, cardiomegaly and congestive cardiac failure, which may be due to ischaemic heart disease, hypertension or cardiomyopathy (all more common in acromegaly).

The back. Inspect for kyphosis.

The abdomen. Examine for hepatic, splenic and renal enlargement, and for testicular atrophy (the latter indicating gonadotrophin deficiency secondary to an enlarging pituitary tumour). Acromegaly

Table 9.9 Causes of Cushing's syndrome

Exogenous administration of excess steroids or
    ACTH (most common)
Adrenal hyperplasia
• Secondary to pituitary ACTH production
  (Cushing's disease)
    Microadenoma
    Macroadenoma
    Pituitary-hypothalamic dysfunction
• Secondary to ACTH-producing tumours—
  e.g. small cell lung carcinoma
Adrenal neoplasia
• Adenoma
• Carcinoma (rare)

GOOD SIGNS GUIDE 9.4
Cushing's syndrome

Sign	Positive LR	Negative LR
Vital signs		
Hypertension	2.3	0.8
Body habitus		
Moon face	1.6	0.1
Central obesity	3.0	0.2
General obesity	0.1	2.5
Skin findings		
Thin skinfold (women)	115.6	0.2
Plethora	2.7	0.3
Hirsutism (women)	1.7	0.7
Ecchymoses	4.5	0.5
Red or purple striae	1.9	0.7
Acne	2.2	0.6
Extremities		
Proximal muscle weakness	NS	0.4
Oedema	1.8	0.7

NS = not significant.
From McGee S, *Evidence-based physical diagnosis*, Saunders, 2001.

can be associated with a mixed pituitary tumour and resultant hyperprolactinaemia can also cause testicular atrophy.

The lower limbs. Look for signs of osteoarthritis in the hips especially, and knees (page 234), and for pseudogout. Foot drop may be present because of common peroneal nerve entrapment (page 343).

The urine and blood pressure. Test the urine for glucose, as excess growth hormone is diabetogenic in 25% of cases. Take the blood pressure to test for hypertension.

Finally decide if the disease is active or not. Signs of active disease include: (i) large numbers of skin tags; (ii) excessive sweating; (iii) presence of glycosuria; (iv) increasing visual field loss; (v) enlarging goitre; and (vi) hypertension. *Note:* Headache also suggests disease activity.

The adrenals

Cushing's syndrome

This is due to a chronic excess of glucocorticoids. Steroids have multiple effects on the body, due to stimulation of the DNA-dependent synthesis of select messenger ribonucleic acids (RNAs). This leads to the formation of enzymes, which alter cell function and result in increased protein catabolism and gluconeogenesis. Remember that Cushing's disease is specifically pituitary ACTH overproduction, while Cushing's syndrome is due to excessive steroid hormone production from any cause (Table 9.9; see *Good signs guide 9.4*).

The hands. Skinfold thickness is best assessed on the backs of the hands and may be reliable only as a sign of Cushing's in young women. The skinfold should be thicker than 1.8 mm.

Standing. Have the patient undress to the underpants and, if possible, stand up (Figure 9.9). Look from the front, back and sides. Note *moon-like facies* and *central obesity*. The limbs appear thin despite sometimes very gross truncal (mostly intra-abdominal rather than subcutaneous fat) obesity.[k] This is the characteristic fat distribution that occurs with steroid excess. *Bruising* may be present (due to loss of perivascular supporting tissue–protein catabolism). Look for excessive *pigmentation* on the extensor surfaces (because of melanocyte-stimulating-hormone-(MSH-)like activity in the ACTH molecule). Ask the patient to squat at this point to test for *proximal myopathy*, due to mobilisation of muscle tissue or excessive urinary potassium loss. Look at the back for the 'buffalo hump', which is due

[k] The enthusiastic student can calculate the central obesity index. This is the sum of three truncal circumferences (neck, chest and waist) divided by six peripheral ones (arms, thighs and legs on both sides). A normal index is less than 1.

Figure 9.9 Buffalo hump and central obesity in Cushing's syndrome

(From FS McDonald, ed., *Mayo Clinic images in internal medicine*, with permission. © Mayo Clinic Scientific Press and CRC Press.)

Table 9.10 Causes of Addison's disease

Chronic

Primary
Autoimmune adrenal disease
Infection (tuberculosis, HIV)
Granuloma
Following heparin therapy
Malignant infiltration
Haemochromatosis
Adrenoleucodystrophy

Secondary
Pituitary or hypothalamic disease

Acute
Septicaemia: meningococcal
Adrenalectomy
Any stress in a patient with chronic hypoadrenalism or abrupt cessation of prolonged high-dose steroid therapy

to fat deposition over the interscapular area. Palpate for bony *tenderness* of the vertebral bodies due to crush fractures from osteoporosis (a steroid anti-vitamin D effect and increased urinary calcium excretion may be responsible in part for disruption of the bone matrix).

Sitting. Ask the patient to sit on the side of the bed, but remember that he or she may be suffering from steroid psychosis and refuse to do anything you ask.

The face and neck. Look for plethora (this occurs in the absence of polycythaemia which, however, may also be present). The face may have a typical moon shape due to fat deposition in the upper part. Inspect for acne and hirsutism (if adrenal androgen secretion is also increased). Telangiectasiae may also be present.

Examine the visual fields for signs of a pituitary tumour, and the fundi for visual field defects, optic atrophy, papilloedema and hypertensive or diabetic changes.

Look for supraclavicular fat pads.

The abdomen. Lay the patient in bed on one pillow. Examine the abdomen for purple striae, which are due to weakening and disruption of collagen fibres in the dermis, leading to exposure of vascular subcutaneous tissues. In patients with Cushing's syndrome these are wider (1 cm) than those seen in people who have gained weight rapidly for other reasons. They may also be present near the axillae on the upper arms or on the inside of the thighs. Palpate for adrenal masses (rarely a large adrenal carcinoma will be palpable over the renal area). Palpate for hepatomegaly due to fat deposition or rarely to adrenal carcinoma deposits.

The legs. Palpate for oedema (due to salt and water retention). Look for bruising and poor wound healing.

The urinalysis and blood pressure. Test the urine for sugar (as steroids are diabetogenic; this is due to an increase in hepatic gluconeogenesis and an anti-insulin effect on peripheral tissues). Hypertension is common due to salt and water retention (an aldosterone effect) and possibly to increased angiotensin secretion or a direct effect on blood vessels.

Synthesis of signs. Certain signs are of some aetiological value in Cushing's syndrome.

- **Signs which suggest that adrenal carcinoma may be the underlying cause:** (i) a palpable abdominal mass; (ii) signs of virilisation in the female; (iii) gynaecomastia in the male.
- **Signs which suggest that ectopic ACTH production may be the cause:** (i) absence of the Cushingoid body habitus; (ii) more prominent oedema and hypertension; (iii) marked muscle weakness. *Note:* When Cushing's is due to ectopic ACTH production from a small cell carcinoma, the patient is much more likely to be male (positive LR 13) and the history to be of more rapid onset of the symptoms and signs (18 months: positive LR 15).

Table 9.11 A classification of conditions found in various combinations in autoimmune polyglandular syndromes

Type I (rare autosomal recessive)	Type II (more common, HLA DRB1, DQA1, DQB1)
1 Chronic mucocutaneous candidiasis 2 Hypoparathyroidism 3 Addison's disease	1 Insulin-requiring diabetes (type 1) 2 Autoimmune thyroid disease 3 Addison's disease 4 Myasthenia gravis 5 Pernicious anaemia 6 Primary gonadal failure

- **Significance of hyperpigmentation:** this suggests an extra-adrenal tumour, or enlargement of an ACTH-secreting pituitary adenoma following adrenalectomy (Nelson's[l] syndrome).

Addison's disease[m]

This is adrenocortical hypofunction with reduction in the secretion of glucocorticoids and mineralocorticoids. It is most often due to autoimmune disease of the adrenal glands. Other causes are listed in Table 9.10.

If this disease is suspected, look for cachexia. Then, with the patient undressed, look for pigmentation in the palmar creases (Figure 9.10), elbows, gums and buccal mucosa, genital areas and in scars. This occurs because of compensatory ACTH hypersecretion in primary hypoadrenalism (when there is adrenal disease) as ACTH has melanocyte-stimulating activity. Also inspect for vitiligo (localised hypomelanosis), an autoimmune disease that is commonly associated with autoimmune adrenal failure.

Take the blood pressure and test for postural hypotension. Remember that the rest of the autoimmune disease cluster may be associated with autoimmune adrenal failure (Table 9.11).

Calcium metabolism

Primary hyperparathyroidism

This is due to excess parathyroid hormone (Table 9.12), which results in an increased serum calcium level, increased renal phosphate excretion and increased formation of 1,25-dihydroxycholecalciferol by activation of adenyl cyclase in the bone and kidneys. Primary hyperparathyroidism causes problems with 'stones' (renal stones), 'bones' (osteopenia and

Figure 9.10 Palmar crease pigmentation in Addison's disease

Table 9.12 Types of hyperparathyroidism

Primary
Adenoma (80%) Hyperplasia Carcinoma (rare)
Secondary
Hyperplasia following chronic renal failure
Tertiary (autonomous)
The appearance of autonomous hyperparathyroidism is a complication of secondary hyperparathyroidism

pseudogout), 'abdominal groans' (constipation, peptic ulcer and pancreatitis) and 'psychological moans' (confusion).

Other causes of hypercalcaemia are listed in Table 9.13.

---

[l] Warren Nelson (1906–64), American endocrinologist.
[m] Thomas Addison (1793–1860) described the disease in 1849. Addison, Bright and Hodgkin made up the famous trio of physicians at Guy's Hospital, London.

Table 9.13 Important causes of hypercalcaemia

Primary hyperparathyroidism
Carcinoma (from bone metastases or humoral
　mediators)
Thiazide diuretics
Vitamin D excess
Excessive production of vitamin D metabolites:
　e.g. sarcoidosis, certain T cell lymphomas
Thyrotoxicosis
Associated with renal failure (e.g. severe
　secondary hyperparathyroidism)
Multiple myeloma
Prolonged immobilisation or space flight

Table 9.14 Causes of hypocalcaemia

Hypoparathyroidism: after thyroidectomy,
　idiopathic
Malabsorption
Deficiency of vitamin D
Chronic renal failure
Acute pancreatitis
Pseudohypoparathyroidism
Magnesium deficiency
Hypocalcaemia of malignant disease

General inspection. Note the mental state of the patient. Severe hypercalcaemia may cause coma or convulsions. Assess hydration (polyuria from hypercalcaemia may cause dehydration).

The face. Look in the eyes for band keratopathy, which is rare (page 185).

The body and lower limbs. Palpate the shoulders, sternum, ribs, spine and hips for bony tenderness, deformity or evidence of previous fractures. Test for proximal muscle weakness. Look for pseudogout. Take the blood pressure, as hypertension may occur.

Urinalysis. Test for blood in the urine (renal stones).

The MEN syndromes

The multiple endocrine neoplasias (MEN), types I and II, are autosomal dominant conditions. Hyperparathyroidism can be associated with both. MEN type I (due to a mutation on chromosome 11) is associated with tumours of the parathyroid, pituitary and pancreatic islet cells. MEN Type IIA (due to a mutation on chromosome 10 involving the c-*ret* proto-oncogene) is associated with medullary carcinoma of the thyroid, hyperparathyroidism and phaeochromocytoma.

Hypoparathyroidism

This results in hypocalcaemia with neuromuscular consequences (tetany). It is usually a postoperative complication after thyroidectomy, but can be idiopathic. Hypocalcaemia can also result from end-organ resistance to parathyroid hormone (pseudohypoparathyroidism) (Table 9.14).

Look first for Trousseau's and Chvostek's signs. *Trousseau's sign* is elicited with a blood pressure cuff placed on the arm with the pressure raised above the patient's systolic pressure. Typical contraction of the hand occurs within two minutes when hypocalcaemia has caused neuromuscular irritability. The thumb becomes strongly adducted, and the fingers are extended, except at the metacarpophalangeal joints. The appearance is that of an obstetrician about to remove the placenta manually and is called the *main d'accoucheur.*

Chvostek's sign is performed by tapping gently over the facial (seventh) cranial nerve under the ear. The nerve is hyperexcitable in hypocalcaemia and a brisk muscular twitch occurs on the same side of the face.

Next test for hyperreflexia, again due to neuromuscular irritability.

Look at the nails for fragility and monilial infection. Note any dryness of the skin. Go to the face and look for deformity of the teeth. Examine the eyes for cataracts or papilloedema. These signs may all occur in idiopathic hypoparathyroidism, an autoimmune disease. Cataracts may also follow surgically induced hypoparathyroidism.

Pseudohypoparathyroidism. In this disease the patients have tetany (due to hypocalcaemia) as well as typical skeletal abnormalities. These include short stature, a round face, a short neck, thin stocky build and very characteristically short fourth or fifth fingers or toes (due to metacarpal or metatarsal shortening; this can be unilateral or bilateral) (Figure 9.11). Ask the patient to make a fist to demonstrate the characteristic clinical signs.

Pseudopseudohypoparathyroidism. This amusing name is given to a disease where there is no tetany (calcium concentration in the blood is normal), but the characteristic skeletal deformities are present.

Figure 9.11 Pseudohypoparathyroidism:
(a) feet; (b) hands

(Figure 9.11(a) from FS McDonald, ed., *Mayo Clinic images in internal medicine*, with permission. © Mayo Clinic Scientific Press and CRC Press.)

Some syndromes associated with short stature

These conditions begin in childhood.

General inspection

First measure the height of the patient; in children this should be compared with percentile charts for age and sex. Look for the classical appearance of Turner's syndrome, Down syndrome, achondroplasia or rickets (Figure 9.12), which may explain the short stature. The height of parents and siblings should be checked as well.

Note any evidence of weight loss, including loose skinfolds, which may suggest a nutritional cause (starvation, malabsorption or protein loss). Look for signs of hypopituitarism or hypothyroidism, or steroid excess. Sexual precocity (early onset of secondary sexual characteristics) causes relative tallness at first but short stature later.

The chest

Examine for evidence of cyanotic congenital heart disease and pulmonary disease, such as cystic fibrosis.

The abdomen

Look for evidence of hepatic failure or renal failure.

Turner's syndrome (45XO)

Sexual infantalism—female genitalia.

Upper limbs. Lymphoedema of the hands; short fourth metacarpal bones; hyperplastic nails; increased carrying angle; hypertension.

Facies. Micrognathia (small chin); epicanthic folds ptosis; fish-like mouth; deformed or low-set ears; hearing loss.

Neck. Webbing of the neck; low hairline; redundant skinfolds on the back of the neck.

Chest. Widely spaced nipples (a shield-like chest); coarctation of the aorta.

Other. Pigmented naevi; keloid formation; lymphoedema of the legs.

Down syndrome (Trisomy 21)

Facies. Oblique orbital fissures; conjunctivitis; Brushfield spots on the iris; small simple ears; flat nasal bridge; mouth hanging open; protruding tongue; narrow high-arched palate.

Hands. Short broad hands; incurving fifth finger; single palmar crease; hyperflexible joints.

Chest. Congenital heart disease; especially endocardial cushion defects.

Other. Straight pubic hair; gaps between the first and second toes; mental deficiency usually present.

Rickets (Figure 9.12)

Defective mineralisation of the *growing* skeleton, due to lack of vitamin D (e.g. nutritional or chronic renal failure) or hypophosphataemia (e.g. renal tubular disorders).

Upper limbs. Tetany; hypotonia, proximal myopathy; bowing of the radius and ulna.

Facies. Frontal bossing; parietal flattening.

Figure 9.12 Rickets (postrachitic patient)
Look for frontal bossing, proximal myopathy of arms and thighs, and bowing of the ulna, femur and tibia.

Chest. 'Rickety rosary'—thickening of costochondral junctions; Harrison's groove—indentation of lower ribs at the diaphragmatic attachment.

Lower limbs. Bowing of femur and tibia; hypotonia, proximal myopathy; fractures.

Achondroplasia

This is an autosomal dominant disease of cartilage caused by mutation of the fibroblast growth factor receptor gene.

Short stature, short limbs, normal trunk, relatively large head, saddle-shaped nose, exaggerated lumbar lordosis and occasionally spinal cord compression are features.

Hirsutism

This is excessive hairiness in a woman beyond what is considered normal for her race (Table 9.15). In the examination of such a patient, it is important to decide whether virilisation is also present. Virilisation is the appearance of male secondary sexual characteristics (clitoromegaly, frontal hair recession, male body habitus and deepening of the voice) and indicates that excessive androgen is present.

General inspection

Ask the patient to undress to her underwear. Note the hair distribution over the face and in the midline,

Table 9.15 Causes of hirsutism

Polycystic ovary syndrome (commonest cause)
Adrenal: Cushing's syndrome, congenital adrenal hyperplasia, virilising tumour (more often a carcinoma than an adenoma)
Ovarian: tumour
Drugs: phenytoin, diazoxide, streptomycin, minoxidil, anabolic steroids
Other: acromegaly, porphyria cutanea tarda

front and back. In general, an obvious male balding pattern (a receding hairline), hair over the beard area or on the back and chest, and hair in the escutcheon (umbilicus to groin in the midline) is usually abnormal. Look for obvious acromegaly or Cushing's syndrome and for the skin changes of porphyria cutanea tarda (page 391).

Ask the patient to remove her underclothing and lie flat. Look for signs of virilism. These include breast atrophy and increased muscle bulk of the arms and legs, male pattern of pubic hair, and enlargement of the clitoris. Look in the axillae; the patient with polycystic ovarian syndrome may have acanthosis nigricans (and associated insulin resistance).

The abdomen

Palpate for adrenal masses, polycystic ovaries or an ovarian tumour (these are rarely palpable).

The blood pressure

Hypertension occurs in the rare C11-hydroxylase deficiency, which is a virilising condition.

Gynaecomastia

This is 'true' enlargement of the male breasts.[4] Virtually no breast tissue is palpable in normal men. Remember that gynaecomastia occurs in up to 50% of adolescent boys, and also in elderly men in whom it is due to falling testosterone levels. Fat deposition ('false' enlargement) in obese men can be confused with gynaecomastia.

Examine the breasts (page 122) for evidence of localised disease (e.g. malignancy, which is rare), tenderness, which indicates rapid growth, and any discharge from the nipple.

Note the general body habitus, looking especially for *Klinefelter's syndrome* (47,XXY). These

Table 9.16 Causes of pathological gynaecomastia

Increased oestrogen production

Leydig cell tumour (oestrogen)
Adrenal carcinoma (oestrogen)
Bronchial carcinoma (human chorionic
  gonadotrophin)
Liver disease (increased conversion of oestrogen
  from androgens)
Thyrotoxicosis (increased conversion of
  oestrogen from androgens)
Starvation

**Decreased androgen production
(hypogonadal states)**

Klinefelter's syndrome
Secondary testicular failure: orchitis, castration,
  trauma

Testicular feminisation syndrome

Drugs

Oestrogen receptor binders: oestrogen, digoxin,
  marijuana
Anti-androgens: spironolactone, cimetidine

Table 9.17 Causes of diabetes mellitus

Criteria for diagnosis of diabetes mellitus: fasting plasma venous blood sugar level of 7.0 mmol/L or more (≥126 mg/dL), or a 2-hour postprandial blood sugar level of 11.1 mmol/L or more (≥200 mg/dL), on more than one occasion.

I. Type 1 (absolute insulin deficiency)

II. Type 2 (insulin deficiency and resistance)

III. Other types of diabetes

  A. Mutations leading to abnormalities of β cell function

  B. Inherited defects of insulin action: e.g. lipoatrophic diabetes (characterised by generalised lipoatrophy, hepatomegaly, hirsutism, acanthosis nigricans, hyperpigmentation and hyperlipidaemia)

  C. Diseases of the exocrine pancreas: e.g. chronic pancreatitis, carcinoma, haemochromatosis

  D. Endocrine abnormalities: e.g. acromegaly, Cushing's syndrome, phaeochromocytoma, glucagonoma

  E. Drug induced: e.g. steroids, the contraceptive pill, streptozotocin, diazoxide, phenytoin, thiazide diuretics

  F. Infections: e.g. cytomegalovirus, coxsackie, congenital rubella

  G. Rare forms of immune-mediated diabetes: e.g. anti-insulin receptor antibodies

  H. Genetic abnormalities associates with diabetes: e.g. Down's syndrome, Klinefelter's syndrome, Turner's syndrome

IV. Gestational diabetes mellitus

patients are tall, have decreased body hair and characteristically small, firm testes.

Look also for signs of panhypopituitarism or chronic liver disease (page 167). Thyrotoxicosis can occasionally be a cause.

Examine the genitalia now for sexual ambiguity and the testes for absence or a reduced size. Note any loss of secondary sexual characteristics.

Finally, examine the visual fields and fundi for evidence of a pituitary tumour.

Causes of pathological gynaecomastia are summarised in Table 9.16.

Diabetes mellitus[n]

Diabetes mellitus is characterised by hyperglycaemia due to an absolute or relative deficiency of insulin.

---

[n] This disease was called diabetes by ancient Greek and Roman physicians because the word diabetes means a siphon, referring to the large urine volume. Rather courageously, they distinguished diabetes mellitus from diabetes insipidus by the sweet taste of the urine: *mellitus*, 'sweet'; *insipidus*, 'tasteless'.

The causes of diabetes are listed in Table 9.17. The disease can present with asymptomatic glycosuria detected on routine physical examination or with symptoms of diabetes (Table 9.1), ranging from polyuria to coma as a result of diabetic ketoacidosis.

General inspection (Figure 9.13)

Assess for evidence of dehydration (page 21) because the osmotic diuresis caused by a glucose load in the urine can cause massive fluid loss. Note obesity

Lying

1. General inspection
Weight—obesity
Hydration
Endocrine facies
Pigmentation—haemochromatosis,
etc

2. Legs
Inspect
- Skin—necrobiosis, hair loss,
infection, pigmented scars,
atrophy, ulceration, injection
sites
Muscle wasting
Palpate
- Temperature of feet (cold, blue
due to 'small' or 'large' vessel
disease)
- Peripheral pulses
Femoral (auscultate)
Popliteal
Posterior tibial
Dorsalis pedis

3. Arms
Inspect
- Injection sites
- Skin lesions
Pulse

4. Eyes
Fundi—cataracts, rubeosis,
retinal disease
III nerve palsy, etc

5. Mouth
Monilia
Infection

6. Neck
Carotid arteries—palpate,
auscultate

7. Chest
Signs of infection

8. Abdomen
Liver—fat infiltration; rarely
haemochromatosis
Neurological assessment
- Femoral nerve mononeuritis
- Peripheral neuropathy

9. Other
Urine analysis—glycosuria,
ketones, proteinuria
Blood pressure—lying and
standing
Oedema

Figure 9.13 Diabetes mellitus

(non-insulin-dependent diabetics are usually obese) or signs of recent weight loss (this can be evidence of uncontrolled glycosuria).

Look for one of the abnormal endocrine facies (e.g. Cushing's syndrome or acromegaly) and for pigmentation (e.g. haemochromatosis—bronze diabetes) as these may cause secondary diabetes.

The patient may be comatose due to dehydra-tion, acidosis or plasma hyperosmolality. Kuss-maul's breathing ('air hunger') (page 97) is present in diabetic ketoacidosis due to the acidosis (this occurs because fat metabolism is increased to com-pensate for the lack of availability of glucose; excess acetyl-CoA is produced, which is converted in the liver to ketone bodies, and two of these are organic acids).

The lower limbs

Unlike most other systematic examinations, assessment of the diabetic can profitably begin with the legs, as many of the major physical signs are found to be here. In particular, vascular and neurological abnormalities in the feet must not be missed.[5]

Inspection. Look at the skin. The *skin* of the feet and lower legs may be hairless and atrophied due to small vessel vascular disease and resultant ischaemia (the mechanism is uncertain, but may be related to lipoprotein alterations in the vessel walls). Note any leg *ulcers*, particularly on the toes or any area of the feet exposed to pressure. These ulcers are due to a combination of ischaemia and peripheral neuropathy (the cause of the neuropathy is unknown, but may be related to small vessel ischaemia and glycosylation of neural proteins). Look for superficial skin *infection*, such as boils, cellulitis and fungal infections. These are more common in diabetics because of a combination of high tissue glucose levels and ischaemia, which provides a favourable environment for the growth of organisms. Note any *pigmented scars* (late diabetic dermopathy). There may be small rounded plaques with raised borders lying in a linear fashion over the shins (diabetic dermopathy).

Necrobiosis lipoidica diabeticorum is a reasonably specific skin manifestation of diabetes mellitus, but is rare (fewer than 1% of diabetics) (Figure 9.15). It is found over the shins, where a central yellow scarred area is surrounded by a red margin when the condition is active. These plaques may ulcerate (Figure 9.15).

Look now at the thighs for insulin injection sites. These may be associated with localised *fat atrophy* and *fat hypertrophy*, and may be related to impure insulin use which causes a localised immune reaction. Note any *quadriceps muscle wasting* due to femoral nerve mononeuropathy, which is called (inaccurately) diabetic amyotrophy.

Inspect the knees for the very rare Charcot's joints (grossly deformed disorganised joints, due to loss of proprioception or pain, or both; this leads to recurrent and unnoticed injury to the joint) (Figure 9.16).

Figure 9.15 Necrobiosis lipoidica diabeticorum

(From FS McDonald, ed., *Mayo Clinic images in internal medicine*, with permission. © Mayo Clinic Scientific Press and CRC Press.)

Figure 9.14 Diabetic (neuropathic) ulcer

(From FS McDonald, ed., *Mayo Clinic images in internal medicine*, with permission. © Mayo Clinic Scientific Press and CRC Press.)

Figure 9.16 Charcot's joint of left knee

Note: This is very rare.

Palpation. Palpate any injection sites for fat atrophy or hypertrophy. Feel all the peripheral pulses and the temperature of the feet, and test the capillary return. Absent peripheral pulses, cold extremities and reduced capillary return are all evidence of peripheral vascular disease.

Neurological examination. Assess formally for peripheral neuropathy, including dorsal column loss (diabetic pseudotabes), and tap the reflexes. Test proximal muscle power (diabetic amyotrophy).

The upper limbs

Look at the nails for signs of *Candida* infection. Inspect and feel for injection sites over the upper arms. Take the blood pressure lying and standing, as diabetic autonomic neuropathy can cause postural hypotension.

The face

The eyes. Test visual acuity. This may be permanently impaired because of retinal disease or temporarily disturbed because of changes in the shape of the lens associated with hyperglycaemia and water retention. Look for Argyll Robertson pupils[o], which are a rare complication of diabetes.

Using the ophthalmoscope, begin by examining for rubeosis (new blood vessel formation over the iris, which can cause glaucoma) (Figure 9.17). Then note any cataracts, which are related to sorbitol deposition in the lens (when glucose is present in high concentrations in the tissues it is converted to sorbitol by aldose reductase).

Now examine the retina, where many exciting changes await the fundoscopist. There are two main types of retinal change in diabetes, non-proliferative and proliferative.

Non-proliferative changes (Figure 9.18) are directly related to ischaemia of blood vessels and include: (i) two types of haemorrhages—*dot haemorrhages,* which occur in the inner retinal layers, and *blot haemorrhages,* which are larger and which occur more superficially in the nerve fibre layer; (ii) *microaneurysms,* which are due to vessel wall damage; and (iii) two types of exudates—*hard exudates,* which have straight edges, and *soft exudates* (cottonwool spots), which have a fluffy appearance.

Proliferative changes (Figure 9.19) are changes in blood vessels in response to ischaemia of the

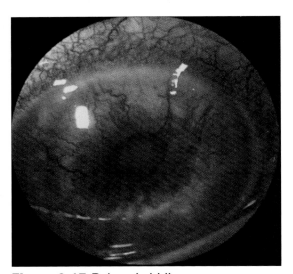

Figure 9.17 Rubeosis iridis
Shows new vessels on the anterior surface of the iris. These are secondary to ischaemia (often due to diabetes).

retina. They are characterised by new vessel formation, which can lead to vitreal haemorrhage, scar formation and eventually retinal detachment. The *detached retina* appears as an opalescent sheet that balloons forwards into the vitreous. The underlying choroid is visible through the detached retina as a bright red-coloured sheet. Look also for *laser scars* (small brown or yellow spots), which are secondary to photocoagulation of new vessels by laser therapy.

Assess the third, fourth and sixth cranial nerves. In particular examine for a diabetic third nerve palsy from ischaemia, which usually spares the pupil (as infarction of the third nerve affects the inner pupillary fibres more than the outer fibres; in this way it differs from compressive lesions, which have the opposite effect).

Other cranial nerves may be affected sometimes because of cerebrovascular accidents (large vessel atheroma). *Rhinocerebral mucormycosis* may rarely develop in very poorly controlled diabetic patients, causing periorbital and perinasal swelling and cranial nerve palsies.

The ears. Look in the ears for evidence of infection. The rare *malignant otitis externa,* usually due to *Pseudomonas aeruginosa,* causes a mound of granulation tissue in the external canal, and facial nerve palsy in 50%.

The mouth. Look for evidence of *Candida* infection.

---

[o] Douglas Argyll Robertson (1837–1909), a Scottish ophthalmic surgeon and President of the Royal College of Surgeons, described these in 1869. The pupils are small, irregular and unequal, and react briskly to accommodation but not to light. Tertiary syphilis is another cause (page 301).

Figure 9.18 Diabetic retinopathy

(a) Soft exudate (arrow) and small haemorrhages. (b) Microaneurysms (dots), retinal haemorrhages (blots) and hard yellow exudates.

Figure 9.19 Proliferative diabetic retinopathy

The neck and shoulders

Examine the carotid arteries for evidence of vascular disease.

Rarely there may be thickening of the skin of the upper back and shoulders (scleroedema diabeticorum—this diffuse cutaneous infiltration has a very different distribution from scleroderma, with which it is sometimes confused). Look for acanthosis nigricans—associated with insulin resistance.

The abdomen

Palpate for hepatomegaly (fatty infiltration, or due to haemochromatosis).

Urinalysis

Test for glucose and protein. Diabetic nephropathy (from glomerulonephritis, renal arterial disease or pyelonephritis) can cause proteinuria. The presence of nitrite and/or blood is of value as asymptomatic urinary tract infections can occur. In advanced disease there may be signs of renal failure.

Paget's[P] disease (osteitis deformans)

This disease is characterised by excessive reabsorption of bone by osteoclasts and compensatory disorganised deposition of new bone. It is possibly a disease of viral origin.

General inspection

Note short stature (due to bending of the long bones of the limbs) and any obvious deformity of the head and lower limbs.

Head and face

Inspect the scalp for enlargement in the frontal and parietal areas and measure the head circumference (greater than 55 cm is usually abnormal). There may be prominent skull veins. Palpate for increased bony warmth and auscultate over the skull for systolic bruits. Both of these are due to increased vascularity of the skull vault. Oddly enough bronchial breath sounds may be audible over the pagetic skull through the stethoscope. These are due to increased bone conduction of air. An area of very localised bony swelling and warmth may indicate development of a bony

---

[P] Sir James Paget (1814–99), a surgeon at St Bartholomew's Hospital, London, was also Queen Victoria's doctor.

sarcoma (1% of cases of Paget's disease may develop this complication).

Examine the eyes. Assess visual acuity and visual fields, and look in the fundi for angioid streaks (page 267) and optic atrophy. Retinitis pigmentosa occurs rather more rarely (page 300). Test for hearing loss (due to bony ossicle involvement or eighth nerve compression by bony enlargement).

Examine the remaining cranial nerves (page 293); all may be involved because of bony overgrowth of the foramina or be caused by basilar invagination (platybasia; where the posterior fossa becomes flat and the basal angle increased).

The neck

Patients with basilar invagination have a short neck and low hairline. The head is held in extension and neck movements are decreased. Assess the jugular venous pressure, as a high output cardiac failure may be present, particularly if there is coexistent ischaemic heart disease.

The heart

Examine for signs of cardiac failure.

The back

Inspect for kyphosis (due to vertebral involvement causing collapse of the vertebral bodies). Tap for localised tenderness, feel for warmth and auscultate for systolic bruits over the vertebral bodies.

Figure 9.20 Paget's disease, showing bowing of the tibia

The legs

Inspect for anterior bowing of the tibia and lateral bowing of the femur (Figure 9.20). Feel for bony warmth and tenderness. Note any changes of osteoarthritis in the hips and knees, which often coexist with Paget's disease. Note any localised warm swelling, which may indicate sarcoma.

Examine for evidence of paraplegia (page 350), which is uncommon but can occur due to cord compression by bone or vascular shunting in the spinal cord. Cerebellar signs may rarely be present due to platybasia.

Urinalysis

Check for blood (there is an increased incidence of renal stones in Paget's disease).

Summary

The endocrine system: a suggested method of examination (Figure 9.21)

Inspect the patient for one of the diagnostic facies or body habituses. If the diagnosis is obvious, proceed with the specific examination outlined previously. If not, examine as follows.

Pick up the hands. Look at the overall size (acromegaly), length of the metacarpals (pseudo-hypoparathyroidism and pseudopseudohypoparathyroidism), for abnormalities of the nails (hyperthyroidism and hypothyroidism, and hypoparathyroidism), tremor, palmar erythema and sweating of the palms (hyperthyroidism).

Take the pulse (thyroid disease) and the blood pressure (hypertension in Cushing's syndrome, or postural hypotension in Addison's disease). Look for Trousseau's sign (tetany). Test for proximal muscle weakness (thyroid disease, Cushing's syndrome).

Go to the axillae. Look for loss of axillary hair (hypopituitarism), or acanthosis nigricans and skin tags (acromegaly).

Examine the eyes (hyperthyroidism) and the fundi (diabetes, acromegaly). Look at the face for hirsutism, or fine-wrinkled hairless skin (panhypopituitarism). Note any skin greasiness, acne or plethora (Cushing's syndrome).

Look at the mouth for protrusion of the chin and enlargement of the tongue (acromegaly) or buccal pigmentation (Addison's disease).

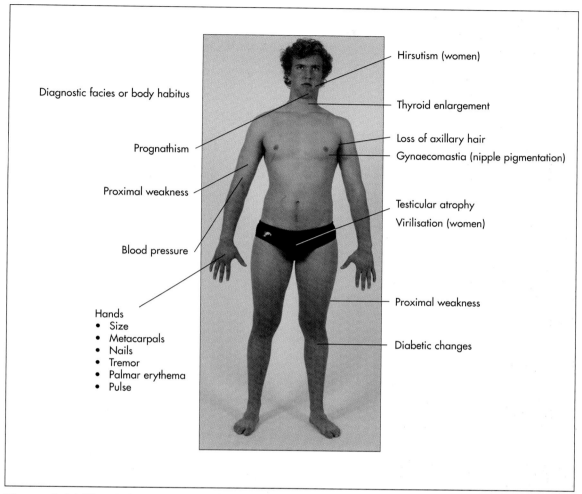

Figure 9.21 The endocrine examination

Examine the neck for thyroid enlargement. Note any neck webbing (Turner's syndrome). Palpate for supraclavicular fat pads (Cushing's syndrome).

Inspect the chest wall for hirsutism or loss of body hair, reduction in breast size in women (panhypopituitarism) or gynaecomastia in men. Look for nipple pigmentation (Addison's disease).

Examine the abdomen for hirsutism, central fat deposition, purple striae (Cushing's syndrome) and the external genitalia for virilisation or atrophy. Look at the legs for diabetic changes.

Measure the body weight and height, and examine the urine.

References

1. Alvi A, Johnson JT. The neck mass. A challenging differential diagnosis. *Postgrad Med* 1995; 97:87–90, 93–94. Reviews how the history and examination narrow the differential diagnosis.
2. Siminoski K. Does this patient have a goiter? *JAMA* 1995; 273:813–817. A guide to examining the thyroid.
3. Wallace C, Siminoski K. The Pemberton sign. *Ann Intern Med* 1996; 125:568–569. Describes the sign, due to a retrosternal goitre compressing cephalic venous inflow (and in some tracheal airflow).
4. Braunstein GD. Gynecomastia. *N Engl J Med* 1993; 328:490–495. A good review.

5. Edelson GW, Armstrong DG, Lavery LA, Ciacco G. The acutely infected diabetic foot is not adequately evaluated in an inpatient setting. *Arch Intern Med* 1996; 156:2372–2378. All patients evaluated had undergone a less than adequate foot examination. Of admitted patients, 31% did not have their pedal pulses documented; 60% of the admitted patients were not evaluated for the presence or absence of protective sensation.

Suggested reading

Original and review articles

Bull RH, Coburn PR, Mortimer PS. Pretibial myxoedema: a manifestation of lymphoedema? *Lancet* 1993; 341:403–404.

Clark CM, Lee DA. Prevention and treatment of the complications of diabetes mellitus. *N Engl J Med* 1995; 332:1210–1217.

Hegedus L. Clinical practice. The thyroid nodule. *N Engl J Med* 2004;351:1764–1771.

Utiger RD. Pathogenesis of Graves' ophthalmopathy. *N Engl J Med* 1992; 326:1772–1773.

Textbooks

Besser GM, Thorner MO. *Comprehensive clinical endocrinology*, 3rd edn. Edinburgh: Mosby-Wolfe, 2002.

Greenspan FS, Gardner DG, eds. *Basic and clinical endocrinology*, 7th edn. New York: Lange Medical/ McGraw Hill, 2004.

Hall R, Evered D, Greene R. *Color atlas of endocrinology*, 2nd edn. Chicago: Mosby-Year Book, 1990.

Larsen PR, Kronenberg HM, Melmed S, Polonsky KS. *Williams textbook of endocrinology*, 10th edn. Philadelphia: Saunders, 2003.

chapter 10

The nervous system

Who could have foretold, from the structure of the brain, that wine could derange its functions?

Hippocrates (460–375 BC)

The neurological history

The neurological history begins in detail with the presenting problem or problems (Table 10.1). The patient should be allowed to describe the symptoms in his or her own words to begin with, and then the clinician needs to ask questions to clarify information and obtain more detail. It is particularly important to ascertain the *temporal course of the illness*, as this may give important information about the underlying aetiology.

An acute onset of symptoms (within minutes to an hour) is suggestive of a vascular or convulsive problem (e.g. the explosive severe headache of subarachnoid haemorrhage or the rapid onset of a seizure). For these episodes of sudden onset, a precipitating event (e.g. exercise) or warning (*aura*) may be present. The aura that precedes a seizure may be localising (e.g. auditory hallucinations, an unusual smell or taste, loss of speech, or motor changes) or non-localising (e.g. a feeling of apprehension). The occurrence of an aura followed by sudden unconsciousness is very suggestive of the diagnosis of a major seizure or complex partial seizure.

The sudden onset of weakness on one side of the body followed by resolution and a severe headache is characteristic of hemiplegic migraine. Sudden resolution without headache suggests a transient ischaemic episode. The very gradual onset of muscle weakness suggests a muscle abnormality such as myopathy rather than a vascular event.

A subacute onset (hours to days) occurs with inflammatory disorders (e.g. meningitis, cerebral abscess or the Guillain-Barré[a] syndrome—acute inflammatory polyradiculoneuropathy).

A more chronic symptom course suggests that the underlying disorder may be related to either a tumour (weeks to months) or a degenerative process (months to years). Metabolic or toxic disorders may present with any of these time courses.

Based on the history (and physical examination), a judgment is made as to whether the disease process is *localised or diffuse*, and which *levels of the nervous system* are involved (the nervous system may be thought of as having four different levels: the peripheral nervous system, the spinal cord, the posterior fossa, and the cerebral hemispheres). Consideration of the time course and the levels of involvement will usually lead to a logical differential diagnosis of the patient's symptoms.

Headache and facial pain

Headache is a very common symptom. It is important, as with any type of pain, to determine the character, severity, site, duration, frequency, radiation, aggravating and relieving factors and associated symptoms.[1,2] Unilateral headache that is preceded by flashing lights or zig-zag lines and is associated with

---

[a] Georges Guillain (1876–1961), Jean Alexandre Barré (1880–1967) and A Strohl described the syndrome in 1916; Strohl's name was dropped because of anti-German feeling during World War I.

Table 10.1 Neurological history

Presenting symptoms*

Headache, back or neck pain
Facial pain
Fits, faints or funny turns
Dizziness or vertigo
Disturbances of vision, hearing or smell
Disturbances of gait
Loss of or disturbed sensation, or weakness in
    limb(s)
Disturbances of sphincter control (bladder,
    bowels)
Involuntary movements or tremor
Speech and swallowing disturbance
Altered cognition

Risk factors for cerebrovascular disease

Hypertension
Smoking
Diabetes mellitus
Hyperlipidaemia
Atrial fibrillation, bacterial endocarditis,
    myocardial infarction (emboli)
Haematological disease
Family history of stroke

* Note particularly the temporal course of the illness,
  whether symptoms suggest focal or diffuse disease, and
  the likely level of involvement of the nervous system.

light hurting the eyes (photophobia) is likely to be a *migraine with an aura* ('classical migraine'). Pain over one eye lasting for minutes to hours, associated with lacrimation, rhinorrhoea and flushing of the forehead, and occurring in bouts that last several weeks a few times a year or less, is suggestive of *cluster headache*. This occurs predominantly in males. Headache over the occiput and associated with neck stiffness may be from *cervical spondylosis*.

A generalised headache that is worse in the morning and is associated with drowsiness or vomiting may reflect *raised intracranial pressure*, while generalised headache associated with photophobia and fever as well as with a stiff neck of more gradual onset may be due to *meningitis*. A persistent unilateral headache over the temporal area associated with tenderness over the temporal artery and blurring of vision suggests *temporal arteritis*.[3,4] This condition (Table 10.2) is often associated with jaw claudication, or jaw pain during eating, which can lead to considerable loss of weight. Headache with pain or fullness behind the eyes or over the cheeks

or forehead occurs in *acute sinusitis*. The dramatic and usually instantaneous onset of severe headache that is initially localised but becomes generalised and is associated with neck stiffness may be due to a *subarachnoid haemorrhage*.

Finally, the most frequent type of headache is episodic or chronic *tension-type headache*; this is commonly bilateral, occurs over the frontal, occipital or temporal areas, and may be described as a sensation of tightness that lasts for hours and recurs often. There are usually no associated symptoms such as nausea, vomiting, weakness or paraesthesiae (tingling in the limbs), and the headache does not usually wake the patient at night from sleep.

Pain in the face can result from trigeminal neuralgia (page 307), temporomandibular arthritis (page 232), glaucoma (page 297), cluster headache, temporal arteritis, psychiatric disease, aneurysm of the internal carotid or posterior communicating artery, or the superior orbital fissure syndrome (page 306).

Faints and fits (see also page 30)

It is important to try to differentiate syncope (transient loss of consciousness) from *epilepsy*. However, primary syncopal events can cause a few clonic jerks in a significant number of cases. With generalised tonic-clonic seizures (grand mal epilepsy) there is abrupt loss of consciousness, which may be preceded by an aura. Often the patient is incontinent of urine and faeces, and the tongue may be bitten. A witness may be able to describe the type of attack that occurred. It is important to try to determine whether any seizure is generalised or localised to one side of the body: a seizure affecting part of the body may indicate a focal lesion in the central nervous system such as a tumour or abscess. If consciousness is impaired, these partial seizures are described as 'complex'; if consciousness is unimpaired they are termed 'simple'. Idiopathic absence seizures ('petit mal') occur in children. These are frequent brief episodes of loss of awareness often associated with staring. Major motor movements do not occur with this type of epilepsy.

Transient ischaemic attacks affecting the brainstem can occasionally cause blackouts. Use of the term 'drop attacks' means the patient falls but there is no loss of consciousness. In either case the patient falls to the ground without premonition and the attacks are of brief duration. *Hypoglycaemia* can lead to episodes of loss of consciousness. Patients with hypoglycaemia may also report sweating, weakness and confusion before losing consciousness. Bizarre attacks of loss of consciousness occur with *hysteria*.[b] During such attacks the patient may slump

Table 10.2 Symptoms and signs of temporal arteritis

Symptoms	Frequency (%)	Positive LR	Negative LR
Headache often present for 2 or 3 months	77	1.5	0.82
Jaw claudication (pain in proximal jaw near TMJ after brief chewing of tough food)	51	4.2	0.72
Malaise	48	1.2	0.94
Polymyalgia rheumatica (shoulder girdle pain and stiffness)	34	0.97	0.99
Visual disturbance (often sudden monocular blindness)	29	0.85	1.2
Examination findings			
Fever	26	–	–
Tender temporal artery (palpated just anterior and superior to the tragus of the ear).	53	2.6	0.82
Enlarged temporal artery		4.3	0.67
There can be ischaemic changes of the tongue or scalp.			

TMJ = temporomandibular joint.

to the ground without sustaining any injury and there may be apparent fluctuations in the level of consciousness for a prolonged period.

Dizziness

If a patient complains of dizziness, it is important to determine what is meant by this term. In true *vertigo*, there is actually a sense of motion, usually of the surroundings but also of the head itself (page 30).[5] When vertigo is severe it may not be possible for the patient to stand or walk, and associated symptoms of nausea, vomiting, pallor, sweating and headache may be present. 'Peripheral vestibular lesions' including benign positioning vertigo, vestibular neuronitis and acute labyrinthitis can cause vertigo; there is usually no deafness or ringing in the ears (tinnitus) in such cases. Other causes of vertigo include:

- ototoxic drugs (e.g. aminoglycosides), associated with deafness or tinnitus;
- Ménière's disease,[c] which occurs in those over 50 years of age and presents with the triad of episodic vertigo and tinnitus with progressive deafness;
- acoustic neuroma (where patients may also have deafness and tinnitus);
- central causes such as vertebrobasilar transient ischaemic attacks—these may be associated with diplopia (double vision), visual loss and ataxia; and
- rarely, internal auditory artery occlusion.

Visual disturbances and deafness

Problems with vision can include double vision (diplopia), blurred vision (amblyopia), light intolerance (photophobia) and visual loss (page 297). The causes of deafness are summarised on page 313.

Disturbances of gait

Many neurological conditions can make walking difficult. These are described on page 344. Walking may also be abnormal when orthopaedic disease affects the lower limbs or spine. A bizarrely abnormal gait can sometimes be a sign of a hysterical reaction.

Disturbed sensation or weakness in the limbs

Pins and needles in the hands or feet may indicate nerve entrapment or a peripheral neuropathy (page 348) but can result from sensory pathway involvement at any level. The carpal tunnel syndrome is common; here there is median nerve entrapment,

[b] Hysteria is an old but still popular term that refers to a presumed psychogenic condition.

[c] Prosper Ménière (1799–1862), director of the Paris Institution for Deaf-Mutes, characterised this condition just before he died of post-influenzal pneumonia. He was an expert on orchids and a friend of Victor Hugo and Honoré de Balzac. He added the grave accent on the second 'e' in his name himself; the acute accent on the first 'e' was added by his son.

and patients experience pain and paraesthesiae in the hand and wrist. Sometimes pain may extend to the arm and even to the shoulder, but paraesthesiae are felt only in the fingers. These symptoms are usually worse at night and may be relieved by dangling the arm over the side of the bed or shaking the hand.

Nerve root, spinal cord and cerebral abnormalities can all cause disturbance of sensation and weakness.

Limb weakness can be caused by lesions at different levels in the motor system. There are a number of patterns of limb and muscle weakness:

- Upper motor neurone (UMN) weakness (page 322) is due to interruption of a neural pathway at a level above the anterior horn cell. The result is an increase in tone and peripheral reflexes. Interruption of this pathway has the greatest effect on the antigravity muscles and is called *pyramidal weakness*. There is little or no muscle wasting.
- Lower motor neurone (LMN) weakness (page 348) is due to a lesion that interrupts the reflex arc between the anterior horn cell and the muscle. There is a reduction in tone and reflexes, fasciculation (irregular contractions of small areas of muscle) may be seen and muscle wasting is prominent.
- Muscle disease causes weakness in a particular muscle or group of muscles. There is wasting, decreased tone, and the reflexes are reduced or absent.
- Disease at the neuromuscular junction (e.g. myasthenia gravis, page 356) causes generalised weakness, which worsens with repetition. The reflexes and tone are often normal.
- Non-organic weakness (e.g. due to hysteria) causes a non-anatomical pattern of weakness in association with normal tone and power and, unless there has been prolonged disuse, normal muscle bulk.

Tremor and involuntary movements

Tremor is a rhythmical movement (Table 10.3). A slow tremor has, by definition, a rate between 3 Hz and 5 Hz. Rapid tremors are faster than 10 Hz. *Resting* tremors are present mostly during relaxation of the muscles, while *intention* tremors occur with deliberate movement and become more pronounced towards the end of the action. Tremors become worse with fatigue or anxiety. Shivering is a type of tremor brought on by cold. It is normal for there to be a fine tremor associated with holding a posture or per-

Table 10.3 Rates of tremors

Parkinson's disease	3 to 5 Hz
Essential/familial	4 to 7 Hz
Physiological	8 to 13 Hz

forming a movement slowly. This is called a *physiological* tremor. It becomes more obvious with fright and fatigue. It is often increased by the beta-agonist drugs used to treat asthma. Thyrotoxicosis is a cause of exaggeration of physiological tremor. These movements are very fine and may be difficult to see unless looked for specifically. *Benign essential (familial)* tremor is an inherited disorder which causes tremor, but no other signs. The tremor is most easily seen when the patient's arms are stretched out; it can become worse during voluntary movements. It usually disappears when the muscles are at complete rest. Parkinson's disease[d] may present with a resting tremor (page 360). Intention (or target-seeking) tremor is due to cerebellar disease (page 357). *Chorea* involves involuntary jerky movements (page 362). Definitions of the terms used to describe movement disorders are shown in Table 10.4.

Speech and mental status

Speech may be disturbed by many different neurological diseases and is discussed on page 288. A number of different diseases can also result in delirium or dementia, as described on page 288 and in Chapter 11.

Past health

Inquire about a past history of meningitis or encephalitis, head or spinal injuries, a history of epilepsy or convulsions and any previous operations. Any past history of sexually transmitted disease (e.g. risk factors for HIV infection or syphilis) should be obtained. Treatment with anticonvulsants, the contraceptive pill, antihypertensive agents, steroids, anticoagulants, antiplatelet agents or drugs for other disorders needs to be documented. Ask about risk factors that may predispose to the development of cerebrovascular disease (Table 10.1). A previous diagnosis of peripheral vascular disease or

---

[d] James Parkinson (1755–1824), English general practitioner, published an essay on 'The Shaking Palsy' in 1817. He was nearly transported to Australia for reformist activities.

Table 10.4 Definitions of terms used to describe movement disorders.

Akithesia	Motor restlessness; constant semi-purposeful movements of the arms and legs
Asterixis	Sudden loss of muscle tone during sustained contraction of an outstretched limb
Athetosis	Writhing, slow sinuous movements, especially of the hands and wrists
Chorea	Jerky small rapid movements, often disguised by the patient with a purposeful final movement: e.g the jerky upward arm movement is transformed into a voluntary movement to scratch the head
Dyskinesia	Purposeless and continuous movements, often of the face and mouth; often a result of treatment with major tranquillisers for psychotic illness
Dystonia	Sustained contractions of groups of agonist and antagonist muscles, usually in flexion or extremes of extension; it results in bizarre postures
Hemiballismus	An exaggerated form of chorea involving one side of the body: there are wild flinging movements which can injure the patient (or bystanders)
Myoclonic jerk	A brief muscle contraction which causes a sudden purposeless jerking of a limb
Myokymia	A repeated contraction of a small muscle group; often involves the orbicularis oculi muscles
Tic	A repetitive irresistible movement which is purposeful or semi-purposeful
Tremor	A rhythmical alternating movement

of coronary artery disease indicates an increased risk of cerebrovascular disease. Chronic or frequent paroxysmal atrial fibrillation is associated with a greatly increased risk of embolic stroke.

Social history

As smoking predisposes to cerebrovascular disease, the smoking history is relevant. It is useful to ask about occupation and exposure to toxins (e.g. heavy metals). Alcohol can also result in a number of neurological diseases (see Table 1.3).

Family history

Any history of neurological or mental disease should be documented.

The neurological examination

As a preliminary to the neurological assessment, the clinician should obtain some biographical information from the patient, including the age, place of birth, handedness (page 288), occupation and level of education.

The examination of the nervous system and the interpretation of findings require a lot of practice. In a viva voce examination, this system more than any other system requires a polished technique. The signs need to be elicited carefully because the precise anatomical localisation of any lesions can often be determined this way. It is important, therefore, to remember some elementary neuroanatomy.

Examination can be long and difficult and it is said to take much of a day if absolutely everything that can be done (including psychometric assessment) is done. This is obviously impractical, but a screening examination that will uncover most signs takes only a relatively short time.

In brief, the following aspects of the examination must be attended to:

1   General, including examination for neck stiffness, assessment of the higher centres, speech, and abnormal movements.
2   The cranial nerves II to XII.
3   The upper limbs. Motor system: inspection, tone, power, reflexes, coordination. Sensory system: pinprick sensation, proprioception, vibration sense, light touch.

4   The lower limbs: as for the upper limbs, but including assessment of walking (gait).
5   The skull and spine for local disease.
6   The carotid arteries for bruits.

General signs

Consciousness

Note the level of consciousness. If the patient is unconscious look for responses to various stimuli (page 363).

Neck stiffness

Any patient with an acute neurological illness or who is febrile must be assessed for signs of meningism.[6]

With the patient lying flat in bed, the examiner slips a hand under the occiput and gently flexes the neck passively (i.e. without assistance from the patient). The chin is brought up to approach the chest wall. Meningism may be caused by pyogenic or other infection of the meninges, or by blood in the subarachnoid space secondary to subarachnoid haemorrhage. There is resistance to neck flexion due to painful spasm of the extensor muscles of the neck. Other causes of resistance to neck flexion are characterised by an equal resistance to head rotation. They include: (i) cervical spondylosis; (ii) after cervical fusion; (iii) Parkinson's disease; and (iv) raised intracranial pressure, especially if there is impending tonsillar herniation.

Kernig's sign[e] should also be elicited if meningitis is suspected. Flex each hip in turn, then attempt to straighten the knee while keeping the hip flexed. This is greatly limited by spasm of the hamstrings (which in turn causes pain) when there is meningism due to an inflammatory exudate around the lumbar spinal roots.

Although the diagnostic value has been questioned (combined meningeal signs had a positive LR of 0.92 and a negative LR of 0.88),[6] we have found these signs useful clinically and the quality of the data remains suboptimal.

Higher centres and speech

Handedness

Shake the patient's hand and ask if he or she is right- or left-handed. This is polite and allows the examiner to assess the likely dominant hemisphere. Ninety-four per cent of right-handed people and about 50% of left-handed people have a dominant

left hemisphere. There is division of function between the two hemispheres, the most obvious distinction being that the dominant hemisphere controls language and mathematical functions.

Orientation

Test orientation in *person*, *place* and *time* by asking the patient his or her name, present location and the date (normal patients who have been in hospital for long periods often get the day wrong as one day seems very much like another in hospital). Disorientation is not a specific localising sign and may be acute and reversible (delirium) or chronic and irreversible (dementia). The mini-mental state examination (Table 11.5) is a useful way to document the progress of a confusional state or dementia over time.

Speech

At this stage dysarthria (difficulty with articulation), dysphonia (altered quality of the voice with reduction in volume as a result of vocal cord disease) or dysphasia (dominant higher centre disorder in the use of symbols for communication—language) may be obvious. If not, before going on to compartmentalised tests, the clinician should get the patient to talk freely—*propositional* or *free* speech. In a normal clinical encounter this comes from history taking. In viva voce or observed standardised clinical examinations (OSCEs), ask the patient to describe the room, his or her clothes, or job or daily activities, in order to promote flowing speech. Then test *comprehension*. This is done first without eliciting language—for example, 'Touch your chin, then your nose and then your ear'; and then with yes and no questions—for example, 'Do you put your shoes on before your socks?' Then test *repetition*—for example, 'Repeat the phrase "no ifs, ands or buts"'.

To complete the screening, ask the patient to *name two objects* pointed at, and to *say a phrase* such as 'British Constitution' or 'West Register St' (page 358).

There is no need to examine further if no abnormality of speech is detected in this way.

If there is an abnormality, proceed as outlined in Table 10.5.

Dysphasia. There are four main types of dysphasia:[7] receptive, expressive, nominal and conductive. The expressive aphasias are forms of motor *apraxia*. This means the inability to perform deliberate actions in the absence of paralysis.

1   **Receptive (posterior) dysphasia.** This is where the patient cannot understand the spoken (*auditory dysphasia*) or written word (*alexia*). This condition is suggested when the patient is unable

---

[e] Vladimir Kernig (1840–1917), St Petersburg neurologist, described this in 1882.

Table 10.5 Examination of a patient with dysphasia

Fluent speech (receptive, conductive or nominal aphasia, usually)

1 Name objects. Patients with nominal, conductive or receptive aphasia will name objects poorly.
2 Repetition. Conductive and receptive aphasic patients cannot repeat 'no ifs, ands or buts'.
3 Comprehension. Only receptive aphasic patients cannot follow commands (verbal or written): 'Touch your nose, then your chin and then your ear'.
4 Reading. Conductive and receptive aphasic patients may have difficulty (dyslexia).
5 Writing. Conductive aphasic patients have impaired writing (dysgraphia) while receptive aphasic patients have abnormal content of writing. Patients with dominant frontal lobe lesions may also have dysgraphia.

Non-fluent speech (expressive aphasia, usually)

1 Naming of objects. This is poor but may be better than spontaneous speech.
2 Repetition. May be possible with great effort. Phrase repetition (e.g. 'No ifs, ands or buts') is poor.
3 Comprehension. Often mildly impaired despite popular belief, but written and verbal commands are followed.
4 Reading. Patients may have dyslexia.
5 Writing. Dysgraphia may be present.
6 Look for hemiparesis. The arm is more affected than the leg.
7 As patients are usually aware of their deficit they are often frustrated and depressed.

to understand any commands or questions or to recognise written words in the absence of deafness or blindness. Speech is fluent but disorganised. It occurs with a lesion (infarction, haemorrhage or space-occupying tumour) in the dominant hemisphere in the posterior part of the first temporal gyrus (Wernicke's area[f]).

2 **Expressive (anterior) dysphasia.** This is present when the patient understands, but cannot answer appropriately. Speech is non-fluent. This occurs with a lesion in the posterior part of the dominant third frontal gyrus (Broca's area[g]). Certain types of speech may be retained by these patients. These include *automatic speech*. The patient may be able to recite word series such as the days of the week or letters of the alphabet. Sometimes *emotional speech* may be preserved so that when frustrated or upset the patient may be able to swear fluently. In the same way the patient may be able to sing familiar songs while unable to speak the words. It is important to remember that unless the lesion responsible for these defects is very large there may be no reduction in the patient's higher intellectual functions, memory or judgment. Some of these patients may incorrectly be considered psychotic, because of their disorganised speech.

3 **Nominal dysphasia.** All types of dysphasia cause difficulty naming objects. There is also a specific type of nominal dysphasia. Here objects cannot be named (e.g. the nib of a pen) but other aspects of speech are normal. The patient may use long sentences to overcome failure to find the correct word (circumlocution). It occurs with a lesion of the dominant posterior temporoparietal area. Other causes include encephalopathy or the intracranial pressure effects of a distinct space-occupying lesion; it may also occur in the recovery phase from any dysphasia. Its localising value is therefore doubtful.

4 **Conductive dysphasia.** Here patients repeat statements and name objects poorly, but can follow commands. This is thought to be caused by a lesion of the arcuate fasciculus and/or other fibres linking Wernicke's and Broca's areas.

To examine for dysphasia in more detail refer to Table 10.5. If the speech is fluent, but conveys information with paraphasic errors, such as 'treen' for 'train' (i.e. a word of similar sound or spelling to the one intended is used),[h] the main possibilities are nominal, receptive and conductive dysphasia. Test for these by asking the patient to name an object, repeat a statement after you, and then follow commands. Then, if the above are abnormal, ask the patient to read and write, but remember that the occasional patient may be illiterate.

---

[f] Karl Wernicke (1848–1904), Professor of Neurology at Breslau, described receptive aphasia in 1874. He was killed while riding his bicycle.

[g] Pierre Broca (1824–1880), Professor of Surgery at Paris, described this area in 1861. He described muscular dystrophy before Duchenne.
[h] Sometimes a word of similar meaning is used (e.g. 'go' for 'start'): this is called *semantic paraphrasia*.

If the speech is slow, hesitant and non-fluent, expressive dysphasia is more likely and exactly the same procedure is followed. It is important to note that many dysphasias will have mixed elements. Large lesions in the dominant hemisphere may cause global dysphasia.

Dysarthria. Here there is no disorder of the content of speech but a difficulty with articulation. It can occur because of abnormalities at a number of levels. Upper motor neurone lesions of the cranial nerves, extrapyramidal conditions (e.g. Parkinson's disease, page 360) and cerebellar lesions cause disturbances to the rhythm of speech.

Table 10.6 Symptoms and signs in higher centre dysfunction

Parietal lobe

Dysphasia (dominant)
Acalculia,* agraphia,* left–right disorientation,* finger agnosia*
Sensory and visual inattention,† construction and dressing apraxia,† spatial neglect and inattention,† lower quadrantic hemianopia,‡ astereognosis‡
Seizures

Temporal lobe

Memory loss
Upper quadrantic hemianopia
Dysphasia (receptive if dominant lobe)
Seizures

Frontal lobe

Personality change
Primitive reflexes, e.g. grasp, pout
Anosmia
Optic nerve compression (optic atrophy)
Gait apraxia
Leg weakness (parasagittal)
Loss of micturition control
Dysphasia (expressive), dysgraphia
Seizures

Occipital lobe

Homonymous hemianopia
Alexia (inability to read; word blindness)
Seizures (flashing light aura)

---
* Gerstmann's syndrome: dominant hemisphere parietal lobe only.
† Non-dominant parietal lobe signs.
‡ Non-localising parietal lobe signs.

Ask the patient to say a phrase such as 'British Constitution' or 'Peter Piper picked a peck of pickled peppers'.

Pseudobulbar palsy is an upper motor neurone weakness that causes a spastic dysarthria (it sounds as if the patient is trying to squeeze out words from tight lips). *Bulbar palsies* (page 317) cause a nasal speech, while *facial muscle* weakness causes slurred speech. *Extrapyramidal disease* can be responsible for monotonous speech, as it causes bradykinesia and muscular rigidity (page 362). Other causes of dysarthria include alcohol intoxication and *cerebellar disease*. These result in loss of coordination and slow, slurred and often explosive speech, or speech broken up into syllables, called scanning speech (page 357).

Mouth ulceration or disease may occasionally mimic dysarthria. Each of these causes must be considered and examined for as appropriate.

Dysphonia. This is alteration of the sound of the voice, such as huskiness of the voice with decreased volume. It may be due to laryngeal disease (e.g. following a viral infection or a tumour of the vocal cord), or to recurrent laryngeal nerve palsy.

The cerebral hemispheres

Parietal, temporal and frontal lobe functions are tested if the patient is disoriented or has dysphasia, or if dementia is suspected. If the patient has a receptive aphasia, however, these tests cannot be performed. Their examination is otherwise not routine (Table 10.6). Students should now turn to page 293 and read how to examine the cranial nerves and limbs; return to this section once you have completed that task.

Parietal lobe function

The parietal lobe is concerned with the reception and analysis of sensory information.

Dominant lobe signs. A lesion of the dominant parietal lobe in the angular gyrus causes a distinct clinical syndrome called Gerstmann's syndrome. Test for this in the following manner.

1 Ask the patient to perform simple arithmetical calculations. The inability to do this at least with partial accuracy is called *acalculia*.
2 Ask the patient to write—inability is called *agraphia*.
3 Test for left–right disorientation by asking the patient to show you his or her right and then left hand. If this is correctly performed, ask the patient to touch his or her left ear with the right hand and vice versa. Inability to do this is called *left–right disorientation*.

4 Ask the patient to name his or her fingers—inability to do this is called *finger agnosia*. This inability may extend to identification of the examiner's fingers. The *agnosias* are receptive defects involving the inability to understand the meaning of stimulations of different types.

A mnemonic for these four dominant parietal lobe signs is **AALF**. Remember that Gerstmann's syndrome can be diagnosed only if the higher centres are intact. A demented patient would not be able to perform many of these tests.

Non-dominant and non-localising parietal lobe signs *(cortical sensation)*. Cortical sensations are those that require processing at a higher level than simple sensation. They rely on an intact simple sensation, especially touch and pinprick.

■ *Graphaesthesia* is the ability to recognise numbers or letters drawn on the skin. Use a pointed object or pencil to draw numbers on the skin (Figure 10.1).
■ *Tactile extinction* is the ability to feel a stimulus when it is applied to each side separately, but not on one side when both sides are stimulated. The patient (with eyes shut) is touched first on one hand and then on the other, and then on both together. Ask on which side the touch is felt. The normal response is 'both' when stimulation is applied to each side. It is important that the hands be touched simultaneously.

Now test for general signs of parietal lobe dysfunction.

■ Look for *sensory* and *visual inattention*. When one arm or leg is tested at a time, sensation is normal (page 328), but when both sides are tested simultaneously the sensation is appreciated only on the normal side. A right-sided parietal lesion will lead to inattention on the left side and vice versa.
■ Formal *visual field testing* is also important (page 295), as parietal, temporal and occipital lesions can give distinctive defects.
■ Examine now for *astereognosis (tactile agnosia)*, which is the inability, with eyes closed, to recognise an object placed in the hand when the ordinary sensory modalities are intact. A parietal lobe lesion results in astereognosis on the opposite side.
■ *Agraphaesthesia* may also be present; this is the inability to appreciate a number drawn on the hand on the opposite side to a parietal lesion (Figure 10.1). Avoid the use of an indelible pencil.
■ *Two-point discrimination* testing involves the ability to distinguish a single point, from two points close together (Fig 10.2). The minimal separation that can be distinguished is about 3 cm on the hand or foot and 0.6 cm on the fingertips. A compass can be used for this test. Ask the patient to shut the eyes and then whether one or two points can be felt. Bring the compass points closer together and test intermittently with just one point (Figure 10.2).
■ Examine for *dressing* and *constructional apraxia*. Dressing apraxia is tested by taking the patient's pyjama top or cardigan, turning it inside out and asking him or her to put it back on. Patients with a non-dominant parietal lobe lesion may find this impossible to do. Constructional apraxia is tested by asking the patient to copy an object that you have drawn (e.g. a flower or a house—Figure 10.3).
■ Next test *spatial neglect* by asking the patient to fill in the numbers on an empty clock face. Patients with a right parietal lesion may fill in numbers only on the left side (the other side of the clock face is ignored). Spatial neglect also occurs with dominant parietal lobe lesions but is less common.

Figure 10.1 Agraphaesthesia: 'What number have I drawn?' Patient's reply: 'One.'

Figure 10.2 Two-point discrimination: 'Can you feel one point or two?'

Figure 10.3 Constructional apraxia

Temporal lobe function

This lobe is concerned with short-term and long-term memory. Test short-term memory by the name, address, flower test—ask the patient to remember a name, address and the names of three flowers, and repeat them immediately. Then ask the patient five minutes later to repeat the names again. Test long-term memory by asking, for example, what year World War II ended. Memory may be impaired in dementia from any cause.

An alert patient with a severe memory disturbance may make up stories to fill any gaps in his or her memory. This is called *confabulation*, and is typical of the syndrome of Korsakoff's psychosis[i] (amnesic dementia). Confabulation can be tested by asking the patient whether he or she has met you before. However, be prepared for the very long, detailed and completely false story that may follow.

Korsakoff's psychosis occurs most commonly in alcoholics (where there is loss of nerve cells in the thalamic nuclei and mammillary bodies), and rarely with head injury, tumour, anoxic encephalopathy or encephalitis. It is characterised by retrograde amnesia (memory loss for events before the onset of the illness) and an inability to memorise new information, in a patient who is alert, responsive and capable of problem-solving.

Frontal lobe function

Frontal lobe damage as a result of tumours or surgery (or both), or diffuse disease such as dementia, may cause changes in emotion, memory, judgment, carelessness about personal habits, and disinhibition. There may be persistent or alternating irritability and euphoria.[j] These features may be clear when the history is taken but may need to be reinforced by interviewing relatives or friends. Changes of this sort in a previously reserved personality may be obvious and very distressing to relatives.

Assess first the *primitive reflexes*. There is controversy concerning their significance; they are not normally present in adults but may reappear in normal old age.[8] The presence of an isolated primitive reflex may not be abnormal, but multiple primitive reflexes are usually associated with diffuse cerebral disease involving the frontal lobes and frontal association areas more than other parts of the brain. Dementia, encephalopathy and neoplasms are all possible causes.

1 Grasp reflex: the examiner runs his or her fingers across the palm of the patient's hand, which will grasp the examining fingers involuntarily on the side contralateral to the lesion.
2 Palmomental reflex: ipsilateral contraction of the orbicularis oris muscle occurs when the examiner strokes the thenar eminence.

---

i Sergei Sergeyevich Korsakoff (1853–1900), Russian psychiatrist and great humanitarian, described the syndrome in 1887.

j Euphoria may cause a lack of seriousness, and the repetition of bad jokes and puns (*witzelsucht*).

3   Pout and snout reflexes: stroking or tapping with the tendon hammer over or above the upper lip induces pouting movements of the lips. This can occur with many intracranial lesions. The sucking reflex is an extension of this. The stimulation may produce sucking, chewing and swallowing movements. It is not a localising sign.

Next ask the patient to *interpret a proverb*, such as 'A rolling stone gathers no moss'. Patients with frontal lobe disease give concrete explanations of proverbs. Test for loss of smell (*anosmia*) and for *gait apraxia*, where there is marked unsteadiness in walking, which can be bizarre—the feet typically behave as if glued to the floor, causing a strange shuffling gait (page 344). Look in the *fundi*; you may rarely see optic atrophy on the side of a frontal lobe space-occupying lesion caused by compression of the optic nerve, and papilloedema on the opposite side due to secondarily raised intracranial pressure (Foster Kennedy[k] syndrome).

The cranial nerves[l]

If possible, position the patient so that he or she is sitting over the edge of the bed. Look at the head, face and neck. If hydrocephalus has occurred in infancy—before closure of the cranial sutures—the head and face may resemble an inverted triangle. Acromegaly (page 267), Paget's disease (page 279) or basilar invagination (page 280) may be obvious. A careful *general inspection* may reveal signs easily missed when each cranial nerve is examined separately. This is particularly true of ptosis (page 320), proptosis (page 263), pupillary inequality (page 320), skew deviation of the eyes (page 303) and facial asymmetry (page 307). Inspect the whole scalp for craniotomy scars and the skin for neurofibromas (Figure 10.4). Look for skin lesions: for example, a capillary or cavernous haemangioma is seen on the face in the distribution of the trigeminal (V) nerve in the Sturge-Weber syndrome.[m] It is associated with an intracranial venous haemangioma of the leptomeninges and with seizures.

Figure 10.4 Subcutaneous neurofibromas in neurofibromatosis type I, associated with optic nerve and pontine gliomas (acoustic neuromas occur in type II)

The cranial nerves are usually tested in approximately the order of their number.[9]

The first (olfactory) nerve[n]

Anatomy. This is a purely sensory nerve, whose fibres arise in the mucous membrane of the nose and pass through the cribriform plate of the ethmoid bone to synapse in the olfactory bulb. From here the olfactory tract runs under the frontal lobe and terminates in the medial temporal lobe on the same side.

Examination of the nose and sense of smell. Note the external appearance of the nose. Look for rash or deformity. Then examine the nasal vestibule by elevating the tip of the nose (in adults a speculum is usually needed to give an adequate view).

The first nerve is not tested routinely. If the patient complains of loss of smell (anosmia) or there are other signs suggesting a frontal or temporal lobe lesion, then it should be examined. Anosmic patients sometimes complain of loss of taste rather than of smell because the sense of smell plays a large part in the appreciation of taste. Test each nostril separately with a series of bottles containing essences of familiar smells, such as coffee, vanilla and peppermint (this is traditional, but not very reliable). Pungent substances such as ammonia should not be used, first because they

---

k   Robert Foster Kennedy (1884–1952), a New York neurologist.
l   The anatomy and function of the cranial nerves was well established by the late 19th century. Galen identified at least seven of the cranial nerves in the 2nd century. These were probably the optic, oculomotor, the sensory part of the trigeminal, the motor part of the trigeminal, facial, vestibular, the glossopharyngeal (including the vagus and accessory) and the hypoglossal.
m   William Allen Sturge (1850–1919), British physician, described this in 1879, and Frederick Parkes Weber (1863–1962), London physician, described it in 1922.

n   Samuel von Sommerring (1755-1830) is responsible for the modern classification of 12 cranial nerves. He separated the vestibular from the facial, and the glossopharyngeal from the vagus and accessory.

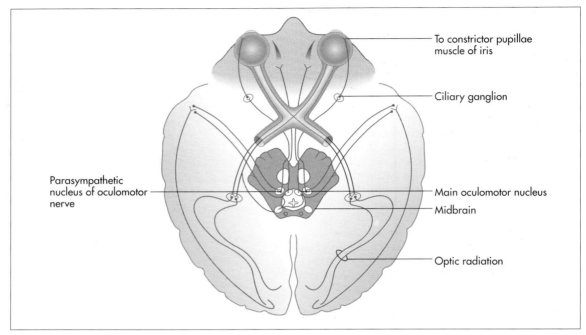

Figure 10.5 The optic pathways and visual reflexes

(Adapted from Snell RS, Westmoreland BF, *Clinical neuroanatomy for medical students*, 4th edn. Boston: Little Brown, 1997.)

upset the patient and second because noxious stimuli of this sort are detected by sensory fibres of the fifth (trigeminal) nerve.

Examination of the nasal passages must be performed if anosmia is present. Polyps and mucosal thickening may be seen and may explain the findings.

Causes of anosmia. Most cases of anosmia are bilateral. Causes include: (i) upper respiratory tract infection (commonest); (ii) smoking and increasing age; (iii) ethmoid tumours; (iv) basal skull fracture or frontal fracture, or after pituitary surgery; (v) congenital—for example, Kallmann's syndrome (hypogonadotrophic hypogonadism); (vi) meningioma of the olfactory groove; and (vii) following meningitis. The main unilateral causes are head trauma without a fracture, or an early meningioma of the olfactory groove.°

° Other abnormalities of smell are hyperosmia and parosmia. *Hyperosmia* is an increase in the sensitivity of the sense of smell. It is often a sign of psychosis or hysteria but may occur with migraine, during menstruation and in cases of encephalitis. *Parosmia* is a perversion of the sense of smell. It can occur following trauma to the head and in some psychoses. Olfactory hallucinations are more often than not a result of an organic lesion and suggest an irritating lesion in the olfactory cortex.

The second (optic) nerve

Anatomy. The optic nerve is not really a nerve but an extension of fibres of the central nervous system that unites the retinas with the brain. It is purely sensory, contains about a million fibres and extends for about 5 cm (Figure 10.5), passing through the optic foramen close to the ophthalmic artery and joining the nerve from the other side at the base of the brain to form the optic chiasm. The spatial orientation of fibres from different parts of the fundus is preserved so that fibres from the lower part of the retina are found in the inferior part of the chiasm and vice versa. Fibres from the temporal visual fields (the nasal halves of the retinas) cross in the chiasm, whereas those from the nasal visual fields do not. Fibres for the light reflex from the optic chiasm finish in the superior colliculus, whence connections occur with both third nerve nuclei. The remainder of the fibres leaving the chiasm are concerned with vision, and travel in the optic tract to the lateral geniculate body. From here the fibres form the optic radiation and pass through the posterior part of the internal capsule, finishing in the visual cortex of the occipital lobe. In their course they splay out so that fibres serving the lower quadrants course through the parietal lobe, while those for the upper quadrants traverse the temporal lobe. The result of the decussation of fibres in the optic chiasm is that fibres from the left visual field terminate in the right occipital lobe and vice versa.

History. The majority of visual symptoms involve reduction in visual acuity. These are discussed in detail with the physical examination findings. Some patients notice a more specific change, which will help direct the examination. Ask about the time course of the visual disturbance and whether it seems to involve the vision of one eye or one visual field. Sudden loss of vision in one eye (often described as the awareness of a curtain being drawn across the eye) may be due to an embolus to the retina. There is usually, but not always, spontaneous return of vision. This is called *amaurosis fugax.* Migraine attacks may be preceded by subjective visual changes, including scintillating scotomas, photophobia, blurred vision or hemianopia (page 297). Visual hallucinations such as flashing lights and distortions of vision can occur in psychotic states or as the aura of an epileptic seizure.

More gradual loss of vision has many possible causes (Table 10.7).

Examination. Assess visual acuity, visual fields and the fundi.

Visual acuity is tested with the patient wearing his or her spectacles, if used for reading or driving, as refractive errors are *not* considered to be cranial nerve abnormalities. Use a hand-held eye chart or a Snellen's chart[p] on the wall. Each eye is tested separately, while the other is covered by a small card.

Formal testing with a standard Snellen's chart requires the patient to be 6 metres from the chart. Unless a very large room is available, this is done using a mirror. Normal visual acuity is present when the line marked 6 can be read correctly with each eye (6/6 acuity). A patient who is unable to read even the largest letter of the chart should be asked to count fingers held up in front of each eye in turn, and if this is not possible, then perception of hand movement is tested. Failing this, light perception only may be present.

Any abnormality of the lens, cornea, fundus or optic nerve pathway can cause reduction in visual acuity:

- *Causes of bilateral blindness of rapid onset* include bilateral occipital lobe infarction; bilateral occipital lobe trauma; bilateral optic nerve damage, as with methyl alcohol poisoning; and hysteria.
- *Sudden blindness in one eye* can be due to retinal artery or vein occlusion, temporal arteritis,

Figure 10.6 Visual field testing: 'Tell me when you first see the red pin come into view'

non-arteritic ischaemic optic neuropathy and occasionally optic neuritis or migraine.
- *Bilateral blindness of gradual onset* may be caused by cataracts; acute glaucoma; macular degeneration; diabetic retinopathy (vitreous haemorrhages); bilateral optic nerve or chiasmal compression; and bilateral optic nerve damage—for example, tobacco *amblyopia* (blindness due to retinal disease).

Visual fields are examined by *confrontation* (Figure 10.6). Always remove a patient's spectacles first. The examiner's head should be level with the patient's head. Use a white- or red-tipped hat pin or pen. Test each eye separately. The examiner holds the pin at arm's length with the coloured head upwards. It should be positioned halfway between the patient

---

Table 10.7 Causes of eye abnormalities

Cataracts
1 Old age (senile cataract)
2 Endocrine—e.g. diabetes mellitus, steroids
3 Hereditary or congenital—e.g. dystrophia myotonica, Refsum's disease*
4 Ocular disease—e.g. glaucoma
5 Radiation
6 Trauma

Papilloedema vs papillitis

Papilloedema	*Papillitis*
Optic disc swollen without venous pulsation	Optic disc swollen
Acuity normal (early)	Acuity poor
Large blind spot	Large central scotoma
Peripheral constriction of visual fields	Pain on eye movement
Colour vision normal	Onset usually sudden and unilateral
Usually bilateral	Colour vision affected (particularly red desaturation)

Causes of papilloedema
1 Space-occupying lesion (causing raised intracranial pressure) or a retro-orbital mass
2 Hydrocephalus (large cerebral ventricles)
   Obstructive (a block in the ventricle, aqueduct or outlet to the fourth ventricle)—e.g. tumour
   Communicating
   Increased formation of CSF—e.g. choroid plexus papilloma (rare)
   Decreased absorption of CSF—e.g. tumour causing venous compression, subarachnoid space
      obstruction from meningitis
3 Benign intracranial hypertension (pseudotumour cerebri) (small or normal-sized ventricles)
   (a) Idiopathic
   (b) The contraceptive pill
   (c) Addison's disease
   (d) Drugs—e.g. nitrofurantoin, tetracycline, vitamin A, steroids
   (e) Head trauma
4 Hypertension (grade 4)
5 Central retinal vein thrombosis

Causes of optic atrophy
1 Chronic papilloedema or optic neuritis
2 Optic nerve pressure or division
3 Glaucoma
4 Ischaemia
5 Familial—e.g. retinitis pigmentosa, Leber's disease,[†] Friedreich's ataxia

Causes of optic neuritis
1 Multiple sclerosis
2 Toxic—e.g. ethambutol, chloroquine, nicotine, alcohol
3 Metabolic—e.g. vitamin B_{12} deficiency
4 Ischaemia—e.g. diabetes mellitus, temporal arteritis, atheroma
5 Familial—e.g. Leber's disease
6 Infective—e.g. infectious mononucleosis

Causes of retinitis pigmentosa
1 Congenital (associated with cataract and deaf-mutism)
2 Laurence-Moon-Biedl syndrome[‡]
3 Hereditary ataxia
4 Familial neuropathy, i.e. Refsum's disease

CSF = cerebrospinal fluid.
* Sigvald Refsum, 20th century Norwegian physician.
[†] Theodor von Leber (1840–1917), Göttingen and Heidelberg ophthalmologist.
[‡] John Laurence (1830–1874), London ophthalmologist; Robert Charles Moon (1844–1914), American ophthalmologist; and Arthur
   Biedl (1869–1933), Professor of Physiology, Prague.

and the examiner, and brought in from just outside the examiner's peripheral vision until the patient can see it. Make sure the patient is staring directly at the examiner's eye and explain that he or she is looking for the first sight of the pin out of the corner of the eye. When the right eye is being tested the patient should look straight into the examiner's left eye. The patient's head should be at arm's length and the eye not being tested should be covered. The pin should be brought into the visual field from the four main directions, diagonally towards the centre of the field of vision.

Next the blind spot can be mapped out by asking about disappearance of the pin around the centre of the field of vision of each eye. The pin is moved slowly across the field of vision. A large central scotoma (page 298) will lead to its apparent temporary disappearance and then reappearance. Only a gross enlargement may be detectable.

If a patient has such poor acuity that a pin is difficult to see, the fields should be mapped with the fingers. The examiner's fingers can also be used to perform a quick screening test of the visual fields. Usually two fingers are held up and brought into the centre of vision in the four quadrants. The examiner wriggles the fingers and asks the patient to say 'yes' when movement of the fingers is first seen. The following patterns of visual field loss may be detected (Figures 10.7 and 10.8):

- *Concentric diminution of the field (tunnel vision)* may be caused by glaucoma; retinal abnormalities such as chorioretinitis or retinitis pigmentosa; papilloedema; or acute ischaemia, as with migraine. Normally even a reduced field of vision widens as objects are moved further away. Tubular diminution of the visual fields suggests

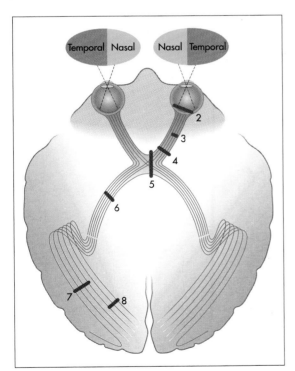

Figure 10.7 The visual fields and optic pathways

Numbers indicate sites of lesions producing field defects shown in Figure 10.8.
(Adapted from Snell RS, Westmoreland BF, *Clinical neuroanatomy for medical students*, 4th edn. Boston: Little Brown, 1997.)

1. TUNNEL VISION
   Concentric diminution, e.g. glaucoma, papilloedema, syphilis

2. ENLARGED BLIND SPOT
   Optic nerve head enlargement

3. CENTRAL SCOTOMATA
   Optic nerve head to chiasmal lesion, e.g. demyelination, toxic, vascular, nutritional

4. UNILATERAL FIELD LOSS
   Optic nerve lesion, e.g. vascular tumour

5. BITEMPORAL HEMIANOPIA
   Optic chiasm lesion, e.g. pituitary tumour, sella meningioma

6. HOMONYMOUS HEMIANOPIA
   Optic tract to occipital cortex, e.g. vascular, tumour (NB: incomplete lesion results in macular (central) vision sparing)

7. UPPER QUADRANT HOMONYMOUS HEMIANOPIA
   Temporal lobe lesion, e.g. vascular, tumour

8. LOWER QUADRANT HOMONYMOUS HEMIANOPIA
   Parietal lobe lesion

Figure 10.8 Visual field defects with lesions at various levels along the optic pathway, at sites indicated in Figure 10.7

(Adapted from Bickerstaff ER, Spillane JA. *Neurological examination in clinical practice*, 5th edn. Oxford: Blackwell, 1989.)

hysteria. There is always a small area close to the centre of the visual fields where there is no vision (the blind spot). This is the area where the optic disc is seen on fundoscopy and is the point where the optic nerve joins the retina. The blind spot enlarges with papilloedema.

- *Central scotomata, or loss of central (macular) vision,* may be due to demyelination of the optic nerve (multiple sclerosis causes unilateral or asymmetrical bilateral scotomata); toxic causes, such as methyl alcohol (symmetrical bilateral scotomata); nutritional causes, such as tobacco or alcohol amblyopia (symmetrical central or centrocecal scotomata); vascular lesions (unilateral); and gliomas of the optic nerve (unilateral).
- *Total unilateral visual loss* is due to a lesion of the optic nerve or to unilateral eye disease.
- *Bitemporal hemianopia* is due to a lesion that affects the centre of the optic chiasm, damaging fibres from the nasal halves of the retinas as they decussate. This will result in loss of both temporal halves of the visual fields. Causes include a pituitary tumour, a craniopharyngioma and a suprasellar meningioma.
- *Binasal hemianopia* is very rare and is due to bilateral lesions affecting the uncrossed optic fibres, such as atheroma of the internal carotid siphon.
- *Homonymous hemianopia* is due to a lesion that damages the optic tract or radiation, affecting the visual field on the right or left side. For example, left temporal and right nasal field loss will occur with a right-sided lesion. The exact nature of the defect depends on the site of interruption of the fibres. In the optic tract the defect is usually complete—there is no macular sparing. In the more posterior optic radiation the macular vision is usually spared if the cause is ischaemia, but not if a destructive process such as tumour or haemorrhage is responsible. The macular cortical area is thought to have some additional blood supply from the anterior and middle cerebral arteries.
- *Homonymous quadrantanopia* is loss of the upper or lower homonymous quadrants of the visual fields. This may be due to temporal lobe lesions (e.g. vascular lesions or tumours), which cause upper quadrantanopia, or parietal lobe lesions (e.g. vascular lesions or tumours), which cause lower quadrantanopia.

The presence of an abnormality has diagnostic value (positive LRs 4.2 to 6.8), but absence is largely unhelpful.

Fundoscopy does not begin with the examination of the fundus, but rather with visualisation of the cornea with the ophthalmoscope. Use the right eye to look in the patient's right eye and vice versa. This prevents contact between the noses of the patient and the examiner in the midline. Keep your head vertical so that the patient can fix with the other eye.

Begin with the ophthalmoscope on the +20 lens setting, with the patient gazing into the distance. This prevents reflex pupil contraction, which occurs if the patient attempts to accommodate. Look first at the cornea and iris, and then at the lens. Large corneal ulcers may be visible, as may undulation of the rim of the iris, which is due to previous lens extraction and is called iridodonesis.

By racking the ophthalmoscope down towards 0, the focus can be shifted towards the fundus. Opacities in the lens (cataracts) may prevent inspection of the fundus. When the retina is in focus, search first for the optic disc. This is done by following a large retinal vein back towards the disc. All these veins radiate from the optic disc.

The margins of the disc must be examined with care. The disc itself is usually a shallow cup with a clearly outlined rim. Loss of the normal depression of the optic disc will cause blurring at the margins and is called papilloedema (Figure 10.9a). It indicates raised intracranial pressure. If papilloedema is suspected, the retinal veins should be examined for spontaneous pulsations. When these are present raised intracranial pressure is excluded, but their absence does not prove the pressure is raised.[10] If the appearance of papilloedema is associated with demyelination in the anterior part of the optic nerve, it is called papillitis (Table 10.7). These two can be distinguished because papillitis causes visual loss but papilloedema does not.

Next note the colour of the optic disc. Normally it is a rich yellow colour in contrast to the rest of the fundus which is a rich red colour. The fundus may be pigmented in some diseases and in patients with pigmented skin. When the optic disc has a pale insipid white colour, optic atrophy is usually present (Figure 10.9b).

Each of the four quadrants of the retina should be examined systematically for abnormalities. Look especially for diabetic (page 278) and hypertensive changes (Figure 10.9c; see also page 64). Note haemorrhages or exudates.

There are four types of *haemorrhages*: streaky haemorrhages near the vessels (linear or flame-shaped); large ecchymoses that obliterate the vessels; petechiae, which may be confused with micro-aneurysms; and subhyaloid haemorrhages (large effusions of blood which have a crescentic shape and well-marked borders; a fluid level may be seen). The

Figure 10.9 Fundoscopy in the neurological patient

(a) Papilloedema. (b) Optic atrophy. (c) Grade 4 hypertensive retinopathy, with papilloedema, a 'macular star' of hard exudates collecting around the fovea, and retinal oedema. (d) Retinitis pigmentosa. (e) Central retinal artery occlusion.

first two types of haemorrhage occur in hypertensive and diabetic retinopathy. They may also result from any cause of raised intracranial pressure or venous engorgement, or from a bleeding disorder. The third type occurs in diabetes mellitus, and the fourth is characteristic of subarachnoid haemorrhage.

Look for signs of *retinal detachment*. Note the presence of *retinitis pigmentosa,* where there is a scattering of black pigment in a criss-cross pattern. This will be missed if the periphery of the retina is not examined (Figure 10.9d). Retinitis pigmentosa is the most common form of retinal dystrophy; it causes loss of peripheral vision and therefore night blindness, because the periphery of the retina is concerned with night vision. In *choroidal inflammation* (page 318) there are white patches behind the retinal vessels that may be associated with discrete areas of black pigmentation.

When there is a *central retinal artery occlusion* the whole fundus appears milky-white because of retinal oedema, and the arteries become greatly reduced in diameter (Figure 10.9e).

Central retinal vein thrombosis causes tortuous retinal veins, and haemorrhages scattered over the whole retina, particularly occurring alongside the veins. The differential diagnosis is retinal vasculitis, where there is haemorrhage, new vessel formation, oedema and the presence of retinal vessels of irregular calibre.

Causes of abnormalities seen on ophthalmoscopy are summarised in Table 10.7.

The third (oculomotor), fourth (trochlear) and sixth (abducens) nerves—the ocular nerves

Anatomy. The size of the pupils depends on a balance of parasympathetic and sympathetic innervation. The parasympathetic innervation to the eyes is supplied by the Edinger-Westphal nucleus[q] of the third nerve (stimulation of these fibres causes pupillary constriction: *miosis*). The sympathetic innervation to the eye (stimulation causes pupillary dilatation: *mydriasis*) (see page 320) is as follows: fibres from the hypothalamus go to the ciliospinal centre in the spinal cord at C8, T1 and T2, synapse, and second-order neurones exit via the anterior ramus in the thoracic trunk and synapse in the superior cervical ganglion in the neck. Third-order neurones travel from here with the internal carotid

artery to the eye. In addition, the pupillary reflexes (Figure 10.10) depend for their afferent limb on the optic nerve (Figure 10.5). Constriction of the pupil in response to light is relayed by the optic nerve and tract to the superior colliculus and then to the Edinger-Westphal nucleus of the third nerve in the midbrain. Efferent motor fibres from the oculomotor nucleus (Figure 10.11) travel in the wall of the cavernous sinus, where they are in association with the fourth, ophthalmic division of the fifth, and the sixth cranial nerves (see Figure 9.7 and page 268). These nerves leave the skull together through the superior orbital fissure. The iridoconstrictor fibres terminate in the ciliary ganglion, whence postganglionic fibres arise to innervate the iris. The rest of the third nerve supplies all the ocular muscles except the superior oblique (fourth nerve) and the lateral rectus (sixth nerve) muscles. The third nerve also supplies the levator palpebrae superioris, which elevates the eyelid (Figure 10.12).

Examination. Assess the pupils and eye movements.

The pupils. With the patient looking at an object at an intermediate distance, examine the pupils for size, shape, equality and regularity. Slight differences in pupil size (up to 20%) may be normal.[r] Look for ptosis (drooping) of one or both eyelids.

Test the *light reflex*. Using a pocket torch, shine the light from the side (so the patient does not focus on the light and accommodate) into one of the pupils to assess its reaction to light. Inspect both pupils and repeat this procedure on the other side. Normally the pupil into which the light is shone constricts briskly— this is the *direct* response to light. Simultaneously, the other pupil constricts in the same way. This is called the *consensual* response to light.

Move the torch in an arc from pupil to pupil. If an eye has optic atrophy or severely reduced visual acuity from another cause, the affected pupil will dilate paradoxically after a short time when the torch is moved from the normal eye to the abnormal eye. This is called an *afferent pupillary defect* (or the Marcus Gunn pupillary sign[s]). It occurs because an eye with severely reduced acuity has reduced afferent impulses so that the light reflex is markedly

---

[q] Ludwig Edinger (1855–1918), Frankfurt neurologist, and Carl Friedrich Otto Westphal (1833–90), Berlin neurologist.

[r] Gross differences are abnormal and called *anisocoria*. A small amount of fluctuation in the size of the pupils is normal and called *pupillary unrest*. More pronounced rhythmical contraction and dilatation of the pupils is called *hippus*; this may follow recovery from a third nerve palsy or occur during sleepiness. This is not often of any significance and is not a localising sign.

[s] Robert Marcus Gunn (1850–1909), London ophthalmologist, described the defect in 1883.

Figure 10.10 Cranial nerves II and III

(a) The pupils: inspect for size and symmetry. (b)Testing the pupillary reflex.

Superior colliculus

Aqueduct

Cranial nerve III nucleus

Medial lemniscus and lateral spinothalamic tract

Red nucleus

Peduncle (pyramidal tract)

Substantia nigra

Figure 10.11 Anatomy of the midbrain

decreased. When the light is shone from the normal eye to the abnormal one the pupil dilates, as reflex pupillary constriction in the abnormal eye is so reduced that relaxation after the consensual response dominates.

Now test *accommodation*. Ask the patient to look into the distance and then to focus his or her eyes on an object such as a finger or a white-tipped hat pin brought to a point about 30 cm in front of the nose. There is normally constriction of both pupils— the accommodation response. It depends on a pathway from the visual association cortex descending to the third nerve nucleus. Causes of an absent light reflex with an intact accommodation reflex include a midbrain lesion (e.g. the Argyll Robertson pupil of syphilis, see page 278), a ciliary ganglion

Superior rectus
CRANIAL NERVE III

Inferior oblique
CRANIAL NERVE III

lateral rectus
CRANIAL NERVE VI

Medial rectus
CRANIAL NERVE III

Inferior rectus
CRANIAL NERVE III

Superior oblique
CRANIAL NERVE IV

Figure 10.12 The eye muscles and nerve innervation

Figure 10.13 The cranial nerves III, IV & VI: voluntary eye movements.

(a) 'Look to the left.' (b) 'Look to the right.' (c) 'Look up.' (d) 'Look down.'

lesion (e.g. Adie's pupil[t]) or Parinaud's syndrome[u] (page 304). Failure of accommodation alone may occur occasionally with a midbrain lesion or with cortical blindness.

Eye movements. Here failure of eye movement, double vision (diplopia) and nystagmus are assessed. Ask the patient to look at the invaluable hat pin. (The presence of these pins in the lapel of a well-cut white coat or expensive suit often indicates that the wearer is a neurologist.) Assess voluntary eye movements in both eyes first. Ask the patient to look laterally right and left, then up and down (Figure 10.13a, b, c, d). Remember the lateral rectus (sixth nerve) only moves the eyes horizontally outwards, while the medial rectus (third nerve) only moves the eyes horizontally inwards. The remainder of the muscle movements are a little more complicated. When the eye is abducted, the elevator is the superior rectus (third nerve), while the depressor is the inferior rectus (third nerve). When the eye is adducted, the elevator is the inferior oblique (third nerve) while the depressor is the superior oblique (fourth nerve) (Figure 10.12). The practical upshot of all this is that the testing of pure movement (that is, one muscle only) for elevation and depression is performed first with the eye adducted and then with it abducted. Therefore, ask the patient to follow the moving hat pin, held by the examiner 30–40 cm from the patient and moved in an H pattern, with both eyes and to say if double images are seen in any direction.

Diplopia (see also page 320) can be an early sign of ocular muscle weakness because the light falls on different parts of the corresponding retinas due to slight movement differences. If diplopia is present, further testing is necessary. The false image is usually paler, less distinct and always more peripheral than the real one. Ask the patient whether the two images lie side by side or one above the other. If they are side by side, only the lateral or medial recti can be responsible. If they lie one above the other, then either of the obliques or the superior or inferior recti may be involved. To decide which pair of muscles is responsible, ask in which direction there is maximum image separation. Separation is greatest in the direction in which the weak muscle has its purest action. At the point of maximum separation, cover one eye and find out which image disappears. Loss of the lateral image indicates that the covered eye is responsible. Diplopia that persists when one eye is covered can be due to astigmatism, a dislocated lens or hysteria.

---

[t] William Adie (1886–1935), Australian neurologist working in Britain, described this in 1931.

[u] Henri Parinaud (1844–1905), French ophthalmologist, described this in 1889.

Note failure of movement of either eye in any direction. This indicates ocular muscle involvement. If any abnormality is detected, then each eye must be tested separately. The other eye is covered with a card or with the examiner's hand. Abnormal eye movement may be due to III, IV or VI nerve palsy, or to an abnormality of conjugate gaze.

Features of a third nerve lesion. These are complete ptosis (partial ptosis may occur with an incomplete lesion); divergent strabismus (eye 'down and out'); and dilated pupil which is unreactive to direct light (the consensual reaction in the opposite normal eye is intact) and unreactive to accommodation. Always try to exclude a fourth (trochlear) nerve lesion when a third nerve lesion is present. One way to do this is by tilting the head to the same side as the lesion. The affected eye will intort if the fourth nerve is intact (remember SIN—the superior oblique intorts the eye).

Aetiology of a third nerve palsy. Third nerve lesions are most commonly related to trauma or are idiopathic. Central causes include vascular lesions in the brainstem, tumours and rarely demyelination.

Peripheral causes include: (i) compressive lesions, such as an aneurysm (usually on the posterior communicating artery), tumour, basal meningitis, nasopharyngeal carcinoma or orbital lesions—for example, Tolosa-Hunt syndrome (superior orbital fissure syndrome—painful lesions of III, IV, VI and the first division of V); and (ii) ischaemia or infarction, as in arteritis, diabetes mellitus and migraine.

Features of a fourth nerve lesion. Test this nerve by asking the patient to turn the eye in and then to try to look down: a lesion results in paralysis of the superior oblique with weakness of downward (and outward) movement. The patient may walk around with his or her head tilted away from the lesion—that is, to the opposite shoulder (this allows the patient to maintain binocular vision).

An isolated fourth nerve palsy is rare and is usually idiopathic or related to trauma. It may occasionally occur with lesions of the cerebral peduncle.

Features of a sixth nerve lesion. These are failure of lateral movement, convergent strabismus and diplopia. These signs are maximal on looking to the affected side, and the images are horizontal and parallel to each other. The outermost image from the affected eye disappears on covering this eye (this image is usually also more blurred).

Aetiology of sixth nerve palsy. Bilateral lesions may be due to trauma or Wernicke's encephalo-pathy (a syndrome of ophthalmoplegia, confusion and ataxia which is often associated with Korsakoff's psychosis, page 292). Korsakoff's psychosis is usually due to thiamine deficiency. Mononeuritis multiplex and raised intracranial pressure are also causes of sixth nerve palsy.

Unilateral sixth nerve lesions are most commonly idiopathic or related to trauma. They may have a central (e.g. vascular lesion or tumour) or peripheral (e.g. raised intracranial pressure or diabetes mellitus) origin.

Abnormalities of conjugate gaze. Normal eye movements occur in an organised fashion so that the visual axes remain in the same plane throughout eye movements. There are centres for conjugate gaze in the frontal lobe for saccadic movements and in the occipital lobe for pursuit movements. Conjugate movement to the right is controlled from the left side of the brain. From these centres fibres travel to the region of the sixth nerve nucleus, from which area the medial longitudinal fasciculus coordinates movement with the contralateral third nerve (medial rectus) nucleus (Figure 10.14). A brainstem lesion causes ipsilateral paralysis of horizontal conjugate gaze and a frontal lobe lesion causes contralateral paralysis of horizontal conjugate gaze.

There are a number of possible causes for deviation of the eyes to one side. For example, *deviation of the eyes to the left* can result from: (i) a destructive lesion (usually vascular or neoplastic), which involves the pathways between the *left* frontal lobes and the oculomotor nuclei; (ii) a destructive lesion of the *right* side of the brainstem; or (iii) an irritative lesion, such as an epileptic focus, of the *right* frontal lobe, which stimulates deviation of the eyes to the left.

Supranuclear palsy is loss of vertical or horizontal gaze or both (Figure 10.14). The clinical features that distinguish this from third, fourth and sixth nerve palsies include: (i) both eyes are affected; (ii) pupils may be fixed and are often unequal; (iii) there is usually no diplopia; and (iv) the reflex eye movements—for example, on flexing and extending the neck—are usually intact.

- *Progressive supranuclear palsy* (or Steele Richardson Olszewski syndrome[v]): here there is loss of vertical and later of horizontal gaze, which is associated with extrapyramidal signs (page 288), neck rigidity and dementia. Reflex eye movements on neck flexion and extension are preserved until late in the course of the disease.

---

[v] J Steele and J Richardson, Canadian neurologists, described this in 1964.

Figure 10.14 Horizontal (a) and vertical (b) eye movements

(Adapted from Lance JW, McLeod JG. *A physiological approach to clinical neurology*, 3rd edn. London: Butterworths, 1981.)

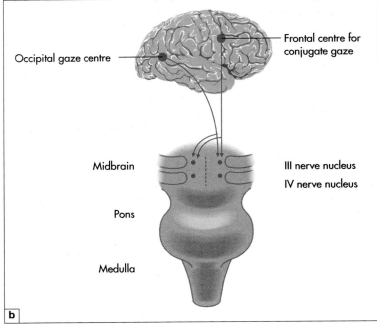

- *Parinaud's syndrome* is loss of vertical gaze often associated with nystagmus on attempted convergence (see below). There are pseudo-Argyll Robertson pupils (page 278).

    The causes of Parinaud's syndrome include a pinealoma, multiple sclerosis and vascular lesions.

- Involuntary upward deviation of the eyes (*oculogyric crises*) occurs with post-encephalitic Parkinson's disease and may be seen in patients sensitive to phenothiazine derivatives or in patients on levodopa therapy.

    One-and-a-half syndrome is rare but important to recognise. These patients have a horizontal gaze

Figure 10.15 Anatomy of the pons

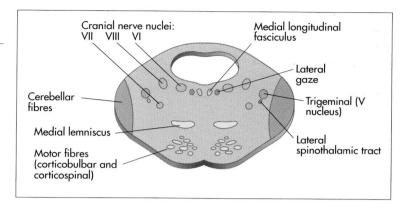

palsy when looking to one side (the 'one') plus impaired adduction on looking to the other side (the 'and-a-half'). Other features often include turning out (exotropia) of the eye opposite the side of the lesion (paralytic pontine exotropia). One-and-a-half syndrome can be caused by a stroke (infarct), plaque of multiple sclerosis or tumour in the dorsal pons.

Nystagmus. The eyes are normally maintained at rest in the middle line by the balance of tone between opposing ocular muscles. Disturbance of this tone, which depends on impulses from the retina, the muscles of the eyes themselves and various vestibular and central connections, allows the eyes to drift in one direction. This drift is corrected by a quick movement (saccadic) back to the original position. When these movements occur repeatedly nystagmus is said to be present. The direction of the nystagmus is defined as that of the fast (correcting) movement, although it is the slow drift that is abnormal. Nystagmus from any cause tends to be accentuated by gaze in a direction away from the middle line. In many instances nystagmus is not present when the eyes are at rest, and is only detected when the eyes are deviated (gaze-evoked nystagmus). At the extremes of gaze, fine nystagmus is normal (physiological). Therefore test for nystagmus by asking the patient to follow your pin out to 30 degrees from the central gaze position.

Nystagmus may be jerky or pendular.

Jerky horizontal nystagmus may be due to (i) a vestibular lesion (acute lesions cause nystagmus away from the side of the lesion while chronic lesions cause nystagmus to the side of the lesion); (ii) a cerebellar lesion (unilateral diseases cause nystagmus to the side of the lesion); (iii) toxic causes, such as phenytoin and alcohol (may also cause vertical nystagmus but less often); and (iv) *internuclear ophthalmoplegia*. Internuclear ophthalmoplegia is present when there is nystagmus in the abducting eye

and failure of adduction of the other (affected) side. This is due to a lesion of the medial longitudinal fasciculus. The most common cause in young adults with bilateral involvement is multiple sclerosis; in the elderly, vascular disease is an important cause.

Jerky vertical nystagmus may be due to a brainstem lesion. (Vertical nystagmus means nystagmus where the oscillations are in a vertical direction.) Upbeat nystagmus suggests a lesion in the midbrain or floor of the fourth ventricle, while downbeat nystagmus suggests a foramen magnum lesion. Phenytoin or alcohol can also cause this abnormality.

With **pendular nystagmus** the nystagmus phases are equal in duration. Its cause may be retinal (decreased macular vision, e.g. albinism) or congenital. This condition is thought to occur as a result of poor vision or increased sensitivity to light. It develops in childhood and occurs as the patient performs searching movements in an attempt to fixate or improve the visual impulses.

A summary of how to approach the medical eye examination is provided on page 318.

The fifth (trigeminal) nerve

Anatomy. This nerve contains both sensory and motor fibres. Its motor nucleus and its sensory nucleus for touch lie in the pons (Figure 10.15), its proprioceptive nucleus lies in the midbrain, while its nucleus serving pain and temperature sensation descends through the medulla to reach the upper cervical cord. It is the largest of the cranial nerves.

The nerve itself leaves the pons from the cerebellopontine angle and runs over the temporal lobe in the middle cranial fossa. At the petrous temporal bone the nerve forms the trigeminal (Gasserian[w]) ganglion and from here the three sensory divisions arise. The first (ophthalmic) division

[w] Johann Laurenz Gasser (1723–65), Professor of Anatomy, Vienna.

runs in the cavernous sinus with the third nerve and emerges from the superior orbital fissure to supply the skin of the forehead, the cornea and conjunctiva. The second (maxillary) division emerges from the infraorbital foramen and supplies skin in the middle of the face and the mucous membranes of the upper part of the mouth, palate and nasopharynx. The third and largest (mandibular) division runs with the motor part of the nerve, leaving the skull through the foramen ovale to supply the skin of the lower jaw and mucous membranes of the lower part of the mouth (Figures 10.16 and 10.17).

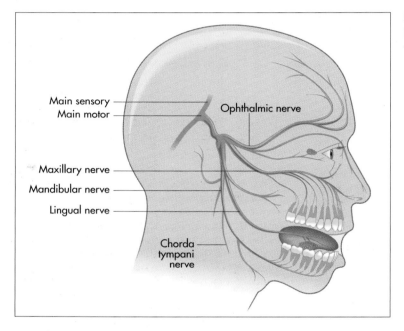

Figure 10.16 The trigeminal nerve (cranial nerve V)

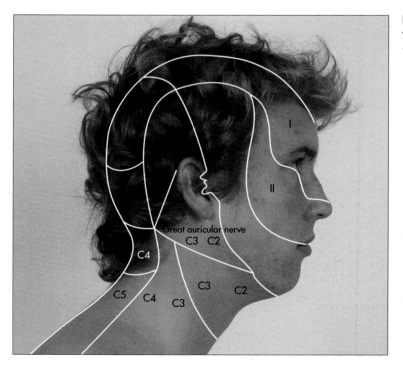

Figure 10.17 Dermatomes of the head and neck

Pain and temperature fibres from the face run from the pons through the medulla as low as the upper cervical cord, terminating in the spinal tract nucleus as they descend. The second order neurones arise in this nucleus and ascend again as the ventral trigeminothalamic tract. Touch and proprioceptive fibres terminate in the pontine or main sensory and mesencephalic nuclei, respectively, to form the dorsal and ventral mesencephalic tracts. Because of this segregation in the brainstem, lesions of the medulla or upper spinal cord can cause a *dissociated sensory loss of the face*—loss of pain and temperature sensation, but retention of touch and proprioception.

The motor part of the nerve supplies the muscles of mastication.

History. Pain in the distribution of part of the trigeminal nerve is common. *Tic douloureux (trigeminal neuralgia)* is a sudden severe shooting pain in one of the divisions of the nerve. It is more common in elderly people. The occurrence in a young woman suggests multiple sclerosis. The pain is brief but very distressing. It may be precipitated by an activity such as eating or brushing the teeth. The pain is caused by a pontine lesion or by compression of the trigeminal nerve by a vascular abnormality. Pain due to sinusitis, dental abscess, malignant disease of the sinuses and herpes zoster may be felt in a trigeminal nerve distribution. Muscle weakness of the trigeminal nerve may lead the patient to complain of difficulty eating or talking.

Examination. Test the *corneal reflex.* Lightly touch the cornea (*not* the conjunctiva) with a wisp of cottonwool brought to the eye from the side. Reflex blinking of *both* eyes is a normal response. Ask the patient whether he or she feels the touch of the cottonwool. The sensory component of the reflex is mediated by the ophthalmic division of the fifth nerve, while the reflex blink (motor) results from facial nerve innervation of the orbicularis oculi muscles. Absence of corneal sensation is associated with corneal ulceration.

Note: If blinking occurs only with the contralateral eye this indicates an ipsilateral seventh nerve palsy. The patient will then still feel the touch of the cottonwool on the cornea.

Test *facial sensation* in the three divisions of the nerve, comparing each side with the other (Figure 10.18). Test first with the sharp end of a new neurological pin for pain sensation (never use an old pin in these days of hepatitis B, HIV etc).[11] The pin is applied lightly to the skin and the patient is asked whether it feels sharp or dull. Some examiners ask patients to shut their eyes. Loss of pain sensation will result in the pinprick feeling dull. An area of dull sensation should be

Figure 10.18 Facial sensation V, maxillary division: 'Does this feel sharp or blunt?'—test all three divisions on each side

mapped by testing pinprick sensation progressively: testing should go *from the dull to the sharp area.* Test also above the forehead progressively back over the top of the head. If the ophthalmic division is affected sensation will return when the C2 dermatome is reached (Figure 10.17). It is important to exercise caution: too sharp a pin will leave a little trail of bloody spots, which is embarrassing. Temperature is not tested routinely unless syringobulbia is suspected, as temperature loss usually accompanies loss of pain sensation.

The patient keeps the eyes closed and a new piece of cottonwool is used to test light touch in the same way. The patient should be instructed to say 'yes' each time the touch of the cottonwool is felt (do *not* stroke the skin). Proprioception loss is not routinely tested on the face (and indeed it would be rather a difficult thing to do!).

Now examine the *motor division* of the nerve. Begin by inspecting for wasting of the temporal and masseter muscles. Ask the patient then to clench the teeth and palpate for contraction of the masseter above the mandible (Figure 10.19). The strength of these muscles can be tested by asking the patient to bite forcefully onto a wooden tongue depressor with the molar teeth. The depth of the teeth marks on each side give an indication of the relative strengths of the muscles. The examiner can attempt to withdraw the tongue depressor as the patient bites it. A bite of normal strength will prevent this. Then get the patient to open the mouth (pterygoid muscles) and hold it open while the examiner attempts to force it shut. A unilateral lesion of the motor division causes the jaw to deviate towards the weak (affected) side.

Test the *jaw jerk* or *masseter reflex.* The patient lets the mouth fall open slightly and the examiner's finger is placed on the tip of the jaw and tapped lightly with

Figure 10.19 Cranial nerve V (motor): 'Clench your jaw'—feel the masseter muscles

Figure 10.20 Cranial nerve V: the jaw jerk

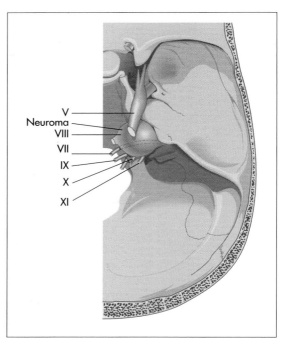

Figure 10.21 Cerebellopontine angle tumour

A neuroma arising from the acoustic (VIII) nerve compresses adjacent structures, including the trigeminal (V) and facial (VII) nerves and the brainstem and cerebellum (removed to permit the cranial nerves to be seen).

(Adapted from Simon RP, Aminoff MJ, Greenberg DA, *Clinical neurology 1989.* Appleton & Lange, 1989.)

a tendon hammer (Figure 10.20). Normally there is a slight closure of the mouth or no reaction at all. In an upper motor neurone lesion above the pons the jaw jerk is greatly exaggerated. This is commonly seen in pseudobulbar palsy (page 317).[x]

Causes of a fifth nerve palsy. Central (pons, medulla and upper cervical cord) causes include a vascular lesion, tumour or syringobulbia.

Peripheral (middle fossa) causes include an aneurysm, tumour (secondary or primary) or chronic meningitis.

Trigeminal ganglion (petrous temporal bone) causes include a trigeminal neuroma, meningioma, or fracture of the middle fossa.

Cavernous sinus causes involve the ophthalmic division only and are usually associated with third, fourth and sixth nerve palsies. They include aneurysm, tumour or thrombosis.

Remember, if there is total loss of sensation in all three divisions of the nerve, this suggests that the level of the lesion is at the ganglion or the sensory root—for example, an acoustic neuroma (Figure 10.21). If there is total sensory loss in one division only, this suggests a postganglionic lesion. The ophthalmic division is most commonly affected because it runs in the cavernous sinus and through the orbital fissure, where it is vulnerable to a number of different insults.

---

[x] Testing of the sneeze reflex is not routine. Here stimulation or irritation of the nasal mucosa with a hair or small piece of string is followed by contraction of the muscles of the nasopharynx and thorax. The afferent limb of this arc is through the trigeminal nerve and the efferent limb through the facial, glossopharyngeal, vagus and trigeminal nerves, and the motor nerves of the cervical spine. The reflex centre is in the brainstem and upper spinal cord.

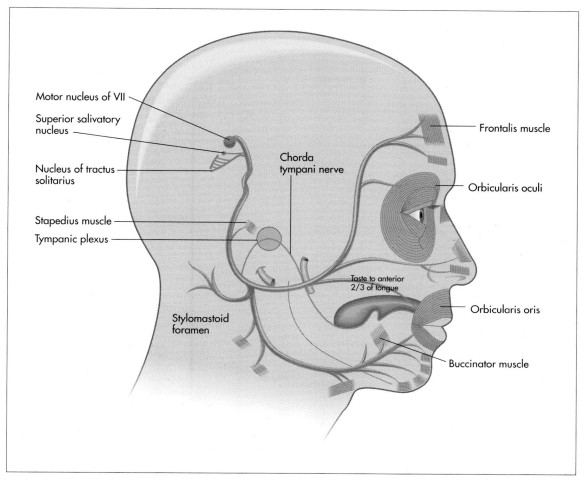

Figure 10.22 The facial nerve (cranial nerve VII)

Note: The branches of the facial nerve: 'Two zebras bit my car'—**t**emporal, **z**ygotic, **b**uccal, **m**andibular, **c**ervical.

If there is dissociated sensory loss (loss of pain, but preservation of touch sensation) this suggests a brainstem or upper cord lesion, such as syringobulbia, foramen magnum tumour, or infarction in the territory of the posterior inferior cerebellar artery. If touch sensation is lost but pain sensation is preserved, this is usually due to an abnormality of the pontine nuclei, such as a vascular lesion or tumour. Motor loss can also be central or peripheral.

Irritative motor changes. Convulsive seizures that involve the precentral gyrus can include clenching of the jaw and biting of the tongue. Parkinson's disease (page 360) and essential tremor can cause a rhythmic tremor of the lips or jaw. *Trismus* is a forceful clenching of the jaw that can occur in tetanus and encephalitis. The patient may be unable to open the mouth. Repetitive chewing and yawning movements can occur as an effect of antipsychotic drugs (*tardive orofacial dyskinesias*).

The seventh (facial) nerve

Anatomy. The seventh nerve nucleus lies in the pons next to the sixth cranial nerve nucleus (Figure 10.15). The nerve leaves the pons with the eighth nerve through the cerebellopontine angle (Figure 10.22). After entering the facial canal it enlarges to become the geniculate ganglion. The branch that supplies the stapedius muscle is given off from within the facial canal. The chorda tympani (containing taste fibres from the anterior two-thirds of the tongue) joins the nerve in the facial canal. The seventh nerve leaves the skull via the stylomastoid foramen. It then passes through the middle of the parotid gland and supplies the muscles of facial expression.

History. The patient may have noticed the onset of difficulty with speaking and keeping liquids in the mouth or may have noticed facial asymmetry in the mirror. He or she may be aware of dryness of the eyes (decreased lacrimation) or the mouth (decreased salivary production).

Examination. Inspect for *facial asymmetry*, as a seventh nerve palsy can cause unilateral drooping of the corner of the mouth, and smoothing of the wrinkled forehead and the nasolabial fold (Figure 10.23). However, with bilateral facial nerve palsies symmetry can be maintained.

Test the *muscle power*. Ask the patient to look up so as to wrinkle the forehead (Figure 10.24). Look for loss of wrinkling and feel the muscle strength by pushing down against the corrugation on each side. This movement is relatively preserved on the side of an upper motor neurone lesion (a lesion that occurs above the level of the brainstem nucleus) because of bilateral cortical representation of these muscles. The remaining muscles of facial expression are usually affected on the side of an upper motor neurone lesion, although occasionally the orbicularis oculi muscles are preserved. Ask the patient to puff out the cheeks (Figure 10.25). Look for asymmetry.

In a lower motor neurone lesion (at the level of the nucleus or nerve root), all muscles of facial expression are affected on the side of the lesion.

Next ask the patient to shut the eyes tightly (Figure 10.26). Compare how deeply the eyelashes are buried on the two sides and then try to force open each eye. Check whether Bell's phenomenon[y] is evident. Bell's phenomenon is present in everyone, although not usually visible unless a person has a VII nerve palsy. In this case, when the patient attempts to shut the eye on the side of a lower motor neurone VII nerve palsy, there is upward movement of the eyeball and incomplete closure of the eyelid. Next ask the patient to grin (Figure 10.27) and compare the nasolabial grooves, which are smooth on the weak side.

If a lower motor neurone lesion is detected, check quickly for the ear and palatal vesicles of herpes zoster of the geniculate ganglion—the Ramsay Hunt[z] syndrome.

A facial paralysis due to a cortical lesion may spare facial movements due to emotion such as crying or smiling and indeed these movements may be exaggerated. The opposite abnormality (preservation of voluntary but loss of emotional movements) can also occur as a result of lesions in a number of areas, including the frontal lobes.

Examining for taste on the anterior two-thirds of the tongue is not usually required. If necessary, it can be tested by asking the patient to protrude the tongue to one side: sugar, vinegar, salt and quinine (sweet, sour, saline and bitter) are placed one at a time on each side of the tongue. The patient indicates the taste by pointing to a card with the various tastes listed on it. The mouth is rinsed with water between each sample.

Causes of a seventh (facial) nerve palsy. Vascular lesions or tumours are the common causes of **upper motor neurone lesion (supranuclear)**. Note that lesions of the frontal lobes may cause weakness of the emotional movements of the face alone; voluntary movements are preserved.

In **lower motor neurone lesion**, *pontine* causes (often associated with V and VI lesions) include vascular lesions, tumours, syringobulbia or multiple sclerosis. *Posterior fossa* lesions include an acoustic neuroma, a meningioma or chronic meningitis. At the level of the *petrous temporal bone*, Bell's palsy (an idiopathic acute paralysis of the nerve), a fracture, the Ramsay Hunt syndrome or otitis media may occur,

Figure 10.23 Left upper motor neurone facial weakness, showing drooping of the corner of the mouth, flattened nasolabial fold, and sparing of the forehead

[y] Sir Charles Bell (1774–1842), Professor of Anatomy at London's Royal College of Surgeons, later Professor of Surgery at Edinburgh, described facial nerve palsy in 1821.
[z] James Ramsay Hunt (1874–1937), American neurologist.

Figure 10.24 Cranial nerve VII: 'Look up to wrinkle your forehead'

Figure 10.25 Cranial nerve VII: 'Puff out your cheeks'

Figure 10.27 Cranial nerve VII: 'Show me your teeth' (before asking this question, make sure the patient's teeth are not in a container beside the bed)

Figure 10.26 Cranial nerve VII: 'Shut your eyes tight and stop me opening them'

while the parotid gland may be affected by a tumour or sarcoidosis. Remember, Bell's palsy is the most common cause (up to 80%) of a facial nerve palsy.[aa]

aa A patient with an old Bell's palsy may exhibit *synkinesis*. When the patient blinks the corner of the mouth twitches; when the lips are protruded the affected eye closes.

Bilateral facial weakness may be due to the Guillain-Barré syndrome, sarcoid, bilateral parotid disease, Lyme disease or rarely mononeuritis multiplex. Myopathy and myasthenia gravis can also cause bilateral facial weakness, but in these cases it is not due to facial nerve involvement.

Unilateral **loss of taste**, without other abnormalities, can occur with middle-ear lesions involving the chorda tympani or lingual nerve, but these are very rare.

Irritative changes. Tonic and clonic movements of the facial muscles can occur in seizures. Various abnormal movements of the facial muscles can occur as a result of basal ganglia or extrapyramidal abnormalities (page 362). These include athetoid and dystonic (page 363) movements. Irritative lesions in the brainstem can cause increased secretion of saliva (*sialorrhoea*). This can also occur in Parkinson's disease or accompany attacks of nausea.

The eighth (acoustic) nerve

Anatomy. The eighth (acoustic) nerve has two components: the cochlear, with afferent fibres subserving hearing; and the vestibular, containing afferent fibres subserving balance. Fibres for hearing originate in the organ of Corti[bb] and run to the cochlear nuclei in the pons. From here there is bilateral transmission to the medial geniculate bodies and thence to the superior gyrus of the temporal lobes. Fibres for balance begin in the utricle and semicircular canals, and join auditory fibres in the facial canal. They then enter the brainstem at the cerebellopontine angle. After entering the pons, vestibular fibres run widely throughout the brainstem and cerebellum.

History. Loss of hearing may have been noticed by the patient or complained of by his or her relatives or friends. Unilateral hearing loss is much more likely to be due to a nerve lesion and must be identified. One should also find out if this has been of gradual or sudden onset, whether there is a family history of deafness, and whether there has been an occupational or recreational exposure to loud noise (e.g. boilermaker, retired rock musician) without hearing protection. There may be a history of trauma or recurrent ear infections.

Examination of the ear and hearing. Look to see if the patient is wearing a hearing aid; remove it. Examine the pinna and look for scars behind the ears. Pull on the pinna gently (it is tender if the patient has external ear disease or temporomandibular joint disease). Feel for nodes (pre- and post-auricular) that may indicate disease of the external auditory meatus.

Inspect the patient's external auditory meatus. The adult canal angulates, so in order to see the eardrum it is necessary to pull up and backwards on the auricle before inserting the otoscope. The normal eardrum (tympanic membrane) is pearly grey and concave. Look for wax or other obstructions, and inspect the eardrum for inflammation or perforation.

Next test hearing. A simple test involves covering the opposite auditory meatus with a finger, moving this about as a distraction while whispering a number in the other ear. This should be standardised by the use of set numbers for different tones. For example, the number 68 is used to test high tone and 100 to test low tone. Whispering should be performed towards the end of expiration in an attempt to standardise the volume and at about 60 cm from the ear. The examiner's larynx should not vibrate if

Figure 10.28 Cranial nerve VIII, Rinné's test: 'Where does it sound louder?'

Figure 10.29 Cranial nerve VIII, Weber's test: 'Is the buzzing louder on one side'

the whispering is soft enough. If partial deafness is suspected, perform Rinné's and Weber's tests:

- In **Rinné's test**[cc] a 256 Hz vibrating tuning fork is placed on the mastoid process, behind the ear, and when the sound is no longer heard it is placed in line with the external meatus (Figure 10.28). Normally the note is audible at the external meatus. If a patient has nerve deafness the note is audible at the external meatus, as air and bone conduction are reduced equally, so that air conduction is better (as is normal). This is termed Rinné-positive. If there is a conduction (middle ear) deafness, no note is audible at the external meatus. This is termed Rinné-negative.
- In **Weber's**[dd] test a vibrating 256 Hz tuning fork is positioned on the centre of the forehead

[bb] Alfonso Corti (1822–1888), Italian anatomist, described this in 1851.

[cc] Heinrich Adolf Rinné (1819–1868), German ear specialist, described his test in 1855.
[dd] Sir Hermann Weber (1832–1918), London physician.

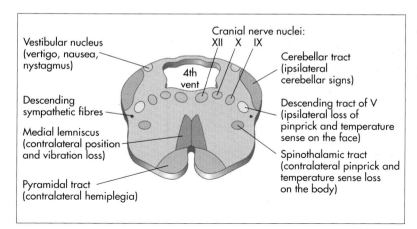

Figure 10.30 Anatomy of the medulla

Shows correlation between lesions and clinical features.

(Figure 10.29). Normally the sound is heard in the centre of the forehead. Nerve deafness causes the sound to be heard better in the normal ear. A patient with a conduction deafness finds the sound louder in the abnormal ear.

Causes of deafness. Unilateral nerve deafness may be due to (i) tumours, such as an acoustic neuroma; (ii) trauma, such as fracture of the petrous temporal bone; or (iii) vascular disease of the internal auditory artery (rare).

Bilateral nerve deafness may be due to (i) environmental exposure to noise; (ii) degeneration, such as presbyacusis; (iii) toxicity, such as aspirin, streptomycin or alcohol; (iv) infection, such as congenital rubella syndrome, congenital syphilis; or (vi) Ménière's disease.

Brainstem disease is a rare cause of bilateral deafness.

Conduction deafness may be due to (i) wax; (ii) otitis media; (iii) otosclerosis; or (iv) Paget's disease of bone.

Examination of vestibular function. If a patient complains of vertigo, the *Hallpike*[ee] *manoeuvre* should be performed. The patient sits up; having warned him or her what is about to occur, the examiner grasps the patient's head between the hands and gets him or her to lie back quickly so that the head lies 30 degrees below the horizontal. At the same time, the head is rotated 30 degrees towards the examiner. Ask the patient to keep the eyes open. If the test is positive, after a short latent period vertigo and nystagmus (rotatory) towards the affected (lowermost) ear occur for several seconds and then abate

and are not reproducible for 10 to 15 minutes. This result is seen in the condition called *benign paroxysmal positioning vertigo (BPPV)*. It occurs with repositioning of the head and then abates so that the old name, *benign positional vertigo*, is not really appropriate. It is due to a disorder in the utricle and occurs, for example, following infection, trauma or vascular disease. It is caused by the presence of concretions in the semicircular canals. Inertia of these concretions following movement of the head causes the illusion of movement and nystagmus. If there is no latent period, no fatiguability or the nystagmus persists or is variable, this suggests that there is a lesion of the brainstem (e.g. multiple sclerosis) or cerebellum (e.g. metastatic carcinoma).

Causes of vestibular abnormalities. Labyrinthine causes include acute labyrinthitis, motion sickness, streptomycin toxicity or, rarely, Ménière's disease.

Vestibular causes include vestibular neuronitis as well as many of the causes of nerve deafness.

In the brainstem, vascular lesions, tumours of the cerebellum or fourth ventricle, demyelination or vasospastic conditions such as migraine may involve the central connections of the vestibular system.

Vertigo may be associated with temporal lobe dysfunction (e.g. ischaemia or complex partial seizures).

The ninth (glossopharyngeal) and tenth (vagus) nerves

Anatomy. These nerves have motor, sensory and autonomic functions. Nerve fibres from nuclei in the medulla (Figure 10.30) form multiple nerve rootlets as they exit the medulla. These join to form the ninth and tenth nerves, and also contribute to the eleventh nerve. The nerves emerge from the skull

---

[ee] Charles Hallpike (1900–1979), English ear, nose and throat surgeon.

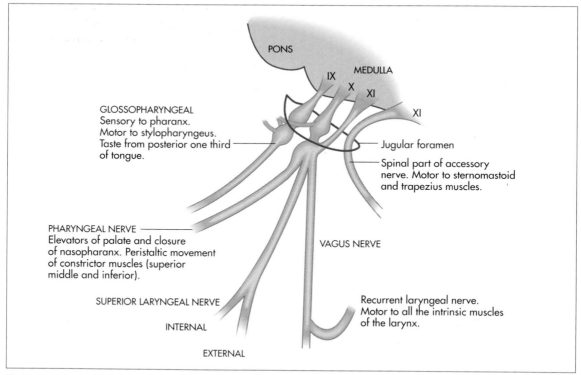

Figure 10.31 The lower cranial nerves—glossopharyngeal (IX), vagus (X) and accessory (XI)

(Adapted from Walton JN, *Brain's diseases of the nervous system*, 10th edn. Oxford: Oxford University Press, 1993.)

through the jugular foramen (Figure 10.31). The ninth nerve receives sensory fibres from the naso-pharynx, pharynx, middle and inner ear and from the posterior third of the tongue (including taste fibres). It also carries secretory fibres to the parotid gland. The tenth nerve receives sensory fibres from the pharynx and larynx, and innervates muscles of the pharynx, larynx and palate.

History. A lesion of the glossopharyngeal nerve may cause the patient no definite symptoms, but difficulty in swallowing dry foods may have been noticed. *Glossopharyngeal neuralgia* is a tic doulour-eux of the ninth nerve. The patient experiences sudden shooting pains which radiate from one side of the throat to the ear. There may be trigger areas in the throat and attacks can be brought on by chewing or swallowing.

Unilateral vagus nerve paralysis may cause difficulty in initiating the swallowing of solids and liquids and hoarseness.

Examination. Ask the patient to open the mouth and inspect the palate with a torch. Note any displacement of the uvula. Then ask the patient to say

'Ah!' (Figure 10.32). Normally the posterior edge of the soft palate—the *velum*[ff]—rises symmetrically. If the uvula is drawn to one side this indicates a uni-lateral tenth nerve palsy. Note that the uvula is drawn towards the normal side.

Testing for the *gag reflex* (ninth is the sensory component and tenth the motor component) is traditional but not necessary.[12] A better alternative is to touch the back of the pharynx on each side with a spatula (rather than the soft palate). The patient is asked if the touch of the spatula (ninth) is felt each time. Normally, there is reflex contraction of the soft palate. If contraction is absent and sensation is intact this suggests a tenth nerve palsy. The most common cause of a reduced gag reflex is old age. Of more concern to the examiner is the patient with an exaggerated but still normal reflex. This can lead to vomiting on to the examining clinician.

Ask the patient to speak in order to assess hoarseness (which may occur with a unilateral recurrent laryngeal nerve lesion), and then to cough. Listen for the characteristic bovine cough that occurs

---

[ff] Velum means 'curtain' in Latin.

adduct the arms with the elbows flexed and not allow the examiner to separate them.

Elbow
- *Flexion*—biceps and brachialis—(C5, C6): the patient should bend the elbow and pull so as not to let the examiner straighten it out (Figure 10.44).
- *Extension*—triceps brachii—(C7, C8): the patient should bend the elbow and push so as not to let the examiner bend it (Figure 10.45).

Wrist
- *Flexion*—flexor carpi ulnaris and radialis—(C6, C7): the patient should bend the wrist and not allow the examiner to straighten it.
- *Extension*—extensor carpi group—(C7, C8): the patient should extend the wrist and not allow the examiner to bend it (Figure 10.46).

Fingers
- *Extension*—extensor digitorum communis, extensor indicis and extensor digiti minimi—(C7, C8): the patient should straighten the fingers and not allow the examiner to push them down (push with the side of your hand across the patient's metacarpophalangeal joints).
- *Flexion*—flexor digitorum profundus and sublimis—(C7, C8): the patient squeezes two of the examiner's fingers (Figure 10.47).
- *Abduction*—dorsal interossei—(C8, T1): the patient should spread out the fingers and not allow the examiner to push them together (Figure 10.48).
- *Adduction*—volar interossei—(C8, T1): the patient holds the fingers together and tries to prevent the examiner from separating them further.

Reflexes. The sudden stretching of a muscle usually evokes brisk contraction of that muscle or muscle group. This reflex is usually mediated via a neural pathway synapsing in the spinal cord. It is subject to regulation via pathways from the brain. As the reflex is a response to stretching of a muscle it is correctly called a muscle stretch reflex rather than a tendon reflex. The tendon merely transmits stretch to the muscle.

Tendon hammers are available in a number of designs. Sir William Gowers[mm] used the ulnar side of his hand or part of his stethoscope. In Australia

Figure 10.49 A Queen Square patellar hammer

Table 10.14 Classification of muscle stretch reflexes

0	= absent
+	= present but reduced
++	= normal
+++	= increased, possibly normal
++++	= greatly increased, often associated with clonus (page 335)

and Britain, the Queen Square hammer[nn] is in common use (Figure 10.49). The Taylor hammer is popular in America; it is shaped like a tomahawk and has a broad rubber edge for most tendons and a more pointed side for the cutaneous reflexes.

Reflexes are graded from absent to greatly increased (Table 10.14).

Make sure the patient is resting comfortably with the elbows flexed and hands lying pronated on the lap and not overlapping one another.

To test the **biceps jerk (C5, C6)**, place one forefinger on the biceps tendon and tap this with the tendon hammer (Figure 10.50). The hammer should be held near its end and the head allowed to fall with gravity onto the positioned forefinger. The examiner soon learns not to hit too hard. Normally, if the reflex

---

[mm] Sir William Gowers (1845–1915) Professor of Clinical Medicine at University College Hospital, London, and neurologist to the National Hospital for Nervous Diseases, Queen Square, London. He was also an artist who illustrated his own books and had paintings exhibited at the Royal Academy.

[nn] The Queen Square hammer was invented by Miss Wintle, staff nurse at Queen Square. She made hammers from brass wheels covered by a ring pessary and mounted on a bamboo handle; she sold these to medical students and resident medical officers.

Figure 10.50 The biceps jerk examination

Figure 10.51 The triceps jerk examination

arc is intact, there is a brisk contraction of the biceps muscle with flexion of the forearm at the elbow, followed by prompt relaxation. Practice will help the examiner decide whether the response is within the normal range. When a reflex is greatly exaggerated, it can be elicited away from the usual zone.

If a reflex appears to be absent, always test following a *reinforcement manoeuvre*. For example, ask the patient to clench the teeth tightly just before you let the hammer fall. Supraspinal and fusiform mechanisms have been identified to explain reinforcement, but it works partly as a distraction, especially if the reflex is absent because an anxious patient has contracted opposing muscle groups. Merely talking to the patient may provide enough distraction for the reflex to be elicited. Sometimes normal reflexes can be elicited only after reinforcement, but they should still be symmetrical.

An increased jerk occurs with an upper motor neurone lesion (page 345). A decreased or absent reflex occurs with a breach in any part of the reflex motor arc—the muscle itself (e.g. myopathy), the motor nerve (e.g. neuropathy), the anterior spinal cord root (e.g. spondylosis), the anterior horn cell (e.g. poliomyelitis) or the sensory arc (sensory root or sensory nerve).

To test the **triceps jerk** (C7, C8), support the elbow with one hand and tap over the triceps tendon (Figure 10.51). Normally, triceps contraction results in forearm extension.

To test the **brachioradialis (supinator) jerk** (C5, C6), strike the lower end of the radius just above the wrist (Figure 10.52). To avoid hurting the patient by striking the radial nerve directly, place your own first two fingers over this spot and then strike the fingers, as with the biceps jerk. Normally, contraction of the brachioradialis causes flexion of the elbow.

Figure 10.52 The supinator jerk examination

Figure 10.53 The finger jerk examination

Figure 10.54 Finger–nose test: 'Touch your nose with your forefinger and then reach out and touch my finger'

If elbow extension and finger flexion is the only response when the patient's wrist is tapped, the response is said to be inverted, known as the *inverted brachioradialis (supinator) jerk*. The triceps contraction causes elbow extension instead of the usual elbow flexion. This is associated with an absent biceps jerk and an exaggerated triceps jerk. It indicates a spinal cord lesion at the C5 or C6 level due, for example, to compression (e.g. disc prolapse), trauma or syringomyelia. It occurs because a lower motor neurone lesion at C5 or C6 is combined with an upper motor neurone lesion affecting the reflexes below this level (page 351).

To test **finger jerks (C8)**, the patient rests the hand palm upward, with the fingers slightly flexed. The examiner's hand is placed over the patient's and the hammer struck over the examiner's fingers (Figure 10.53). Normally, slight flexion of all the fingers occurs.

Coordination. The cerebellum has multiple connections (afferent and efferent) to sensory pathways, brainstem nuclei, the thalamus and the cerebral cortex. Via these connections the cerebellum plays an integral role in coordinating voluntary movement. A standard series of simple tests is used to test coordination. Always demonstrate these movements for the patient's benefit.

Finger–nose test. Ask the patient to touch his or her nose with the index finger and then turn the finger around and touch the examiner's outstretched forefinger at nearly full extension of the shoulder and elbow (Figure 10.54). The test should be done both briskly and slowly, and repeated a number of times with the patient's eyes open and later closed. Slight resistance to the patient's movements by the examiner pushing on his or her

Figure 10.55 Testing for dysdiadochokinesis in the upper limbs: 'Turn your hand over, backwards and forwards on the other one, as quickly and smoothly as you can'

forearm during the test may unmask less severe abnormalities.

Look for the following abnormalities: (i) intention tremor, which is tremor increasing as the target is approached (there is no tremor at rest); and (ii) past-pointing, where the patient's finger overshoots the target towards the side of cerebellar abnormality. These abnormalities occur with cerebellar disease.

Rapidly alternating movements. Ask the patient to pronate and supinate his or her hand on the dorsum of the other hand as rapidly as possible (Figure 10.55). This movement is slow and clumsy in cerebellar disease and is called dysdiadochokinesis.[oo]

oo Actually, dysdiadochokinesis is the inability to perform alternating movements of both wrists with the arms and forefingers extended. *Diadochi* is a Greek word meaning succession. The problem here is with successive movements. The Diadochi were the successors of Alexander the Great. They divided his empire.

Figure 10.56 Pain and temperature pathways

(Adapted from Snell RS, Westmoreland BF, *Clinical neuroanatomy for medical students*, 4th edn. Boston: Little Brown, 1997.)

Rapidly alternating movements may also be affected in extrapyramidal disorders (e.g. Parkinson's disease) and in pyramidal disorders (e.g. internal capsule infarction).

Rebound. Ask the patient to lift the arms rapidly from the sides and then stop. Hypotonia due to cerebellar disease causes delay in stopping the arms. This method of demonstrating rebound is preferable to the more often used one where the patient flexes the arm at the elbow against the examiner's resistance. When the examiner suddenly lets go, violent flexion of the arm may occur and, unless prevented, the patient can strike himself or herself in the face. Therefore, only medical students trained in self-defence should use this method.

Muscle weakness may also cause clumsiness, but motor testing should have revealed any impairment of this sort.

The sensory system

To test sensation, which can be a difficult assessment and can be frustratingly time-consuming, use the following routine.[13]

Spinothalamic pathway (pain and temperature). Pain and temperature fibres enter the spinal cord and cross a few segments higher to the

Figure 10.57 Testing for pinprick (pain) sensation with a disposable neurology pin: 'Does this feel sharp or blunt?'

opposite spinothalamic tract (Figure 10.56). This tract ascends to the brainstem.

Pain (pinprick) testing. Using a new pin,[11] demonstrate to the patient that this induces a relatively sharp sensation by touching lightly a normal area, such as the anterior chest wall. Then ask the patient to say whether the pinprick feels sharp or dull. Begin proximally on the upper arm and test in each dermatome—the area of skin supplied by a vertebral

Cerebral cortex

Fasciculus gracilis and cuneatus in white column of spinal cord

Figure 10.58 Vibration and joint position sense pathways

(Adapted from Snell RS, Westmoreland BF, *Clinical neuroanatomy for medical students*, 4th edn. Boston: Little Brown, 1997.)

spinal segment (Figure 10.57). Also compare right with left in the same dermatome. Map out the extent of any area of dullness. Always do this by going from the area of dullness to the area of normal sensation.

Temperature testing. This can be done in a similar fashion, using test tubes filled with hot (40–45 degrees) and cold (5–10 degrees) water. Cold sensation can also be tested with a metal object, such as a tuning fork. Absence of ability to feel heat is almost always associated with inability to feel cold. Temperature differences of 2 to 5 degrees can usually be distinguished. These tests are performed only in special circumstances—for example, for suspected syringomyelia.

Posterior columns (vibration and proprioception[PP]).

These fibres enter and ascend ipsilaterally in the posterior columns of the spinal cord to the nucleus gracilis and nucleus cuneatus in the medulla, where they decussate (Figure 10.58).

[PP] In 1826 Sir Charles Bell recognised that there was a 'sixth sense', which was later called proprioception. Vibration sense had been recognised in the 16th century and tests for it developed in the 19th century by Rinné and others. Rydel and Seiffer found that vibration sense and proprioception were carried in the posterior columns of the spinal cord.

Vibration testing. Use a 128 Hz tuning fork (not a 256 Hz fork). Ask the patient to close the eyes, and then place the vibrating tuning fork on one of the distal interphalangeal joints. The patient should be able to describe a feeling of vibration. The examiner then deadens the tuning fork with the hand, and the patient should be able to say exactly when this occurs. Compare one side with the other. If vibration sense is reduced or absent, test over the ulnar head at the wrist, then the elbows (over the olecranon) and then the shoulders to determine the level of abnormality. Although the tuning fork is traditionally placed only over bony prominences, vibration sense is just as good over soft tissues.

Proprioception testing. Use the distal interphalangeal joint of the patient's little finger. When the patient has his or her eyes open, grasp the distal phalanx from the sides and move it up and down to demonstrate these positions. Then ask the patient to close the eyes while these manoeuvres are repeated randomly. Normally, movement through even a few degrees is detectable, and should be reported correctly. If there is an abnormality, proceed to test the wrists and elbows similarly. As a rule, sense of position is lost before sense of movement, and the little finger is affected before the thumb.

Figure 10.59 Dermatomes of the upper limb and trunk

(a) The dermatomes explained.
(b) The distribution of the dermatomes makes more sense if we are thought of as quadripedal.

Light-touch testing. Some fibres travel in the posterior columns (i.e. ipsilaterally) and the rest cross the middle line to travel in the anterior spino-thalamic tract (i.e. contralaterally). For this reason light touch is of the least discriminating value. Irritation of light-touch receptors is probably responsible for paraesthesiae—for example following ischaemia of a limb.

Test light touch by touching the skin with a wisp of cottonwool. Ask the patient to shut the eyes and say 'yes' when the touch is felt. Do not stroke the skin because this moves hair fibres. Test each dermatome,[qq] comparing left and right sides.

Interpretation of sensory abnormalities. Try to fit the distribution of any sensory loss into a dermatome (due to a spinal cord or nerve root lesion), a single peripheral nerve territory, a peripheral neuropathy pattern (glove distribution, page 349), or a hemisensory loss (due to spinal cord or upper brainstem or thalamic lesion).

Sensory dermatomes of the upper limb (Figure 10.59) can be recognised by memorising the following rough guides: C5 supplies the shoulder tip and outer part of the upper arm; C6 supplies the lateral aspect of the forearm and thumb; C7 supplies the middle finger; C8 supplies the little finger; T1 supplies the medial aspect of the upper arm and elbow.

[qq] The human dermatomes (which he called *pain spots*) were first mapped by Sir Henry Head (1861–1940). He was most famous for his experimental cutting of his own radial nerve. This enabled him to chart the order of return of the sensory modalities.

Examination of the peripheral nerves of the upper limb

A lesion of a peripheral nerve causes a characteristic motor and sensory loss.[14] Peripheral nerve lesions may have local causes, such as trauma or compression, or may be part of a mononeuritis multiplex, where more than one nerve is affected by systemic disease.

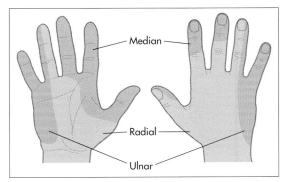

Figure 10.60 Average loss of pain sensation (pinprick) with lesions of the major nerves of the upper limbs

Figure 10.61 Pen-touching test for loss of abductor pollicis brevis: 'Lift your thumb straight up to touch my pen'

Figure 10.62 Ochsner's clasping test

(a) Normal. (b) Abnormal due to loss of function of the flexor digitorum (simulated demonstration).

The radial nerve (C5–C8). This is the *motor nerve* supplying the triceps and brachioradialis and the extensor muscles of the hand. The characteristic deformity that results from radial nerve injury is *wrist drop*. To demonstrate this, if it is not already obvious, get the patient to flex the elbow, pronate the forearm and extend the wrist and fingers. If a lesion occurs above the upper third of the upper arm the triceps muscle is also affected. Therefore, test elbow extension, which will be absent if the lesion is high.

Test *sensation* using a pin over the area of the anatomical snuff box. Sensation here is lost with a radial nerve lesion before the bifurcation into posterior interosseous and superficial radial nerves at the elbow (Figure 10.60).

The median nerve (C6–T1). This nerve contains the *motor* supply to all the muscles on the front of the forearm except the flexor carpi ulnaris and the ulnar half of the flexor digitorum profundus. It also supplies the following short muscles of the hand (LOAF)—the lateral two lumbricals, opponens pollicis, abductor pollicis brevis, and in many people the flexor pollicis brevis.

Lesion at the wrist (carpal tunnel).[15,16] Use the pen-touching test to assess for weakness of the abductor pollicis brevis. Ask the patient to lay the hand flat, palm upwards on the table, and attempt to abduct the thumb vertically to touch the examiner's pen held above it (Figure 10.61). This may be impossible if there is a median nerve palsy at the wrist or above. Remember, however, that most patients with the carpal tunnel syndrome have normal power and may indeed have symptoms but no signs at all.

Lesion in the cubital fossa. Ochsner's clasping test[rr] (for loss of flexor digitorum sublimis). Ask the patient to clasp the hands firmly together (Figure 10.62a)—the index finger on the affected side fails to flex with a lesion in the cubital fossa or higher (Figure 10.62b).

[rr] Albert Ochsner (1858–1925), American surgeon of Swiss extraction, who claimed descent from Andreas Vesalius, the great anatomist.

Figure 10.63 Motor neurone disease
Shows wasting of the small muscles of the hand.

For the *sensory* component of the median nerve, test pinprick sensation over the hand. The constant area of loss includes the palmar aspect of the thumb, index, middle and lateral half of the ring fingers (Figure 10.60). The palm is spared in median nerve lesions in the carpal tunnel.

The ulnar nerve (C8–T1). This nerve contains the *motor* supply to all the small muscles of the hand (except the LOAF muscles), flexor carpi ulnaris and the ulnar half of flexor digitorum profundus. Look for wasting of the small muscles of the hand and for partial clawing of the little and ring fingers (a claw-like hand). Clawing is hyperextension at the metacarpophalangeal joints and flexion of the inter-phalangeal joints. Note that clawing is more pronounced with an ulnar nerve lesion at the wrist, as a lesion at or above the elbow also causes loss of the flexor digitorum profundus, and therefore less flexion of the interphalangeal joints. This is the 'ulnar nerve paradox', in that a more distal lesion causes greater deformity.

Froment's sign.[ss] Ask the patient to grasp a piece of paper between the thumb and lateral aspect of the forefinger with each hand. The affected thumb will flex because of loss of the adductor of the thumb.

Causes of a true claw hand are shown in Table 10.15, while causes of wasting of the small muscles of the hand are shown in Table 10.16 (Figure 10.63).

[ss] Jules Froment (1878–1946), Professor of Medicine, Lyons, France, described the sign in 1915.

Table 10.15 Causes of a true claw hand (all fingers clawed)

Ulnar and median nerve lesion (ulnar nerve palsy alone causes a claw-like hand)
Brachial plexus lesion (C8–T1)
Other neurological disease—e.g. syringomyelia, polio
Ischaemic contracture (late and severe)
Rheumatoid arthritis (advanced, untreated disease)

Table 10.16 Causes of wasting of the small muscles of the hand

Spinal cord lesions
Syringomyelia
Cervical spondylosis with compression of the C8 segment
Tumour
Trauma

Anterior horn cell disease
Motor neurone disease, poliomyelitis
Spinal muscular atrophies, e.g. Kugelberg-Welander* disease

Root lesion
C8 compression

Lower trunk brachial plexus lesion
Thoracic outlet syndromes
Trauma, radiation, infiltration, inflammation

Peripheral nerve lesions
Median and ulnar nerve lesions
Peripheral motor neuropathy

Myopathy
Dystrophia myotonica—forearms are more affected than the hands
Distal myopathy

Trophic disorders
Arthropathies (disuse)
Ischaemia, including vasculitis
Shoulder hand syndrome

Note: Distinguishing an ulnar nerve lesion from a C8 root/lower trunk brachial plexus lesion depends on remembering that sensory loss with a C8 lesion extends proximal to the wrist, and the thenar muscles are involved with a C8 root or lower trunk brachial plexus lesion. Distinguishing a C8 root from a lower trunk brachial plexus lesion is difficult clinically, but the presence of a Horner's syndrome or an axillary mass suggests the brachial plexus is affected.
* E Kugelberg and L Welander described this in 1956.

For the *sensory* component of the ulnar nerve, test for pinprick loss over the palmar and dorsal aspects of the little finger and the medial half of the ring finger (Figure 10.60).

The brachial plexus. Brachial plexus lesions vary from mild to complete; motor and/or sensory fibres may be involved. Nerve roots form trunks, which divide into cords and then form peripheral nerves (see Tables 10.17 and 10.18). The anatomy is shown in Figure 10.64.

Patients with brachial plexus lesions may complain of pain or weakness in the shoulders or arms. Pain is often prominent, especially when

Table 10.17 Nerve roots and brachial plexus trunks

Nerve roots	Trunks	Muscles supplied
C5 and 6	Upper	Shoulder (especially biceps and deltoid)
C7	Middle	Triceps and some forearm muscles
C8 and T1	Lower	Hand and some forearm muscles

Table 10.18 Brachial plexus cords, nerves and their supplied muscles

Cords	Nerves formed	Muscles supplied
Lateral	Musculocutaneous, median	Biceps, pronator teres, flexor carpi radialis
Medial	Median and ulnar	Hand muscles
Posterior	Axillary and radial	Deltoid, triceps and forearm extensors

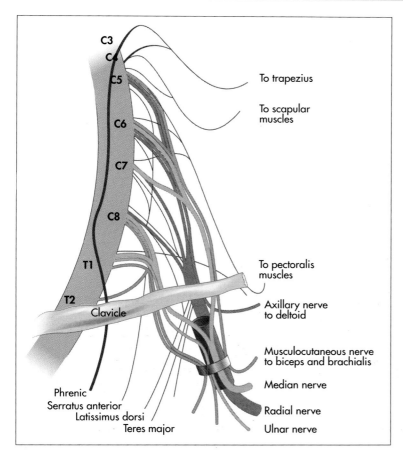

Figure 10.64 The brachial plexus

(Adapted from Chusid JG, *Correlative neuroanatomy and functional neurology*, 19th edn. Los Altos: Lange Medical, 1985.)

there has been nerve root avulsion. A neurological cause is more likely if there is dull pain that is difficult to localise, if the pain is not related to limb movement and is worse at night, and if there is no associated tenderness. The patient may be unable to get comfortable. An orthopaedic or traumatic cause is more likely if the pain is much worse with movement, or there are signs of inflammation, joint deformity or local tenderness. Most plexus lesions are supraclavicular (i.e. proximal), especially when they occur after trauma. When infraclavicular (i.e. distal) lesions occur they are usually less severe.

Examine the arms and shoulder girdle (Table 10.19). Remember that the dorsal scapular nerve (which supplies the rhomboid muscles) comes from the C5 nerve root proximal to the upper trunk, and so rhomboid function is usually spared in upper trunk lesions. Typical lesions of the brachial plexus are described in Table 10.20. The cervical rib syndrome may cause a lower brachial plexus lesion (Table 10.21). Table 10.22 suggests a scheme for distinguishing plexus and nerve root lesions.

Causes of brachial plexus lesions include:

Table 10.19 Shoulder girdle examination

Method

Abnormalities are likely to be due to a muscular dystrophy, single nerve or a root lesion. Inspect each muscle, palpate its bulk and test function as follows:

1 *Trapezius (XI, C3, C4):* ask the patient to elevate the shoulders against resistance and look for winging of the upper scapula.
2 *Serratus anterior (C5–C7):* ask the patient to push the hands against the wall and look for winging of the lower scapula.
3 *Rhomboids (C4, C5):* ask the patient to pull both shoulder blades together with the hands on the hips.
4 *Supraspinatus (C5, C6):* ask the patient to abduct the arms from the sides against resistance.
5 *Infraspinatus (C5, C6):* ask the patient to rotate the upper arms externally against resistance with the elbows flexed at the sides.
6 *Teres major (C5–C7):* ask the patient to internally rotate the upper arms against resistance.
7 *Latissimus dorsi (C7, C8):* ask the patient to pull the elbows into the sides against resistance.
8 *Pectoralis major, clavicular head (C5–C8):* ask the patient to lift the upper arms above the horizontal and push them forward against resistance.
9 *Pectoralis major, sternocostal part (C6–T1) and pectoralis minor (C7):* ask the patient to adduct the upper arms against resistance.
10 *Deltoid (C5, C6) (and axillary nerve):* ask the patient to abduct the arms against resistance.

Table 10.20 Brachial plexus lesions

Complete lesion (rare)

1 Lower motor neurone signs affect the whole arm
2 Sensory loss (whole limb)
3 Horner's syndrome (an important clue)
Note: This is often painful.

Upper lesion (Erb Duchenne*) (C5, C6)

1 Loss of shoulder movement and elbow flexion—the hand is held in the waiter's tip position
2 Sensory loss over the lateral aspect of the arm and forearm

Lower lesion (Klumpke†) (C8, T1)

1 True claw hand with paralysis of all the intrinsic muscles
2 Sensory loss along the ulnar side of the hand and forearm
3 Horner's syndrome

---

* Wilhelm Heinrich Erb (1840–1921), Germany's greatest neurologist.
† Auguste Déjérine-Klumpke (1859–1927), French neurologist, described this lesion as a student. She was an American, but educated in Switzerland. As a final-year student she married the great French neurologist Jules Déjérine.

Table 10.21 Cervical rib syndrome

Clinical features

1 Weakness and wasting of the small muscles of the hand (claw hand)
2 C8 and T1 sensory loss
3 Unequal radial pulses and blood pressure
4 Subclavian bruits on arm manoeuvring (may be present in normal people)
5 Palpable cervical rib in the neck (uncommon)

Table 10.22 Distinguishing brachial plexus lesions and nerve root compression

	Root	Plexus
Previous trauma	Occasionally	Some types
Insidious onset	Usually	Some types
Neck pain	Yes	No
Unilateral interscapular pain	Yes	No
Weakness	Mild–moderate	Often severe
Pattern of weakness	Most commonly triceps (C7 lesions, the most commonly affected root)	Usually shoulder and biceps or hand

1 Inflammation, autoimmune (more often upper plexus).
2 radiotherapy (more often upper plexus).
3 Cancer (more often lower plexus). *Cancer* causes a brachial plexus lesion by local invasion. The lower trunk is usually affected first. These plexus lesions are usually painful and progress rapidly. Weakness and sensory loss are both present.
4 Trauma: direct (motor vehicle accident, surgery including sternotomy, lacerations and gunshots), traction (birth injuries, motor vehicle accidents, sporting injuries such as rugby tackles—more often upper plexus), chronic compression (thoracic outlet, 'backpack palsy', fractures with bone displacement).

The lower limbs

Begin by testing *gait,* if this is possible (see page 344).

Inspect the legs with the patient lying in bed with the legs and thighs entirely exposed (place a towel over the groin). Note whether there is a urinary catheter present, which may indicate that there is spinal cord compression or other spinal cord disease, particularly multiple sclerosis.

The motor system

Fasciculations and muscle wasting. Inspect for fasciculations. Look for muscle wasting. Feel the muscle bulk of the quadriceps and calves. Then run a hand along each shin, feeling for wasting of the anterior tibial muscles.

Tone. Test tone at the knees and ankles. Place one hand under a chosen knee and then abruptly pull the knee upwards, causing flexion. When the patient is relaxed this should occur without resistance. Then, supporting the thigh, flex and extend the knee at increasing velocity, feeling for resistance to muscle stretch (tone). Tone in the legs may also be tested by sitting the patient with legs hanging freely over the edge of the bed. A leg (of the patient) is raised by the examiner to the horizontal and let go of suddenly. The leg will oscillate up to half a dozen times in a normal person who is completely relaxed. If hypotonia is present, as occurs in cerebellar disease, the oscillations will be wider and more prolonged. If increased tone or spasticity is present, the movements will be irregular and jerky.

Next test for *clonus* of the ankle and knee. This is a sustained rhythmical contraction of the muscles when put under sudden stretch. It is due to hypertonia from an upper motor neurone lesion. It represents an increase in reflex excitability (from increased alpha motor neurone activity).

Sharply dorsiflex the foot with the knee bent and the thigh externally rotated. When ankle clonus is present, recurrent ankle plantar flexion movement occurs. This may persist for as long as the examiner sustains dorsiflexion of the ankle. Test for patellar clonus (which is not so common) by resting the hand on the lower part of the quadriceps with the knee extended and moving the patella down sharply. Sustained rhythmical contraction of the quadriceps occurs as long as the downward stretch is maintained.

Power. Test power next.
Hip
- *Flexion*—psoas and iliacus muscles—(L2, L3): ask the patient to lift up the straight leg and not let you push it down (having placed your hand above the knee) (Figure 10.65).
- *Extension*—gluteus maximus—(L5, S1, S2): ask the patient to keep the leg down and not let you pull it up from underneath the calf or ankle (Figure 10.66).
- *Abduction*—gluteus medius and minimus, sartorius and tensor fasciae latae—(L4, L5, S1): ask the patient to abduct the leg and not let you push it in (Figure 10.67).

Figure 10.65 Testing power—hip flexion: 'Lift your leg up and don't let me push it down'

Figure 10.66 Testing power—hip extension: 'Push your heel down and don't let me pull it up'

Figure 10.67 Testing power—hip abduction: 'Don't let me push your knees together'

- *Adduction*—adductors longus, brevis and magnus—(L2, L3, L4): ask the patient to keep the leg adducted and not let you push it out (Figure 10.68).

Knee

- *Flexion*—hamstrings (biceps femoris, semimembranosus, semitendinosus)—(L5, S1): ask the patient to bend the knee and not let you straighten it (Figure 10.69). If there is doubt about the real strength of knee flexion, it should be tested with the patient in the prone position. Here possible help from hip flexion is prevented and the muscles can be palpated during contraction.
- *Extension*—quadriceps femoris (this muscle is three times as strong as its antagonists, the hamstrings)—(L3, L4): with the knee slightly bent, ask the patient to straighten the knee and not let you bend it (Figure 10.70).

Figure 10.68 Testing power—hip adduction: 'Don't let me push your knees apart'

Figure 10.69 Testing power—knee flexion: 'Bend your knee and don't let me straighten it'

Figure 10.70 Testing power—knee extension: 'Straighten your knee and don't let me bend it'

Figure 10.72 Testing power—ankle, dorsiflexion: 'Don't let me push your foot down'

Figure 10.71 Testing power—ankle, plantar flexion: 'Don't let me push your foot up'

Figure 10.73 Testing power—ankle (tarsal joint) eversion: 'Stop me turning your foot inwards'

Ankle

- *Plantar flexion*—gastrocnemius, plantaris, soleus—(S1, S2): ask the patient to push the foot down and not let you push it up (Figure 10.71).
- *Dorsiflexion*—tibialis anterior, extensor digitorum longus and extensor hallucis longus—(L4, L5): ask the patient to bring the foot up and not let you push it down (Figure 10.72). The power of the ankle joint can also be tested by having the patient stand up on the toes (plantar flexion) or on the heels (dorsiflexion); these movements may also be limited if coordination is impaired.

Tarsal joint

- *Eversion*—peroneus longus and brevis, and extensor digitorum longus—(L5, S1): ask the patient to evert the foot against resistance (Figure 10.73).
- *Inversion*—tibialis posterior, gastrocnemius and hallucis longus—(L5, S1): with the foot in complete plantar flexion, ask the patient to invert the foot against resistance (Figure 10.74).

Figure 10.74 Testing power—ankle (tarsal joint) inversion: 'Stop me turning your foot outwards'

Figure 10.75 Quick test of lower limbs power

(a) 'Stand up on your toes.' (b) 'Now lift up on your heels.' (c) 'Now squat and stand up again.'

Quick test of lower limb power. The clinician in a hurry can test lower limb power quickly by asking the patient to:

1　stand up on his or her toes (S1) (Figure 10.75a);
2　stand up on the heels (L4, L5) (Figure 10.75b);
3　squat and stand again (L3, L4) (Figure 10.75c).

This tests ankle, knee and hip power. Inability to perform any of the tests suggests a need to test more formally.

Reflexes. Test the following reflexes.

Knee jerk (L3, L4). Slide one arm under the knees so that they are slightly bent and supported. The tendon hammer is allowed to fall onto the infrapatellar tendon (Figure 10.76). Normally, contraction of the quadriceps causes extension of the knee. Compare the two sides. If the knee jerk appears to be absent on one or both sides, it should be tested again following a reinforcement manoeuvre. Ask the patient to interlock the fingers and then pull apart hard at the moment before the hammer strikes the tendon (Jendrassik's manoeuvre[tt]) (Figure 10.77). This manoeuvre has been shown to restore an apparently absent ankle jerk in 70% of elderly people. A reinforcement manoeuvre such as this, or teeth clenching or grasping an object, should be used if there is difficulty eliciting any of the muscle stretch reflexes.

[tt] Ernst Jendrassik (1858–1921), Budapest physician.

Figure 10.76 The knee jerk examination

Figure 10.77 The knee jerk with reinforcement: 'Grip your fingers and pull your hands apart'

Ankle jerk (S1, S2). Have the foot in the mid-position at the ankle with the knee bent, the thigh externally rotated on the bed, and the foot held in dorsiflexion by the examiner. The hammer is allowed to fall on the Achilles tendon (Figure 10.78). The normal response is plantar flexion of the foot with contraction of the gastrocnemius muscle. Again test with reinforcement if appropriate. This reflex can also be tested with the patient kneeling (page 268) or by tapping the sole of the foot.[17]

Plantar reflex (L5, S1, S2). After telling the patient what is going to happen, use a blunt object (such as the key to an expensive motor car) to stroke up the lateral aspect of the sole, and curve inwards before it reaches the toes, moving towards the middle metatarsophalangeal (MTP) joint (Figure 10.79). The patient's foot should be in the same position as for testing the ankle jerk. The normal response is flexion of the big toe at the MTP joint in patients over one year of age. The extensor (Babinski[uu])[18] response is abnormal and is characterised by extension of the big toe at the MTP joint (the upgoing toe) and fanning of the other toes. This indicates an upper motor neurone (pyramidal) lesion, although the test's reliability can be relatively poor. Bilateral upgoing toes may also be found after a generalised seizure, or in a patient in coma.

Coordination. Test for cerebellar disease with three manoeuvres.

Heel–shin test. Ask the patient to run the heel of one foot up and down the opposite shin at a moderate pace and as accurately as possible (Figure 10.80). In cerebellar disease the heel wobbles all over the place, with oscillations from side to side and overshooting. Closing the eyes makes little difference to this in cerebellar disease, but if there is posterior column loss the movements are made worse when the eyes are shut—that is, there is 'sensory ataxia'.

Toe–finger test. Unfortunately, a toe–nose test is not a practical way of assessing the lower limbs, so a toe–finger test is used. Ask the patient to lift the foot (with the knee bent) and touch the examiner's finger with the big toe. Look for intention tremor.

Foot-tapping test. Rapidly alternating movements are tested by getting the patient to tap the sole of the foot quickly on the examiner's hand or tap the heel on the opposite shin. Look for loss of rhythmicity.

uu Josef Babinski (1857–1932), Parisian neurologist of Polish extraction, described this sign in 1896. (It was probably first described by Remak in 1893.) Babinski was a famous gourmet and assistant to Charcot.

Figure 10.78 The ankle jerk (first method, see also page 268): the examiner dorsiflexes the foot slightly to stretch the tendon

Figure 10.79 The plantar reflex examination

Figure 10.80 The heel–shin test: 'Run your heel down your shin smoothly and quickly'

The sensory system

As for the upper limb, test for pain sensation first in each dermatome, comparing the right with the left side (Figure 10.81). Map out any abnormality and decide on the pattern of loss.

Figure 10.81 Testing pinprick (pain) sensation in the lower limbs (do not draw blood with the pin)

Then test vibration sense over the ankles and, if necessary, on the knees and the anterior superior iliac spines (Figure 10.82). Next test proprioception, using the big toes (Figure 10.83) and, if necessary, the knees and hips.

Finally, test light touch (Figure 10.84).

Dermatomes. Memorise the following rough guide (Figure 10.85): L2 supplies the upper anterior thigh; L3 supplies the area around the front of the knee; L4 supplies the medial aspect of the leg; L5 supplies the lateral aspect of the leg and the medial side of the dorsum of the foot; S1 supplies the heel and most of the sole; S2 supplies the posterior aspect of the thigh; S3, S4 and S5 supply concentric rings around the anus.

Sensory levels. If there is peripheral sensory loss in the leg, attempt to map out the upper level with a pin, moving up at 5 cm intervals initially, from the leg to the abdomen, until the patient reports it is sharp. This may involve testing over the abdominal or even the chest dermatomes. Establishing a sensory level on the trunk indicates the spinal cord level that is affected. Remember, a level of hyperaesthesia (increased sensitivity) often occurs above the sensory

Figure 10.82 Testing vibration sense in the lower limbs

(a) Strike a 128 Hz tuning fork confidently on your thenar eminence. (b) Demonstrate the vibration of the tuning fork on the patient's sternum: 'Can you feel this vibration?' (c) Place the tuning fork on the great toe: 'Can you feel the vibration there? Tell me when it stops.' (d) If vibration sense is absent on the great toe, try testing on the patella. (e) If vibration sense is absent at the knee, try testing on the anterior superior iliac spine.

Figure 10.83 Position sense: 'Shut your eyes and tell me whether I have moved your toe up or down'

Figure 10.84 Testing light-touch sensation (do not stroke the skin with the cottonwool)

Figure 10.85 Dermatomes of the lower limbs

level and it is the upper level of this that should be determined, as it usually indicates the highest affected spinal segment. Also remember that the level of a vertebral body only corresponds to the spinal cord level in the upper cervical cord because the spinal cord is shorter than the spinal canal. The C8 spinal segment lies opposite the C7 vertebra. In the upper thoracic cord there is a difference of about two segments and in the mid-thoracic cord three segments. All the lumbosacral segments are opposite the T11 to L1 vertebrae.

The superficial or cutaneous reflexes

These reflexes occur in response to light touch or scratching of the skin or mucous membranes. The stimulus is more superficial than the tendon (muscle stretch) reflexes. As a rule these reflexes occur more slowly after the stimulus, are less constantly present and fatigue more easily.

Examples include the palmar or grasp reflex (page 292), the cremasteric reflex and the abdominal reflexes and the plantar responses.

The abdominal reflexes (epigastric T6–T9, mid-abdominal T9–T11, lower abdominal T11—L1). Test these by lightly stroking the abdominal wall diagonally towards the umbilicus in each of the four quadrants of the abdomen (Figure 10.86). Reflex contractions of the abdominal wall are *absent* in upper motor neurone lesions above the segmental level and also in patients who have had surgical operations interrupting the nerves. They disappear in coma and deep sleep, and during anaesthesia. They are usually difficult to elicit in obese patients and can also be absent in some normal people (20%). Their absence in the presence of increased tendon reflexes is suggestive of corticospinal tract abnormality.

Figure 10.86 Abdominal reflex: stroke towards the umbilicus from each quadrant and watch for abdominal muscle contraction

The cremasteric reflexes (L1–L2). Stroke the inner part of the thigh in a downward direction; normally contraction of the cremasteric muscle pulls up the scrotum and testis on the side stroked. It may be absent in old men and in those with a hydrocele or varicocele, or after an episode of orchitis.

Saddle sensation and anal reflex. Test now for saddle sensation if a cauda equina lesion is suspected (e.g. because of urinary or faecal incontinence). The only sensory loss may be on the buttocks or around the anus (S3–S5). In this case also test the anal reflex (S2, S3, S4): normal contraction of the external sphincter in response to pinprick of the perianal skin is abolished in patients with a lesion of the sacral segments of the cauda equina. If, however, the lowest sacral segments are spared but the higher ones are involved, this suggests that there is an intrinsic cord lesion.

Spine. Examine the spine and perform the straight-leg raising test (page 233).

Examination of the peripheral nerves of the lower limb

Lateral cutaneous nerve of the thigh. Test for sensory loss (Figure 10.87). A lesion of this nerve usually occurs because of entrapment between the

Figure 10.87 Distribution of the lateral cutaneous nerve of the thigh

Figure 10.88 Sensory distribution of the femoral nerve

inguinal ligament and the anterior superior iliac spine. It causes a sensory loss over the lateral aspect of the thigh with no motor loss detectable. If painful, it is called *meralgia paraesthetica*.

Femoral nerve (L2, L3, L4). Test for weakness of knee extension (quadriceps paralysis) (Figure 10.88). Hip flexion weakness is only slight, and adductor strength is preserved. The knee jerk is absent. The sensory loss involves the inner aspect of the thigh and leg.

Sciatic nerve (L4, L5, S1, S2). This nerve supplies all the muscles below the knee and the hamstrings (Figure 10.89). Test for loss of power below the knee resulting in a footdrop (plantar flexed foot) and for weakness of knee flexion. Test the reflexes: with a sciatic nerve lesion the knee jerk is intact but the ankle jerk and plantar response are absent. Test sensation on the posterior thigh, lateral and posterior calf, and on the foot (lost with a proximal nerve lesion).

Common peroneal nerve (L4, L5, S1). This is a major terminal branch of the sciatic nerve. It supplies the anterior and lateral compartment muscles of the leg (Figure 10.90). On inspection one may notice a footdrop (Table 10.23). Test for weakness of dorsiflexion and eversion. Test the reflexes, which will

Figure 10.89 Sensory distribution of the sciatic nerve

Figure 10.90 Sensory distribution of the common peroneal nerve

Table 10.23 Causes of footdrop

Common peroneal nerve palsy
Sciatic nerve palsy
Lumbosacral plexus lesion
L4, L5 root lesion
Peripheral motor neuropathy
Distal myopathy
Motor neurone disease
Stroke—anterior cerebral artery or lacunar
   syndrome ('ataxic hemiparesis')

Table 10.24 Gait disorders

Hemiplegia: the foot is plantar flexed and the
   leg is swung in a lateral arc
Spastic paraparesis: scissors gait
Parkinson's disease: hesitation in starting
- shuffling
- freezing
- festination
- propulsion
- retropulsion

Cerebellar: a drunken gait which is wide-based
   or reeling on a narrow base; the patient
   staggers towards the affected side if there is a
   unilateral cerebellar hemisphere lesion
Posterior column lesion: clumsy slapping down
   of the feet on a broad base
Footdrop: high stepping gait
Proximal myopathy: waddling gait
Prefrontal lobe (apraxic): feet appear glued to
   floor when erect, but move more easily when
   the patient is supine
Hysterical: characterised by a bizarre,
   inconsistent gait

all be intact. Test for sensory loss. There is only minimal sensory loss over the lateral aspect of the dorsum of the foot. Note that these findings can be confused with an L5 root lesion, but the latter includes weakness of knee flexion and loss of foot inversion, as well as sensory loss in the L5 distribution.

Gait

Method

Make sure the patient's legs are clearly visible. Now ask the patient to walk normally for a few metres and then turn around quickly and walk back. Then ask the patient to walk heel-to-toe to exclude a midline cerebellar lesion (Figure 10.91). Ask the patient to then walk on the toes (an S1 lesion will make this

difficult or impossible) and then on the heels (an L4 or L5 lesion causing footdrop will make this difficult or impossible).

Test for proximal myopathy by asking the patient to squat and then stand up, or sit in a low chair and then stand.

To test *station* (Romberg[vv] test), ask the patient to stand erect with the feet together and the eyes open (Figure 10.92a). Once the patient is stable ask him or her to close the eyes (Figure 10.92b). Compare the steadiness shown with the eyes open, then closed. Even in the absence of neurological disease a person may be slightly unsteady with the eyes closed. Marked unsteadiness with the eyes open is seen with cerebellar or vestibular dysfunction.

The Romberg test is positive when unsteadiness increases with eye closure. This is usually seen with the loss of proprioceptive sensation.

Gait disorders are summarised in Table 10.24.

Figure 10.91 Cerebellar testing—heel–toe walking

[vv] Moritz Heinrich von Romberg (1795–1873), Berlin professor, wrote the first modern neurology textbook.

Figure 10.92 Romberg's test

(a) 'Stand with your feet together.'
(b) 'Now shut your eyes. I won't let you fall.'

Correlation of physical signs and neurological disease

Upper motor neurone lesions

In neurology a clinical diagnosis is made by defining the deficit that is present, deciding on its anatomical level and then considering the likely causes. It is important to be able to distinguish *upper motor neurone* signs (*Good signs guide 10.1*) from *lower motor neurone* signs (Figure 10.93). The former occur when a lesion has interrupted a neural pathway at a level above the anterior horn cell: for example, motor pathways in the cerebral cortex, internal capsule, cerebral peduncles, brainstem or spinal cord. When this occurs there is greater weakness of abductors and extensors in the upper limb, and flexors and abductors in the lower limb, as the normal function of this pathway is to mediate voluntary contraction of the antigravity muscles. All muscles, however, are usually weaker than normal. Muscle wasting is slight or absent, probably because there is no loss of trophic factors normally released from the lower motor neurone. The disuse that results from severe weakness may, however, cause some atrophy.

Spasticity occurs because of destruction of the corticoreticulospinal tract, resulting in stretch reflex hyperactivity.

Monoplegia is paralysis affecting only one limb, when there is a motor cortex or partial internal capsule lesion. *Hemiplegia* affects one side of the body due to a lesion affecting projection of pathways from the contralateral motor cortex.

Paraplegia affects both legs, while *quadriplegia* affects all four limbs, and is the result of spinal cord trauma or, less often, a brainstem lesion (e.g. basilar artery thrombosis).

GOOD SIGNS GUIDE 10.1 Unilateral hemisphere lesion		
Sign	**Positive LR**	**Negative LR**
Upper limb drift	33.0	0.2
Facial weakness	32.3	0.2
Hemiparesis	31.7	0.3
Wrist extensor weakness	29.0	0.3
Babinski response	19.0	0.6
Hemianopia	NS	0.7
Hemisensory disturbance	NS	0.7

NS = not significant.
From McGee S, *Evidence-based physical diagnosis*, Saunders, 2001.

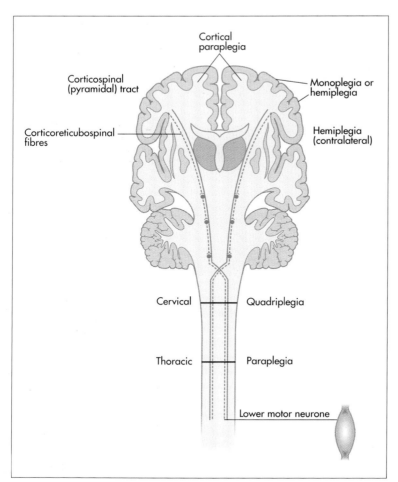

Figure 10.93 Upper and lower motor neurone lesions

(Adapted from Lance JG, McLeod JW, *A physiological approach to clinical neurology*, 3rd edn. London: Butterworths, 1981.)

Table 10.25 Intracerebral thrombosis or embolism: clinical features

Middle cerebral artery	Posterior cerebral artery	Anterior cerebral artery
Main branch Infarction middle third of hemisphere: UMN face, arm>leg; homonymous hemianopia; aphasia or non-dominant hemisphere signs (depends on side); cortical sensory loss	*Main branch** Infarction of thalamus and occipital cortex: hemianaesthesia (loss of all modalities); homonymous hemianopia (complete)	UMN leg>arm; cortical sensory loss leg only; urinary incontinence
Perforating artery Internal capsule infarction: UMN face, UMN arm>leg		

UMN = upper motor neurone lesion.
* Effects variable because of anastomoses with distal middle cerebral artery branches and supply from posterior communicating artery, but one would examine particularly for occipital and temporal lobe dysfunction.

Causes of hemiplegia (upper motor neurone lesion)

Vascular disease. Thrombosis, embolism or haemorrhage occur in specific vascular territories (Figure 10.94).[19] Lesions in the territory of the *internal carotid artery* result in hemiplegia on the opposite side of the body if a large area of the internal capsule or hemisphere is involved. Homonymous hemianopia, hemianaesthesia and dysphasia may occur (Table 10.25). Stenosis of the internal carotid artery in the neck may be associated with a bruit.[20]

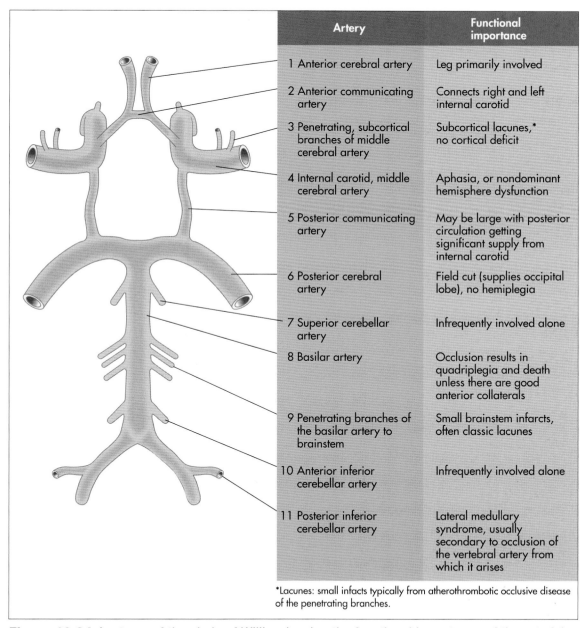

Artery	Functional importance
1 Anterior cerebral artery	Leg primarily involved
2 Anterior communicating artery	Connects right and left internal carotid
3 Penetrating, subcortical branches of middle cerebral artery	Subcortical lacunes,* no cortical deficit
4 Internal carotid, middle cerebral artery	Aphasia, or nondominant hemisphere dysfunction
5 Posterior communicating artery	May be large with posterior circulation getting significant supply from internal carotid
6 Posterior cerebral artery	Field cut (supplies occipital lobe), no hemiplegia
7 Superior cerebellar artery	Infrequently involved alone
8 Basilar artery	Occlusion results in quadriplegia and death unless there are good anterior collaterals
9 Penetrating branches of the basilar artery to brainstem	Small brainstem infarcts, often classic lacunes
10 Anterior inferior cerebellar artery	Infrequently involved alone
11 Posterior inferior cerebellar artery	Lateral medullary syndrome, usually secondary to occlusion of the vertebral artery from which it arises

*Lacunes: small infacts typically from atherothrombotic occlusive disease of the penetrating branches.

Figure 10.94 Anatomy of the circle of Willis, showing the functional importance of the arterial blood supply

(Adapted from Weiner HL, Levitt LP, *Neurology for the house officer*, 6th edn. Baltimore: Williams & Wilkins, 2000.)

Lesions in the territory of the *vertebrobasilar artery* may produce cranial nerve palsies, cerebellar signs, Horner's syndrome and sensory loss, as well as upper motor neurone signs (often bilateral because of the close proximity of structures in the brainstem). For example, a lesion in the midbrain may be associated with a third nerve paralysis and upper motor neurone signs on the opposite side. Hemianaesthesia and homonymous hemianopia may occur if the posterior cerebral arteries are affected. Atheroma in the ascending aorta is increasingly recognised as a source of cerebral emboli.

Compressive and infiltrative lesions. Tumours tend to occur in the lobes of the brain, and focal signs will depend on the tumour site. Signs localised to the parietal, temporal, occipital or frontal lobe suggest this disease process (see Table 10.6).

There may, however, be false localising signs in the presence of raised intracranial pressure: for example, a unilateral or bilateral sixth nerve palsy (because of the nerve's long intracranial path). Papilloedema is usually associated if there is raised intracranial pressure.

Demyelinating disease. Multiple sclerosis results in lesions in different areas usually with a relapsing and remitting course.

Infection. Human immunodeficiency virus (HIV) infection.

Lower motor neurone lesions

Lower motor neurone lesions interrupt the spinal reflex arc and therefore cause muscle wasting, reduced or absent reflexes and sometimes fasciculations. This results from a lesion of the spinal motor neurones, motor root or peripheral nerve (Table 10.26).

Motor neurone disease

This disease of unknown aetiology results in pathological changes in the anterior horn cells, the motor nuclei of the medulla and the descending tracts. It therefore causes a combination of upper motor neurone and lower motor neurone signs, although one type may predominate. Importantly, fasciculations are almost always present. The muscle stretch reflexes are usually present (often increased) until late in the course of the disease, and there are rarely any objective sensory changes (15%–20% of patients report sensory symptoms).

Table 10.26 Upper and lower motor neurone lesions (Figure 10.93)

Signs of upper motor neurone lesions

1 Weakness is present in all muscle groups, but in the lower limb may be more marked in the flexor and abductor muscles. In the upper limb, weakness may be most marked in the abductors and extensors. There is very little muscle wasting.
2 Spasticity: increased tone is present (may be clasp-knife) and often associated with clonus.
3 The reflexes are increased except for the superficial reflexes (e.g. abdominal), which are absent.
4 There is an extensor (Babinski) plantar response (upgoing toe).

Signs of lower motor neurone lesions

1 Weakness may be more obvious distally than proximally, and the flexor and extensor muscles are equally involved. Wasting is a prominent feature.
2 Tone is reduced.
3 The reflexes are reduced and the plantar response is normal or absent.
4 Fasciculation may be present.

Peripheral neuropathy

Distal parts of the nerves are usually involved first because of their distance from the cell bodies, causing a distal loss of sensation or motor function, or both, in the limbs. A typical sensory change is a symmetrical glove and stocking loss to all modalities (see Figure 10.95). This is unlike the pattern found with individual nerve or nerve root disease, which should be suspected if sensory loss is asymmetrical or confined to one limb. Peripheral muscle weakness may be present due to motor nerve involvement. Occasionally motor neuropathy may occur without sensory change. In the latter case, reflexes are reduced but may not be absent in the distal parts of the limbs (Table 10.27).

Guillain-Barré syndrome (acute inflammatory polyradiculoneuropathy)

This disease, thought to have an immune basis, may begin 7 to 10 days after an infective illness. It results in flaccid proximal and distal muscle paralysis,

Table 10.27 Peripheral neuropathy
(Figure 10.95)

Causes of peripheral neuropathy

1 Drugs—e.g. isoniazid, vincristine, phenytoin, nitrofurantoin, cisplatinum, heavy metals, amiodarone
2 Alcohol abuse (with or without vitamin B_1 deficiency)
3 Metabolic—e.g. diabetes mellitus, chronic renal failure
4 Guillain-Barré syndrome
5 Malignancy—e.g. carcinoma of the lung (paraneoplastic neuropathy), leukaemia, lymphoma
6 Vitamin deficiency (e.g. B_{12}) or excess (e.g. B_6)
7 Connective tissue disease or vasculitis—e.g. PAN, SLE
8 Hereditary—e.g. hereditary motor and sensory neuropathy
9 Others, e.g. amyloid, HIV infection
10 Idiopathic

Causes of a predominant motor neuropathy

1 Guillain-Barré syndrome, chronic inflammatory polyradiculoneuropathy
2 Hereditary motor and sensory neuropathy
3 Diabetes mellitus
4 Others—e.g. acute intermittent porphyria, lead poisoning, diphtheria, multifocal conduction block neuropathy

Causes of a painful peripheral neuropathy

1 Diabetes mellitus
2 Alcohol
3 Vitamin B_1 or B_{12} deficiency
4 Carcinoma
5 Porphyria
6 Arsenic or thallium poisoning

PAN = polyarteritis nodosa; SLE = systemic lupus erythematosus; HIV = human immunodeficiency virus.

Figure 10.95 Peripheral neuropathy: glove and stocking sensory loss

Table 10.28 Mononeuritis multiplex

Definition: mononeuritis multiplex refers to the separate involvement of more than one peripheral (or less often cranial) nerve by a single disease

Acute causes (usually vascular)

Polyarteritis nodosa
Diabetes mellitus
Connective tissue disease—e.g. rheumatoid arthritis, systemic lupus erythematosus

Chronic causes

Multiple compressive neuropathies
Sarcoidosis
Acromegaly
HIV infection
Leprosy
Lyme disease
Others—e.g. carcinoma (rare)

which typically ascends from the lower to the upper limbs. Wasting is rare. The cranial nerves can be affected; occasionally disease is confined to these. Sensory loss is minimal or absent. Unlike transverse myelitis, the sphincters are little affected. Weakness of the respiratory muscles can be fatal but the disease is usually self-limiting. HIV infection can cause a similar syndrome.

Thickened peripheral nerves

If there is evidence of a peripheral nerve lesion, peripheral neuropathy or a mononeuritis multiplex (Table 10.28), palpate for thickened nerves. The median nerve at the wrist, the ulnar nerve at the elbow, the greater auricular nerve in the neck and the common peroneal nerve at the head of the fibula are the most easily accessible. If nerves are thickened consider the following diagnoses:

- Acromegaly (page 267)
- Amyloid
- Chronic inflammatory demyelinating poly-radiculoneuropathy
- Leprosy
- Hereditary motor and sensory neuropathy (autosomal dominant) (Table 10.34)
- Other—e.g. sarcoid, diabetes mellitus, neurofibromatosis

Spinal cord compression

(Figures 10.96 to 10.100)

It is important to remember that a spinal cord lesion causes lower motor neurone signs at the level of the lesion and upper motor neurone signs below that level (Table 10.29). Don't forget the spinal cord's anatomy and vascular supply (Figure 10.96). Examine any suspected case as follows.

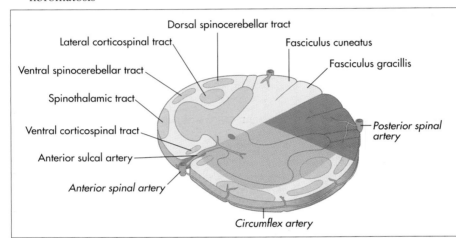

Figure 10.96 Anatomy and vascular supply of the spinal cord

Note: Anterior spinal artery occlusion spares posterior column function.

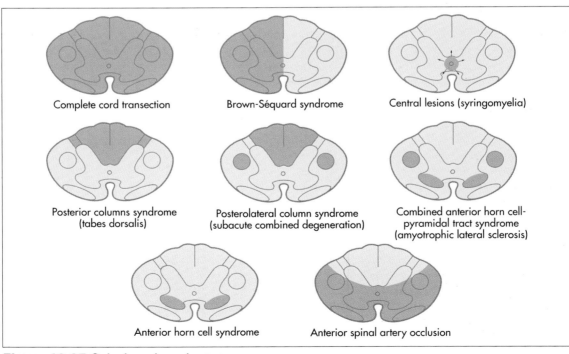

Figure 10.97 Spinal cord syndromes

(Adapted from Brazis PW, *Localisation in clinical neurology*, Philadelphia: Lippincott, Williams & Wilkins, 2001.)

Table 10.29 Important motor and reflex changes of spinal cord compression

See Figures 10.96 to 10.100 for sensory changes.

Upper cervical

Upper motor neurone signs in the upper and lower limbs.

C5
* Lower motor neurone weakness and wasting of rhomboids, deltoids, biceps and brachioradialis.
* Upper motor neurone signs affect the rest of the upper and all the lower limbs. The biceps jerk is lost. The brachioradialis jerk is inverted.

C8
* Lower motor neurone weakness and wasting of the intrinsic muscles of the hand.
* Upper motor neurone signs in the lower limbs.

Midthoracic

Intercostal paralysis.
Upper motor neurone signs in the lower limbs.
Loss of upper abdominal reflexes at T7 and T8.

T10–T11
* Loss of the lower abdominal reflexes and upward displacement of the umbilicus.
* Upper motor neurone signs in the lower limbs.

L1
* Cremasteric reflex is lost (normal abdominal reflexes).
* Upper motor neurone signs in the lower limbs.

L4
* Lower motor neurone weakness and wasting of the quadriceps.
* Knee jerks lost.
* Ankle jerks may be hyperreflexic with extensor plantar response (upgoing toes), but more often the whole conus is involved, causing a lower motor neurone lesion.

L5–S1
* Lower motor neurone weakness of knee flexion and hip extension (S1) and abduction (L5) plus calf and foot muscles.
* Knee jerks present.
* No ankle jerks or plantar responses.
* Anal reflex present.

S3–S4
* No anal reflex.
* Saddle sensory loss.
* Normal lower limbs.

Causes of spinal cord compression

1 Vertebral
  * Spondylosis
  * Trauma
  * Prolapse of a disc
  * Tumour
  * Infection
2 Outside the dura
  * Lymphoma, metastases
  * Infection—e.g. abscess
3 Within the dura but extramedullary
  * Tumour—e.g. meningioma, neurofibroma
4 Intramedullary*
  * Tumour—e.g. glioma, ependymoma
  * Syringomyelia
  * Haematomyelia

* Lower motor neurone signs may extend for several segments, and spastic paralysis occurs late, unlike the situation with extramedullary lesions.

Figure 10.98 Sensory loss with transverse section of the spinal cord

Figure 10.99 Pattern of sensory loss with intrinsic spinal cord disease

For example, central tumour or less commonly with extrinsic compression of the spinal cord—sacrum is spared.

Figure 10.100 Conus medullaris or cauda equina lesion—saddle anaesthesia

After carefully examining the lower limbs (see above) determine the level of any sensory impairment (Table 10.30). Then examine the back for signs of a local lesion. Look for deformity, scars and neurofibromas. Palpate for vertebral tenderness and auscultate down the spine for bruits. Next examine the upper limbs and cranial nerves to determine the upper level if this is not already obvious.

Important spinal cord syndromes

Brown-Séquard syndrome[ww]

Clinical features are shown in Figure 10.101. These signs result from hemisection of the cord.

[ww] Charles Edouard Brown-Séquard (1817–1894) succeeded Claude Bernard at the College de France. He was the son of an American sea captain (pirate) and a French woman. He was born in Mauritius at a time when it was under British rule. With this background he roved around the world, working in Paris, Mauritius, London and New York. His syndrome usually arose from failed murder attempts. Traditionally Mauritian cane cutters, when trying to murder someone, used a very long thin knife which was slipped between the ribs from behind, to cut the aorta or penetrate the heart. Only such a knife could have caused a cord hemitransection.

Figure 10.101 Brown-Séquard sydrome

Loss of pain and temperature on the opposite side to the lesion, with loss of vibration and proprioception on the same side as the lesion.

Table 10.30 Important patterns of abnormal sensation

Sign	Location of lesion
Total unilateral loss of all forms of sensation	Thalamus or upper brainstem (extensive lesion)
Pain and temperature loss on one side of face and *opposite* side of body	Medulla involving descending nucleus of spinal tract of the fifth nerve and ascending spinothalamic tract (lateral medullary lesion) (Figure 10.102)
Bilateral loss of all forms of sensation below a definite level	Spinal cord lesion (if only pain and temperature affected: anterior cord lesion)
Unilateral loss of pain and temperature below a definite level	Partial unilateral spinal cord lesion on opposite side (Brown-Séquard syndrome) (Figure 10.101)
Loss of pain and temperature over several segments but normal sensation above and below	Intrinsic spinal cord lesion near its centre anteriorly (involves the crossing fibres), e.g. syringomyelia, intrinsic cord tumour (*Note:* more posterior lesions cause proprioceptive loss)
Loss of sensation over many segments with sacral sparing	Intrinsic cord compression more likely
Saddle sensory loss (lowest sacral segments)	Cauda equina lesion (touch preserved in conus medullaris lesions)
Loss of position and vibration sense only	Posterior column lesion
Glove and stocking loss (hands and feet)	Peripheral neuropathy
Loss of all forms of sensation over a well-defined body part only	Posterior root lesion (purely sensory) or peripheral nerve (often motor abnormality associated)

- **Motor changes:** (i) upper motor neurone signs below the hemisection on the same side as the lesion; (ii) lower motor neurone signs at the level of the hemisection on the same side.
- **Sensory changes:** (i) pain and temperature loss on the opposite side to the lesion—note that the upper level of sensory loss is usually a few segments below the level of the lesion; (ii) vibration and proprioception loss occur on the same side; (iii) light touch is often normal.
- **Causes:** (i) multiple sclerosis; (ii) angioma; (iii) trauma; (iv) myelitis; (v) post-radiation myelopathy.

Subacute combined degeneration of the cord (vitamin B$_{12}$ deficiency)

Clinical features are (i) posterior column loss symmetrically (vibration and joint position sense), causing an ataxic gait; (ii) upper motor neurone signs in the lower limbs symmetrically with absent ankle reflexes; knee reflexes may be absent or, more often, exaggerated. There may also be (iii) peripheral sensory neuropathy (less common and mild); (iv) optic atrophy; (v) dementia.

Dissociated sensory loss

This usually indicates spinal cord disease but may occur with a peripheral neuropathy.

- **Causes of spinothalamic loss only:** (i) syringomyelia; (ii) Brown-Séquard syndrome (contralateral leg); (iii) anterior spinal artery thrombosis; (iv) lateral medullary syndrome (contralateral to the other signs) (Figure 10.102); (v) small fibre peripheral neuropathy (e.g. diabetes mellitus, amyloid).
- **Causes of dorsal column loss only:** (i) subacute combined degeneration; (ii) Brown-Séquard syndrome (ipsilateral leg); (iii) spinocerebellar degeneration (e.g. Friedreich's ataxia); (iv) multiple sclerosis; (v) tabes dorsalis; (vi) peripheral neuropathy (e.g. diabetes mellitus, hypothyroidism); (vii) sensory neuronopathy (a dorsal root ganglionopathy which may be caused by carcinoma, diabetes mellitus or Sjögren's syndrome).

Syringomyelia (a central cavity in the spinal cord)

- **Clinical triad:** (i) loss of pain and temperature over the neck, shoulders and arms (a 'cape'

Table 10.31 Differentiating intramedullary from extramedullary cord lesions

Intramedullary	Extramedullary
Root pains rare	Root pains common
Late onset of corticospinal signs	Early onset of corticospinal signs
Lower motor neurone signs extend for several segments	Lower motor neurone signs localised
Dissociated sensory loss (pain and temperature) may be present	Brown-Séquard syndrome if lateral cord compression
Normal or minimally altered cerebrospinal fluid findings	Early, marked cerebrospinal fluid abnormalities
May have sacral sparing	

Figure 10.102 Pattern of sensory loss in the lateral medullary syndrome

distribution); (ii) amyotrophy (atrophy and areflexia) of the arms; (iii) upper motor neurone signs in the lower limbs.

There may also be thoracic scoliosis due to asymmetrical weakness of the paravertebral muscles.

An extensor plantar response plus absent knee and ankle jerks

- **Causes:** (i) subacute combined degeneration of the cord (B$_{12}$ deficiency); (ii) conus medullaris lesion; (iii) combination of an upper motor

Table 10.32 Causes of proximal weakness and myopathy

Causes of proximal weakness

Myopathy (qv)
Neuromuscular junction disease, e.g. myasthenia gravis
Neurogenic, e.g. motor neurone disease, polyradiculopathy, Kugelberg-Welander disease (proximal muscle wasting and fasciculation due to anterior horn cell disease—autosomal recessive)

Causes of myopathy

Hereditary muscular dystrophy (Table 10.33)
Congenital myopathies (rare)
Acquired myopathy (mnemonic, PACE, PODS):
  Polymyositis or dermatomyositis (Figure 10.103)
  Alcohol, AIDS (HIV infection)
  Carcinoma
  Endocrine—e.g. hyperthyroidism, hypothyroidism, Cushing's syndrome, acromegaly, hypopituitarism
  Periodic paralysis (hyperkalaemic, hypokalaemic or normokalaemic)
  Osteomalacia
  Drugs—e.g. clofibrate, chloroquine, steroids, zidovudine
  Sarcoidosis
Note: Causes of proximal myopathy with a peripheral neuropathy include:
Paraneoplastic syndrome
Alcohol
Hypothyroidism
Connective tissue diseases

neurone lesion with cauda equina compression or peripheral neuropathy, such as a stroke in a diabetic; (iv) syphilis (taboparesis); (v) Friedreich's ataxia; (vi) motor neurone disease; (vii) diabetes mellitus (uncommon); (viii) human T-cell lymphotropic virus (HTLV-I) infection.

A summary of the features that differentiate intramedullary from extramedullary cord lesions is presented in Table 10.31.

Myopathy

Muscle weakness can be due to individual peripheral nerve lesions, mononeuritis multiplex, peripheral neuropathy or spinal cord disease. Each of these has a characteristic pattern. Primary disease of muscle (myopathy) also causes weakness. There is no sensory loss with myopathy, which is an important clue. The motor weakness is similar to that of the lower motor neurone type. There are two major patterns: proximal myopathy and distal myopathy.

Proximal myopathy is the more common form. On examination there is proximal muscle wasting and weakness (Tables 10.32 and 10.33) (Figure 10.103). Reflexes involving these muscles may be reduced. This can be caused by genetic (e.g. muscular dystrophy) or acquired disease. *Distal myopathy* also occurs and is always genetic, although peripheral neuropathy is a much more common cause of distal muscle weakness. If the distal limbs are affected, consider hereditary motor and sensory neuropathy (Table 10.34). Motor neurone disease also causes weakness without any sensory loss.

Figure 10.103
Dermatomyositis

(a) Gottren's sign in dermatomyositis—heliotrope (lilac-coloured) flat topped papules, which occur over the knuckles, but may also be seen over the elbows or knees and may ulcerate. (b) Dermatomyositis may also cause a heliotrope rash on the face (especially on the eyelids, upper cheeks and forehead), periorbital oedema, erythema, maculopapular eruptions and scaling dermatitis. Dermatomyositis and the closely related condition polymyositis are idiopathic myopathies. Up to 10% of adult patients with dermatomyositis may have an underlying malignancy. (Figure 10.103a from FS McDonald, ed., *Mayo Clinic images in internal medicine*, with permission. © Mayo Clinic Scientific Press and CRC Press.)

Table 10.33 Muscular dystrophies

1 Duchenne's* (pseudohypertrophic)
 • Affects only males (sex-linked recessive)
 • Calves and deltoids: hypertrophied early, weak later
 • Proximal weakness: early
 • Dilated cardiomyopathy
2 Becker†
 • Affects only males (sex-linked recessive)
 • Similar clinical features to Duchenne's except for less heart disease, a later onset and less rapid progression
3 Limb girdle
 • Males or females (autosomal recessive), onset in the third decade
 • Shoulder or pelvic girdle affected
 • Face and heart usually spared
4 Facioscapulohumeral
 • Males or females (autosomal dominant)
 • Facial and pectoral weakness with hypertrophy of deltoids
5 Dystrophia myotonica (autosomal dominant)

* Guillaume Duchenne (1806–75), brilliant eccentric who founded French neurology. He died of a stroke.
† Peter Becker (b. 1908), German professor of genetics.

Table 10.34 Features of hereditary motor and sensory neuropathy (Charcot-Marie-Tooth* disease)

1 Pes cavus (short-arched feet)
2 Distal muscle atrophy due to peripheral nerve degeneration. This does not usually extend above the elbows or above the middle third of the thighs
3 Absent reflexes
4 Slight or no sensory loss in the limbs
5 Thickened nerves
6 Optic atrophy, Argyll Robertson pupils (rare)

* Jean Martin Charcot (1825–93), Parisian physician and neurologist; Pierre Marie (1853–1940), Parisian neurologist and Charcot's greatest pupil; and Howard Henry Tooth (1856–1926), London physician, who described the condition independently in 1886. Type I is usually autosomal dominant.

Dystrophia myotonica

If this disease (which is inherited as an autosomal dominant condition) is suspected because of an inability on the part of the patient to let go when shaking hands (myotonia), or because general inspection reveals the characteristic appearance (Figure 10.104), examine as follows.

Observe the face for frontal baldness (the patient may be wearing a wig), the expressionless triangular facies, atrophy of the temporalis muscle and partial ptosis. Thick spectacles, a traditional sign of this disease, are not often seen now because of lens replacement surgery. The eyes should still be examined, as these patients can develop characteristic iridescent cataracts and subcapsular fine deposits.

Look at the neck for atrophy of the sternomastoid muscles and then test neck flexion (neck flexion is weak while extension is normal).

Go to the upper limbs. Shake hands and test for percussion myotonia. Tapping over the thenar eminence causes contraction and then slow relaxation of abductor pollicis brevis. Examine the arm now for signs of wasting and weakness distally (forearms are usually affected first) and proximally. There are no sensory changes.

Go to the chest and look for gynaecomastia (uncommon). Examine the cardiovascular system for cardiomyopathy. Next palpate the testes for atrophy. Examine the lower limbs. The tibial nerves are affected first. Always ask to test the urine for sugar (diabetes mellitus is associated with this disease).

Note: Muscle myotonia can also occur in the hereditary diseases myotonia congenita (autosomal dominant or recessive) and hereditary paramyotonia (autosomal dominant cold-induced myotonia).

Myasthenia gravis

Myasthenia gravis is an autoimmune disease of the neuromuscular junction. There are circulating antibodies against acetylcholine receptors. It differs from the proximal myopathies in that muscle power decreases with use. There is little muscle wasting and no sensory change.

It is necessary to test for muscle fatigue. Test the oculomotor muscles by asking the patient to sustain upward gaze by looking up at the ceiling for one minute, and watch for progressive ptosis (Figure 10.39). Test the Peek sign for orbicularis oculi weakness. Ask the patient to close the eyes; if positive, within 30 seconds the lid margin will begin to separate, showing the sclera. This test strongly increases the likelihood of myasthenia (positive LR = 30.0).[21] Then test the proximal limb girdle muscles—ask the patient to hold the arms above the head. The examiner can repeatedly press the abducted arms down until they weaken. Power will decrease with repeated muscle contraction.

Partial ptosis cataracts
Subcapsular fine deposits

Temporalis atrophy

Proximal muscle wasting and weakness

Gynaecomastia

Forearm wasting and weakness

Proximal muscle wasting and weakness

Baldness

Triangular facies

Sternomastoid atrophy (weak neck flexion)

Cardiac failure (cardiomyopathy)

Percussion myotonia

Testicular atrophy

Glycosuria

Figure 10.104 Dystrophia myotonica

Look for a thymectomy scar (over the sternum)—thymectomy is often undertaken as treatment for generalised myasthenia.

The cerebellum (Figure 10.105)

If the patient complains of clumsiness or problems with coordination of movement, a cerebellar examination is indicated. Signs of cerebellar disease occur on the same side as the lesion in the brain. This is because most cerebellar fibres cross twice in the brainstem, both on entry to and exit from the cerebellum. Proceed as follows with the examination.

Look first for nystagmus—usually jerky horizontal nystagmus with an increased amplitude on looking towards the side of the lesion. Assess speech next. Ask the patient to say 'British Constitution' or 'West Register Street' (Figure 10.106). Cerebel-lar speech is jerky, explosive and loud, with an irregular separation of syllables (page 288).

Go to the upper limbs. Ask the patient to extend the arms and look for arm drift due to hypotonia of the agonist muscles. Test tone. Hypotonia[xx] is due to loss of a facilitatory influence on the spinal motor neurones.

Next perform the finger–nose test. The patient touches the nose, then rotates the finger and touches the examiner's finger. Note any intention tremor (tremor which increases as the target is

[xx] The concepts of hypotonia, rebound and pendular jerks in cerebellar disease are currently being reassessed. They stem from Gordon Holmes' 1917 description of signs in acute unilateral cerebellar disease. They may well not exist in other cerebellar problems. Students will, however, still be expected to know how to test for these signs.

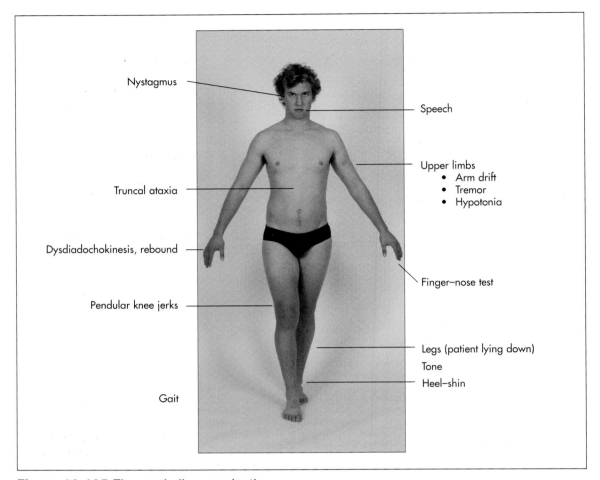

Nystagmus

Truncal ataxia

Dysdiadochokinesis, rebound

Pendular knee jerks

Gait

Speech

Upper limbs
- Arm drift
- Tremor
- Hypotonia

Finger–nose test

Legs (patient lying down)
Tone
Heel–shin

Figure 10.105 The cerebellar examination

Figure 10.106 West Register Street, Edinburgh

approached—this is due to loss of cerebellar connections in the brainstem) and past-pointing (the patient overshoots the target). Test rapidly alternating movements: the patient taps alternately the palm and back of one hand on the other hand or thigh. Inability to perform this movement smoothly is called dysdiadochokinesis. Now test rebound—ask the patient to lift the arms quickly from the sides, then stop (incoordination of antagonist and agonist action causes the patient to be unable to stop the arms). Before testing, always demonstrate these movements for the patient's benefit.

Go on to examine the legs. Again, test tone here. Then perform the heel–shin test looking for accuracy of fine movement when the patient slides the heel down the shin slowly on each side for several cycles. Then ask the patient to lift the big toe up to touch the examiner's finger, and look for intention tremor and past-pointing. Ask the patient then to tap each heel on the other shin.

Look for truncal ataxia by asking the patient to fold the arms and sit up. While the patient is sitting, ask him or her to put the legs over the side of the bed and test for pendular knee jerks (the lower leg continues to swing a number of times before coming to rest—this is evidence of hypotonia).

Test gait (the patient will stagger towards the affected side if there is a unilateral cerebellar hemisphere lesion).

If there is an obvious unilateral cerebellar problem examine the cranial nerves for evidence of a cerebellopontine angle tumour (fifth, seventh and eighth nerves affected) or the lateral medullary syndrome, and auscultate over the cerebellum. Always look in the fundi for papilloedema. Next examine for peripheral signs of malignant disease and for vascular disease (carotid bruits).

If there is evidence of a midline lesion, such as truncal ataxia, abnormal heel–toe walking or abnormal speech, consider either a midline tumour or a paraneoplastic syndrome (Table 10.35). If there is bilateral disease, look for signs of multiple sclerosis,

Friedreich's ataxia (pes cavus is the most helpful initial clue) (Table 10.36) and hypothyroidism (rare). Alcoholic cerebellar degeneration (which affects the anterior lobe of the cerebellar vermis) classically spares the arms. If there are, in addition, upper motor neurone signs, consider the causes in Table 10.37. Remember that there are important reciprocal

Table 10.35 Causes of cerebellar disease

Rostral vermis lesion (only lower limbs affected)

Usually due to alcohol

Unilateral
1 Space-occupying lesion (tumour, abscess, granuloma)
2 Ischaemia (vertebrobasilar disease)
3 Multiple sclerosis
4 Trauma

Bilateral
1 Drugs—e.g. phenytoin
2 Alcohol (both acutely and chronically, possibly due to thiamine deficiency)
3 Friedreich's ataxia
4 Hypothyroidism
5 Paraneoplastic syndrome
6 Multiple sclerosis
7 Trauma ('punch drunk')
8 Arnold-Chiari malformation
9 Large space-occupying lesion, cerebrovascular disease

Midline
1 Paraneoplastic syndrome
2 Midline tumour

Table 10.36 Clinical features of Friedreich's ataxia (autosomal recessive)

This is usually a young person with:
1 Cerebellar signs (bilateral) including nystagmus
2 Pes cavus.* Cocking of the toes. Kyphoscoliosis
3 Upper motor neurone signs in the limbs (although reflexes are absent)
4 Peripheral neuropathy
5 Posterior column loss in the limbs
6 Cardiomyopathy (ECG abnormalities occur in more than 50% of cases)
7 Diabetes mellitus (common)
8 Optic atrophy (uncommon)
9 Normal mentation

* Other causes of pes cavus include hereditary motor and sensory neuropathy, spinocerebellar degeneration or neuropathies in childhood.

Table 10.37 Causes of spastic and ataxic paraparesis (upper motor neurone and cerebellar signs combined)

In adolescence
Spinocerebellar degeneration—e.g. Marie's spastic ataxia

In young adults
Multiple sclerosis
Spinocerebellar degeneration
Syphilitic meningomyelitis
Arnold-Chiari malformation or other lesion at the craniospinal junction

In later life
Multiple sclerosis
Syringomyelia
Infarction (in upper pons or internal capsule on one side—'ataxic hemiparesis')
Lesion at the craniospinal junction—e.g. meningioma

Note: Unrelated diseases that are relatively common (e.g. cervical spondylosis and cerebellar degeneration from alcohol) may cause a similar clinical picture.

connections between the cerebellum and the parietal and frontal lobes. These explain the problems cerebellar abnormalities can cause with functions other than coordination. Loss of verbal fluency, grammatical problems with speech, difficulty with memory and planning can all sometimes be features of cerebellar disease.

Parkinson's disease

This is a common extrapyramidal disease of middle to old age (1% of people older than 65) where there is degeneration of the substantia nigra and its pathways. This results in dopamine deficiency and a relative excess of cholinergic transmission in the caudate nucleus and putamen, which causes excessive supraspinal excitatory drive. There may be a history of insidious and asymmetrical onset. Non-specific symptoms (sleep abnormalities, constipation, depression and dementia) may precede or accompany the classic tremor.

Examine as follows.[22]

Inspection

Note the lack of facial expression, which leads to a mask-like facies. The posture is characteristically flexed and there are few spontaneous movements.

Gait and movements

Ask the patient to rise from a chair, walk, turn quickly, stop and start.

The characteristic gait is described as *shuffling*—there are small steps, and the patient hardly raises the feet from the ground. There is often difficulty in initiating walking, but once it begins the patient hurries (festination) and has difficulty stopping. The Parkinsonian patient seems always to be trying to catch up with the centre of gravity. There is a lack of the normal arm swing. Walking heel to toe will be difficult.

Testing for *propulsion* or *retropulsion* (propulsion involves pushing the patient from behind and retropulsion pushing from in front) is of uncertain value and must be done with some caution because the patient may be unable to stop and may fall over. The examiner can stand behind the patient and pull him or her backwards, but should stand braced to catch the patient.

Bradykinesia (a decrease in the speed and amplitude of complex movements) may be the result of a lesion in the nigrostriatal pathway (a dopaminergic pathway), which affects connections between the caudate nucleus, putamen and the motor cortex, causing abnormal movement programming and abnormal recruitment of single motor units. Two simple tests (Figure 10.107 a and b) for this are *finger tapping* and *twiddling*. Ask the patient to tap the fingers in turn onto a surface repeatedly, quickly and with both hands at once. Twiddling is rotating the hands around each other in front of the body. These movements are slow and clumsy in Parkinsonian patients but obviously depend on motor and cerebellar function as well. Difficulty getting out of a chair can be another sign of bradykinesia and patients often have difficulty turning over in bed.

Kinesia paradoxica is the striking ability of a patient to perform rapid movements (especially if startled) but not slow ones; for example, the patient may be able to run down the stairs in response to a fire alarm but be unable to stop at the bottom—this is *not* a recommended test.

Tremor

Have the patient return to bed. Look for a resting tremor, which is often asymmetrical. The character-

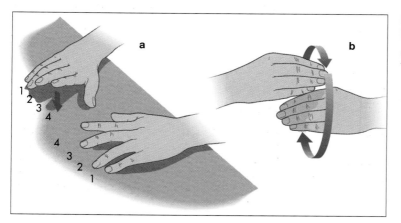

Figure 10.107 Detecting bradykinesia

(a) Tapping the fingers. (b) Twiddling.

istic movement is described as pill-rolling. Movement of the fingers at the metacarpophalangeal joints is combined with the movements of the thumb. Various attending movements may also occur at the wrist. On finger–nose testing the resting tremor decreases, but a faster action tremor may supervene.

Tremor can be facilitated by getting the patient to perform 'serial 7s'—take 7 from 100, then 7 from the answer and so forth (mental stimulation)—or to move the contralateral limb (e.g. by rapidly opposing the contralateral thumb and fingers). Other types of tremor are summarised in Table 10.38.

Tone

Test tone at both wrists. The characteristic increase in tone is called cogwheel or plastic (lead pipe) rigidity. Tone is increased with an interrupted nature, the muscles giving way with a series of jerks. If hypertonia is not obvious, obtain reinforcement by asking the patient to turn the head from side to side or to wave the contralateral arm. Cogwheel rigidity occurs because the exaggerated stretch reflex is interrupted by tremor.

Remember, the signs are often asymmetrical early in the course of Parkinson's disease.

Figure 10.108 The glabellar tap

Face

There may be *titubation* (tremor) of the head, absence of blinking, dribbling of saliva and lack of facial expression. Test the *glabellar tap*—keeping your finger out of the patient's line of vision, tap the middle of the forehead (glabella) with your middle finger (Figure 10.108). This sign is positive when the patient continues to blink as long as the examiner taps. Normal people blink only a couple of times and then stop.

Assess *speech*, which is typically monotonous, soft and faint, lacking intonation. Sometimes palilalia is present; this is repetition of the end of a word (the opposite of stuttering).

Now test the ocular movements, particularly for *weakness of upward gaze*. Isolated failure of upward gaze is a feature of Parkinson's disease. There is a separate group of patients with marked rigidity and paralysis of gaze who should be diagnosed as having progressive supranuclear palsy (page 303) rather than Parkinson's disease. These people develop loss first of downward gaze then of upward gaze and finally of horizontal gaze.

Feel the brow for greasiness (seborrhoea) or sweatiness, due to associated autonomic dysfunction. Orthostatic hypotension may also be present for the same reason.

Writing

Ask the patient to write his or her name and address. *Micrographia* (small writing) is characteristic. The patient may also be unable to do this because of the development of dementia, a late manifestation. Test the higher centres if appropriate. See *Good signs guide 10.2*.

Table 10.38 A classification of non-physiological tremor*

1 Parkinsonian—resting tremor
2 Postural/action tremor; present throughout movement; the following most often cause a static or postural tremor of the outstretched arms:
   (a) idiopathic (most common)
   (b) anxiety
   (c) drugs
   (d) familial
   (e) thyrotoxicosis
3 Essential/familial
4 Intention tremor (cerebellar disease); increases towards the target
5 Midbrain ('red nucleus') tremor—abduction-adduction movements of upper limbs with flexion-extension of wrists (usually associated with intention tremor)

* Tremor is a rhythmic oscillation of a part of the body around a fixed point.
NB: Flapping (asterixis) is not strictly a tremor but a sudden brief loss of tone in hepatic failure, cardiac failure, respiratory failure or renal failure (metabolic encephalopathies).

GOOD SIGNS GUIDE 10.2 Parkinson's disease		
Sign	Positive LR	Negative LR
Rigidity, tremor and bradykinesia all present	2.2	0.5
Difficulty walking (heel–toe)	2.9	0.32
Asymmetrical onset, no atypical features and no alternative diagnosis	4.1	0.4
Glabellar tap	4.5	0.13
From McGee S, *Evidence-based physical diagnosis*, Saunders, 2001.		

Causes of Parkinson's syndrome

These are shown in Table 10.39.

Other extrapyramidal movement disorders (dyskinesia)

Chorea

Here there is a lesion of the corpus striatum, which causes non-repetitive, abrupt, involuntary jerky movements. These may be unilateral or generalised. Often the patient attempts to disguise this by completing the involuntary movements with a voluntary one. In this disease, dopaminergic pathways dominate over cholinergic transmissions.

Chorea can usefully be distinguished from hemiballismus, athetosis and pseudoathetosis. *Hemiballismus* is due to a subthalamic lesion on the side opposite the movement disorder. It causes unilateral wild throwing movements of the proximal joints. There may be skin excoriation due to limb trauma. These movements may persist during sleep.

Athetosis or *dystonia* is due to a lesion of the outer segment of the putamen and causes slow sinuous

Table 10.39 Causes of Parkinson's syndrome

Idiopathic: Parkinson's disease
Drugs: e.g. phenothiazines, methyldopa
Post-encephalitis (now very rare)
Other: toxins (carbon monoxide, manganese), Wilson's disease, progressive supranuclear palsy, Steele-Richardson syndrome, Shy-Drager syndrome, syphilis, tumour (e.g. giant frontal meningioma)
Atherosclerosis is a controversial cause.

Table 10.40 Causes of chorea

Drugs: e.g. excess levodopa, phenothiazines, the contraceptive pill, phenytoin
Huntington's disease (autosomal dominant)
Sydenham's chorea (rheumatic fever) and other postinfectious states (both rare)
Senility
Wilson's disease
Kernicterus (rare)
Vasculitis or connective tissue disease—e.g. systemic lupus erythematosus (very rare)
Thyrotoxicosis (very rare)
Polycythaemia or other hyperviscosity syndromes (very rare)
Viral encephalitis (very rare)

writhing distal movements that are present at rest. *Pseudoathetosis* is a description given to athetoid movements in the fingers in patients with severe proprioceptive loss (these are especially prominent when the eyes are shut).

If the patient has chorea, proceed as follows. First shake hands. There may be tremor and dystonia superimposed on lack of sustained hand grip ('milkmaid's grip'). Ask the patient to hold out the hands, then look for a choreic (dystonic) posture. This typically involves finger and thumb hyperextension and wrist flexion.

Go to the face and look at the eyes for exophthalmos (thyrotoxicosis), Kayser-Fleischer rings (Wilson's disease) and conjunctival injection (polycythaemia). Ask the patient to poke out the tongue and note frequent retraction of the tongue (serpentine movements). Look for skin rashes (e.g. systemic lupus erythematosus, vasculitis). If the patient is young, examine the heart for signs of rheumatic fever (Sydenham's[yy] chorea).

Test the reflexes. The abdominal reflexes are usually brisk, but tendon reflexes are reduced and may be pendular (due to hypotonia).

Assess the higher centres for dementia (Huntington's chorea[zz]).

Causes of chorea are shown in Table 10.40.

[yy] Thomas Sydenham (1624–89). He was a captain in Cromwell's army and became the most famous English physician of his time, providing clinical descriptions of gout (from which he suffered), fevers, hysteria and venereal disease. He was called the Father of English Clinical Medicine.
[zz] George Huntington (1850–1916), American general practitioner. He described this disease in his only clinical paper in 1872, when he was 22.

Dystonia

The patient manifests an involuntary abnormal posture with excessive co-contraction of antagonist muscles. Dystonia may be focal (e.g. spasmodic torticollis), segmental or generalised. Other forms of movement disorder may be present (e.g. myoclonic dystonia). The acute onset of dystonia is seen most commonly as a side-effect of various drugs (e.g. levodopa, phenothiazines, metoclopramide).

The unconscious patient

The rapid and efficient examination of the unconscious patient is important. The word COMA provides a mnemonic for four major groups of causes of unconsciousness.

C CO_2 narcosis (respiratory failure: uncommon).

O Overdose: for example, tranquillisers, alcohol, salicylates, carbon monoxide, antidepressants.

M Metabolic: for example, hypoglycaemia, diabetic ketoacidosis, uraemia, hypothyroidism, hepatic coma, hypercalcaemia, adrenal failure.

A Apoplexy: for example, head injury, cerebrovascular accident (infarction or haemorrhage), subdural or extradural haematoma, meningitis, encephalitis, epilepsy.

Coma occurs when the reticular formation is damaged by a lesion or metabolic abnormality, or when the cortex is diffusely damaged.

General inspection

Look to see if the patient is breathing, as indicated by chest wall movement. If not, urgent attention is required, including clearing the airway and providing ventilation. Note particularly the pattern of breathing (see Table 4.4). Cheyne-Stokes respiration (which may indicate diencephalic injury, but is not specific), irregular ataxic breathing (Biot's breathing, from an advanced brainstem lesion) and deep rapid respiration (e.g. Kussmaul breathing, secondary to a metabolic acidosis, as in diabetes mellitus) are important signs to look for.

Circulation

Look for signs of shock, dehydration and cyanosis. A typical cherry red colour occurs in cases of carbon monoxide poisoning. Take the pulse rate and blood pressure.

Posture

Look for signs of trauma. Note any neck hyperextension (from meningism in children or cerebellar tonsillar herniation).

Look for:

1 A *decerebrate* or extensor posture, which may be held spontaneously or occur in response to stimuli, and which suggests severe midbrain disease. The arms are held extended and internally rotated and the legs are extended.

2 A *decorticate* or flexor posture, which suggests a lesion above the brainstem. It can be unilateral or bilateral. There is flexion and internal rotation of the arms and extension of the legs.

Involuntary movements

Recurrent or continuous convulsions, which may be focal or generalised, suggest status epilepticus. Myoclonic jerks can occur after hypoxic injury and as a result of metabolic encephalopathy. Remember that complex partial seizure status epilepticus can cause a reduced level of consciousness without convulsive movements.

Level of consciousness

Tickle the patient's nose with cottonwool and watch for facial movements. This is less likely to harm the patient than the traditional method of firm pressing of knuckles over the sternum to cause pain. Determine the level of consciousness. *Coma* is unconsciousness with a reduced response to external stimuli. Coma in which the patient responds semi-purposefully is considered light. In deep coma there is no response to any stimuli and no reflexes are present (it is usually due to a brainstem or pontine lesion, though drug overdosage, such as with barbiturates, can be responsible).

Stupor is unconsciousness, but the patient can be aroused. Purposeful movements occur in response to painful stimuli.

Drowsiness resembles normal sleepiness. The patient can be fairly easily roused to normal wakefulness, but when left alone falls asleep again. The Glasgow coma scale (Table 10.41) is used to assess the depth of coma more accurately: record the subscores and total scores.

The neck

If there is no evidence of neck trauma, assess for neck stiffness and Kernig's sign (for meningitis or subarachnoid haemorrhage).

Table 10.41 Glasgow coma scale

Add up the score for 1, 2 and 3. Score of 4 or less = very poor prognosis, score >11 = good prognosis for recovery.

1 Eyes	Open	Spontaneously	4
		To loud verbal command	3
		To pain	2
	No response		1
2 Best motor response	To verbal command	Obeys	6
	To painful stimuli	Localises pain	5
		Flexion—withdrawal	4
		Abnormal flexion posturing	3
		Extension posturing	2
		No response	1
3 Best verbal response		Oriented	5
		Confused, disoriented	4
		Inappropriate words	3
		Incomprehensible sounds	2
		None	1

The head and face

Inspect and palpate for head injuries, including Battle's sign[aaa], bruising behind the ear indicating a fracture of the base of the skull. Look for facial asymmetry (i.e. facial weakness). The paralysed side of the face will be sucked in and out with respiration. A painful stimulus (e.g. pressing the supraorbital notch) may produce grimacing and make facial asymmetry more obvious. Note jaundice (e.g. hepatic coma) or manifestations of myxoedema.

The eyes

Inspect the pupils. Very small pupils occur in pontine lesions and with narcotic overdoses. One dilated pupil suggests a subdural haematoma, raised intracranial pressure (unilateral tentorial herniation) or a subarachnoid haemorrhage from a posterior communicating artery aneurysm. Conjunctival haemorrhage suggests skull fracture. Widely dilated pupils may occur when increased intracranial pressure and coning cause secondary brainstem haemorrhage, or with atropine-like drugs. Look in the fundi for papilloedema, diabetic or hypertensive retinopathy, or subhyaloid haemorrhage.

Look at the position of the eyes. Particular cranial nerve palsies may cause deviation of an eye in various directions. The sixth nerve is particularly vulnerable

to damage because of its long intracranial course. Deviation of both eyes to one side in the unconscious patient may be due to a destructive lesion in a cerebral hemisphere, which causes fixed deviation towards the side of the lesion. An irritative (epileptic) focus causes the direction of gaze to be away from the lesion. Upward or downward eye deviation suggests a brainstem problem. Trapping of the globe or extraocular muscles by fracture may also lead to an abnormal eye position or to an abnormal eye movement.

Perform *doll's eye testing* by lifting the patient's eyelids and rolling the head from side to side. When vestibular reflexes are intact (i.e. an intact brainstem), the eyes maintain their fixation as if looking at an object in the distance, but change their position relative to the head. This is the normal 'doll's eye phenomenon'. Brainstem lesions or drugs affecting the brainstem cause the eyes to move with the head, so that fixation is not maintained.

Ears and nostrils

Look for any bleeding or drainage of cerebrospinal fluid (the latter indicating a skull fracture). A watery discharge can be simply tested for glucose. The presence of glucose confirms that it is cerebrospinal fluid.

The tongue and mouth

Trauma may indicate a previous seizure, and corrosion around the mouth may indicate ingestion of a corrosive poison. Gum hyperplasia suggests that the patient may be taking phenytoin for epilepsy. Smell the breath for evidence of alcohol ingestion,

---

[aaa] William Battle (1855–1936), surgeon, St Thomas's Hospital, London.

diabetic ketosis, hepatic coma or uraemia. Remember that alcohol ingestion may be associated with head injury. Test the gag reflex; its absence may indicate brainstem disease or deep coma, but is not a specific sign.

The upper and lower limbs

Look for injection marks (drug addiction, diabetes mellitus). Test tone in the normal way and by picking up the arm and letting it fall. Compare each side, assessing for evidence of hemiplegia. In coma and acute cerebral hemiplegia, the muscle stretch reflexes may be normal or reduced at first on the paralysed side. Later the muscle stretch reflexes become increased and the cutaneous reflexes are absent.

Test for pain sensation by placing a pen over a distal finger or toe just below the nail bed. Press firmly and note if there is arm or leg withdrawal. Test all limbs. There will be no response to pain if sensation is absent or if the coma is deep. If sensation is intact but the limb is paralysed, there may be grimacing with movement of the other limbs.

The presence of grimacing or purposeful movements is important. Segmental reflexes alone can cause the limb to move in response to pain.

The body

Look for signs of trauma. Examine the heart, lungs and abdomen.

The urine

Note whether there is incontinence. Test the urine for glucose and ketones (diabetic ketoacidosis), protein (uraemia) and blood (trauma).

The blood glucose

Always prick the finger, place a drop of blood on an impregnated test strip, and test for hypoglycaemia or hyperglycaemia. If this cannot be done immediately, give the patient a bolus of intravenous glucose anyway (which will not harm the patient in diabetic ketoacidosis, but will save the life of a patient with hypoglycaemia). If there is any suspicion of Wernicke's encephalopathy, thiamine must be given as well.

The temperature

Hypothermia (e.g. exposure or hypothyroidism) or fever (e.g. meningitis) must be looked for.

Stomach contents

While protecting the airway, examine stomach contents by inserting a nasogastric tube and washing out the stomach if a drug overdose is suspected, or if no other diagnosis is obvious.

Coma scale

It is most useful to score the depth of coma, as changes in the level of consciousness can then be judged more objectively (Table 10.41).

Summary
Examining the nervous system: a suggested method (Figure 10.109)

Handedness, orientation and speech

Ask the patient if he or she is right- or left-handed. As a screening assessment, ask for the patient's name, present location and the date. Next ask the patient to name an object pointed at and have him or her point to a named object in the room, to test for dysphasia. Ask the patient to say 'British Constitution' to test for dysarthria.

Neck stiffness and Kernig's sign

Ask the patient to lie flat and attempt gently to flex the head by placing a hand under the occiput. Flex the patient's hip with the knee bent and then attempt to straighten the leg.

Cranial nerves

The patient should sit over the edge of the bed if possible. Begin by general inspection of the head and neck looking for craniotomy scars, neurofibromas, facial asymmetry, ptosis, proptosis, skew deviation of the eyes or inequality of the pupils.

The second nerve. Test visual acuity with the patient wearing his or her spectacles. Each eye is tested separately, while the other is covered with a small card.

Examine the visual fields by confrontation using a hat pin or fingers. The examiner's head should be level with the patient's head. Each eye is tested separately. If visual acuity is very poor, the fields are mapped using the fingers.

Look into the fundi.

The third, fourth and sixth nerves. Look at the pupils, noting the shape, relative sizes and any associated ptosis. Use a pocket torch and shine the light from the side to gauge the reaction of the pupils to

1 Handedness and conscious level

2 Neck stiffness and Kernig's sign

3 Cranial nerves
- II Visual acuity and fields; fundoscopy
- III IV VI Pupils and eye movements
- V Corneal reflexes
- VII Facial muscles
- VIII Hearing
- IX X Palate and gag
- XI Trapezius and sternomastoids
- XII Tongue

4 Upper limbs
- Motor system (tone, power, reflexes)
- Coordination
- Sensation

5 Lower limbs
- Motor system (tone, power, reflexes)
- Coordination
- Sensation

6 Saddle region

7 Back

8 Gait

Figure 10.109 The nervous system examination

Assess eye movements with both eyes first, getting the patient to follow the pin in each direction. Look for failure of movement and for nystagmus. Ask about diplopia in each direction.

The fifth nerve. Test the corneal reflexes gently and ask the patient if the touch of the cottonwool on the cornea can be felt. The sensory component of this reflex is V and the motor component VII.

Test facial sensation in the three divisions: ophthalmic, maxillary and mandibular. Test pain sensation with the pin first and map any area of sensory loss from dull to sharp. Test light touch as well so that sensory dissociation can be detected if present.

Examine the motor division of the fifth nerve by asking the patient to clench the teeth while you feel the masseter muscles. Then get the patient to open the mouth while you attempt to force it closed; this is not possible if the pterygoid muscles are working. A unilateral lesion causes the jaw to deviate towards the weak (affected) side.

Test the jaw jerk. This is increased in cases of pseudobulbar palsy.

The seventh nerve. Test the muscles of facial expression. Ask the patient to look up and wrinkle the forehead. Look for loss of wrinkling and feel the muscle strength by pushing down on each side. This is preserved in upper motor neurone lesions because of bilateral cortical representation of these muscles.

Next ask the patient to shut the eyes tightly and compare the two sides. Tell the patient to grin and compare the nasolabial grooves.

The eighth nerve. Softly whisper a number 60 cm away from each ear. Examine the external auditory canals and the eardrums if this is indicated.

The ninth and tenth nerves. Look at the palate and note any uvular displacement. Ask the patient to say 'Ah' and look for symmetrical movement of the soft palate. With a unilateral lesion the uvula is drawn towards the unaffected (normal) side. Test gently for sensation on the palate (the ninth nerve). Ask the patient to speak to assess hoarseness, and to cough. A bovine cough suggests bilateral recurrent laryngeal nerve lesions.

The twelfth nerve. While examining the mouth, inspect the tongue for wasting and fasciculation. Next ask the patient to protrude the tongue. With a unilateral lesion the tongue deviates towards the weaker (affected) side.

The eleventh nerve. Look for torticollis. Ask the patient to shrug the shoulders and feel the trapezius as you push the shoulders down. Then ask the

light. Assess quickly both the direct and consensual responses. Look for an afferent pupillary defect by moving the torch in an arc from pupil to pupil. Test accommodation by asking the patient to look into the distance and then at the hat pin or finger held about 30 cm from the nose.

patient to turn the head against resistance and also feel the bulk of the sternomastoid. Then examine the skull and auscultate for carotid bruits.

Upper limbs

Shake the patient's hand firmly. Ask him or her to sit over the side of the bed facing you, if possible.

Examine the *motor system* systematically every time. Inspect first for wasting (both proximally and distally) and fasciculations. Don't forget to include the shoulder girdle in your inspection.

Ask the patient to hold both hands out (palms up) with the arms extended and close the eyes. Look for drifting of one or both arms (upper motor neurone weakness, cerebellar lesion or posterior column loss). Also note any tremor, or pseudoathetosis due to proprioceptive loss.

- Feel the muscle bulk next, both proximally and distally, and note any muscle tenderness.
- Test tone at the wrists and elbows by passively moving the joints at varying velocities.
- Assess power at the shoulders, elbows, wrists and fingers.
- If indicated, test for an ulnar nerve lesion (Froment's sign) and a median nerve lesion (pen-touching test).
- Examine the reflexes: biceps (C5, C6), triceps (C7, C8) and brachioradialis (C5, C6).
- Assess coordination with finger–nose testing and look for dysdiadochokinesis and rebound.

Motor weakness can be due to an upper motor neurone lesion, a lower motor neurone lesion or a myopathy. If there is evidence of a lower motor neurone lesion, consider anterior horn cell, nerve root or brachial plexus lesions, peripheral nerve lesions or a motor peripheral neuropathy.

Examine the *sensory system* after motor testing, because this can be time-consuming.

First test the spinothalamic pathway (pain and temperature). Demonstrate to the patient the sharpness of a pin on the anterior chest wall or forehead. Then ask him or her to close the eyes and tell you if the sensation is sharp or dull. Start proximally and test each dermatome. Map the abnormal area. As you are assessing, try to fit any sensory loss into dermatomal (cord or nerve root lesion), peripheral nerve, peripheral neuropathy (glove) or hemisensory (cortical or cord) distribution. It is not usually necessary to test temperature.

Next test the posterior column pathway (vibration and proprioception). Use a 128 Hz tuning fork to assess vibration sense. Place the vibrating fork on a distal interphalangeal joint when the patient has the eyes closed and ask whether it can be felt. If so, ask the patient to tell you when the vibration ceases and then, after a short wait, stop the vibrations. If the patient has deficient sensation, test at the wrist, then elbow, then at the shoulder.

Examine proprioception first with the distal interphalangeal joint of the little finger. When the patient has the eyes open grasp the distal phalanx from the sides and move it up and down to demonstrate, then ask the patient to close the eyes; repeat the manoeuvre. Normally, movement through even a few degrees is detectable, and the patient can tell whether it is up or down. If there is an abnormality, test larger movements and then proceed to test the wrist and elbows similarly if necessary.

Test light touch with cottonwool. Touch the skin lightly (do not stroke) in each dermatome.

Feel for thickened nerves—the ulnar at the elbow, the median at the wrist and the radial at the wrist—and feel the axillae if there is evidence of a proximal lesion. Note any scars, and finally examine the neck if relevant.

Lower limbs

Test the stance and gait first if possible. Then put the patient in bed with the legs entirely exposed. Place a towel over the groin—note whether a urinary catheter is present.

Look for muscle wasting and fasciculations. Note any tremor. Feel the muscle bulk of the quadriceps and run your hand up each shin, feeling for wasting of the anterior tibial muscles.

Test tone at the knees and ankles. Test clonus at this time. Push the lower end of the quadriceps sharply down towards the knee. Sustained rhythmical contractions indicate an upper motor neurone lesion. Also test the ankle by sharply dorsiflexing the foot with the knee bent and the thigh externally rotated.

Assess power next at the hips, knees and ankles.

Elicit the reflexes: knee (L3, L4), ankle (S1, S2) and plantar response (L5, S1, S2).

Test coordination with the heel–shin test, toe–finger test and tapping of the feet.

Examine the sensory system as for the upper limbs: pinprick, then vibration and proprioception, and then light touch. If there is a peripheral sensory loss, attempt to establish a sensory level by moving the pin up the leg and onto the abdomen and, if necessary, onto the chest. Examine sensation in the saddle region and test the anal reflex (S2, S3, S4).

Go to the back. Look for deformity, scars and neurofibromas. Palpate for tenderness over the vertebral bodies and auscultate for bruits. Perform the straight leg-raising test.

References

1. Sturm JW, Donnan GA. Diagnosis and investigation of headache. *Aust Fam Phys* 1998; 27:587–589. An accurate clinical history is the key to diagnosing the cause of headache.
2. Marks DR, Rapoport AM. Practical evaluation and diagnosis of headache. *Seminars in Neurology* 1997; 17:307–312. The history should include information about the onset, intensity, associated autonomic symptoms and trigger factors of headache. Special attention must be paid to the frequency of analgesic use, both prescription and over-the-counter, to identify analgesic rebound headache.
3. Hellmann D. Temporal arteritis: a cough, headache and tongue infarction. *JAMA* 2002; 287:2996–3000.
4. Smetana GW, Shmerling RH. Does this patient have temporal arteritis? *JAMA* 2002; 287:92–101.
5. Froehling DA, Silverstein MD, Mohr DN, Beatty CW. Does this dizzy patient have a serious form of vertigo? *JAMA* 1994; 271:385–388. Helps the clinician distinguish vertigo from other causes of dizziness.
6. Thomas KE, Hasbun R, Jekel J et al. The diagnostic accuracy of Kernig's sign, Brudzinski's sign, and nuchal rigidity in adults with suspected meningitis. *Clin Infect Dis* 2002; 35:46–52.
7. Damasio AR. Aphasia. *N Engl J Med* 1992; 326:531–539. A very detailed review.
8. Anonymous. Forgotten symptoms and primitive signs. *Lancet* 1987; 1:841–842. This puts many of the frontal lobe signs into perspective and suggests they are sometimes only of historical interest.
9. Steinberg D. Scientific neurology and the history of the clinical examination of the cranial nerves. *Semin Neurol* 2002; 22:349–356. An interesting historical review that explains the background to the modern understanding of cranial nerve function and structure.
10. Levin DE. The clinical significance of spontaneous pulsations of the retinal vein. *Arch Neurol* 1978; 35:37–40. Elevated intracranial pressure is excluded if pulsations are observed in the retinal veins. However, the absence of pulsations in the retinal veins does not necessarily mean that intracranial pressure is elevated.
11. Nelson KR. Use new pins for each neurologic examination [Letter]. *New Engl J Med* 1986; 314:581. A cautionary tale.
12. Ruffin et al. Gag reflex in disease [Letter]. *Chest* 1987; 92:1130. This suggests that many normal people may have an absent gag reflex.
13. Freeman C, Okun MS. Origins of the sensory examination in neurology. *Semin Neurol* 2002; 22:399–407
14. Medical Research Council. *Aids to the investigation of peripheral nerve injury*. London: Her Majesty's Stationery Office, 1972. Presents, in a clear and straightforward manner, bedside methods for testing the innervation of all important muscles. An invaluable guide.
15. Katz JN, Larson MG, Sabra A et al. The carpal tunnel syndrome: diagnostic utility of the history and physical examination findings. *Ann Intern Med* 1990; 112:321–327. Unfortunately, individual symptoms and signs have limited diagnostic usefulness. Tinel's sign appears to be of little value.
16. D'Arcy DA, McGee S. The rational clinical examination. Does this patient have carpal tunnel syndrome? *JAMA* 2000; 283:3110–3117. Weak thumb abduction and self-reported sensory symptoms (drawn on a diagram) are useful to predict abnormal median nerve conduction testing.
17. Schwartz RS et al. A comparison of two methods of eliciting the ankle jerk. *Aust NZ J Med* 1990; 20:116–119. The ankle jerk can be tested by tapping the sole of the foot.
18. Lance JW. The Babinski sign. *J Neurol Neurosurg Psychiatry* 2002; 73(4):360–362 A clear explanation of the history and clinical relevance of this most important of neurological signs.
19. Goldstein LB, Matchar DB. Clinical assessment of stroke (the Rational Clinical Examination). *JAMA* 1994; 271:1114–1120. Discusses the limitations of physical examination in identifying the lesion.
20. Sauve JS, Laupacis A, Ostbyte T et al. Does this patient have a clinically important carotid bruit? (The Rational Clinical Examination.) *JAMA* 1993; 270:2843–2846. Describes how to interpret the findings of a carotid bruit. Distinguishing high grade from moderate symptomatic carotid stenosis based on the bruit itself is difficult and the absence of a bruit does not mean the absence of a significant carotid stenosis.
21. Scherer K, Bedlack RS, Simel DL. Does this patient have myasthenia gravis? *JAMA* 2005; 293:1906–1914. Speech failure when speaking over a prolonged period and the Peek test increased the likelihood of myasthenia; their absence was unhelpful.
22. Rao G. Fisch L, Srinivason S et al. Does this patient have Parkinson disease? *JAMA* 2003; 289:347–353. Rigidity, the glabella tap and walking (heel–toe) seem to be useful signs of Parkinsonism.

Suggested reading

Review article

Gates P. The rule of 4 of the brainstem: a simplified method for understanding brainstem anatomy and brainstem vascular syndrome for the non-neurologist. *Intern Med J* 2005; 35:263–266. A simple method is described to localise brainstem vascular syndromes.

Textbooks

Fuller G. *Neurological examination made easy*, 3rd edn. Edinburgh: Churchill Livingstone, 2004.

Khaw PT, Elkinton AR, eds. *ABC of eyes*, 3rd edn. London: BMJ Publishing Group, 1999.

Kritzinger EE, Wright BE. *Color atlas of the eye and systemic disease*. Chicago: Wolfe Medical Year Book, 1984.

Morris JGL. *The neurological short case*. London: Edward Arnold, 1992.

Spillane JA. *Bickerstaff's neurological examination in clinical practice*, 6th edn. Oxford: Blackwell, 1996.

Weiner HL, Levitt LP, Rae-Grant AD. *Neurology: house officer series*, 7th edn. Philadelphia: Lippincott, Williams & Wilkins, 2004.

chapter 11

The psychiatric history and mental state examination

Law number four: the patient is the one with the disease.

House of God: Samuel Shem

This chapter deals with the psychiatric history and the mental state examination. The practising clinician must have an understanding of psychiatric illness and know how to perform a psychiatric interview and a mental state examination. This is because there is considerable overlap between psychiatric and physical illness.

Psychiatric disorders (especially anxiety and depression) are common, and people suffering from these conditions often have medical problems. Appropriate management of these patients will require an understanding of the intercurrent psychiatric disorder and the effect of that disorder on the primary medical problem. A medical illness may, in some instances, present as a psychiatric illness. For example, some endocrine disorders, such as myxoedema, may present with depression. On the other hand, some psychiatric disorders may present medically. Panic disorder (or acute anxiety) may be mistaken for an acute myocardial infarction. Furthermore, a patient's psychological state may interfere with the course of a medical illness; it may lead in some cases to exaggeration of the symptoms and in others to denial of the severity of physical symptoms.

The psychiatric history generally follows the same format as the standard medical history, and the principles described in Chapter 1 apply just as much here as in any history taking.[1] One should inquire about the history of the present illness, the past psychiatric and medical history, and the social and family history. However, the psychiatric history aims to elicit more detail about the patient's illness from a broad perspective, focusing not only on symptoms but also on the patient's social background, psychological functioning and life circumstances (a biopsychosocial approach). There is, therefore, more attention paid to the developmental, personal and social history than is normal for a standard medical history.

The method of psychiatric history taking is somewhat different from the standard medical interview. The psychiatric interview aims to be therapeutic as well as diagnostic. In the course of the interview it is hoped that the patient will be able to talk about his or her problems and their context. In doing so, patients will gain some relief from their distress by airing their problems. For this to take place, the clinician's attitude needs to be unhurried, patient and understanding. The psychiatric history also aims to gain an understanding of how the patient's problem arose from a biological, interpersonal, social and psychological perspective, so that the best management plan can be worked out.

Obtaining the history

The clinician taking a psychiatric history wants the patient to tell his or her story in his or her own words. In this way the patient will be more likely to report the most important aspects of the illness. This is best achieved using a non-directive approach with open-ended questions. Open-ended questions are those to which the patient will respond with narrative (or a description about what has been happening) rather than a simple factual response. They give the patient an opportunity to talk about his or her problems. Closed questions are more likely to elicit 'yes' or 'no' responses. For example, in the assessment of a patient with depression, a closed question would be: 'Have you been depressed?'. An open-ended question would be: 'Tell me about how you have been feeling'. At first glance it might appear that the open-ended question is less efficient, as it could take a longer time to find out about a range of symptoms. However, with a careful and judicious approach, open-ended questioning—by permitting the patient to tell the story—will enable the clinician to get a comprehensive history efficiently. This is not to say that targeted, more closed questions must not be used—they are necessary to elicit certain symptoms.

While the patient is telling his or her story, the clinician should begin to formulate hypotheses about the problem or diagnosis. These hypotheses are tested by asking more focused questions later in the interview, at which point a diagnostic hypothesis can be rejected or pursued further. For example, a patient may describe tiredness and lethargy, an inability to concentrate and loss of appetite. These symptoms will suggest a diagnosis of depression. Follow-up questions should focus on this possibility. The clinician should ask questions about other symptoms of depression such as: 'How have you been feeling in yourself?', 'What has your mood been like?' and 'How have you been sleeping?'.

Introductory questions

The psychiatric interview should start off with non-threatening questions. After introducing yourself, it can be useful to begin by asking about basic demographic information (age, marital state, occupation, whom the patient lives with) and then making the patient feel at ease by discussing some neutral topic.

History of the presenting illness

In assessing the history of the presenting illness one needs to cover a number of areas.

1. The problem

Find out the nature of the patient's problem, and the patient's perception of his or her difficulties. This can, of course, be difficult if the patient is psychotic and does not believe a problem exists at all. In these cases a corroborative history must be taken. For example, a manic patient may consider that there is nothing wrong and that his or her behaviour is reasonable, whereas his or her partner is able to recognise that ordering an expensive new sports car when the family is impoverished is a problem.

A range of symptoms commonly found in psychiatric disorders needs to be reviewed in the course of assessing the history of the present illness. These include mood change, anxiety, worry, sleep pattern, appetite, hallucinations and delusions. A set of simple screening questions for each of the major diagnoses is listed in Table 11.1. It is especially useful to ask about symptoms of anxiety and depression (the most common psychiatric disorders). The definitions of other symptoms are given in Table 11.2. It is important to ask about drug usage (legal and illegal) as well as alcohol and caffeine (which may be associated with anxiety disorders).

2. Precipitating events

Psychiatric illness rarely occurs for no reason and there is generally an event that has precipitated the illness. Such events include a range of experiences which may have affected the patient, or a member of the patient's social network. Events such as physical illness, drug treatment or treatment non-compliance may be implicated as precipitants. The last-mentioned is important, as patients with psychiatric illness are often non-compliant, a major contribution to relapse.

3. Risk

An assessment of the patient's risk of harm, either to others or to him- or herself, is essential: this will indicate whether the patient needs to be treated involuntarily. Patients with psychotic illness may, in some circumstances, need to be treated involuntarily under the *Mental Health Act*. While the exact details for involuntary treatment are different under

Table 11.1 Screening questions for the common psychiatric disorders

MOOD DISORDERS

Mood disorders have a pathological disturbance in mood (depression or mania) as the predominant feature. They are distinguished from 'normal' mood changes by their persistence, duration and severity, together with the presence of other symptoms and impairment of functioning.

1. Manic-depressive illness—bipolar disorder

Bipolar disorder is a broad term to describe a recurrent illness characterised by episodes of either mania or depression, with a return to normal functioning between episodes of illness.

a. Mania	*Questions*
A disorder demonstrated by change in mood (*elation*), thought form (*grandiosity*) and behaviour disturbance (*increased energy and disinhibition*). Frequently associated symptoms: increased talkativeness, distractability, decreased need for sleep, loss of inhibition (e.g. engaging in reckless behaviour such as spending sprees, sexual indiscretion or social overfamiliarity).	Have you felt especially good about yourself? Have you been needing less sleep than usual? Do you feel that you are special or that you have special powers? Have you been spending more than usual?

b. Depression	*Questions*
A disorder characterised by depressed mood (or loss of pleasure) and the presence of somatic (*sleep disturbance, change in appetite, fatigue and weight*), psychological (*low self-esteem, worry-anxiety, guilt, suicidal ideation*), affective (*sadness, irritability, loss of pleasure and interest in activities*) and psychomotor (*retardation or agitation*) symptoms.	How have you been feeling in yourself? What has your mood been like? Have you been feeling sad, blue, down or depressed? Have you lost interest in things you usually enjoy? How have you been sleeping?

ANXIETY DISORDERS

Anxiety disorders are those in which the person experiences excessive levels of anxiety. Anxiety may be somatic (*palpitations, difficulty breathing, dry mouth, nausea, frequency of micturition, dizziness, muscular tension, sweating, abdominal churning, tremor, cold skin*) or psychological (*feelings of dread and threat, irritability, panic, anxious anticipation, inner (psychic) tension, worrying over trivia, difficulty concentrating, initial insomnia, inability to relax*).

1. Generalised anxiety disorder (GAD)	*Questions*
A chronic disorder characterised by a tendency to worry excessively about everyday things. It is accompanied by: symptoms of anxiety or tension; mental tension (*feeling tense or nervous, poor concentration, on edge*); physical tension.	Have you been feeling nervy or tense? Do you worry a lot about things? Do you worry about things most other people would not worry about?

Table 11.1 Screening questions for the common psychiatric disorders (continued)

2. Panic disorder	**Questions**
A disorder characterised by episodes of panic occurring spontaneously in situations where most people would not be afraid. A panic attack is characterised by the presence of physical symptoms (*palpitations, chest pain, a choking feeling, a churning stomach, dizziness, feelings of unreality*) or fear of some disaster (*losing control or going mad, heart attack, sudden death*). They begin suddenly, build up rapidly, and may last only a few minutes.	Have you ever had an attack of acute anxiety or panic? Did this occur in a situation in which most people would not feel afraid? Can these attacks happen at any time?
3. Agoraphobia	**Questions**
A disorder in which an individual avoids places (such as supermarkets or trains) in which they fear they may have a panic attack and cannot escape.	Do you avoid going out? Do you avoid going to places because you fear you may have an anxiety attack?
4. Obsessive compulsive disorder	**Questions**
A disorder in which the person has either obsessions or compulsions which interfere with everyday life.	Are there any rituals or habits that you have to carry out every day? Do they cause you problems? Do you ever have a thought going round in your head that you can't get rid of?
5. Severe stress disorders	**Questions**
Individuals may present shortly after a traumatic event with a range of symptoms, such as *anxiety, depression, disturbed sleep, problems with memory or concentration*. Images, dreams or flashbacks of the traumatic event may also occur.	Have you been having any problems following ...? Have you been feeling worried? ... or depressed? Have you had trouble sleeping? Do you have bad memories?
6. Post-traumatic stress disorder (PTSD)	**Questions**
Onset of persistent problems within 6 months of a traumatic event of exceptional severity. The individual experiences *repetitive and intrusive re-enactments* of the trauma in images, dreams or flashbacks. *Sleep, concentration, memory, mood and attention may be disturbed*. Individuals may feel emotionally detached and avoid things that act as reminders of the traumatic event.	Since ... happened, have you been troubled by bad memories of it? Have you been having nightmares? Have you had trouble with sleep? Have you had trouble with your memory? Are you jumpy?

Table 11.1 Screening questions for the common psychiatric disorders (continued)

SCHIZOPHRENIA	*Questions*
A disorder characterised by disorders of content (*presence of delusions*), thought form (*shown by difficulty understanding the connections between the patient's thoughts*), perception (*hallucinations—predominantly auditory*), behaviour (*erratic or bizarre*) and/or volition (*apathy and withdrawal*).	Have you ever heard people speaking when there is no-one around? Do you ever hear voices? Have you heard your thoughts out loud? Do you have any thoughts or beliefs that others might find unusual or strange? Have you felt people may be against you? Have you felt that the TV or radio sends you messages? Do you ever feel as if someone is spying on you or plotting to hurt you? Do you have any ideas that you don't like to talk about because you're afraid other people will think you're mad?

ORGANIC BRAIN DISORDERS

These are disorders in which there is brain dysfunction manifested by cognitive disturbances such as memory loss or disorientation; there may be behavioural disturbance as well.

1. Delirium (acute brain syndrome)	*Questions*
A disorder characterised by the acute onset of disturbed consciousness plus changes in cognition that are not due to a pre-existing dementia. It is a direct physiological consequence of a *general medical condition* (*substance intoxication or withdrawal, use of a medication, exposure to a toxin, or a combination of these factors*). Delirium is characterised by *confusion* and *clouding of consciousness*. This may be accompanied by *poor memory, disorientation, inattention, agitation, emotional upset, hallucinations, visions or illusions, suspiciousness and disturbed sleep* (*reversal of sleep pattern*).	What day is it today? How long have you been here? What is the name of the place we are in? Do you remember my name? Mental state examination

2. Dementia (chronic brain syndrome)	*Questions*
A generalised impairment of intellect, memory and personality with no impairment of consciousness. Characterised by *loss of memory* (especially short-term memory), *loss of orientation and deterioration in social functioning and behaviour and emotional control* (may be easily upset—tearful or irritable).	What day is it today? How long have you been here? What is the name of the place we are in? Do you remember my name? Mental state examination

---

Table 11.1 Screening questions for the common psychiatric disorders (continued)

OTHER DISORDERS

There are a number of other psychiatric disorders which may present with physical problems, or may be seen in an emergency department with some complication (particularly after attempted suicide).

1. Eating disorders (anorexia nervosa and bulimia nervosa)	*Questions*
Here the sufferer (generally female) has a disturbed body image with an unreasonable fear of being fat, and makes extensive efforts to lose weight (strict dieting, vomiting, use of purgatives, excessive exercise). She may deny that weight or eating habits are problems. *Bulimia nervosa* is characterised by binge eating followed by vomiting or purging. *Anorexia nervosa* is characterised by excessive dieting, but there may also be binges followed by vomiting or purging. Anorexic patients will be grossly underweight and may show signs of malnutrition. Amenorrhoea is generally present.	Do you worry about your weight? Do you think that you are fat? Do you diet? Have you ever made yourself sick after a meal?
2. Somatisation disorder	*Questions*
A disorder characterised by multiple physical complaints that cannot be satisfactorily explained by physical disease. An individual with this disorder will have complaints in several bodily systems (e.g. gastrointestinal, cardiac, respiratory, musculoskeletal, menstrual).	Do you have any other medical problems? Have you had symptoms that your doctor has not been able to find a cause for? Are you often sick?
3. Personality disorders	*Questions*
In these disorders the individual, while not having specific symptoms, has behavioural disturbances and problems with impulse control, interpersonal relationships and mood. Individuals who repeatedly attempt suicide often have a personality disorder. They may also have stormy illnesses, causing frequent problems for staff.	Have you ever tried to harm yourself? Have you ever had problems with relationships?

individual mental health acts, the essential features are generally that: (a) a person has a mental illness; and (b) the person is a danger to self or to others. Assessment of danger to others is difficult, with the best predictor being a history of past threat or harm to others. It is best to err on the side of caution in such cases. Assessment of suicide risk needs to be made with sensitivity and using a direct approach, as shown in Table 11.3.

Table 11.2 Symptoms of psychiatric illness

Affect	The observable behaviour by which a person's internal emotional state is judged.
Agitation (psychomotor agitation)	Excessive motor activity associated with a feeling of inner tension. The activity is usually non-productive and repetitious and consists of such behaviour as pacing, fidgeting, wringing the hands, pulling the clothes and inability to sit still.
Anxiety	The apprehensive anticipation of future danger or misfortune. It is associated with feelings of tension and symptoms of autonomic arousal.
Conversion symptom (hysteria)	A loss of, or alteration in, motor or sensory function. Psychological factors are judged to be associated with the development of the symptom, which is not fully explained by anatomical or pathological conditions. The symptom is the result of unconscious conflict and is not feigned.
Delusion	A false unshakable idea or belief that is out of keeping with the patient's educational, cultural and social background.
Depersonalisation	An alteration in the awareness of the self—the individual feels as if he or she is unreal.
Derealisation	An alteration in the perception or experience of the external world so that it seems unreal.
Disorientation	Confusion about the time of day, date or season (time), where one is (place) or who one is (person).
Flight of ideas	A nearly continuous flow of accelerated speech with abrupt changes from topic to topic that are usually based on understandable associations, distracting stimuli, or plays on words. When severe, speech may be disorganised or incoherent.
Grandiosity	An inflated appraisal of one's worth, power, knowledge, importance or identity. When extreme, grandiosity may be of delusional proportions.
Hallucination	A sensory perception that seems real, but occurs without external stimulation of the relevant sensory organ. The term *hallucination* is not ordinarily applied to the false perceptions that occur during dreaming, while falling asleep (*hypnagogic*) or when awakening (*hypnopompic*).
Ideas of reference	The feeling that casual incidents and external events have a particular significance and unusual meaning that is specific to the person.
Illusion	A misperception or misinterpretation of a real external stimulus.
Mood	A pervasive and sustained emotion that colours the perception of the world.
Overvalued idea	An unreasonable belief that is held, but not as strongly as a delusion (i.e. the person is able to acknowledge the possibility that the belief may not be true). The belief is not one that is ordinarily accepted by other members of the person's culture or subculture.
Personality	Enduring patterns of perceiving, relating to, and thinking about the environment and oneself.
Phobia	A persistent irrational fear of a specific object, activity or situation (the phobic stimulus) that results in a compelling desire to avoid it.
Pressured speech	Speech that is increased in amount, accelerated, and difficult or impossible to interrupt. Usually it is also loud and emphatic. Frequently the person talks without any social stimulation and may continue to talk even though no-one is listening.
Psychomotor retardation	Visible generalised slowing of movements and speech.
Psychotic	Psychotic can be used to mean a loss of contact with reality, but is generally used to imply the presence of delusions or hallucinations.

Based on DSM-IV, APA 1994.[2]

Table 11.3 Assessment of suicide risk

Suicide is the unfortunate outcome of psychiatric illness. Assessing the risk of suicide is an essential part of the psychiatric interview. Asking about this does not increase the risk or put the idea into the patient's head. It may reduce the risk, as the patient may feel relief in talking about his or her fears. The risk of suicide is assessed by asking directly whether the person has ever contemplated it.

Have you thought that life was not worth living?
Or
Have you felt so bad that you have considered ending it all?

If 'yes'...
Have you thought of killing yourself?
Have you thought how you might do this?
Have you made any plans for doing this?

The past history

Both the past psychiatric and medical history should be assessed. The past medical history should be evaluated in the same way as in the general medical history. For the past psychiatric history, it is important to obtain not only the diagnosis but also the treatment the patient has had, and its outcome. An assessment should be made of stresses that may have contributed to past episodes of illness, and that may have led to relapse.

The family history

There is a familial component in many psychiatric disorders. Two aspects must be assessed in the family history.

First, the patient should be asked tactfully if anyone in the family has had any psychiatric or mental illness or has committed suicide. He or she should also be asked if anyone in the family has had any treatment for psychological problems, such as anxiety, depression, agoraphobia, eating disorders or drug and alcohol problems (these last few areas are often not considered by patients to be psychiatric or mental illnesses).

Second, one should try to determine what sort of family the patient grew up in. Drawing up a family tree is a useful way of finding this out. Factual details about each family member can be included in this family tree (age, mental state, health). In the psychiatric history we also need to know about what type of person each family member is, and how family members get on with each other. It is worth exploring how much care (or neglect) the patient received from each parent, and how controlling or protective each was. These two things have been shown to be important in contributing to psychiatric illness. One needs to ask about the quality of the parental relationship and the general family atmosphere.

Childhood abuse (physical or sexual)[3] may be an important predisposing event for many illnesses, and should be inquired about. This can be elicited by saying something like 'Sometimes children can have had some unpleasant experiences—I wonder if you had any? Did anyone ever harm you? ... or hit you? ... How about interfering with you sexually? ... Could you tell me more about that and what happened?'.

Taking a detailed family history in this way sets the scene for the patient's developmental history, which should be taken next.

The social and personal history

Open-ended questions are again the best way to obtain the personal and social history. Ask the patient something like 'Could you tell me a bit about your background, your development, what sort of childhood you had, what are the important things you remember from your childhood?', and then allow the patient to tell his or her own story. During the course of this narrative, the patient may require some prompting to add information about important issues such as the birth history (schizophrenia is known to be associated with perinatal morbidity) and early development, and whether there were significant problems in early childhood, such as head injuries or serious infections. How did the patient cope with early separations, particularly when starting primary school and going on to secondary school (difficulty in separation may be a risk factor for panic disorder or abnormal illness behaviour). The patient should be asked about peer relationships, friendships, school, academic ability, adolescence and teenage relationships. The adult history should focus predominantly on the quality of intimate relationships and the social support network, especially whether there are people in whom the patient can confide.

The patient's living circumstances should be asked about in the same way as for a medical history. There should also be a focus on the patient's occupation: not only on the type of job but also on how he or she copes with work or, if he or she does not work, how that is coped with.

Premorbid personality

An assessment should be made of the patient's premorbid personality. Ask the patient to describe him- or herself. The personality can be described using the predominant trait, such as obsessional, nervy or highly strung; it is not necessary to use official systems to describe a patient's personality. In the assessment of premorbid personality it is important to evaluate both positive and negative aspects of the person, how he or she copes adaptively and maladaptively to life stress, what type of interests he or she has, and what other strengths and weaknesses are present.

The mental state examination

While assessing the patient, one should carefully make observations about appearance, behaviour, patterns of speech, attitude to the examiner and ways of interacting. These observations are brought together in a systematic fashion in the mental state examination. This is not something that is 'done' at the conclusion of taking a history; it is an essential part of the total process of assessing the patient.[4]

However, there are a number of tests that need to be conducted in a formalised way as part of the mental state examination. These include assessing the cognitive state (orientation, memory, attention, registration) and inquiring about perceptual disturbances and, in some cases, disorders of thought. The mental state examination provides valuable diagnostic information; with some disorders, it is this examination which gives most of the diagnostic clues.

The headings under which the mental state is recorded are shown in Table 11.4, together with some simple bedside tests for assessing cognitive function. Also shown in Table 11.4 are some abnormal features of the mental state examination that are commonly found in psychiatric disorders.

When cognitive dysfunction is suspected, as in patients with dementia,[5] a more detailed examination of cognitive function should be carried out. A widely used tool for doing this is the mini-mental state examination,[6] which assesses aspects of orientation, memory and concentration. Details of this examination are shown in Table 11.5. Some of the common causes of delirium and dementia are listed in Tables 11.6 and 11.7.

The diagnosis

At the conclusion of the psychiatric history, which should include a general physical examination, a provisional diagnosis and formulation should be made. Essentially, the diagnostic formulation is a means of pulling together, in a succinct yet comprehensive manner, your understanding of the patient's problem. Psychiatric disorders generally arise through a combination of biological, psychological and psychosocial factors, and each of these needs to be considered when a patient's problem is being assessed (a biopsychosocial approach). The patient's problem needs to be understood longitudinally, by defining biophysical factors that may have predisposed to the illness and, more immediately, may have precipitated the illness, and factors that may be contributing to the person remaining ill (perpetuating factors). A simple grid can be used for assessing the patient in this manner (Table 11.8). Here biological, psychological or psychosocial factors that predispose to, precipitate or perpetuate the psychiatric illness are identified. Perpetuating factors are very important, particularly among medically ill patients, as it may be the medical or physical illness that maintains the patient's psychiatric problem. By the same token, psychological factors may perpetuate a patient's medical illness.

An example of such a grid is shown for a 53-year-old man who becomes depressed after a myocardial infarction. He has a family history of depression (a genetic predisposing factor) and chronic low self-esteem (a psychological predisposing factor), which he coped with by succeeding in business. He has few friends and his marriage is unsatisfactory (a psychosocial factor). He had his infarct one week after he heard that he would not be promoted at work (a psychological factor) and his job was at risk (a psychosocial precipitant). His insecurity about work and his failing marriage, together with his low self-esteem, is maintaining his illness, as are the biological changes to the neurotransmitter system. A formulation grid for this patient is shown in Table 11.9.

Understanding the patient in this manner helps to plan an effective management approach that will focus on all the relevant factors, so that, for example, a combination of antidepressants, marital counselling and assertiveness training (to build self-esteem) can be organised.

A good psychiatric history will provide a comprehensive understanding of the patient and will permit appropriate management to be planned. This is immensely rewarding for the clinician, and will also be of considerable benefit to the patient.

Table 11.4 The mental state examination

	What is assessed, described or observed	Common findings indicating psychopathology	Types of illness
General description			
Appearance	A general description of the patient's appearance, including body build, posture, clothing (appropriateness), grooming (e.g. make-up) and hygiene. Note any physical stigmata (e.g. tattoos) and facial expression (depression, apprehension, worry etc).	Bizarre appearance	Psychotic disorders (schizophrenia, mania), personality disorder
		Unkempt, poorly groomed	Schizophrenia, depression
		Apprehensive, anxious	Anxiety disorders
		Over bright clothing	Mania, personality disorder
		Scarred wrists, tattoos	Personality disorder
Behaviour	All aspects of the patient's behaviour. Note the appropriateness of the patient's behaviour within the interview context.	Uncooperative behaviour	Psychotic disorder, personality disorder
	Abnormal motor behaviour: mannerisms, stereotyped movements, tics.	Manneristic behaviour	Psychotic disorder
	Variants of normal motor behaviour: restlessness, psychomotor change (agitation, retardation).	Stereotypic behaviour	Psychotic disorders, developmental disability, organic syndromes
		Bizarre behaviour	Psychotic disorders
		Assaultive, threatening	Personality disorders, intoxication, neurological disorders
		Restlessness	Akathisia from antipsychotic medication
		Psychomotor change	Depression
Attitude towards examiner	The way the patient responds to the interviewer, the level of cooperation, willingness to disclose information. A range of attitudes and deviation from appropriateness may occur, ranging from hostility to seductiveness.	Uncooperative attitude, belligerence	Psychotic disorder, personality disorder
		Seductiveness	Personality disorder
Mood and affect			
Mood	A relatively persistent emotional state: describe the depth, intensity, duration and fluctuations of mood. Mood may be neutral, euphoric, depressed, anxious or irritable.	Depressed	Depression
		Anxious/irritable	Depression/anxiety disorders
Affect	The way a patient conveys his or her emotional state. Affect may be full, blunted, restricted or inappropriate.	Depressed	Depression
		Blunted, restricted	Schizophrenia

Table 11.4 The mental state examination (continued)

	What is assessed, described or observed	Common findings indicating psychopathology	Types of illness
Mood and affect (continued)			
Appropriateness	Are the patient's responses appropriate to the matter being discussed?	Inappropriate	Schizophrenia
Speech	The tempo, modulation and quality of the patient's speech should be described here. Note should be made of dysphasia or dysarthria (see Chapter 10).	Increased tempo / Slowed	Mania, acute schizophrenia / Depression
Perceptual disturbances	The presence of hallucinations (auditory, visual, gustatory or tactile) should be noted. It is important to check whether they occurred with a clear sensorium. Hypnagogic or hypnopompic hallucinations are normal experiences. Other perceptual disturbances (e.g. illusions, depersonalisation or derealisation) should be noted.	Visual hallucinations / Auditory / Tactile/gustatory	Acute brain syndrome, epilepsy, alcohol withdrawal, drug intoxication / Schizophrenia / Epilepsy, schizophrenia
Thought			
Thought form	The process of the patient's thinking. This involves the quantity of ideas (pressured thought, poverty of ideas) and the way in which the ideas (thoughts) are produced. Are they logical and relevant, or are they fragmented and irrelevant? The link between ideas should be assessed—do they flow logically, or are they disconnected and 'fragmented'? Are ideas connected by spurious concepts (rhyming, the way they sound—'clang' associations)?	Disorder of thought form / Flight of ideas / Poverty of ideas	Schizophrenia / Mania, schizophrenia / Schizophrenia, mania, depression
Thought content	The content of the patient's thought. Abnormalities range from preoccupation, obsessions, overvalued ideas to delusions. Themes should also be assessed: suicidal or homicidal thoughts or paranoid ideas. In the medical setting, preoccupation with illness (hypochondriacal thoughts) should be assessed, as well as thoughts of omnipotence—denying illness when it is present.	Delusions	Schizophrenia, mania, depression

Table 11.4 The mental state examination (continued)

	What is assessed, described or observed	Common findings indicating psychopathology	Types of illness
Sensorium and cognition			
	Listed below are bedside tests for a basic assessment of cognitive function. If abnormalities are detected, a full mini-mental state examination (Table 11.5) should be carried out.		
Alertness and level of consciousness	The level of consciousness should be assessed. Clouding or fluctuating levels of consciousness should be noted.	Clouding	Delirium
Orientation	Orientation to time, place and person. Ask the day, date, month and year. Ask where he or she is, and if he or she knows who he or she is.	Disorientation	Dementia, delirium
Short-term memory	Short-term memory refers to the ability to retain information over a period of 3–5 minutes. Less than this refers to immediate recall. Ask the patient to recall a list of three objects after 3–5 minutes.	Loss of short-term memory	Dementia, delirium
Long-term memory	This refers to memory of remote events. Ask the patient to recall events of the previous few days, as well as events of a year ago.	Loss of long-term memory	Dementia
Concentration	Subtract 7 from 100 and keep subtracting 7, or spell 'world' backwards.	Poor concentration	Delirium, acute psychosis
General knowledge and intelligence	Ask about some recent events. Intelligence can be gauged from the language used. Ask the patient to do some simple arithmetical tasks. Literacy should be assessed.	Poor general knowledge	Dementia, delirium
Judgment and insight			
Judgment	The capacity to behave appropriately. Describe a hypothetical situation, and ask how the patient would behave in it (e.g. 'What would you do if you smelt smoke while sitting in a cinema?').	Impaired judgment	Psychoses, dementia, personality disorders
Insight	Determine whether the patient is aware that he or she has a problem, and the level of understanding of this.	Lack of insight	Psychoses, dementia

Table 11.5 The mini-mental state examination

	Score	Max
Orientation		
'What is the (year) (season) (date) (day) (month)?' Ask for the date, then specifically inquire about parts omitted (e.g. season). Score 1 point for each correct answer.	☐	5
'Where are we (country) (state) (town) (hospital) (ward)?' Ask in turn for each place. Score 1 point for each correct answer.	☐	5
Registration		
'May I test your memory?' Repeat three objects (e.g. pen, watch, book). Score 1 point for each correct answer.	☐	3
Then repeat until the patient learns all three. Count trials and record (up to six).		
Attention and calculation		
'Count backwards from 100 by sevens' (serial 7s). One point for each answer, up to five (93, 86, 79, 72, 65) *Or* Spell 'world' backwards. Score 1 point for each letter in correct order.	☐	5
Recall		
Ask the patient to recall the three objects in 'registration', above. Score 1 point for each correct answer.	☐	3
Language		
Ask the patient to name two objects shown (e.g. pen and watch). Score 0–2 points.	☐	2
'Repeat the following: "No ifs, ands or buts".' Score 1 point.	☐	1
Ask the patient to follow a three-stage command: e.g. 'Take this paper in your right hand, fold it in half and put it on the table.' Score 1 point for each step.	☐	3
Read and obey the following: CLOSE YOUR EYES. Score 1 point.	☐	1
WRITE A SENTENCE. Do not dictate—must be sensible, but punctuation and grammar not essential. Score 1 point.	☐	1
'Copy this design.' All ten angles must be present, and the two must intersect. Score 1 point.	☐	1
TOTAL	☐	30

Assess patient's level of consciousness along a continuum

Alert	Drowsy	Stuporose	Coma

Scores of 21–29 indicate mild cognitive impairment. Scores below 20 indicate more severe cognitive impairment, and are likely to be due to dementia, especially if obtained on repeated examinations.

Table 11.6 Some common causes of delirium

Delirium	
Drug intoxication	Anxiolytics Digoxin L-dopa Alcohol 'Street drugs'
Withdrawal states	Alcohol (delirium tremens) Anxiolytic sedatives
Metabolic disturbance	Uraemia Liver failure Anoxia Cardiac failure Electrolyte imbalance Postoperative states
Endocrine disturbance	Diabetic ketosis Hypoglycaemia
Systemic infections	Pneumonia Urinary tract infection Septicaemia Viral infections
Intracranial infection	Encephalitis Meningitis
Other intracranial causes	Space-occupying lesions Raised intracranial pressure
Head injury	Subdural haemorrhage Cerebral contusion Concussion
Nutritional and vitamin deficiency	Thiamine (Wernicke's encephalopathy) Vitamin B_{12} Nicotinic acid
Epilepsy	Status epilepticus Post-ictal states

Table 11.7 Some common causes of dementia

Dementia	
Degenerative	Senile dementia of Alzheimer's type Pick's disease Huntington's chorea Parkinson's disease Normal-pressure hydrocephalus Multiple sclerosis
Intracranial space-occupying lesions	Tumour Subdural haematomas
Traumatic	Head injuries Boxing encephalopathy
Infections and related conditions	Encephalitis Neurosyphilis HIV (AIDS dementia) Jacob-Creutzfeldt disease
Vascular	Multi-infarct dementia Carotid artery occlusion
Metabolic	Uraemia Hepatic failure
Toxic	Alcoholic dementia Heavy metal poisoning
Anoxia	Anaemia Carbon monoxide poisoning Cardiac arrest Chronic respiratory failure
Vitamin deficiency	Vitamin B_{12} Folic acid Thiamine (Wernicke–Korsakoff's syndrome)
Endocrine	Myxoedema Addison's disease

Table 11.8 A formulation grid

	Predisposing	Precipitating	Perpetuating
Biological			
Psychological			
Psychosocial			

Table 11.9 A completed formulation grid

	Predisposing	Precipitating	Perpetuating
Biological	Genetic predisposition	Acute myocardial infarct	Neurotransmitter changes
Psychological	Low self-esteem	Not promoted	Low self-esteem and insecurity
Psychosocial	Poor social support Dysfunctional marriage		Dysfunctional marriage

References

1. Kopelman MD. Structured psychiatric interview: psychiatric history and assessment of the mental state. *Br J Hosp Med* 1994; 52:93–98.
2. American Psychiatric Association. *Diagnostic and Statistical Manual of Mental Disorders*, 4th edn. Washington, DC: APA, 1994.
3. Drossman DA, Talley NJ, Lesserman J et al. Sexual and physical abuse and gastrointestinal illness. *Ann Intern Med* 1995; 123:782–794. A good clinical summary of the relevance of abuse to illness.
4. Davies T. The ABC of mental health. Mental health assessment. *BMJ* 1997; 314:1536–1539.
5. Johnson J, Sims R, Gottlieb G. Differential diagnosis of dementia, delirium and depression. Implications for drug therapy. *Drugs and Aging* 1994; 5:431–445. The differential diagnosis hinges on a careful clinical evaluation. Dementia is defined as a chronic loss of intellectual or cognitive function of sufficient severity to interfere with social or occupational function. Delirium is an acute disturbance of consciousness marked by an attention deficit and a change in cognitive ability.
6. Folstein MF, Folstein SE, McHugh PR. Mini Mental State. A practical method for grading the cognitive state of patients for the clinician. *J Psychiatr Res* 1975; 12:189–198.

Suggested reading

Review articles

Gleason OC. Delirium. *Am Fam Physician* 2003; 67:1027–1034.
Morgan H, Blashki G. Fits, faints and funny turns. Could it be a mental disorder? *Aust Fam Physician* 2003; 32:211–213, 216–219.
Zun LS. Evidence-based evaluation of psychiatric patients. *J Emerg Med* 2005; 28:35–39.

Textbooks

Balint M. *The doctor, his patient and the illness*. Millennium Edition. New York: Churchill Livingstone, 2000.
Kaplan HI, Sadock BJ. *Synopsis of psychiatry and study guide/self examination review CD-ROM*, 8th edn. Baltimore: Williams & Wilkins, 1998.
Stern TA, Fricchione GL, Cassem NH et al. *Massachusetts General Hospital handbook of general hospital psychiatry*, 5th edn. St Louis: Mosby Year Book, 2004.

chapter 12

The skin and nails

For one mistake made for not knowing, ten mistakes are made for not looking.

JA Lindsay

The dermatological history

With any rash or skin condition, it is important to determine when and where it began, its distribution, whether it has changed over time, its relationship to sun exposure or heat or cold, and any response to treatment.[1] Ask if pruritus is associated; localised pruritus is usually due to dermatological disease. Determine if pain or disturbed sensation has occurred; for example, inflammation and oedema can produce pain in the skin, while disease involving neurovascular bundles or nerves can produce anaesthesia (e.g. leprosy, syphilis). Constitutional symptoms such as fever, headache, fatigue, anorexia and weight loss also need to be documented.

It is important to obtain a past history of rashes or allergic reactions. A past history of asthma, eczema or hay fever suggests atopy. Similarly, evidence of systemic disease in the past may be important in a patient with a rash (e.g. diabetes mellitus, connective tissue disease, inflammatory bowel disease).

A detailed social history needs to be obtained regarding occupation and hobbies, as chemical exposure and contact with animals or plants can all induce dermatitis. All medications that have been taken must be documented. Orally ingested or parenteral medications can cause a whole host of cutaneous lesions and can mimic many skin diseases (Table 12.1). Similarly, a family history of atopic dermatitis, hay fever or skin infestation can be helpful.

General principles of physical examination of the skin

The aim of this chapter is to provide an approach to the diagnosis of skin diseases.[2,3] Particular emphasis will be placed on cutaneous signs as indications of systemic disease. Other chapters have included the usual clues that can be used to arrive at a particular diagnosis. This chapter tries to unify the concept of 'inspection' as a valuable starting point in the examination of the patient.

Ask the patient to undress. The whole surface of the skin and its appendages should be carefully inspected (Table 12.2).

When one is examining actual skin lesions, a number of features should be documented. First, each lesion should be *described* precisely, including colour and shape. Use the appropriate dermatological terminology (Table 12.3), even though this may seem to make dermatological diseases more, rather than less, mysterious. As many dermatological diagnoses are purely descriptive, a good description will often be of considerable help in making the diagnosis. Second, the *distribution* of the lesions should be noted, as certain distributions suggest specific diagnoses. Third, the *pattern* of the lesions—such as linear, annular (ring-shaped), reticulated (net-like), serpiginous (snake-like) or grouped—also helps establish the diagnosis. Then *palpate* the lesions, noting consistency, tenderness, temperature,

Table 12.1 Types of cutaneous drug reactions

1 Acne, e.g. steroids
2 Hair loss (alopecia), e.g. cancer chemotherapy
3 Pigment alterations: hypomelanosis (e.g. hydroxyquinone, chloroquine, topical steroids), hypermelanosis (page 393)
4 Exfoliative dermatitis or erythroderma (page 391)
5 Urticaria (hives), e.g. non-steroidal anti-inflammatory drugs, radiographic dyes, captopril, penicillin
6 Maculopapular (morbilliform) eruptions, e.g. ampicillin, allopurinol
7 Photosensitive eruptions, e.g. sulphonamides, sulphonylureas, chlorothiazides, phenothiazines, tetracycline, nalidixic acid, anticonvulsants
8 Drug-induced lupus erythematosus, e.g. procainamide, hydralazine
9 Vasculitis, e.g. propylthiouracil, allopurinol, thiazides, penicillin, phenytoin
10 Skin necrosis, e.g. warfarin
11 Drug-precipitated porphyria, e.g. alcohol, barbiturates, sulphonamides, contraceptive pill
12 Lichenoid eruptions, e.g. gold, antimalarials, beta-blockers, captopril
13 Fixed drug eruption, e.g. sulphonamides, tetracycline, phenylbutazone, barbiturates
14 Bullous eruptions, e.g. frusemide, nalidixic acid, penicillamine, clonidine
15 Erythema nodosum or erythema multiforme (page 392)
16 Toxic epidermal necrolysis, e.g. allopurinol, phenytoin, sulphonamides, non-steroidal anti-inflammatory drugs
17 Pruritus (page 388)

Table 12.2 Considerations when examining the skin

1 Hair
2 Nails
3 Sebaceous glands—oil-producing and present on the head, neck and back
4 Eccrine glands—sweat-producing and present all over the body
5 Apocrine glands—sweat-producing and present in the axillae and groin
6 Mucosa

Table 12.3 Dermatological terms

Term	Definition
Atrophy	Thinning of epidermis with loss of normal skin markings
Bulla	A large collection of fluid below the epidermis
Crust	Dried serum and exudate
Ecchymoses	Bruises
Excoriations	Lesions caused by scratching that results in loss of the epidermis
Keloid	Hypertrophic scarring
Macule	A circumscribed alteration of skin colour
Nodule	A circumscribed palpable mass, greater than 1 cm diameter
Papule	A circumscribed palpable elevation, less than 1 cm diameter
Petechiae	Red, non-blanching spots <5 mm
Pigment alterations	Increased (hyperpigmentation) or decreased (hypopigmentation)
Plaque	A palpable disc-shaped lesion
Purpura	Red, non-blanching spots >5 mm
Pustule	A visible collection of pus
Scales	An accumulation of excess keratin
Sclerosis	Induration of subcutaneous tissues, which may involve the dermis
Ulcer	A circumscribed loss of tissue
Vesicle	A small collection of fluid below the epidermis
Wheal	An area of dermal oedema

Descriptive terms

Annular	Ring-shaped (hollow centre), e.g. tinea infection
Arcuate	Curved, e.g. secondary syphilis
Circinate	Circular
Confluent	Lesions that have run together, e.g. measles
Discoid	Circular without a hollow centre, e.g. lupus
Eczematous	Inflamed and crusted, e.g. allergic eczema
Keratotic	Thickened from increased keratin, e.g. psoriasis
Lichenified	Thickening and roughening of the epidermis associated with accentuated skin markings
Linear	In lines, e.g. contact dermatitis
Nodule	Raised solid lesion >10 mm, e.g. erythema nodosum
Papule	Raised solid lesion <10 mm, e.g. wart
Papulosquamous	Plaques associated with scaling
Reticulated	In a network pattern, e.g. cutaneous parasite
Serpiginous	Sinuous
Zosteriform	Following a nerve distribution

depth and mobility. A clinical algorithm for diagnosis is presented in Figure 12.1.

How to approach the clinical diagnosis of a lump

First, determine the lump's site, size, shape, consistency and tenderness. Next, evaluate in what tissue layer the lump is situated. If it is in the *skin* (e.g. sebaceous cyst, epidermoid cyst, papilloma), it should move when the skin is moved, but if it is in the *subcutaneous tissue* (e.g. neurofibroma, lipoma), the skin can be moved over the lump. If it is in the *muscle* or *tendon* (e.g. tumour), then contraction of the muscle or tendon will limit the lump's mobility. If it is in a *nerve*, pressing on the lump may result in pins and needles being felt in the distribution of the nerve, and the lump cannot be moved in the

longitudinal axis but can be moved in the transverse axis. If it is in *bone*, the lump will be immobile.

Determine if the lump is *fluctuant* (i.e. contains fluid). Place one forefinger (the 'watch' finger) halfway between the centre and periphery of the lump. The forefinger from the other hand (the 'displacing' finger) is placed diagonally opposite the 'watch' finger at an equal distance from the centre of the lump. Press with the displacing finger and keep the watching finger still. If the lump contains fluid, the watching finger will be displaced in *both* axes of the lump (i.e. fluctuation is present). Place a small torch behind the lump to determine whether it can be *transilluminated*.

Note any associated signs of *inflammation* (i.e. redness, swelling, heat and tenderness).

Look for similar lumps elsewhere, such as multiple subcutaneous swellings from neurofibromas or lipomas.

If an inflammatory or neoplastic lump is suspected, remember always to examine the regional lymphatic field and the other lymph node groups.

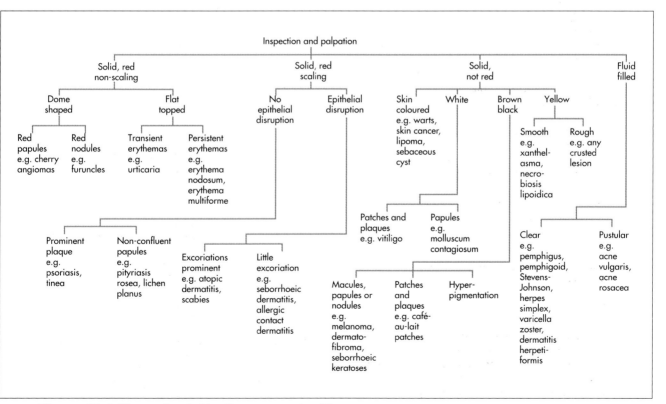

Figure 12.1 Diagnosis of skin disease: an algorithm

(Adapted from Lynch PJ. *Dermatology for the house officer*, 2nd edn. Baltimore: Williams & Wilkins, 1987.)

Correlation of physical signs and skin disease

There are many different skin diseases with varied physical signs. With each major sign the groups of common important diseases that should be considered will be listed.

Pruritus

Pruritus simply means itching. It may be either generalised or localised. Scratch marks are usually present. Localised pruritus is usually caused by a dermatological condition such as dermatitis or eczema. Generalised pruritus may be caused by primary skin disease, systemic disease or psychogenic factors.

To determine the cause of the pruritus it is essential to examine the skin in detail (Table 12.4).

Table 12.4 Primary skin disorders causing pruritus

1 Asteatosis (dry skin)
2 Atopic dermatitis
3 Urticaria
4 Scabies
5 Dermatitis herpetiformis

Excoriations are caused by scratching, regardless of the underlying cause. Specific features of cutaneous diseases such as dermatitis, scabies (Figure 12.2) or the blisters of dermatitis herpetiformis (page 136) should be looked for.

When primary skin diseases have been excluded, a detailed history and examination should be undertaken to consider the various systemic diseases listed in Table 12.5.

Erythrosquamous eruptions

Erythrosquamous eruptions are made up of lesions that are red and scaly. They may be well demarcated or have diffuse borders. They may be itchy or asymptomatic.

Table 12.5 Systemic conditions causing pruritus

1 Cholestasis, e.g. primary biliary cirrhosis
2 Chronic renal failure
3 Pregnancy
4 Lymphoma and other internal malignancies
5 Iron deficiency, polycythaemia rubra vera
6 Endocrine diseases, e.g. diabetes mellitus, hypothyroidism, hyperthyroidism, carcinoid syndrome

Figure 12.2 Scabies

Scattered fine papules with severe itching. Finger web involvement is common.

Figure 12.3 Lichen planus

With polygonal flat-topped violaceous lesions.

When one is attempting to establish a diagnosis of an erythrosquamous eruption, the history is very important. First ask about the time course of the eruption, about a family history of similar skin diseases and whether or not there is a family history of atopy.

The presence or absence of itching and the distribution of the lesions also give clues about the diagnosis.

Asymptomatic lesions on the palms and soles are suggestive of secondary syphilis, whereas itchy lesions in the same location would be more suggestive of lichen planus (Figures 12.3 and 12.4). Lichen planus

is occasionally associated with primary biliary cirrhosis and other liver diseases, chronic graft-versus-host disease and drugs (e.g. gold, penicillamine). Scattered lesions of recent origin on the trunk would be more suggestive of pityriasis rosea (Figure 12.5), whereas more widespread diffuse intensely itchy lesions would be more suggestive of nummular eczema (Figure 12.6) (Table 12.6).

Figure 12.4 Lichen planus

With development of lesions in an area of trauma—the 'Koebner' phenomenon.

Table 12.6 Causes of erythrosquamous eruptions

1 Psoriasis (bright pink plaques with silvery scale)
2 Atopic eczema (diffuse erythema with fine scaling)
3 Pityriasis rosea (paler pink, scaly, macular lesions)
4 Nummular eczema (round patches of subacute dermatitis)
5 Contact dermatitis (irritant or allergic)
6 Dermatophyte infections (ringworm)
7 Lichen planus (violet-coloured, small, polygonal papules)
8 Secondary syphilis (flat, red, hyperkeratotic lesions)

Figure 12.5 Pityriasis rosea

With scattered scaly oval lesions on the trunk and a larger 'herald' patch.

Figure 12.6 Nummular eczema

Typical scattered coin-like lesions of indolent dermatitis.

Figure 12.7 Psoriasis

Typical bright red, scaly plaque with silvery scale over a joint.

Figure 12.8 Acute widespread pustular psoriasis

Often the eruption is bright red with bizarre patterns and pustules predominantly at the margins.

Scaly lesions with a well-demarcated edge over the extensor surfaces are usually due to psoriasis (Figures 12.7 and 12.8).

Blistering eruptions

There are a number of different diseases which will present with either vesicles or blisters. Dermatitis can present as a blistering eruption, particularly acute contact dermatitis (Figure 12.9) (Table 12.7).

Clinical features of bullous eruptions

Viral blisters such as those of herpes simplex virus infection (Figure 12.10) have a distinctive morphology (grouped vesicles on an erythematous background).

Bullous pemphigoid is a rare disease usually affecting older patients. Blisters are widespread, have a thick roof and tend not to rupture easily.

Pemphigus vulgaris is much more severe. It has thin-roofed blisters that readily rupture and form crusts. The affected superficial skin can be moved over the deeper layer (Nikolsky's[a] sign). Oral ulcers are common.

[a] Pyotr Vasilyevich Nikolsky (1855–1940), Kiev and Warsaw dermatologist.

Figure 12.9 Allergic contact dermatitis

From over-the-counter topical medication rubbed over congested sinuses.

Table 12.7 Causes of blistering eruptions	
1	Traumatic blisters and burns
2	Bullous impetigo
3	Viral blisters (e.g. herpes simplex, varicella)
4	Bullous erythema multiforme
5	Bullous pemphigoid
6	Dermatitis herpetiformis
7	Pemphigus
8	Porphyria
9	Epidermolysis bullosa
10	Dermatophyte infections
11	Acute contact dermatitis

Figure 12.10 Primary herpes simplex virus infection in an adult

Shows typical widespread distribution around the mouth.

Dermatitis herpetiformis is characterised by a very itchy widespread vesicular or bullous eruption.

Porphyria cutanea tarda is characterised by clear or haemorrhagic blisters on the hands (page 138).

Erythroderma

Erythroderma is best thought of as the end-stage of numerous skin conditions (Table 12.8). The erythrodermic patient has involvement of nearly all the skin with an erythematous inflammatory process, often with exfoliation. There is usually associated oedema and loss of muscle mass. This represents that most unusual occurrence, a dermatological emergency.

An attempt should be made to determine the underlying cause of the erythroderma and this is best done based on history and examination. Specific treatment can then be directed at the underlying cause. Some patients with erythroderma will develop

profound metabolic changes (including hypo-albuminaemia and extrarenal water loss), and these patients require constant supervision and monitoring until they have recovered from the acute phase of their illness.

The most common cause is eczema, which is usually of the atopic variety. These patients often have an intense pruritus. Some of them will develop a chronic unremitting erythroderma.

Pustular and crusted lesions

The clinical appearance of a *pustular* lesion results from accumulation of neutrophils. Such collections usually indicate an infectious process; however, sterile pustules may form as part of a number of skin diseases due to the release of chemotactic factors following an immunological reaction.

A *crust* is a yellowish crystalline material that is found on the skin; it is made up of desiccated serum.

It is essential to determine whether or not a pustular lesion (or a group of pustular lesions) represents a primarily infectious process or an inflammatory dermatological condition.

For example, pustular lesions on the hands and feet may either be due to tinea infection or be a primary pustular psoriasis or palmoplantar pustulosis (Table 12.9).

Dermal plaques

Plaques are localised thickenings of the skin which are usually caused by changes in the dermis or subcutaneous fat. These may be due to chronic inflammatory processes or scarring sclerotic processes (Table 12.10).

The pattern of involvement of the plaques, the age of the patient and other clinical features should enable a diagnosis to be established.

Table 12.8 Causes of erythroderma
1 Eczema
2 Psoriasis
3 Drugs, e.g. phenytoin, allopurinol
4 Pityriasis rubra pilaris
5 *Mycosis fungoides*, leukaemia, lymphoma
6 Lichen planus
7 Pemphigus foliaceus
8 Hereditary disorders
9 Dermatophytosis

Table 12.9 Causes of pustular and crusted lesions
1 Acne vulgaris
2 Impetigo
3 Folliculitis
4 Acne rosacea
5 Viral lesions
6 Pustular psoriasis
7 Drug eruptions
8 Dermatophyte infections

Table 12.10 Causes of dermal plaques

1 Granuloma annulare
2 Necrobiosis lipoidica
3 Sarcoidosis
4 Erythema nodosum
5 Lupus erythematosus
6 Morphoea and scleroderma
7 Tuberculosis
8 Leprosy

Table 12.11 Causes of erythema nodosum

1 Streptococcal infections (β-haemolytic)
2 Drugs, e.g. sulphonamides, penicillin, sulphonylurea, oestrogen, iodides, bromides
3 Inflammatory bowel disease
4 Sarcoidosis
5 Tuberculosis
6 Other infections, e.g. lepromatous leprosy, toxoplasmosis, histoplasmosis, *Yersinia, Chlamydia*
7 Systemic lupus erythematosus
8 Behçet's syndrome

Figure 12.11 Erythema multiforme
Shows classic iris or target lesions, secondary to herpes simplex virus infection of the lips.

Erythema nodosum

This is the best known of the group of diseases classified as nodular vasculitis. The lesions of erythema nodosum are usually found below the knee in the pretibial area and are erythematous, palpable and tender (Figure 5.33). There may be an associated fever (Table 12.11).

Erythema multiforme

This is a distinctive inflammatory reaction of skin and mucosa. It is not a systemic disease. Characteristic discrete target lesions occur, particularly on the distal extremities (Figure 12.11). The periphery of these lesions is red, whereas the centre becomes bluish or even purpuric. The lesions can become bullous, and severe cases of this syndrome involve widespread desquamation of the mucosal surfaces (the Stevens-Johnson[b] syndrome). In many cases the condition is precipitated by clinical or subclinical herpes simplex virus infection. Other causes include *Mycoplasma*

pneumoniae, histoplasmosis, malignancy, sarcoidosis and drugs (including those that can cause toxic epidermal necrolysis). Sometimes no underlying cause of the erythema multiforme will be established.

Erythema multiforme is not the same as toxic epidermal necrolysis, which is a systemic condition and usually secondary to a drug reaction. The major causes include penicillin, sulphonamides, phenytoin and non-steroidal anti-inflammatory drugs.

Hyperpigmentation

The presence of hyperpigmentation can be a clue to underlying systemic disease (Table 12.12).

Flushing and sweating

Flushing of the skin may sometimes be observed, especially on the face, by the examiner. Some of the causes of this phenomenon are presented in Table 12.13.

Excessive sweating (hyperhidrosis) can occur with thyrotoxicosis, phaeochromocytoma, acromegaly, hypoglycaemia, autonomic dysfunction, stress, fever and menopause.

Skin tumours

Skin tumours are very common and are usually benign (Table 12.14).[4] Most malignant skin tumours can be cured if they are detected early and treated appropriately (Table 12.15).

---

[b] Albert Mason Stevens (1884–1945), New York paediatrician, and Frank C Johnson (1894–1934), American physician.

Table 12.12 Causes of diffuse hyperpigmentation

Endocrine disease

Addison's disease (excess ACTH)
Ectopic ACTH secretion (e.g. carcinoma)
The contraceptive pill or pregnancy
Thyrotoxicosis, acromegaly,
    phaeochromocytoma

Metabolic

Malabsorption or malnutrition
Liver diseases, e.g. haemochromatosis, primary
    biliary cirrhosis, Wilson's disease
Chronic renal failure
Porphyria
Chronic infection, e.g. bacterial endocarditis
Connective tissue disease, e.g. systemic lupus,
    scleroderma, dermatomyositis

Racial or genetic

Other

Drugs, e.g. chlorpromazine, busulphan,
    arsenicals
Radiation

Table 12.13 Causes of facial flushing

1 Menopause
2 Drugs and foods, e.g. nifedipine, monosodium glutamate (MSG)
3 Alcohol after taking the drug disulfiram (or alcohol alone in some people)
4 Systemic mastocytosis
5 Rosacea
6 Carcinoid syndrome (secretion of serotonin and other mediators by a tumour may produce flushing, diarrhoea and valvular heart disease)
7 Autonomic dysfunction
8 Medullary carcinoma of the thyroid

Table 12.14 Benign skin tumours

1 Warts
2 Molluscum contagiosum
3 Seborrhoeic keratoses
4 Dermatofibroma
5 Neurofibroma
6 Angioma
7 Xanthoma

Table 12.15 Malignant skin tumours

1 Basal cell carcinoma
2 Squamous cell carcinoma
3 Bowen's* disease (squamous cell carcinoma confined to the epithelial layer of the skin— carcinoma *in situ*)
4 Malignant melanoma
5 Secondary deposits

* John Templeton Bowen (1857–1941), Boston dermatologist.

Skin cancer often occurs in those predisposed individuals (with the fair skin of Celtic or Northern European origin) who undergo chronic exposure to ultraviolet light.

Skin cancers may present as flat scaly lesions or as raised scaly or smooth lesions. They may be large or small and they may eventually ulcerate. All non-healing ulcers should be considered to be skin cancer, until proven otherwise.

The earliest lesions are actinic (solar) keratoses, which are pink macules or papules surmounted by adherent scale (Figure 12.12). Basal cell carcinoma is characteristically a translucent papule with a depressed centre and a rolled border with ectatic capillaries (Figure 12.13). Squamous cell carcinoma

Figure 12.12 Actinic keratosis, slightly eroded and scaly

Higher on the forehead additional granular keratosis could be easily palpated.

is typically an opaque papule or plaque which is often eroded or scaly (Figure 12.14).

Malignant melanomas are usually deeply pigmented lesions that are enlarging and have an irregular notched border (Figure 12.15). There is often variation of pigment within the lesion. Malignant melanoma is likely if the lesion is asymmetrical, has an irregular border, has an irregular colour and is large (diameter >6 mm), referred to as the ABCD checklist.[5,6] Patients with numerous large and unusual pigmented naevi (dysplastic naevus syndrome) are at an increased risk of developing malignant melanoma.

Figure 12.13 Pigmented basal cell carcinoma

With pearly quality and depressed centre, in a patient with sun-damaged skin.

Figure 12.14 Squamous cell carcinoma

The nails

Systemic disease is commonly associated with changes in the patient's finger (and toe) nails and in the nail beds. The slow growth of the nails means that the temporal course of an illness may be seen in nail changes. Many of these findings have been described in other chapters but important features of nail changes are dealt with here.

Fungal infection of the nails (onychomycosis) (Figure 12.16) is their most common abnormality. It makes up 40% of all nail disorders and 30% of all cutaneous fungal infections. The characteristic findings are pitting, thickening, ridging and deformity. The changes can be indistinguishable from those of psoriasis. Candidal nail infections are less common than those due to dermatophytes. Candidal nail infection (diagnosed by microscopy and culture) suggests the possibility of chronic mucocutaneous candidiasis, which is a rare condition associated with polyendocrinopathies.

Nail involvement occurs in about 25% of patients with psoriasis (Figure 12.17). The characteristic abnormality is pitting. This can also occur in fungal infections, chronic paronychia, lichen planus and alopecia areata. Psoriasis is also the most common cause of onycholysis (page 22). Rarer changes in psoriatic nails include longitudinal ridging (onychorrhexis), proximal transverse ridging, subungual hyper-keratosis and yellow-brown discoloration.

Nailfold telangiectasia is an important sign in a number of systemic disorders, including systemic lupus erythematosus, scleroderma and Raynaud's phenomenon. These changes are not very specific

Figure 12.15 Superficial spreading melanoma, still confined to the upper dermis

Figure 12.16 Onychomycosis: fungal infection of the nails

Figure 12.17 Nail involvement occurs in about 25% of patients with psoriasis

and considerable variation in nailfold capillary shape is present in normal people. In patients with dermatomyositis, nailfold telangiectasiae are associated with hypertrophy of the cuticle and small haemorrhagic infarcts.

Raynaud's is also associated with nail changes caused by the inadequate blood supply. These include brittleness, longitudinal ridging, splitting, flattening, onycholysis, koilonychia and a redder than normal nail bed.

Clubbing is an important nail abnormality (page 99). It has been described in patients with HIV infection, and its severity seems proportional to the degree of immunosuppression. HIV infection is also associated with onychomycosis and longitudinal melonychia (dark line in the nail), secondary to treatment with zidovudine.

Summary

The dermatological examination in internal medicine: a suggested method (Figure 12.18)

Even if the patient shows the examiner only a small single area of abnormality, proceed to examine all the skin.

After obtaining good lighting conditions and asking the patient to disrobe, begin by looking at the *nails and hands*. Paronychia is an infection of the skin surrounding the nails. Other changes to note include pitting (psoriasis, fungal infections) and onycholysis (e.g. thyrotoxicosis, psoriasis). Dark staining under the nail may indicate a subungual melanoma. Linear splinter haemorrhages (e.g. vasculitis) or telangiectasiae (e.g. systemic lupus erythematosus) may be seen in the nail bed.

A purplish discoloration in streaks over the knuckles may indicate dermatomyositis. Also look at the backs of the hands and forearms for the characteristic blisters of porphyria, which occur on the exposed skin. Papules and scratch marks on the backs of the hands, between the fingers and around the wrists may indicate scabies. Viral warts are common on the hands.

Look at the palms for Dupuytren's contracture, pigmented flat junctional moles (which have a high risk of becoming malignant) and xanthomata in the palmar creases.

Go on to look at the *forearms*, where lichen planus may occur on the flexor surfaces (characterised by small shiny, purple-coloured papules) and psoriasis may be present on the extensor surfaces. Palpable purpura—raised bruising that indicates bleeding into the skin—may be seen on the arms where they have been exposed to trauma. Acanthosis nigricans can occur in the axillae.

Inspect the patient's *hair and scalp*. Decide whether or not the hair is dry and whether the distribution is normal. Alopecia may indicate male pattern baldness, recent severe illness, hypothyroidism or thyrotoxicosis. Patches of alopecia occur in the disease alopecia areata. Short broken-off hairs occur typically in systemic lupus erythematosus. In psoriasis there are silvery scales, which may be seen on the skin of the scalp. Metastatic deposits may rarely be felt as firm nodules within the skin of the scalp. Sebaceous cysts are

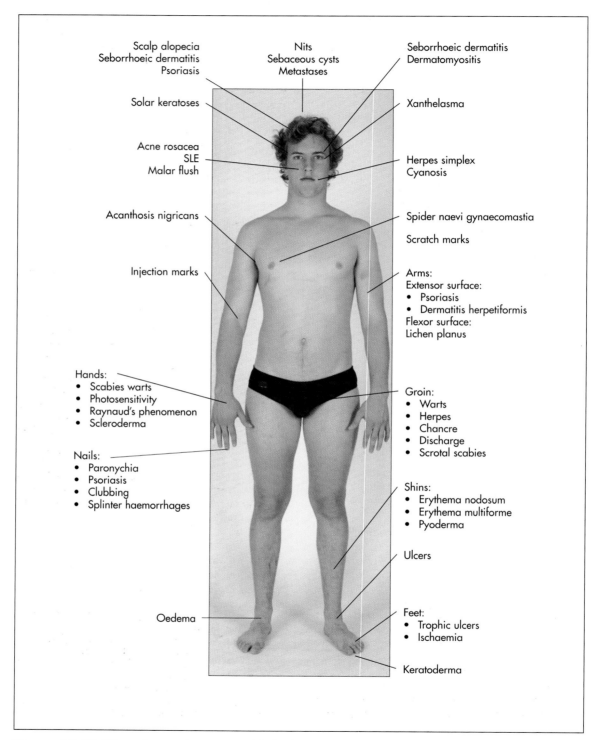

Figure 12.18 Sites of some important skin lesions of the limbs, face and trunk

SLE = systemic lupus erythematosus.

common. The unfortunate examiner may find nits sticking to the head hairs.

Move down now to the *eyebrows* and look for scaling and greasiness, which are found in seborrhoeic dermatitis. A purplish erythema occurs around the eyelids in dermatomyositis. Xanthelasmata are seen near the eyelid.

Look at the *face* for rosacea, which causes bright erythema of the nose, cheeks, forehead and chin, and occasionally pustules and rhinophyma (disfiguring swelling of the nose). Acne causes papules, pustules and scars involving the face, neck and upper trunk. The butterfly rash of systemic lupus erythematosus occurs across the cheeks but is rare. Spider naevi may be present. Ulcerating lesions on the face may include basal cell carcinoma, squamous cell carcinoma or rarely tuberculosis (lupus vulgaris).

Benign tumours of the face include keratoacanthoma (a volcano-like lesion from a sebaceous gland) and congenital haemangiomas.

Look for the blisters of herpes zoster, which may occur strictly in the distribution of one of the divisions of the trigeminal nerve.

Inspect the *neck*, which is prone to many of the lesions that occur on the face. Rarely, the redundant loose skin of pseudoxanthoma elasticum will be seen around the neck.

Go on to inspect the *trunk*, where any of the childhood exanthems produce their characteristic rashes.

Look for spider naevi. Campbell de Morgan spots are commonly found on the abdomen (and chest), as are flat, greasy, yellow-coloured seborrhoeic warts. Erythema marginatum (rheumatic fever) occurs on the chest and abdomen. Herpes zoster may be seen overlying any of the dermatome distributions. Metastases from internal malignancies may rarely occur anywhere on the skin. Neurofibromas are soft flesh-coloured tumours; when associated with more than five 'café-au-lait' spots (brownish, irregular lesions), they suggest neurofibromatosis (von Recklinghausen's disease). Pigmented moles are seen on the trunk and evidence of malignancy must be looked for with these. The patient's buttocks and sacrum must be examined for bedsores, and the abdomen and thighs may have areas of fat atrophy or hypertrophy from insulin injections.

Go to the *legs*, where erythema nodosum or erythema multiforme may be seen on the shins.

Necrobiosis lipoidica diabeticorum affects the skin over the tibia in diabetics. Pretibial myxoedema also occurs over the shins. Look for ulcers on either side of the lower part of the leg.

Inspect the *feet* for the characteristic lesion of Reiter's disease called keratoderma blennorrhagica, where crusted lesions spread across the sole because of the fusion of vesicles and pustules. Look at the foot for signs of ischaemia, associated with wasting of the skin and skin appendages. Trophic ulcers may be seen in patients with peripheral neuropathy (e.g. diabetes mellitus).

References

1. Marks R. A diagnostic approach to common dermatology problems. *Aust Fam Phys* 1982; 11:696–702.
2. Ashton RE. Teaching non-dermatologists to examine the skin: a review of the literature and some recommendations. *Brit J Derm* 1995; 132:221–225.
3. Schwarzenberger K. The essentials of the complete skin examination. *Med Clin Nth Am* 1998; 82:981–999.
4. Preston DS, Stern RS. Nonmelanoma cancers of the skin. *N Engl J Med* 1992; 327:649–662. Provides useful information on discriminating between worrying and non-worrying lesions, and includes colour photographs.
5. Whitehead JD, Gichnik JM. Does this patient have a mole or a melanoma? *JAMA* 1998; 279:696–701. The ABCD checklist (asymmetry, border irregularity, irregular colour, diameter >6 mm) has a sensitivity over 90% and a specificity over 95% for identifying malignant melanoma.
6. Abbasi NR, Shaw HM, Rigel DS et al. Early diagnosis of cutaneous melanoma: rewriting the ABC criteria. *JAMA* 2004;292:2771–2776. Changes (evolving) of symptoms or signs (size, shape; pruritus, tenderness, bleeding or colour) are additional evidence for the presence of melanoma.

Suggested reading

Textbooks

Buxton PK. *ABC of dermatology*, 4th edn. London: BMJ Publishing Group, 2003.
Callen JP, Paller AS, Greer K. eds. *Color atlas of dermatology*, 2nd edn. Philadelphia: WB Saunders, 2000.
Fitzpatrick TB, Johnson RA, Polano MK, Suurmond D, Wolff K. *Color atlas and synopsis of clinical dermatology*, 4th edn. New York: McGraw-Hill, 2001.
Gawkrodger DJ. *Dermatology. An illustrated color text*, 3rd edn. New York: Churchill Livingstone, 2002.

chapter 13

A system for the infectious diseases examination

As it takes two to make a quarrel, so it takes two to make a disease, the microbe and its host.

Charles Chaplain (1856–1941)

We have selected two important diseases to be covered in this chapter to show how infectious diseases can be approached in a systematic manner.

Pyrexia of unknown origin (PUO)

This condition is defined as documented fever (>38°C) of more than 3 weeks' duration, where no cause is found despite basic investigations.[1,2] The most frequent causes to consider are tuberculosis, occult abscess (usually intra-abdominal), osteomyelitis, infective endocarditis, lymphoma or leukaemia, systemic onset juvenile rheumatoid arthritis, giant cell arteritis and drug fever. In studies of fever of unknown origin, infection is found to be the cause in 30%, neoplasia in 30%, connective tissue disease in 15% and miscellaneous causes in 15%; in 10% the aetiology remains unknown (Table 13.1). Remember, the longer the duration of the fever, the less likely there is an infectious aetiology. The majority of patients do not have a rare disease but rather a relatively common disease presenting in an unusual way.[3]

History

The history may give a number of clues in these puzzling cases. In some patients a careful history may give the diagnosis where expensive tests have failed.

The time course of the fever and any associated symptoms must be uncovered. Symptoms from the various body systems should be sought methodically. Examples include:

1 The gastrointestinal system—diarrhoea, abdominal pain, recent abdominal surgery (inflammatory bowel disease, diverticular disease, cholangitis).
2 The cardiovascular system—heart murmurs, dental procedures (infective endocarditis), chest pain (pericarditis).
3 Rheumatology—joint symptoms, rashes.
4 Neurology—headache (meningitis, cerebral abscess).
5 Genitourinary system—history of renal disease or infection, dysuria.
6 Respiratory system—old tuberculosis (TB) or recent TB contact, chest symptoms.

Details of any recent overseas travel are important. Find out also about hobbies and exposure to

Table 13.1 Common causes of pyrexia of unknown origin

1 Neoplasms
- Hodgkin's and non-Hodgkin's lymphoma, leukaemia, malignant histiocytosis
- Other tumours: hepatic, renal, lung, disseminated carcinoma, atrial myxoma

2 Infections
- Bacterial: e.g. tuberculosis, brucellosis and other bacteraemias, abscess formation (especially pelvic or abdominal), endocarditis, pericarditis, osteomyelitis, cholangitis, pyelonephritis, pelvic inflammatory disease, prostatitis, syphilis, Lyme disease, borreliasis, cat scratch disease, dental abscess
- Viral: e.g. infectious mononucleosis, cytomegalovirus infection, hepatitis B or C, human immunodeficiency virus (HIV) infection, Ross River virus
- Parasitic, rickettsial and others: e.g. malaria, Q fever, toxoplasmosis
- Fungal: e.g. histoplasmosis, cryptococcosis, blastomycosis

3 Connective tissue diseases
- Juvenile rheumatoid arthritis, systemic lupus erythematosus
- Vasculitis, e.g. giant cell arteritis, polyarteritis nodosa

4 Drug fever

5 Miscellaneous
Inflammatory bowel disease, alcoholic liver disease, granulomatous disease (e.g. sarcoid), multiple pulmonary emboli, thyroiditis, adrenal insufficiency, phaeochromocytoma, familial Mediterranean fever and other hereditary periodic fever syndromes, factitious fever

6 Uncertain

Table 13.2 Some causes of prolonged fever and rash

1 Viral: e.g. infectious mononucleosis, rubella, dengue fever
2 Bacterial: e.g. syphilis, Lyme disease
3 Non-infective: e.g. drugs, systemic lupus erythematosus, erythema multiforme (which may also be related to an underlying infection)

pets. Occupational exposure may be important. Take a drug history. Find out if the patient is involved in behaviour posing a risk of HIV infection. Patients who are already in hospital may have infected cannulas or old cannula sites.

Examination

General

Look at the temperature chart to see whether there is a pattern of fever that is identifiable (page 23). Inspect the patient and decide how seriously ill he or she appears. Look for evidence of weight loss (indicating a chronic illness). Note any skin rash (Table 13.2).

Hands

Look for the stigmata of infective endocarditis or vasculitic changes. Note whether there is clubbing. The presence of arthropathy or Raynaud's phenomenon may point to a connective tissue disease.

Arms

Inspect for drug injection sites suggesting intravenous drug abuse (see Figure 3.35). Feel for the epitrochlear and axillary nodes (e.g. lymphoma, other malignancy, sarcoidosis, focal infections).

Head and neck

Feel the *temporal arteries* (over the temples). In temporal arteritis these may be tender and thickened.

Examine the *eyes* for iritis or conjunctivitis (connective tissue disease—e.g. Reiter's syndrome) or jaundice (e.g. ascending cholangitis, blackwater fever in malaria). Look in the fundi for choroidal tubercles in miliary tuberculosis, Roth's spots in infective endocarditis, and retinal haemorrhages or the infiltrates of leukaemia or lymphoma.

Inspect the *face* for a butterfly rash (systemic lupus erythematosus, see Figure 8.41) or seborrhoeic dermatitis, which is common in patients with HIV infection.

Examine the *mouth* for ulcers, gum disease or candidiasis, and the teeth and tonsils for infection (e.g. abscess). Look in the *ears* for otitis media. Feel the *parotid glands* for evidence of infection.

Palpate the cervical lymph nodes. Examine for thyroid enlargement and tenderness (subacute thyroiditis).

Chest

Examine the chest. Palpate for bony tenderness. Carefully examine the respiratory system (e.g. for signs of pneumonia, tuberculosis, empyema, carcinoma) and the heart for murmurs (e.g. infective endocarditis, atrial myxoma) or rubs (e.g. pericarditis).

The abdomen

Examine the abdomen. Inspect for rashes, including rose-coloured spots (in typhoid fever—2 to 4 mm flat red spots, which blanch on pressure and occur on the upper abdomen and lower chest). Examine for evidence of hepatomegaly and ascites (e.g. spontaneous bacterial peritonitis, hepatic carcinoma, metastatic deposits), splenomegaly (e.g. haemopoietic malignancy, infective endocarditis, malaria), renal enlargement (e.g. renal cell carcinoma) or localised tenderness (e.g. collection of pus). Palpate for testicular enlargement (e.g. seminoma, tuberculosis). Feel for inguinal lymphadenopathy.

Perform a rectal examination, feeling for a mass or tenderness in the rectum or pelvis (e.g. abscess, carcinoma, prostatitis). Sigmoidoscopy should also be performed for evidence of inflammatory bowel disease or carcinoma. Perform a vaginal examination to detect collections of pelvic pus or evidence of pelvic inflammatory disease. Look at the penis and scrotum for a discharge or rash.

Central nervous system

Examine the central nervous system for signs of meningism (e.g. chronic tuberculous meningitis, cryptococcal meningitis) or focal neurological signs (e.g. brain abscess, mononeuritis multiplex in polyarteritis nodosa).

HIV infection and the acquired immunodeficiency syndrome (AIDS)

This syndrome, first described in 1981, is caused by the human immunodeficiency virus (HIV).[4,5] This is a T-cell lymphotrophic virus, which results in T4 cell destruction and therefore susceptibility to opportunistic infections and the development of tumours, notably Kaposi's sarcoma[a] and non-Hodgkin's lymphoma. The current US Centers for Disease Control criteria for the diagnosis of AIDS are presented in Table 13.3.

[a] Moritz Kohn Kaposi (1837–1902), Professor of Dermatology, Vienna, described the sarcoma in 1892.

HIV infection should be suspected particularly if the patient falls into a high-risk group (e.g. male homosexual, intravenous drug abuser, haemophiliac, blood transfusion or blood product recipient, prostitute, or sexual contact with one of these). Examine the patient as follows.

Examination

General inspection

Take the temperature. The patient may appear ill and wasted due to chronic ill-health or chronic opportunistic infection.

Look at the skin for rashes:

- The maculopapular rash of acute infection (5 to 10 mm maculopapular lesions on the face and trunk and rarely on the palms and soles).
- Herpes zoster (shingles, which may involve more than one dermatome in this disease and is more commonly seen in early rather than in advanced HIV infection).
- Oral herpes simplex (cold sores) or genital herpes (20%).
- Oral and flexural candidiasis (once the CD4 level is below 200/mm^3).
- Molluscum contagiosum (10%), impetigo, seborrhoea (occurs in up to 80% of patients at some time) or other non-specific exanthems.
- Kaposi's sarcoma: red-purple vascular nontender tumours. These present typically on the skin but can occur anywhere.
- Skin lesions resembling Kaposi's sarcoma may also be seen. These are called bacillary angiomatosis and are caused by *Bartonella henselae* and *Bartonella quintana* (Figures 13.1 and 13.2).

Figure 13.1 Angry red nodule of bacillary angiomatosis

Table 13.3 US Centers for Disease Control case definition for surveillance of AIDS in adults and adolescents, 2004

Definitive AIDS diagnoses (with or without laboratory evidence of HIV infection)

1 Candidiasis of the oesophagus, trachea bronchi or lungs
2 Cryptococcosis, extrapulmonary
3 Cryptosporidiosis with diarrhoea persisting >1 month
4 Cytomegalovirus disease of an organ other than liver, spleen or lymph nodes
5 Herpes simplex virus infection causing a mucocutaneous ulcer that persists longer than a month; or bronchitis, pneumonitis or oesophagitis of any duration
6 Kaposi's sarcoma in a patient <60 years
7 Lymphoma of the brain (primary) in a patient <60 years
8 *Mycobacterium avium* complex or *Mycobacterium kansasii* disease, disseminated (at a site other than or in addition to the lungs, skin, or cervical or hilar lymph nodes)
9 *Pneumocystis jiroveci* pneumonia
10 Progressive multifocal leukoencephalopathy
11 Toxoplasmosis of the brain

Definitive AIDS diagnoses (with laboratory evidence of HIV infection)

1 Coccidioidomycosis, disseminated (at a site other than or in addition to lungs or cervical or hilar lymph nodes)
2 HIV encephalopathy
3 Histoplasmosis, disseminated (at a site other than, or in addition to, lungs, or cervical or hilar lymph nodes)
4 Isosporiasis with diarrhoea persisting >1 month
5 Kaposi's sarcoma at any age
6 Lymphoma of the brain (primary) at any age
7 Other non-Hodgkin's lymphoma of B cell or unknown immunological phenotype
8 Any mycobacterial disease caused by mycobacteria other than *Mycobacterium tuberculosis*, disseminated (at any site other than or in addition to lungs, skin, or cervical or hilar lymph nodes)
9 Disease caused by extrapulmonary *M. tuberculosis*
10 Salmonella (non-typhoid) septicaemia, recurrent
11 HIV wasting syndrome
12 CD4 lymphocyte count below 200 cells/μL or a CD4 lymphocyte percentage below 14%
13 Pulmonary TB
14 Recurrent pneumonia
15 Invasive cervical cancer

Presumptive AIDS diagnoses (with laboratory evidence of HIV infection)

1 Candidiasis of the oesophagus: (a) recent onset of retrosternal pain on swallowing; and (b) oral candidiasis
2 Cytomegalovirus retinitis: a characteristic appearance on ophthalmoscopic examinations
3 Mycobacteriosis: specimen from stool or normally sterile body fluids or tissue from a site other than lungs, skin, or cervical or hilar lymph nodes, showing acid-fast bacilli of a species not identified by culture
4 Kaposi's sarcoma: erythematous or violaceous plaque-like lesion on skin or mucous membrane
5 *Pneumocystis jiroveci* pneumonia: (a) a history of dyspnoea on exertion or non-productive cough of recent onset (within the past 3 months); (b) chest X-ray evidence of diffuse bilateral infiltrates or gallium scan evidence of diffuse bilateral pulmonary disease; (c) arterial blood gas analysis showing an arterial oxygen partial pressure of <70 mm/Hg, or low respiratory diffusing capacity of <80% of predicted values, or an increase in the alveolar-arterial oxygen tension gradient; and (d) no evidence of bacterial pneumonia
6 Toxoplasmosis of the brain: (a) recent onset of a focal neurological abnormality consistent with intracranial disease or a reduced level of consciousness; (b) brain imaging evidence of a lesion having a mass effect or the radiographic appearance of which is enhanced by injection of contrast medium; and (c) serum antibody to toxoplasmosis or successful response to therapy for toxoplasmosis
7 Recurrent pneumonia: (a) more than one episode in a 1-year period; and (b) acute pneumonia (new symptoms, signs or radiological evidence not present earlier) diagnoses on clinical or radiological grounds by the patient's physician
8 Pulmonary TB: (a) apical or miliary infiltrates and (b) radiographic and clinical response to anti-tuberculous therapy

Figure 13.2 Late nodules of Kaposi's sarcoma

Adverse drug reactions are more common in patients with HIV infection and may be the cause of a rash. Look for hyperpigmentation. Patients taking the drug clofamizine for *Mycobacterium avium* complex infection usually become deeply pigmented. Areas of peripheral fat atrophy (limbs, cheeks and buttocks) may be seen in 20% to 30% of patients treated with the protease inhibitor drugs. Some of these patients have fat redistribution with central obesity.

Hands and arms

Look for nail changes including onycholysis. Feel for the epitrochlear nodes; a node 0.5 cm or larger may be characteristic.[6] Note any injection marks.

Face

Inspect the mouth for:

- candidal plaques (Figure 13.3),
- angular stomatitis,
- aphthous ulcers,
- tongue ulceration (e.g. herpes simplex, cytomegalovirus or candidal infections) or gingivitis.[7]

Periodontal disease is very common. Kaposi's sarcoma (Figure 13.4) may also occur on the hard or soft palate (in which case associated lesions are almost always present elsewhere in the gastrointestinal tract). Oral squamous cell carcinoma and non-Hodgkin's lymphoma are more common in AIDS.

Parotidomegaly is sometimes seen as a result of HIV-associated Sjögren's syndrome. These patients may have dry eyes and mouth for this reason.

Hairy leucoplakia is a unique raised or flat, white, painless, and often hairy-looking lesion typically present on the lateral surface of the tongue; it is associated with Epstein-Barr virus infection in HIV-infected persons and is almost diagnostic of HIV infection.

Palpate over the sinuses for tenderness (sinusitis). Examine the cervical and axillary nodes. There may be generalised lymphadenopathy, and all lymph node groups should be examined.

Chest

Note any tachypnoea or dry cough. Chronic cough, either dry or productive of purulent sputum, is common. On auscultation crackles may be present at the bases due to bronchiolitis obliterans. There are

Figure 13.3 Kaposi's sarcoma

(From FS McDonald, ed., *Mayo Clinic images in internal medicine*, with permission. © Mayo Clinic Scientific Press and CRC Press.)

Figure 13.4 Oral candidiasis

(From FS McDonald, ed., *Mayo Clinic images in internal medicine*, with permission. © Mayo Clinic Scientific Press and CRC Press.)

often, however, no chest signs despite the presence of pulmonary infiltrates on chest X-ray due to *Pneumocystis carinii* or other opportunistic infections.

Abdomen

Examine for hepatosplenomegaly (e.g. infection, lymphoma). Perform a rectal examination (e.g. perianal ulceration from herpes simplex) and a sigmoidoscopy looking for Kaposi's sarcoma or proctitis (e.g. cytomegalovirus, herpes simplex, amoebic dysentery or pseudomembranous colitis (from antibiotic use). Examine the genitals for herpes simplex, warts, discharge or chancre.

Nervous system

Look for signs of meningism (e.g. cryptococcal meningitis). There may be focal signs due to a space-occupying intracranial lesion (e.g. toxoplasmosis, non-Hodgkin's lymphoma).

A syndrome similar to Guillain-Barré and a pure sensory neuropathy can occur. HIV infection itself, opportunistic infection or the drugs used in treatment can be responsible for peripheral sensorimotor neuropathy, polymyositis, radiculopathy, mononeuritis multiplex or a myelopathy.

Look in the fundi for cottonwool spots (common in AIDS patients), scars (e.g. toxoplasmosis—Figure 13.5) or retinitis (e.g. cytomegalovirus-induced retinitis with perivascular haemorrhages and fluffy exudates, which can cause blindness of rapid onset—Figure 13.6).[8] There may be signs of dementia (AIDS encephalopathy).

Figure 13.5 Retinal toxoplasmosis—old chorioretinal scar

Figure 13.6 Cytomegalovirus retinitis

References

1. Knockaert DC, Vanneste LJ, Vanneste SB, Bobbaers HJ. Fever of unknown origin in the 1980s. An update of the diagnostic spectrum. *Arch Intern Med* 1992; 152: 51–55.
2. Whitby M. The febrile patient. *Aust Fam Phys* 1993; 22:1753–1755, 1758–1761.
3. Mourad O, Palda V, Detsky AS. A comprehensive evidence based approach to fever of unknown origin. *Arch Intern Med* 2003; 163:545.
4. American College of Physicians and Infectious Diseases Society of America. Human immunodeficiency virus (HIV) infection. *Ann Intern Med* 1994; 120:310–319.
5. Nandwani R. Human immunodeficiency virus medicine for the MRCP short cases. *Br J Hosp Med* 1994; 51:353–356.
6. Malin A, Ternouth I, Sarbah S. Epitrochlear nodes as marker of HIV disease in sub-Saharan Africa. *BMJ* 1994; 309:1550–1551.
7. Weinert ML, Grimes RM, Lynch DP. Oral manifestations of HIV infection. *Ann Intern Med* 1996; 125:485–496. Details the 16 leading oral complications, based on an extensive literature review.
8. De Smet MD, Nessenbatt RB. Ocular manifestations of AIDS. *JAMA* 1991; 266:3019–3022. Provides a very good review of eye changes.

Suggested reading

Textbooks

Adler MW, ed. *ABC of AIDS*, 5th edn. London: BMJ Publishing Group, 2001.
Edmond RTD, Rowlard HAK. *A color atlas of infectious diseases*, 3rd edn. New York: Harcourt Brace, 1995.

Writing and presenting the history and physical examination

Experience is never limited, and it is never complete.

Henry James

It is important that the medical record be kept short and simple. The following approach is one recommended by the authors.

History

Personal information

Record the name, sex, date of birth and address. Write down the date and time of the examination.

Presenting (principal) symptoms (PS)

A short sentence identifies the *major* symptoms and their duration; it is often useful to quote the patient's own words.

History of present illness (HPI)

Don't record every detail; rather, prepare short prose paragraphs telling the story of the illness in chronological order. Describe the characteristics of each symptom. Note why the patient presents at this time. Also, describe any past medical problems which are related to the current symptoms. Include the relevant positive and negative findings on the system review here. If there are many seemingly unrelated problems, summarise these in an introductory paragraph and present the history of each problem in separate paragraphs.

List **current medications** and doses and the indications for their use, if they are known, and any side-effects or known or measured therapeutic effects. For example, if the patient takes anti-hypertensive drugs ask whether blood pressure control has been satisfactory as far as the patient knows. Finally, record your impression of the reliability of the historian and, if the patient was unable to give the history, describe who was the source.

Past history (PH)

List in chronological order past medical or surgical problems (sometimes called *inactive* problems), past medication use, if relevant, and any history of allergy (particularly drug allergy) or of drug intolerance. Find out what the problem with the drug was. The patient may know the results of certain previous important investigations (e.g. the scan showed I had clots in my lung). A history of blood transfusions should be noted.

Social history (SH)

This may include recording the patient's occupation, schooling, hobbies, marital status, family structure, personal support system, living conditions and recent travel. The number and sex of sexual partners may be relevant. Analgesic use, smoking, alcohol and other recreational drug use should also be described. Ask about ability to perform the activities of daily living (ADL). If a patient has a chronic illness, ask about the affect of this on his or her life.

Family history (FH)

Describe causes of mortality in the first-degree relatives and, if indicated, draw a family tree.

Systems review (SR)

All directly relevant information should be incorporated in the HPI or PH.

Physical examination (PE)

Under each of the major systems, list the relevant positives and negatives using brief statements. See Appendix II.

Provisional diagnosis

Ask yourself these questions when considering the diagnosis of a patient's major complaint.

1 What is the likely diagnosis based on the patient's age, sex and background?
2 Are there other conditions that resemble the likely diagnosis but can present in the same way?
3 Is there a serious disorder, even if rare, that must not be missed?
4 Could the patient have a specific condition that often masquerades (or mimics) other conditions (e.g. depression, drugs, diabetes mellitus, thyroid dysfunction, anaemia, malignancy, spinal cord disease, urinary infection, renal failure,

alcoholism, syphilis, tuberculosis, HIV, infective endocarditis or connective tissue disease)?
5 Is the patient trying to really tell me that there is an emotional or psychological problem?

Problem list and plans

Using a sentence or two, summarise the most important findings and then give a provisional diagnosis (PD) and differential diagnosis (DD).

Remember Occam's razor: choose the simplest hypothesis to explain observations. Also remember Sutton's law: the famous bank robber said he robbed banks because 'that's where the money is'—that is, consider a common diagnosis before resorting to a rare one to explain the symptoms and signs.

It is often useful to ask yourself if the patient's problem is a diagnostic or treatment one (or both). For example, a patient with the new onset of dyspnoea presents a diagnostic problem (What is the cause of the breathlessness?) and a treatment problem (How should the condition be treated?). The patient who presents with a worsening of previously diagnosed angina presents a treatment problem—How should the symptoms be treated?

List all the active problems that require management. Outline the diagnostic tests and therapy planned for each problem.

Sign your name and then write your name and position clearly underneath your signature.

Continuation notes

Date (and time) each progress note in the record. The SOAP format can be useful (subjective, objective, assessment and plans).

Subjective data refer to what the patient tells you: list relevant current problems and note any new problems. Have the patient's previous symptoms improved on the current treatment?

Objective data are physical or laboratory findings: relevant data for each active problem are summarised.

Assessment refers to the interpretation of any relevant findings for each problem.

Plans describe any interventions that will be started for each problem.

Many patient records are now kept on a computer file. Parts of this can be used to provide referral information for the patient to take to a specialist or if he or she is travelling. It is important that such files be kept up to date and especially that lists of medications that are no longer used are deleted from the current list before it is given to the patient.

Presentation

In their formal examinations and less formally on the wards, students and resident medical officers will often be expected to present the history and physical examination of a patient to a senior colleague. This is excellent training for clinical practice, as the need to discuss patients with colleagues or specialists arises frequently in both hospital and non-hospital practice.

A successful case presentation is both *succinct* and *relevant*. The examiner is most interested in what the patient's problems are now. One should aim to convey basic biographical information and an assessment of the patient's presenting problem in the first few sentences. It is often helpful to present the case as a diagnostic or treatment problem, or both.

The information will have been obtained from the patient by taking the history as set out above. The examination of the patient should be performed, with particular attention to the areas most likely to be abnormal. This information must then be assembled into a form that can be conveyed easily to others. The following is a suggested method.

1 Begin with a sentence that tells your colleague something about the patient and the clinical problem. For example, one might say: 'Mr Jones is a 72-year-old retired cabinet minister who presents with two hours of chest pain that is not typically ischaemic'. This gives an idea about the patient himself and indicates that the problem is likely to be a diagnostic one.
2 One should then go on to explain in what way the pain is atypical of ischaemia and whether it has features suggestive of any other diagnosis.
3 Once the presenting symptom or problem has been described, relevant current and past history should be discussed. In a patient with chest pain this would include any previous cardiac history or investigations, and a summary of the patient's risk factors for ischaemic heart disease.
4 Present a list of the patient's current medications.
5 Important previous health problems should be outlined briefly. This retired cabinet minister might also have a history of intermittent claudication and of chronic obstructive pulmonary disease. These facts will affect possible treatment for ischaemic heart disease (e.g. the use of beta-blockers).
6 Present the physical examination in two parts.
  (a) Abnormal and *important* normal examination findings in the presenting system. In this patient's case, this would mean giving the pulse rate and blood pressure but not details of normal heart sounds. If there has been a history of claudication, as in this case, the examination of the peripheral pulses should be presented, even if it is normal.
  (b) Abnormal findings in the rest of the examination.
7 Offer the most likely diagnosis and the differential diagnosis.
8 Suggest a plan for investigation and treatment.
9 Much more detail will have been obtained in the assessment of the patient than should be presented routinely, but further details may be asked for by your colleague. These may include information about the patient's living conditions and the availability of support from the family. This may determine how soon the patient can be sent home from hospital after treatment.

By the end of your presentation your colleague should know what you think is wrong with the patient and what you intend to do about it.

Suggested reading

Kroenke K. The case presentation: stumbling blocks and stepping stones. *Am J Med* 1985; 79:605–608.

A suggested method for a rapid screening physical examination

To all students of medicine who listen, look, touch and reflect: may they hear, see, feel and comprehend.

John B Barlow (1986)

Begin by positioning the appropriately undressed patient in bed at 45 degrees. Use this opportunity to make a spot diagnosis if this is possible. Look particularly for any of the diagnostic facies or body habituses. Decide also whether the patient looks ill or well. Note if there is any dyspnoea or other distress. Take the blood pressure. Repeat the measurement a few minutes later if the first reading is high.

The hands and arms

Begin by picking up the patient's right hand and examine the nails for clubbing (RESP, CVS, GIT) and for the stigmata of infective endocarditis (CVS) or chronic liver disease (GIT). The nail changes suggesting chronic renal disease or iron deficiency must also be spotted (RENAL, HAEM). Note any evidence of arthropathy (RHEUM). Examine the other hand.

Take the patient's pulse, and note the rate and regularity or irregularity (CVS). While this is being done the arms can be inspected for bruising or scratch marks (GIT, HAEM, RENAL). Determine the state of hydration (GIT, RENAL, CVS). Go on and examine for axillary lymphadenopathy (HAEM).

The face

Look at the eyes for jaundice (GIT, HAEM) or exophthalmos (ENDO). Look at the face for evidence of a vasculitic rash (RHEUM). Inspect the mouth for mucosal ulcers (RHEUM, GIT, HAEM, INF) and the tongue for glossitis (nutritional deficiencies) or cyanosis (RESP, CVS).

Key to Appendix II	
CNS	central (and peripheral) nervous system
CVS	cardiovascular system
ENDO	endocrine system
GIT	gastrointestinal system
HAEM	haematological system
INF	infectious diseases
RENAL	renal system
RESP	respiratory system
RHEUM	rheumatological system

The front of the neck

Feel the carotid pulses and pay careful attention to the state of the jugular venous pressure (CVS). Feel gently for the position of the trachea (RESP). Then palpate the supraclavicular lymph nodes (HAEM, GIT).

The chest

Examine the front of the chest for scars and deformity. Note any spider naevi (GIT) or hair loss (GIT, ENDO). Palpate the chest wall and auscultate the heart (CVS). Then percuss and auscultate the chest (RESP) and examine the breasts.

The back of the chest and neck

Sit the patient up and lean him or her forward. After inspection test chest expansion of the upper and lower lobes of the lungs. Percuss and auscultate the back of the chest (RESP). Feel for cervical lymphadenopathy (RESP, GIT, HAEM). Then examine formally for a goitre from behind (ENDO). Test for sacral oedema (CVS, RENAL).

The abdomen

Lay the patient flat on one pillow. Inspect the abdomen from the side and then palpate for organomegaly and other abdominal masses. Percuss for shifting dullness if this is appropriate, and auscultate over the abdomen. Palpate for inguinal lymphadenopathy and hernias, and in men palpate the testes (GIT, RENAL).

The legs

Look for peripheral oedema (CVS, RENAL) and leg ulcers (HAEM, RHEUM, CVS, CNS). Feel all the peripheral pulses (CVS).

Neurological examination

Find out if the patient is right- or left-handed.

Begin with examination of the higher centres and cranial nerves. Test orientation and note any speech defect. Ask about any noticed problem with the sense of smell (I). Then examine the visual acuity, visual fields, the fundi (II), the pupils and eye

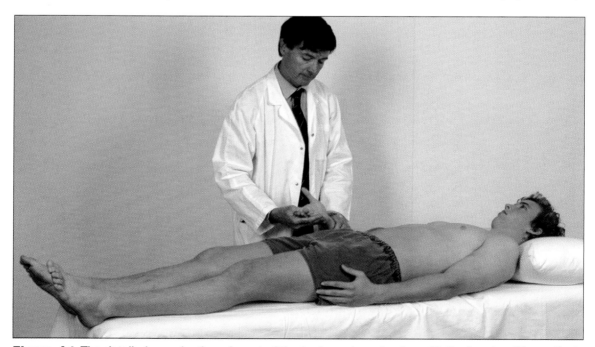

Figure A1 The detailed examination of most of the body systems begins with the hands of the patient.

movements (III, IV, VI). Screen for the other cranial nerves by testing pain sensation over the face (V), the strength of upper and lower facial muscles (VII), whispered voice hearing (VIII), the palatal movement ('Ah') (IX, X), poking out the tongue (XII) and rotation of the head (XI).

Next look for wasting and fasciculation in the upper limbs. Test tone, power (shoulders, elbows, wrists and fingers), and the biceps, triceps and brachioradialis reflexes. Assess finger–nose movements. Then test pinprick sensation on the tip of the shoulder, outer and inner forearms, and on the median, ulnar and radial areas of the hands.

Go to the lower limbs. Test gait fully: ask the patient to walk away several paces, turn around rapidly and walk back. Then test heel–toe walking (cerebellum), ability to stand on the toes (S1) and heels (L4, L5), and squatting (proximal muscles). Finally look for Romberg's sign (posterior columns). Next, test hip and knee flexion and extension, and dorsiflexion and plantar flexion of the feet in bed. Then do knee, ankle and plantar reflexes, and heel–shin tests. Test pinprick sensation on the middle third of the thighs, both sides of the tibia, the dorsum of the feet, the little toes, on the buttocks, and three levels on the trunk on both sides.

Completing the examination

Thorough physical examination requires consideration of a rectal and pelvic examination, analysis of the patient's urine, a temperature reading, measurement of height and weight, and calculation of the BMI.

Specific details of the examination will be altered depending on what is found. An important guide to the areas where examination should be particularly directed, apart from the history, is the general inspection. A minute or two spent standing back to inspect the patient before the detailed examination begins is never wasted.

The pre-anaesthetic medical evaluation (PAME)

An appropriate medical evaluation of the patient who has been admitted for elective surgery is always required. It includes a history and examination that is sufficient to uncover any likely major problems with anaesthesia or the procedure itself.

The history

The first thing to find out, of course, is the presenting problem, what operation is intended, and whether the surgery is expected to be performed under general or local anaesthesia. Clearly the assessment of a patient having a small lesion removed under local anaesthesia can be briefer than the assessment of a patient undergoing extensive bowel resection under general anaesthesia. As a rule, before any patient undergoes surgery under general anaesthesia or spinal anaesthesia, careful attention must be given to identifying whether he or she is at higher risk.

Cardiovascular history

The most important questions here relate to a history of ischaemic heart disease. Patients who have had a myocardial infarct in the preceding six months should not usually undergo elective surgery; the risks of further infarction or malignant arrhythmia and death are high during this period. A patient who has symptoms of angina which have recently become unstable is also at greater risk. A history of stable angina which has not changed for months or years is not a contraindication to most forms of surgery. Symptoms of cardiac failure should be sought. Any

patient with uncontrolled cardiac failure is at considerable risk of severe cardiac failure postoperatively. This is particularly true if large amounts of intravenous fluids are given during and after surgery while the patient's anti-failure drugs (e.g. diuretics) are omitted.

Cardiac drugs should be asked about, particularly anti-anginal and anti-failure drugs. It is important to attempt to ensure that the patient receives these drugs, particularly beta-blockers, on the day of the operation. The surgeon will often require the patient to stop aspirin a week or more before surgery. This is usually a safe thing for the patient to do but may be a problem in the first month at least after a coronary angioplasty because of the risk of thrombosis of the stent in this early period. Previous coronary artery bypass grafting or angioplasty is not a contraindication to surgery.

A history of infective endocarditis or the presence of an abnormal or prosthetic cardiac valve is an indication for antibiotic prophylaxis for any procedure that may result in bacteraemia—the circulation of bacteria in the blood stream. These procedures include most types of dental work, colonoscopy and polypectomy, oesophageal dilatation, and surgery on the bowel or bladder and some gynaecological operations and vaginal delivery. Patients who take the anticoagulant drug warfarin are a special problem. When the drug is being used to protect the patient from embolic events associated with atrial fibrillation it may be reasonable, on the balance of risks, to have the drug stopped 4 days before surgery and resumed as soon as practical afterwards. If the patient takes the drug to protect a mechanical heart valve from clot, the drug should, in general be replaced with intravenous unfractionated or sub-cutaneous fractionated heparin. The last dose of fractionated heparin can be given about 12 hours before surgery and the drug recommenced as soon as the surgeon feels it is safe. Many patients can administer the drug themselves at home. Patients with mechanical valves, especially in the mitral position, are at high risk of embolic events if their warfarin is stopped without replacement with some form of heparin.

The respiratory history

Inquire about a history of respiratory disease, particularly chronic obstructive pulmonary disease or severe asthma. Patients who have continued to smoke up to the time of their surgery have a much higher risk of postoperative chest infections than those who have not. Even stopping a few weeks before will reduce this risk. Severe respiratory disease is a relative contraindication to surgery. It may be difficult to reverse the anaesthetic and muscle relaxant drugs in such a patient, and he or she may require ventilation postoperatively. Doctors in charge of intensive care units are always happier to be warned that a patient may require ventilation postoperatively than to have it come as a surprise. Drug therapy for respiratory disease must be asked about. Steroids may impair wound healing, and steroid doses may need to be increased during the operative period because of steroid-induced adrenal suppression.

Other

Inquire about any history of bleeding diathesis, diabetes mellitus, renal disease, hepatitis, jaundice and drug abuse. The blood sugar control in diabetic patients can be difficult in the perioperative period, especially while normal diet is impossible. The fasting preoperative diabetic on insulin may need to be advised to have half the normal insulin dose on the morning of surgery, possibly with a very early light breakfast. This may be important to avoid ketoacidosis.

Specific inquiries about *previous operations and anaesthetics*, particularly with reference to any complications, should be made. *Allergies* to anaesthetic agents or other drugs must be asked about. Attempt to distinguish a true allergy or anaphylaxis from an adverse effect such as vomiting after a morphine injection. Some operations involve the use of contrast media, and an allergy to iodine may be a contraindication to their use. This risk is now much less with the new non-ionic contrast media. There may occasionally be a *family history of anaesthetic complications* or deaths. This raises the possibility of malignant hyperthermia, which is an inherited disorder leading to fever and muscle destruction after administration of muscle relaxants.

The examination

Examination according to the rapid screening method outlined in Appendix II represents the best approach. Record height, weight and vital signs (pulse rate, blood pressure, respiratory rate). The cardiovascular and respiratory systems must be fully examined. Patients with a short thick neck may be difficult to ventilate and intubate. It is better for the anaesthetist to be aware of this possible problem before the patient is given a muscle relaxation and is unable to breath spontaneously. The presence of loose or fragile teeth must also be noted because of the risk of their dislodgment during attempted intubation.

If a previously undiagnosed symptom or sign of significance is uncovered, some further investigations may be required before surgery, and the operation may have to be deferred. For example, the discovery of a new and significant heart murmur, uncontrolled hypertension, respiratory failure, a bleeding diathesis, uncontrolled diabetes mellitus or renal failure should be brought to the attention of the surgeon and anaesthetist.

Now this is not the end.
It is not even the beginning of the end.
But it is, perhaps, the end of the beginning.

Winston Churchill,
Speech at the Lord Mayor's Day Luncheon,
London, 10 November 1942

Index

A

abdominal
  bloating/swelling 132
  masses 152–4
  pain 127–8
  reflexes 341–2
abdominal examination 56
  for cardiovascular disease
  for respiratory disease 109
  for rheumatological system 242
  for pyrexia of unknown origin 401
  rapid screening 412
abdominal examination for gastrointestinal system 145–7
  acute 164–7
  auscultation 156–8
  gallbladder 149–5
  general abdominal masses 152–4
  kidneys 152
  liver 149
  palpation 148
  percussion 155–6
  spleen 150–2
abdominal examination for genitourinary system 186–7
abdominojugular reflux test 43
abducens nerve 300–5
acanthosis nigricans 137–8
accessory nerve 315–16
Achilles tendon 240, 265
achondroplasia 274
acoustic nerve 312–13
acromegaly 267–8
actinic keratosis 393
activities of daily living (ADL) 8
acute
  aortic dissection 63
  aortic regurgitation 73
  arterial occlusion 57
  cardiac dyspnoea 29
  cardiac tamponade 64
  leukaemia 207–9
  mitral regurgitation 69
  pericarditis 63
  pulmonary oedema 29
  sinusitis 284
acute inflammatory polyradiculoneuropathy see
    Guillain-Barré syndrome
acute renal failure see renal failure
acyanotic congenital heart disease 78–81
Addison's disease 145, 270–1, 280

adrenal examination 269–71
agoraphobia 372
AIDS 96, 401–4
alcohol and hypertension 65
alcohol, history taking 6–7, 24
alcoholic hepatitis 157
alcoholism 98, 129–9, 132–3, 139–40, 144–5, 162
allergic contact dermatitis 390
Alport's syndrome 184
alveolar pulmonary oedema X-ray 86
amyloidosis 114, 142, 144, 170–1, 211, 243, 254
anaemia 5, 19, 34, 98, 116, 132, 140, 168, 197
  and renal failure 185
  causes of 208
  peripheral blood film analysis for 203–5
anal fissure 160
    see also rectal examination
anal reflex 342
aneurysm 153–5, 165
  abdominal aortic 56, 65, 96, 146, 174
  dissecting 29–30
  ventricular 87
angina 27
angioid streaks 267–8, 280
angiotensin-converting enzyme inhibitor 93
ankle examination 239–40, 337
ankle jerk 339, 354–5
ankle swelling 30
ankylosing spondylitis 69, 72–3, 95, 116, 124, 243
anorexia nervosa 257, 374
anxiety 28, 94, 96, 109, 375
  disorders 371–2
aortic coarctation X-ray 87
aortic regurgitation 38, 72–4
aortic stenosis 30, 69–72
aphthous ulceration 144
apical thrills 46
appendicitis 167
appetite and weight change 128, 257
Argyll-Robertson pupils 278, 301
arm examination for gastrointestinal system 140–2
arm examination for genitourinary system 185
arms see joint examination
arterial occlusion 57
arterial pulse character 42
arterial pulse examination 36–8
arterial ulcer 59
artery transposition 81–2
arthritis
  enteropathic 244

arthritis (*continued*)
  gouty 240, 244–5
  monoarthritis 216
  osteoarthritis 222–3
  polyarthritis 216
  psoriatic 244
  rheumatoid 198–9, 217, 240–3
  subcutaneous nodules of 227–8
  see also rheumatological system
ascites 155–6, 174, 186
assessment principles 12–13
associated symptoms 4
asterixis 100, 140
asthma, bronchial 114–15
ataxic paraparesis 359
atrial fibrillation 30
  see also cardiovascular presenting symptoms
atrial septal defect 78–9
  X-ray 87
auscultation, abdomen 156–7, 187
auscultation, chest 105–8
auscultation, thyroid 261
auscultatory percussion 186–7
Austin Flint murmur 72–3
autoagglutination 204
axillary nodes 200, 211–12, 242, 246

B

Babinski response 339
bacillary angiomatosis 401
back examination for cardiovascular system 56
back pain, arthritic 217
bacterial pneumonia 96
balloting 186
band keratopathy 185
Bartholin cyst 193
basal cell carcinoma 394
basilar invagination 293, 316
Battle's sign 364
bedside manner 1
Behçet's syndrome 191
benign paroxysmal positioning vertigo (BPPV) 313
biceps jerk 325–6
biliary pain 128
bilirubin pathway 163–4
bipolar disorder 371
bladder examination
  by palpation 154–5
  by percussion 155
bleeding, gastrointestinal 131, 169
blistering skin eruptions 390–1
blood
  analysis for genitourinary system 190
  analysis for haematological system 203–6
  cells 190–1
  glucose level 189, 365
  in stools 131, 162
  in urine 190–1

blood pressure examination
  for cardiovascular system 38–40
  for hydration 21
  for renal disease 188
  see also systemic hypertension
body habitus 20
bone tenderness 202
  see also joint examination
bowel
  dilation 172
  disease, inflammatory 170–1
  examination by palpation 154
  gas pattern examination 172
  habit change 257
  irritable 163
  obstruction 128, 173
  sounds 157
brachial plexus examination 333–5
brachioradialis jerk 326–7
bradycardia 36–7
bradykinesia 360
breast examination 122–4
breath sounds 105–8
breathing patterns, abnormal 97
breathlessness 94–5
bronchial asthma 114–15
bronchiectasis 114
bronchitis 115–16
Brown-Séquard syndrome 350, 352–3
bruising 185, 198
bruits 157–8
  carotid artery 185–6
  renal 187
bulimia nervosa 374
bursitis 253

C

cachectic appearance 32
calcium arthropathy 245
calcium metabolism 271–3
Campbell de Morgan spots 141, 397
Candida albicans 193
candidiasis 144–5, 404
capsulitis of the shoulder 250
carcinoid syndrome 136, 258
carcinoma 393–4
carcinoma of the lung 117
cardiac cycle 49
cardiac murmurs 51
cardiovascular disease
  acyanotic congenital 78–81
  cardiac failure 60–2
  cardiomyopathy 76–8
  chest pain 62–3
  murmurs and 51–5, 66
  pulmonary hypertension 66
  systemic hypertension 64–6
  see also valve diseases of left heart; valve diseases of
    right heart

cardiovascular presenting symptoms
  ankle swelling 30
  chest pain 27–9
  dyspnoea 29–30
  fatigue 31
  intermittent claudication 31
  palpitations 30
  risk factors 31–2
  syncope, presyncope and dizziness 30–1
cardiovascular system examination 89
  acute arterial occlusion 57
  arterial pulse 36–8
  chest X-rays for 84–7
  deep venous thrombosis 58–9
  general appearance 32–3
  method 88–9
  of abdomen 56
  of back 56
  of blood pressure 38–40
  of face 40–1
  of hands 33–5
  of lower limbs 56–7
  of neck 41–4
  patient positioning for 32
  peripheral vascular disease 57
  varicose veins 60
  see also praecordium examination
cardiovascular system history 32
  for pre-anaesthetic evaluation 415–16
carotid arteries 41–2
carotid artery bruits 185–6
carpal tunnel syndrome 185, 224–5, 241, 254, 285, 331
casts, urinary 191
central sleep apnoea 96
cerebellum disease 357–60
cerebral hemisphere examination 290–3
cervical nodes 201
cervical rib syndrome 334
Charcot's joints 277
chest examination
  for cardiovascular system 84–7
  for gastrointestinal system 145
  for genitourinary system 186
  rapid screening 412
chest examination for respiratory system 101–8
  auscultation 105–8
  palpation 103
  percussion 104–5
  shape and symmetry 101–2
chest pain
  causes of 28
  in cardiovascular examination 27–9, 62–3
  in respiratory examination 96
chest signs in respiratory disorders 112
chest X-rays
  checklist 121
  examples in cardiovascular diseases 84–7
  examples in respiratory diseases 119–21
  frontal film 82
  interpretation 82–4
  lateral film 84

cholecystitis 29
chorea 362
chronic leukaemia 209
chronic obstructive pulmonary disease (COPD) 115
Chvostek's sign 272
claw hand 332
clinical examination see examination
clinical methods, historical perspective xiii
clubbing 33–4, 99–100, 139
coarctation of the aorta 80
collapse, lung 112
coma scale 363–5
common peroneal nerve test 343–4
condylomata acuminata 161
congenital heart disease
  acyanotic 78–80
  adult 81–2
  cyanotic 80–1
Conn's syndrome 65
consolidation 110, 119
constipation 130
coordination test 327–8, 339
COPD see chronic obstructive pulmonary disease
coronary artery disease risk factors 31–2
cortical sensation 291
crackles in breath sounds 107–8
cranial nerve examination 293, 365
  eighth nerve 312–13
  eleventh nerve 315–16
  fifth nerve 305–9
  first nerve 293–4
  ninth and tenth nerves 313–15
  second nerve 294–300
  seventh nerve 309–11
  third, fourth and sixth nerves 300–5
  twelfth nerve 316–17
cremasteric reflexes 342
Crohn's disease 132, 160, 170–1, 244
cross-cultural history taking 12
Cruveilhier-Baumgarten syndrome 157
cubital fossa lesion 331
Cushing's syndrome 64–5, 257–8, 266, 269–70, 280
cutaneous drug reactions 386
cyanosis 19
cyanotic congenital heart disease 80–1
cytomegalovirus retinitis 404

D

deep venous thrombosis 58–9
deformity, joint 219
  see also joint examination
dehydration 21
delirium 373, 382
dementia 373, 382
demyelinating disease 348
depression 371
dermal plaques 391–2
dermatitis 390
dermatitis herpetiformis 136

dermatological disease
blistering eruptions 390–1
crusted lesions 391
dermal plaques 391–2
erythema multiforme 392
erythema nodosum 392
erythroderma 391
erythrosquamous eruptions 388–90
flushing 392
hyperpigmentation 392
pruritus 388
pustular lesions 391
sweating 392
tumours 392–4
dermatological examination 385–6
lumps in 387
method 395–7
dermatological history taking 385
dermatological terms 386
dermatomyositis 355
dermatones 340
dextrocardia in X-rays 82
diabetes and heart disease 31
diabetes mellitus 275–9
diabetic ulcer 59
diarrhoea 129
difficult patients 9, 12
digital infarction 198
dilated cardiomyopathy 77–8
diplomacy in history taking 5
diplopia 302, 320
dissecting aneurysm of the aorta 29
distal interphalangeal joints 222
dizziness 30–1, 285
dorsal column loss 353
Down syndrome 33, 88, 273
drug abuse 64, 75, 192
drug history 4
drugs and lung toxicity 96
Dupuytren's contracture 140
dynamic manoeuvre testing 54–5
dysarthria 290
dyskinesia 362–3
dysphagia 129, 168–9
dysphasia 288–90
dysphonia 290
dyspnoea 29–30, 94–5
dystonia 363
dystrophia myotonica 356

E

Eaton-Lambert syndrome 117
Ebstein's anomaly 80
ecchymoses 198
eczema 389
education of patients 5
Ehlers-Danlos syndrome 29, 63, 169
eighth nerve 312–13, 366
Eisenmenger's syndrome 81

elbow epicondylitis 252–3
elbow joint examination 228, 325
eleventh nerve 315–16, 366–7
embolism 29, 63, 117, 345–6
emphysema 115, 121
endocrine system examination
adrenals 269–71
calcium metabolism 271–3
diabetes mellitus 275–9
gynaecomastia 274–5
hirsutism 274
hyperthyroidism 261–5
method 280–1
Paget's disease 279–80
pituitary 266–9
short stature syndromes 273–4
thyroid 259–61
endocrine system history 259
endocrine system presenting symptoms 257–9
enteropathic arthritis 244
epilepsy 284
epitrochlear nodes 200
erectile dysfunction 258
erythema 171, 219, 392
erythroderma 391
erythrosquamous eruptions 388–90
essential thrombocythaemia 210
ethanol abuse 7
examination principles 15–16
evidence-based 16–17
facial 18–20
first impressions 18
of body habitus/posture/weight 20
of hands and nails 22
of hydration 21–2
of smell 23–4
of temperature 23
preparing patients for 24
vital signs in 18
expansile impulse 155
exposure of X-ray film 82
extramedullary cord lesions 354
extrapyramidal disease 290
extrapyramidal movement disorders 362–3
eye abnormality, cause of 296
eye examination
for endocrine system 263, 276
for gastrointestinal disease 141–2
for neurological disease 318–21, 364
for rheumatological disease 242

F

facial examination 18–20
for cardiovascular system 40–1
for endocrine system 264–8, 272–3, 278–80
for gastrointestinal system 141–5
for genitourinary system 185
for haematological system 200–1
for Parkinson's disease 361

for respiratory system 100
rapid screening 411
see also cranial nerve examination
facial flushing 392–3
facial nerve 309–11
facial pain 284
faeces and jaundice 164–5
Fagan's nomogram 17
fainting 284–5
family history 8–9
    and endocrine system disease 259
    and gastrointestinal disease 133
    and genitourinary disease 184
    and haematological system 198
    and heart disease 31
    and nervous system 287
    and psychiatric illness 376
    and respiratory disease 98
    and rheumatological system 219
fasciculations 322–3, 335
fatigue 31
Felty's syndrome 242
femoral hernia 159–60
femoral nerve test 343
fetor hepaticus 143
fever 23
    pyrexia of unknown origin (PUO) 399–401
fibromyalgia syndrome 251
fifth nerve 305–9, 366
film interpretation, X-ray 82–4
finger examination 325
finger jerks 327
finger–nose test 327, 357
Finkelstein's test 253–4
first impressions in examinations 18
first nerve 293–4, 365
fits 284–5
flapping tremor of the hands 100
flow volume curve 110–11
flushing, skin 392
foot joint examination 239–40
foot-tapping test 339
formulation grid 382
fourth nerve 300–5, 365–6
friction rubs 157
Friedreich's ataxia 359
Froment's sign 332
frontal chest X-ray film 82–4
frontal lobe function 292–3
frozen shoulder 252
fundoscopy 298
fungal infection of nails 394

G

gait 285, 344
galactorrhoea 258
gallbladder examination by palpation 149–51
gastro-oesophageal reflux 29, 128, 139, 169
gastrointestinal disease

bleeding 169
Crohn's disease 170–1
dysphagia 168–9
hepatic encephalopathy 168
inflammatory bowel disease 170–1
liver disease 167
malabsorption 169–70
portal hypertension 167–8
ulcerative colitis 170
gastrointestinal polyposis syndromes 134
gastrointestinal system examination 175
    general appearance 133
    jaundice 133
    method 174–6
    of hernias 158–60
    of mental state 139
    of the arms 140–1
    of the chest 145
    of the face 141–5
    of the gastrointestinal contents 162–3
    of the hands 139–40
    of the neck 145
    of the rectum 160–1
    of the skin 133–9
    patient positioning for 133
    proctosigmoidoscopy 161–2
    urinalysis 163–4
    weight and wasting 133
    X-rays 171–4
    see also abdominal examination for gastrointestinal
        system
gastrointestinal system presenting symptoms 127–33
    abdominal pain 127–8
    appetite and weight change 128
    bleeding 131
    bloating/swelling 132
    constipation 130
    diarrhoea 129
    dysphagia 129
    heartburn/regurgitation 128–9
    jaundice 131
    lethargy 132
    mucus 130
    nausea and vomiting 128
    pain pattern 128
    postprandial fullness 128
    pruritus 132
    satiation 128
gastrointestinal system treatment history 132
genitalia examination, male 191–2
genitourinary system examination
    abdominal 186–7
    blood pressure and 188
    general appearance 184
    method 194–5
    of male genitalia 191–2
    of the arms 185
    of the back 187
    of the chest 186
    of the face 185

genitourinary system examination (*continued*)
 of the fundi 188
 of the hands 184–5
 of the legs 187–8
 of the neck 185–6
 of the pelvis 187, 192–4
 of urine 188–91
genitourinary system history 183–4
genitourinary system presenting symptoms
 change in urine appearance 179
 chronic renal failure 180–3
 urinary incontinence 180
 urinary obstruction 180
 urinary tract infection (UTI) 180
Gerstmann's syndrome 290–1
gingival hyperplasia 185
Glasgow coma scale 363–4
glaucoma 284, 295, 297
glossitis 144
glossopharyngeal nerve 313–15
glossopharyngeal neuralgia 314
glucagonoma 136
glucose analysis 189, 365
glycosuria 190
goitre 261–2
golfer's elbow 252–3
Goodpasture's syndrome 97
gouty arthritis 240, 244–5
grades of evidence 16
Graves' disease 263
groin lumps 158
Guillain-Barré syndrome 283, 315–17, 348–9, 404
gynaecomastia 274–5

H

haematemesis 131
haematological disease
 acute leukaemia 207
 anaemia 207
 chronic leukaemia 209
 essential thrombocythaemia 210
 Hodgkin's disease 211
 lymphoma 210–11
 multiple myeloma 211
 myelofibrosis 205, 210
 myeloproliferative 209
 pancytopenia 207
 polycythaemia 209–10
haematological system examination 212
 abdominal 202
 axillary nodes 200
 bone tenderness 202
 cervical nodes 201
 epitrochlear nodes 200
 general appearance 198
 inguinal nodes 202
 method 211–13
 of the face 200–1
 of the forearms 199–200

 of the fundi 203
 of the hands 198–9
 of the legs 203
 peripheral blood film 203–6
 supraclavicular nodes 201–2
haematological system history 197–8
haematological system infiltration 207
haematological system presenting symptoms 197
haemoptysis 94
haemorrhagic telangiectasia 138–9
haemorrhoids 160
hair distribution changes 257
hair examination 20
Hallpike manoeuvre 313
hand examination 22, 220–8
 for cardiovascular system 33–5
 for endocrine system 262–4, 267, 269, 273
 for gastrointestinal system 139–40
 for genitourinary system 184–5
 for haematological system 198–9
 for respiratory system 99–100
 rapid screening 411
 see also joint examination
handedness and neurological disease 288, 365
headache 283–4
heart disease *see* cardiovascular disease
heart examination for respiratory disease 108–9
 see also praecordium examination
heart murmurs 51–5
 innocent 66
 systolic-click murmur syndrome 69
 ventricular septal defect 78
heart sounds 49–51
heart valve prosthesis 76–7
heartburn/regurgitation 128–9
Heberden's nodes 223
heel–shin test 339, 358
hemiplegia 345–8
Henoch-Schönlein purpura 203
hepatic encephalopathy 168
hepatic flap 140
hepatosplenomegaly 152
hernias 158, 165
 femoral 159–60
 incisional 160
 inguinal 158–9
herpes simplex 390–2
herpes zoster 146–7, 167, 307, 310, 322, 397
high blood pressure 40
hip joint examination 234–6, 335–6
Hippocratic oath xv
Hirschsprung's disease 163
hirsutism 274
history
 cardiovascular system 27–32, 415–16
 dermatological 386
 gastrointestinal system 127–33
 genitourinary system 179–84
 haematological system 197–8
 psychiatric illness 369–77
 respiratory system 93–8

history taking principles 1
  activities of daily living (ADL) and 8
  cross-cultural 12
  difficult/uncooperative patients and 9, 12
  family 8
  for current treatment 4
  for menstrual history 5
  for sexual history 4–5
  for social/personal history 5–8
  for the past 5
  for the presenting illness 3–5
  for writing/presenting 407–9
  initial questions for 2–3
  sequence 2
  skills 12
  systems review in 8–11
HIV infection 401–4
Hodgkin's disease 201, 210–11
hormone-secreting tumours 134
Horner's syndrome 100, 320–1, 348
hydration 21–2
hydropneumothorax X-ray 120
hypercalcaemia 272
hypercholesterolaemia 31
hyperparathyroidism 271–2
hyperpigmentation 392–3
hypertension 31
  portal 168
  systemic 64–6
hypertensive retinopathy 65
hyperthyroidism 261–5
hypertrophic cardiomyopathy 30, 76
hypertrophic pulmonary osteoarthropathy 99–100
hyperventilation 96, 184
hypocalcaemia 272
hypoglossal nerve 316–17
hypoglycaemia 257, 284–5
hypoparathyroidism 272
hypopituitarism 266

I

ileus 172
immunisation 8
incisional hernias 160
infectious disease examination
  HIV infection and AIDS 401–4
  pyrexia of unknown origin (PUO) 399–401
infective endocarditis 64
inflammatory bowel disease 170–1
information extraction see history taking
inguinal hernia 158–9
inguinal nodes 202
intermittent claudication 31
interphalangeal joint examination 240
interstitial pulmonary oedema X-ray 85
intracerebral thrombosis 346
intramedullary cord lesions 354
intravenous drug users 64, 75, 98

involuntary movements 363
  see also tremor
irritable bowel syndrome 163

J

Janeway lesions 35
jaundice 18–19, 40, 131, 133, 185
joint examination 219–20
  ankles and feet 239–40
  elbows 228, 325
  hands and wrists 220–8, 325
  hips 234–6
  knees 235, 237–9
  neck 232–3
  sacroiliac 233–4
  shoulders 228–31
  temporomandibular 232
  thoracolumbar spine 233–4
  see also lower limb examination; upper limb
    examination
jugular venous pressure (JVP) 42–4, 185

K

Kallman's syndrome 294
Kaposi's sarcoma 403
Kayser-Fleischer rings 141
Keith-Wegerer hypertensive changes 188
Kernig's sign 363
ketones 189–90
kidney examination
  by palpation 152, 186–7
  by percussion 155
Killip Class 62–3
Klebsiella pneumonia 98
knee examination 235, 237–9, 366
knee jerk 338, 354–5
knee joint examination 235, 237–9
Korotkoff sounds 38–9

L

Lachman test 237
laryngeal carcinoma 99
laryngeal nerve involvement 94, 96, 99, 116
lateral chest X-ray film 84
lateral cutaneous nerve, thigh 344–5
left ventricular failure (LVF) 61
leg ulcers 59–60
lethargy 132, 257
leucoerythroblastic film 205
leuconychia 139
leukaemia 207, 209
lichen planus 388–9
light-touch testing 330
limb examination 321–2
  see also lower limb examination; upper limb
    examination
limb pain, arthritic 217

liver disease 167
liver examination
    by palpation 149, 151
    by percussion 155
liver palms 140
living conditions 8
lobar pneumonia 110
lower limb examination 335–44, 367
    cardiovascular disease 56–7
    coordination 339
    motor system 335–9
    peripheral nerves 342–4
    power 335–8
    reflexes 338–9
    sensory system 340–1
    superficial/cutaneous reflexes 341–2
    tone 335
lower motor neurone (LMN) weakness 286
lower motor neurone lesions 348
lumps
    breast 122–3
    dermatological 387
    groin 158
lung collapse 112
lung function assessment 109–10
lymph nodes 200–2
lymphadenopathy 202
lymphoma 210–11

M

malabsorption 169–70
malaria 206
malignant hypertension 66
mania 371
Marfan's syndrome 29, 33–4, 41, 44, 63, 69,
    72–3, 84, 88, 102
marital status 8
McMurray's test 239
median nerve examination 331–2
mediastinal compression 116–17
Mees' lines 184–5
megaloblastic anaemia 204
Meigs' syndrome 113
melanoma 393–4
Ménière's disease 285, 313
meningism 288
menstrual history 5
    for endocrine system examination 258–9
    for genitourinary system examination 183
mental state examination 378–80
meralgia paraesthetica 254
metacarpophalangeal joints 222, 224, 240
metatarsalgia 239, 255
microangiopathic haemolysis 205
migraine 283–4
mini-mental state examination 381
mitral
    facies 41, 66
    regurgitation 68–9

stenosis 66–7
    valve disease X-ray 86
    valve prolapse 69–70
mode of symptoms 3
monoarthritis 216
mononeuritis multiplex 349
mood disorders 371
Morton's metatarsalgia 255
motor neurone disease 348
motor neurone lesions 310, 317, 345–8
motor neurone weakness 286
motor system examination 322–8, 335–9
mouth examination 143–5, 201
mouth ulcers 144
mucosal ulcers 185
mucus 130
multiple endocrine neoplasia (MEN) 259, 272
multiple myeloma 211
murmurs *see* heart murmurs
Murphy's kidney pinch 187
muscle wasting 220
muscular dystrophy 355–6
myasthenia gravis 356–7
myelofibrosis 205, 210
myeloproliferative 209
myocardial infarction 27, 62–3
myopathy 355–6
myotonia 322
myxoedema 264–5

N

nail disease 139, 223, 394–5
nail examination 11, 22
    for gastrointestinal disease 139
    for haematological disease 199
    for respiratory disease 113–14
    for rheumatological disease 223
nailfold telangiectasia 394–5
natural remedies 4
nausea and vomiting 128
neck examination 232–3
    for cardiovascular system 41–4
    for gastrointestinal system 145
    for genitourinary system 185–6
    for nervous system 288
    for neurological disease 318, 363–4
neck, rapid screening 412
neck swelling 260
necrobiosis lipoidica diabeticorum 277
nephrotic syndrome 186–7, 190–2, 247
nerve entrapment syndromes 254–5
neurological disease
    cerebellum 357–60
    dystrophia myotonica 356
    extrapyramidal movement disorders 362–3
    Guillain-Barré syndrome 283, 315–17, 348–9, 404
    lower motor neurone lesions 348
    motor neurone disease 348
    myasthenia gravis 356–7

myopathy 355–6
Parkinson's disease 360–62
peripheral neuropathy 348
spinal cord compression 350–2
spinal cord syndromes 352–5
upper motor neurone lesions 345–8
neurological examination 287–8
method 365–7
of gait 344
of higher centres and speech 288–93
of limbs and trunk 321–44, 365
of the eyes 318–21, 364
of the head and neck 318, 363–4
of unconscious patients 363–5
rapid screening 412–13
see also cranial nerve examination; lower limb
examination; upper limb examination
neurological history 283–7
ninth nerve 313–15, 366
nitrate in urine 190
non-verbal clues 2
nummular eczema 389
nystagmus 305, 357

O

obesity 20, 270
obsessive compulsive disorder 372
obstructive ventilatory defect 109
occupation of patients 5
and respiratory disease 97
oculomotor nerve 300–5
odour of patients 23–4
oedema 56–7
oesophageal
cancer 168–9
perforation 129
reflux 29, 93–4, 127, 139, 169
spasm 28
olfactory nerve 293–4
one-and-a-half syndrome 304–5
onycholysis 262
onychomycosis 395–6
optic nerve 294–300
oral candidiasis 404
organic brain disorders 373
orthopnoea 29
Osler's nodes 35
osteoarthritis 222–3
overseas travel and immunisation 8

P

Paget's disease 122, 279–80, 313
pain
abdominal 127–8
arthritic 217
biliary 128
chest 27–9, 62–3, 96
facial 284

history taking of 3–4
pancreatic 128, 153
pleuritic 29
testing 328–9
pallor 19
palmar erythema 140
palmar tendon crepitus 224
palpation of the abdomen 148–9, 152–4
to examine gallbladder 149–50
to examine genitourinary system 186
to examine kidneys 152, 186
to examine liver 149
to examine spleen 150, 152
palpation of the breasts 122
palpation of the chest 103
palpation of the thyroid 260–1
palpitations 30
pancreatic calcification 173–4
pancreatic disease 147, 153, 165, 170
pancreatic pain 128, 153
pancytopenia 207
panic disorder 372
paraesthesiae 239
parietal lobe function 290–1
Parinaud's syndrome 304
Parkinson's disease 286, 304, 311, 316, 323, 360–62
parotid enlargement 142, 242
paroxysmal nocturnal dyspnoea (PND) 29
patent ductus arteriosus 79–80
Paterson–Brown-Kelly syndrome 168
pathological gynaecomastia 24–5
patient assessment see assessment
patient information see history taking
patient odour 23–4
patient positioning 32, 98, 133
patient preparation 24
patients, questions by 13
peak flow meter 109
pelvic examination 187, 192–4
Pemberton's sign 109, 261
peptic ulcer disease 128
percussion in genitourinary examination 186–7
percussion of the chest 104–5
percussion of the thyroid 261
pericardial disease 63–4, 186
peripheral blood film analysis 203–6
peripheral nerve
lower limb examination 342–4
thickening 349–50
upper limb examination 330–5
peripheral neuropathy 348
peripheral vascular disease 57
peritonitis 166
peroneal nerve test 343–4
personal history taking principles 5–8
personality disorders 374
Perthes' test 60
petechiae 199
Peutz-Jeghers' syndrome 137–8
pH analysis of urine 189

Phalen's sign 224, 241, 254
physical examination *see* examination
pigmentation 133
piles 160
pinprick testing 328–9
pituitary examination 266–9
pityriasis rosea 389
plantar reflex 339
    extensor response 354–5
pleural effusion 112–13, 119
pleuritic pain 29
Plumber's nails 262
Plummer-Vinson syndrome 168
pneumonia 96, 98, 110
pneumothorax 29, 113, 119
polyarthritis 216
polycystic kidney disease 186–7
polycystic ovarian syndrome 258–9
polycythaemia 209–10
polyradiculoneuropathy 348–9
polyuria 259
porphyria cutanea tarda 138–9
portal hypertension 168
post-traumatic stress disorder 372
positioning *see* patient positioning
posterior columns testing 329–30
postprandial fullness 128
postsplenectomy 206
postural hypertension 40
posture 20, 363
power testing 323, 335, 338
praecordium examination 44–56
    abnormality sounds 48–51
    auscultation 47–8
    auscultation of the neck 55–6
    dynamic manoeuvre testing 54–5
    inspection 44–5
    murmurs 51–5
    palpitation 45–6
    percussion 46
pre-anaesthetic evaluation 415–16
premorbid personality assessment 377
presentation of physical examination 409
presenting illness, history taking 3–5
presenting symptoms
    cardiovascular examination 27–31
    endocrine system 257–9
    gastrointestinal examination 127–32
    genitourinary examination 179–84
    nervous system 283–6
    psychiatric examination 370–5
    respiratory examination 94–6
    rheumatological examination 216–19
presyncope 30–1
principles *see* examination principles; history taking
        principles
proctosigmoidoscopy 161–2
proprioception testing 329
prosthetic heart valves 76–7
protein analysis of urine 189

Proteus mirabilis 189
proximal interphalangeal joints 222
proximal myopathy 355
pruritus 132, 388
pseudobulbar palsy 290
Pseudomonas aeruginosa 278
psoriasis 389–90, 394–5
psoriatic arthritis 244
psoriatic nails 223
psychiatric history 376–7
psychiatric illness 369–70
    diagnosis 377
    mental state examination for 378–80
    mini-mental state examination for 381
    presenting symptoms 370, 374–5
    screening questions for 371–4
ptosis 100, 109, 124, 149, 319–20
pulmonary
    embolism 29, 63, 117
    fibrosis 94, 116
    mass X-ray 120
    metastases X-ray 121
    regurgitation 76
    stenosis 75
    venous congestion X-ray 85
pulmonary hypertension 66
    right-to-left shunt 81
pulse rate and rhythm 36, 38
pulsus alternans 38
pulsus paradoxus 39
pustular skin lesions 391
pyoderma gangrenosum 171
pyrexia of unknown origin (PUO) 399–401

Q

Queen Square hammer 325
questions by patients 13
questions for psychiatric assessment 371–4
questions, initial 2–3

R

radial artery examination 38
radial nerve examination 331
radiofemoral delay 38
radiography for gastrointestinal disease 172
radiotherapy 102
Ramsay Hunt syndrome 310
rapid screening physical examination 411–13
rapport with patients 1
Raynaud's phenomenon 217
rectal examination 160–1, 187
red blood cells (RBCs) 190–1
red eye 318
reflex test 325–7, 338–9
reflux 29, 93–4, 127, 139, 169
    abdominojugular 43
regurgitation
    aortic regurgitation 72–4

mitral regurgitation 68–9
pulmonary regurgitation 76
tricuspid regurgitation 75
Reiter's syndrome 191, 223, 243–4, 397, 400
renal bruits 187
renal colic 128
renal calculus 181
renal failure 32, 180–2, 184, 194
see also genitourinary system
renal masses 186
respiratory diseases
bronchial asthma 114–15
bronchiectasis 114
bronchitis 115–16
carcinoma of the lung 117
chronic obstructive pulmonary disease (COPD) 115
collapse 112
consolidation 110
emphysema 115, 121
mediastinal compression 116–17
plural effusion 112–13
pneumothorax 113
pulmonary embolism 117
pulmonary fibrosis 116
sarcoidosis 117
tension pneumothorax 114
tuberculosis 96, 98, 102, 116, 118, 121
respiratory rate on exercise 109
respiratory system examination 125
chest X-rays for 118–21
cough character 99
cyanosis 98
dyspnoea 98
general appearance 98
hoarseness 99
method 124–6
of lung function 109–10
of the abdomen 109
of the chest 101–8
of the face 100
of the hands 99–100
of the heart 108–109
of the trachea 100–1
sputum 99
stridor 99
respiratory system presenting symptoms 93–6
breathlessness 94–5
chest pain 96
cough and sputum 93–4
wheeze 94, 107
respiratory system treatment history 96
restrictive cardiomyopathy 78
restrictive ventilatory defect 110
retinal detachment 300
retinal toxoplasmosis 404
retinitis pigmentosa 300
rheumatological system disease
calcium arthropathy 245
gouty arthritis 244–5
nerve entrapment syndromes 254–5

rheumatic fever 249–50
rheumatoid arthritis 198–9, 217, 240–3
scleroderma 247–9
seronegative spondyloarthropathies 243–4
soft tissue rheumatism 250, 251–4
systemic lupus erythematosus (SLE) 245–7
vasculitides 250–1
rheumatological system examination 219–20
see also joint examination
rheumatological system history 218–9
rheumatological system presenting symptoms 215–18
back pain 217
dry eyes/mouth 217–18
limb pain 217
peripheral joints 215–17
Raynaud's phenomenon 217
red eyes 218
systemic 218
rhinocerebral mucormycosis 278
rhomboid function 334
rickets 273–4
right ventricular failure (RVF) 61–2
Rinné's test 312
Romberg test 344
rotator cuff syndrome 252
Roth's spots 64
rubeosis 278

S

sacroiliac joint examination 233–4
saddle sensation 342
salivary gland examination for gastrointestinal disease 142–3
sarcoidosis 117
satiation, early 128
scabies 388
schizophrenia 373
sciatic nerve test 343
scleral icterus 141
scleroderma 247–9
sclerosis 139
screening questions for psychiatric disorders 371–4
scrotal mass diagnosis 192–3
second nerve 294–300, 365
sediment in urine 190–1
sensory system examination 328–30, 340–1
septal defects 78–9
seronegative spondyloarthropathies 243–4
seventh nerve 309–11, 366
sexual history 4–5
for genitourinary system examination 183
short stature syndromes 273–4
shoulder girdle examination 334
shoulder joint examination 228–31, 323–4
shoulder syndromes, arthritic 150
sickle cell anaemia 205
sinusitis 284
sixth nerve 300–5, 365–6
Sjögren's syndrome 116, 218, 403

skills in history taking 12
skin cancer 393–4
skin examination for endocrine system 258
skin examination for gastrointestinal system 133–9
skin tags 160
skin tumours 392–4
sleep apnoea 96
smell, examination indications 23–4
smoking 6, 100
    and heart disease 31
    and respiratory disease 97–8
social habits 6
social history
    cardiovascular disease 32
    endocrine system disease 259
    gastrointestinal disease 133
    genitourinary disease 184
    haematological system 198
    nervous system 287
    psychiatric illness 376–7
    respiratory disease 97–8
    rheumatological system 219
social/personal information about patients 5–8
soft tissue rheumatism 251–4
somatisation disorder 374
spastic paraparesis 359
speech analysis and neurological disease 286,
    288–90, 365
spherocytic anaemia 204
sphygmomanometer 38
spider naevi 141
spinal cord compression 350–2
spinal cord syndromes 352–5
spinothalamic loss 353
spinothalamic pathway 328–9
spirometry 109–10
spleen examination
    by palpation 150, 152
    by percussion 155
splenomegaly 202
splinter haemorrhages, finger 35
splitting heart sounds 49–50
spontaneous pneumothorax 29
squamous cell carcinoma 394
staining of the hands 100
station test 344
stools, blood in 131, 162
stress disorders 372
stupor 363
Sturge-Weber syndrome 293
subcutaneous emphysema 102
subcutaneous nodules of arthritis 227–8
subluxation 220
submandibular gland enlargement 143
suicide risk assessment 376
superficial/cutaneous reflex test 341–2
supraclavicular nodes 201–2
supranuclear palsy 303
supraspinatus tendonitis 252
supra-ventricular tachycardia 30

sweating 257, 392
symptoms analysis 3–5
syncope 30–1
syringomyelia 353–4
systemic hypertension 64–6
systemic lupus erythematosus (SLE) 245–7
systems review in history taking 8–11
systolic-click murmur syndrome 69
    see also valve diseases of left heart

T

tachycardia 30, 36–7
Tanner stages, sexual development 266
tarsal joint examination 337
tarsal tunnel syndrome 255
teeth examination for coronary artery disease 32
temperature test for sensory system 329
temperature, initial examination of 23
temporal arteritis 285
temporal lobe function 292
temporomandibular joint examination 232
tennis elbow 252–3
tenosynovitis, wrist 253
tension pneumothorax 114
tenth nerve 313–15, 366
Terry's nails 139
testes examination by palpation 154, 192
tetralogy of Fallot 81
third nerve 300–5, 365–6
thoracolumbar spine examination 233–4
thrombocythaemia 210
thrush 193–4
thyroid examination 259–61
thyrotoxicosis 262–4
toe–finger test 339
Tolosa-Hunt syndrome 303
tone testing 323, 335, 361
tongue examination 144
tracheal examination 100–1
tracheo-oesophageal fistula 94
transient ischaemic attacks 284
transposition of great arteries 81–2
treatment history 4
    cardiovascular system 32
    endocrine system 259
    gastrointestinal system 132
    genitourinary system 183
    haematological system 197–8
    nervous system 287
    respiratory system 96
    rheumatological system 218–9
tremor of the hands 100
tremor, Parkinson's 360
tremor/involuntary movements 286
Trendelenburg test 60
triceps jerk 326
Trichomonas vaginalis 193–4
tricuspid regurgitation 75
tricuspid stenosis 74

trigeminal nerve 305–9
trochlear nerve 300–5
Trousseau's sign 272
truncal ataxia 359
trunk examination 321–2
tuberculosis 96, 98, 102, 116, 118, 121
tuboeruptive xanthomata, knee 36
tumours, hormone-secreting 134
tumours, skin 392–4
Turner's syndrome 80, 88, 258, 273
twelfth nerve 316–17, 366

U

ulcerative colitis 170
ulcers
    leg 59–60, 277
    mouth 144–5
    mucosal 185
ulnar nerve examination 332–3
unconscious patient examination 363–5
uncooperative patients 9, 12
unilateral hemisphere lesion 345
upper limb examination 322–35, 367
    coordination 327–8
    for pyrexia of unknown origin 401
    motor system 322–8
    peripheral nerves 330–5
    posterior columns 329–30
    power 323
    reflexes 325–7
    sensory system 328–30
    spinothalamic pathway 328–9
    tone 323
upper motor neurone lesions 345–8
upper motor neurone weakness 286
urinalysis 163–4, 188–91, 279–80, 365
urinary incontinence 180
urinary obstruction 180
urinary tract infection (UTI) 180
uveitis 318

V

vagus nerve 313–15
valve diseases of left heart
    aortic regurgitation 72–4
    aortic stenosis 69–72
    mitral regurgitation 68–9
    mitral stenosis 66–7
    mitral valve prolapse 69–70
valve diseases of right heart
    pulmonary regurgitation 76
    pulmonary stenosis 75
    tricuspid regurgitation 75
    tricuspid stenosis 74

varicose veins 60
vascular disease 134–5, 346–8
vascular heart disease *see* coronary artery disease
vasculitides 250–1
venous hums 157
venous pressure, jugular 42–4, 185
venous ulcer 59
ventilatory defects 109–10
ventricular aneurysm X-ray 87
ventricular failure *see* valve diseases
ventricular septal defect 78
vertigo 313
vertebrobasilar artery lesions 348
vibration testing 329
viral pneumonia 96
visual acuity 295
vital signs in initial examination 18
vitamin B_{12} deficiency 353
vocal resonance 108

W

Waldeyer's ring 201
Weber's test 312–13
weight change/wasting 128, 133
weight examination 20, 128, 257
    for hydration 21
wheezing 94, 107
white blood cells (WBCs) 191
Willebrand's disease 198
Wilson's disease 139–40
wrist joint examination 220–8, 325
    see also carpal tunnel syndrome
wrist tenosynovitis 253
writing and Parkinson's disease 361
writing physical examination 407–9

X

xanthelasmata 40
xanthomata 35
X-ray examples
    for cardiovascular disease 85–7
    for gastrointestinal disease 173
    for respiratory disease 119–21
X-rays, chest
    for cardiovascular disease 82–4
    for respiratory diseases 118
    frontal film 82
    interpretation 82–4
    lateral film 84
X-rays, gastrointestinal 171–2, 174

Y

yellow nail syndrome 113–14

T
5